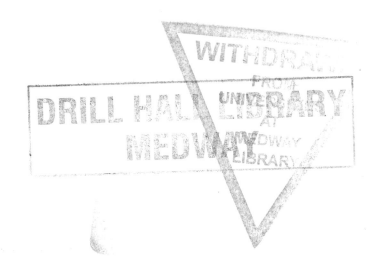

Johannes W. Rohen
Chihiro Yokochi
Elke Lütjen-Drecoll

Color Atlas
of Anatomy

A Photographic Study
of the Human Body

Seventh Edition

Coeditions in 20 Languages

Johannes W. Rohen
Chihiro Yokochi
Elke Lütjen-Drecoll

Color Atlas
of Anatomy

A Photographic Study
of the Human Body

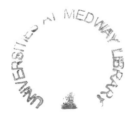

Seventh Edition

With 1211 Figures,
1117 in Color,
and 94 Radiographs, CT and MRI Scans

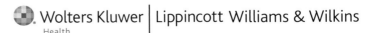
Wolters Kluwer | Lippincott Williams & Wilkins
Health

Philadelphia · Baltimore · New York · London
Buenos Aires · Hong Kong · Sydney · Tokyo

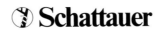
Schattauer

Prof. Dr. med. Dr. med. h.c. Johannes W. Rohen
Anatomisches Institut II der Universität Erlangen-Nürnberg
Universitätsstraße 19, 91054 Erlangen, Germany

Chihiro Yokochi, M.D.
Professor emeritus, Department of Anatomy
Kanagawa Dental College, Yokosuka, Kanagawa, Japan
Correspondence to:
Prof. Chihiro Yokochi, c/o Igaku-Shoin Ltd., 1-28-23 Hongo,
Bunkyo-ku Tokyo 113-8719, Japan

Prof. Dr. med. Elke Lütjen-Drecoll
Anatomisches Institut II der Universität Erlangen-Nürnberg
Universitätsstraße 19, 91054 Erlangen, Germany

With Collaboration of
Kyung W. Chung, Ph.D.
David Ross Boyd Professor & Vice Chairman
Samuel Roberts Noble Foundation Presidential Professor
Director, Advanced Human Anatomy
University of Oklahoma, College of Medicine
Department of Cell Biology

Copyright ©
Fourth Edition, 1998
Fifth Edition, 2002
Sixth Edition, 2006
Seventh Edition, 2011 by
Schattauer GmbH,
Hölderlinstraße 3, 70174 Stuttgart, Germany; http://www.schattauer.de, and
Lippincott Williams & Wilkins, a Wolters Kluwer business

351 West Camden Street   530 Walnut Street
Baltimore, MD 21201   Philadelphia, PA 19106

9 8 7 6 5 4 3 2 1

Library of Congress Cataloging-in-Publication data has been applied for and is available upon request.

DISCLAIMER

To purchase additional copies of this book, call our customer service department at **(800) 638-3030** or fax orders to **(301) 223-2320**. International customers should call **(301) 223-2300**.

Visit Lippincott Williams & Wilkins on the Internet: http://www.lww.com. Lippincott Williams & Wilkins customer service representatives are available from 8:30 am to 6:00 pm, EST.

ISBN: 9781582558561

Preface to the Seventh Edition

This new edition was revised and structured anew in different ways. Each chapter is provided with an introductory front page to give an overview of the topics of the chapter and short descriptions. The whole introductory chapter "General Anatomy" was newly arranged and supported with introductory texts, thus facilitating students to better understand the complicated "world" of gross anatomy. The large chapter 2 "Head and Neck" was split into 5 sub-chapters with an introductory page each. Furthermore, the drawings were revised and improved in many chapters and depicted more consistently. In most of the chapters new photographs taken from newly dissected specimens were incorporated.

The general structure and arrangement of the Atlas were maintained. The chapters of regional anatomy are consequently placed behind the systematic descriptions of the anatomical structures so that students can study – e.g. before dissecting an extremity – the systematic anatomy of bones, joints, muscles, nerves and vessels. For studying the photographs of the specimens the use of a magnifier might be helpful. The enormous plasticity of the photos is surprising, especially at higher magnifications.

In many places new MRI and CT scans were added to give consideration to the new imaging techniques which become more and more important for the student in preclinics. We would like to express our sincere thanks to Prof. Heuck, Munich, who provided us with the MRI scans.

In the underlying seventh edition photographs of the surface anatomy of the human body were included again. We omitted marks and indications in order not to affect the quality of the pictures.

Despite numerous additions and amendments the size of the volume did not increase so that students both in preclinics and in clinics are offered an atlas easy to handle and cope with.

While preparing this new edition, the authors were reminded of how precisely, beautifully, and admirably the human body is constructed. If this book helps the student or medial doctor to appreciate the overwhelming beauty of the anatomical architecture of tissues and organs in the human, then it greatly fulfils its task. Deep interest and admiration of the anatomical structures may create the "love for man", which alone can be considered of primary importance for daily medical work.

We would like to express our great gratitude to all coworkers for their skilled work. Without their help the improvements of the *Color Atlas of Anatomy* would not have been possible. We would also like to express our sincere thanks to those at Schattauer GmbH, Stuttgart, Germany, Lippincott, Williams & Wilkins, Baltimore, Maryland, USA, and Igaku-Shoin, Tokyo, Japan, who always listened to our suggestions and invested again a great deal of their effort into improving this book.

Acknowledgements

We would like to express our great gratitude to all coworkers who helped to make the *Color Atlas of Anatomy* a success. We are particularly indebted to those who dissected new specimens with great skill and knowledge, particularly to Jeff Bryant (member of our staff) and Dr. Martin Rexer (now Klinikum Fürth, Germany), who prepared most of the new specimens of the fifth, sixth and seventh edition. We would also like to thank Dr. K. Okamoto (now Nagasaki, Japan), who dissected many excellent specimens of the fourth edition, also included in the fifth edition. Furthermore, we are greatly indebted to Prof. W. Neuhuber and his coworkers for their great efforts in supporting our work.

The specimens of the previous editions also depicted in this volume were dissected with great skill and enthusiasm by Prof. Dr. S. Nagashima (now Nagasaki, Japan), Dr. Mutsuko Takahashi (now Tokyo, Japan), Dr. Gabriele Lindner-Funk (Erlangen, Germany), Dr. P. Landgraf (Erlangen, Germany), and Miss Rachel M. McDonnell (now Dallas, Texas, USA).

We are greatly indebted to Prof. Kyung Won Chung, Ph.D., Director of Medical Gross Anatomy, University of Oklahoma, USA, Dept. of Cell Biology, for his careful corrections of the proofs of the new edition.

We would also like to express our many thanks to Prof. W. Bautz (Radiologisches Institut, University Erlangen-Nürnberg, Germany) and Prof. A. Heuck (Radiologisches Zentrum, München-Pasing, Germany), who provided the newly included excellent CT and MRI scans.

We are also greatly indebted to Mr. Hans Sommer (SOMSO Co., Coburg, Germany), who kindly provided a number of excellent bone specimens.

Finally, we would like to express our great gratitude to our photographer, Mr. Marco Gößwein, who contributed the very excellent macrophotos. Excellent and untiring work was done by our secretaries, Mrs. Lisa Köhler and Elisabeth Wascher, and as well by our artists, Mr. Jörg Pekarsky and Mrs. Annette Gack, who not only performed excellent new drawings but revised effectively the layout of the new edition.

Last but not least, we would like to express our sincere thanks to all scientists, students, and other coworkers, particularly to the ones at the publishing companies themselves.

Erlangen, Germany; Spring 2010

J. W. Rohen
C. Yokochi
E. Lütjen-Drecoll

Preface to the First Edition

Today there exist any number of good anatomic atlases. Consequently, the advent of a new work requires justification. We found three main reasons to undertake the publication of such a book.

First of all, most of the previous atlases contain mainly schematic or semischematic drawings which often reflect reality only in a limited way; the third dimension, i.e., the spatial effect, is lacking. In contrast, the photo of the actual anatomic specimen has the advantage of conveying the reality of the object with its proportions and spatial dimensions in a more exact and realistic manner than the "idealized", colored "nice" drawings of most previous atlases. Furthermore, the photo of the human specimen corresponds to the student's observations and needs in the dissection courses. Thus he has the advantage of immediate orientation by photographic specimens while working with the cadaver.

Secondly, some of the existing atlases are classified by systemic rather than regional aspects. As a result, the student needs several books each supplying the necessary facts for a certain region of the body. The present atlas, however, tries to portray macroscopic anatomy with regard to the regional and stratigraphic aspects of the object itself as realistically as possible. Hence it is an immediate help during the dissection courses in the study of medical and dental anatomy.

Another intention of the authors was to limit the subject to the essential and to offer it didactically in a way that is self-explanatory. To all regions of the body we added schematic drawings of the main tributaries of nerves and vessels, of the course and mechanism of the muscles, of the nomenclature of the various regions, etc. This will enhance the understanding of the details seen in the photographs. The complicated architecture of the skull bones, for example, was not presented in a descriptive way, but rather through a series of figures revealing the mosaic of bones by adding one bone to another, so that ultimately the composition of skull bones can be more easily understood.

Finally, the authors also considered the present situation in medical education. On one hand there is a universal lack of cadavers in many departments of anatomy, while on the other hand there has been a considerable increase in the number of students almost everywhere. As a consequence, students do not have access to sufficient illustrative material for their anatomic studies. Of course, photos can never replace the immediate observation, but we think the use of a macroscopic photo instead of a painted, mostly idealized picture is more appropriate and is an improvement in anatomic study over drawings alone.

The majority of the specimens depicted in the atlas were prepared by the authors either in the Dept. of Anatomy in Erlangen, Germany, or in the Dept. of Anatomy, Kanagawa Dental College, Yokosuka, Japan. The specimens of the chapter on the neck and those of the spinal cord demonstrating the dorsal branches of the spinal nerves were prepared by Dr. K. Schmidt with great skill and enthusiasm. The specimens of the ligaments of the vertebral column were prepared by Dr. Th. Mokrusch, and a great number of specimens in the chapter of the upper and lower limb was very carefully prepared by Dr. S. Nagashima, Kurume, Japan.

Once again, our warmest thanks go out to all of our coworkers for their unselfish, devoted and highly qualified work.

Erlangen, Germany; Spring 1983   **J. W. Rohen**
C. Yokochi

Contents

1 General Anatomy 1

2 Head and Neck 19

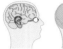

2 Head and Neck

3 Trunk   187

4 Thoracic Organs   243

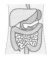

5 Abdominal Organs   291

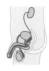

6 Retroperitoneal Organs   323

7 Upper Limb   368

8 Lower Limb   432

Index _____

1 General Anatomy

Three general principles are recognizable in the architecture of the human organism:

1. **The principle of polarity:** Polarity is reflected mainly in the formal and functional contrast between the head (predominantly spherical form) and the extremities (radially arranged skeletal elements). In the phylogenetic development of the upright position of the human body, polarity developed also among the extremities: The lower extremities provide the basis for locomotion whereas the upper extremities are not needed anymore for locomotion, so they can be used for gesture, manual and artistic activities.

2. **The principle of segmentation:** This principle dominates in the trunk. The anatomical structures (vertebrae, pairs of ribs, muscles, and nerves) are arranged segmentally and replicate rhythmically in a similar way.

3. **The principle of bilateral symmetry:** Both sides of the body are separated by a midsagittal plane and resemble each other like image and mirror-image.

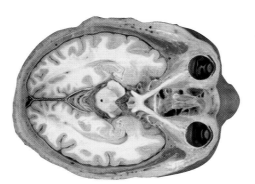

Horizontal section through the head at the level of the eyes.

There are also different principles in the architecture and function of the inner organs:

The **skull** contains the brain and the sensory organs. They are arranged like mirror and mirror-image and are the basis of our consciousness.

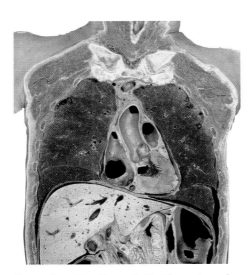

Coronal section through the thoracic and abdominal cavity.

The **thorax** contains the organs of the rhythmic system (heart, lung), which are only to some extent bilaterally organized. The consciousness (feeling, etc.) is located in-between.

In the **abdominal cavity,** the most important abdominal organs (intestinal tract, liver, pancreas) are arranged unpaired. Their functions remain subconscious.

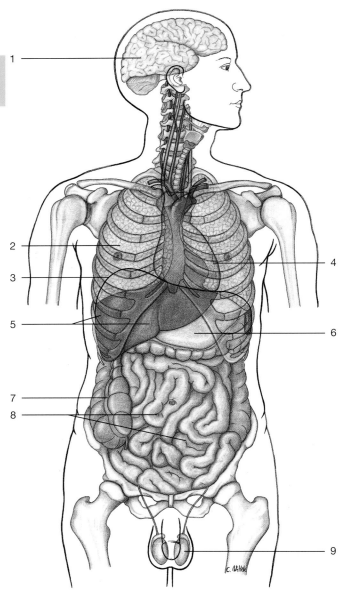

Position of the inner organs of the human body
(anterior aspect). The main cavities of the body and their
contents.

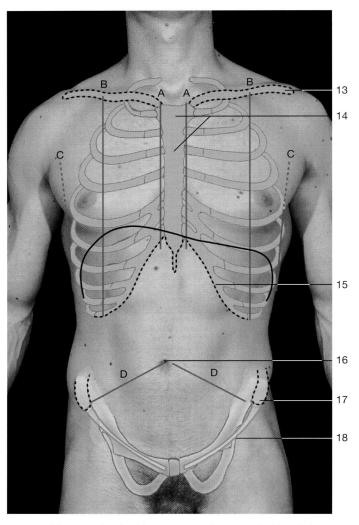

**Regional lines and palpable points at the ventral side of the
human body.**

Regional lines
A = parasternal line
B = midclavicular line
C = anterior axillary line
D = umbilical-pelvic line

The bones of the skeletal system are palpable through the skin at different points. This enables physicians to localize the inner organs. On the **ventral side,** the clavicle, sternum, ribs, and intercostal spaces are palpable. Furthermore, the anterior iliac spine and the symphysis can be localized. For better orientation, several **lines of orientation** are used, e.g., the parasternal line, the midclavicular line, the anterior axillary line, the umbilical-pelvic line.
By means of these lines, the heart and the position of the vermiform process can be localized.

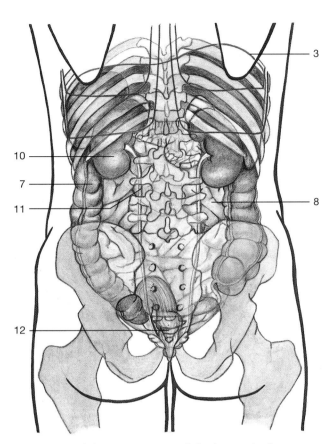

Position of the inner organs of the human body (posterior aspect).

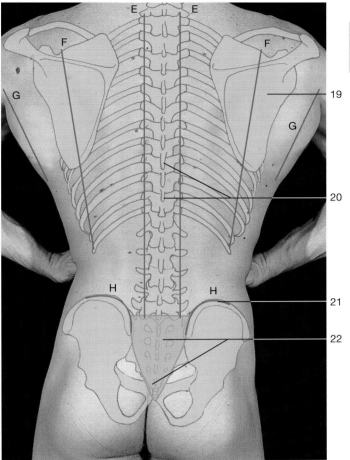

Regional lines and palpable points at the dorsal side of the human body.

Regional lines
E = paravertebral line
F = scapular line
G = posterior axillary line
H = iliac crest

1   Brain
2   Lung
3   Diaphragm
4   Heart
5   Liver
6   Stomach
7   Colon
8   Small intestine
9   Testis
10 Kidney
11 Ureter
12 Anal canal
13 Clavicle
14 Manubrium sterni
15 Costal arch
16 Umbilicus
17 Anterior superior iliac spine
18 Inguinal ligament
19 Scapular spine
20 Spinous processes
21 Iliac crest
22 Coccyx and sacrum

At the **dorsal side** of the body, the posterior spines of the vertebral column, the ribs, the scapula, the sacrum, and the iliac crest are palpable. **Lines of orientation** are the paravertebral line, the scapular line, the posterior axillary line, and the iliac crest.

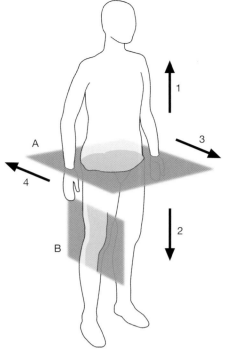

Planes of the body:
A = horizontal or axial or transverse plane
B = sagittal plane (at the level of the knee joint)

Directions:
1 = cranial   3 = anterior (ventral)
2 = caudal   4 = posterior (dorsal)

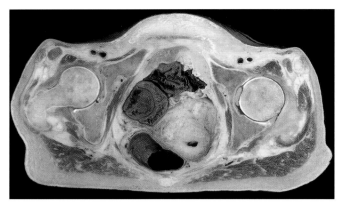

Horizontal section through the pelvic cavity and the hip joints.

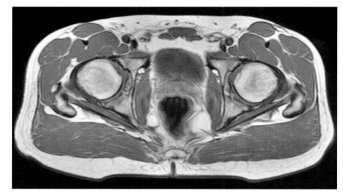

MRI scan through the pelvic cavity and the hip joints (horizontal or axial or transverse plane).

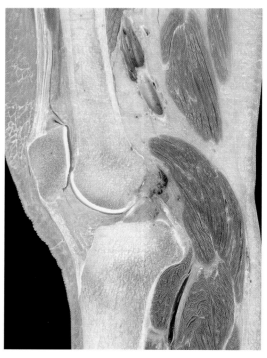

Sagittal section through the knee joint.

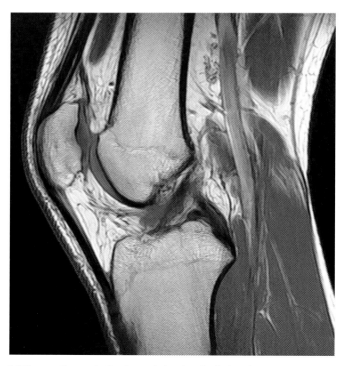

MRI scan through the knee joint (sagittal plane).

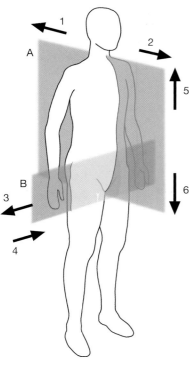

Planes of the body:
A = midsagittal or median plane
B = frontal or coronal plane (through the pelvic cavity)

Directions:
1 = posterior (dorsal)   4 = medial
2 = anterior (ventral)   5 = cranial
3 = lateral   6 = caudal

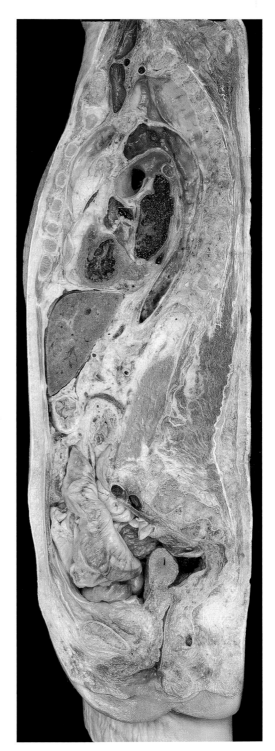

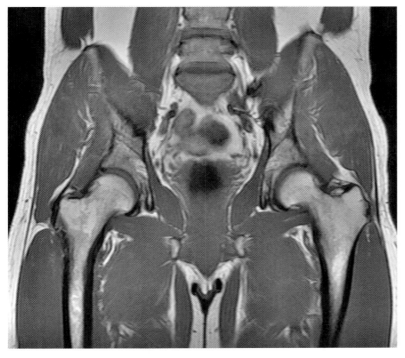

MRI scan through the pelvic cavity and the hip joints (frontal or coronal plane).

Median section through the trunk of a female.

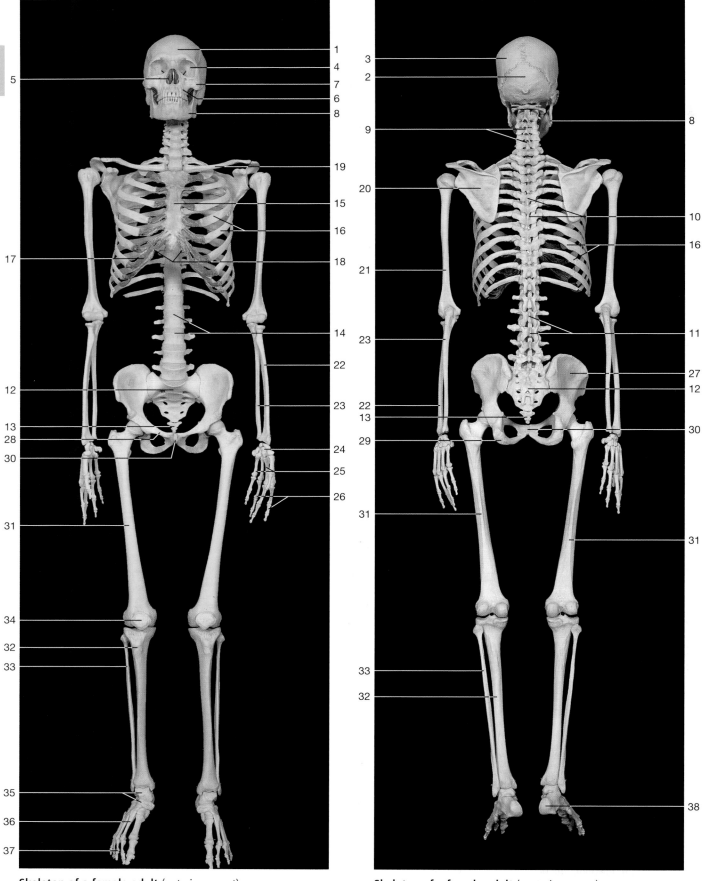

Skeleton of a female adult (anterior aspect).

Skeleton of a female adult (posterior aspect).

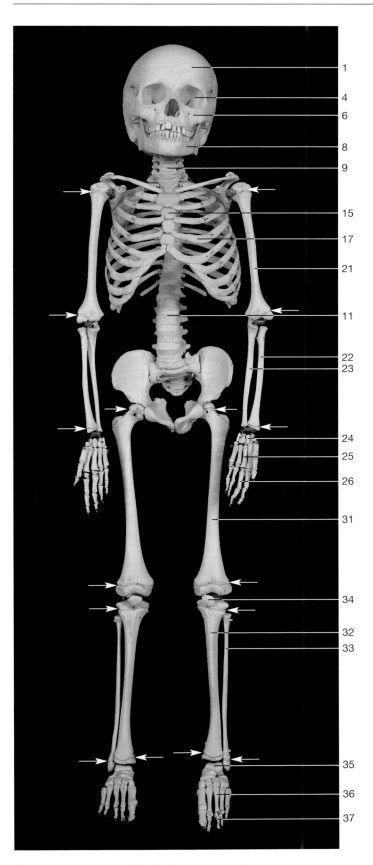

Axial skeleton
Head
1 Frontal bone
2 Occipital bone
3 Parietal bone
4 Orbit
5 Nasal cavity
6 Maxilla
7 Zygomatic bone
8 Mandible

Trunk and thorax
Vertebral column
9 Cervical vertebrae
10 Thoracic vertebrae
11 Lumbar vertebrae
12 Sacrum
13 Coccyx
14 Intervertebral discs
Thorax
15 Sternum
16 Ribs
17 Costal cartilage
18 Infrasternal angle

Appendicular skeleton
Upper limb and shoulder girdle
19 Clavicle
20 Scapula
21 Humerus
22 Radius
23 Ulna
24 Carpal bones
25 Metacarpal bones
26 Phalanges of the hand

Lower limb and pelvis
27 Ilium
28 Pubis
29 Ischium
30 Symphysis pubis
31 Femur
32 Tibia
33 Fibula
34 Patella
35 Tarsal bones
36 Metatarsal bones
37 Phalanges of the foot
38 Calcaneus

Skeleton of a 5-year-old child (anterior aspect).
The zones of the cartilaginous growth plates are seen (arrows).
In contrast to the adult, the ribs show a predominantly
horizontal position.

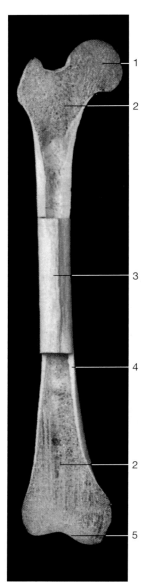

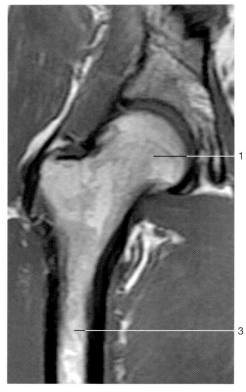

MRI scan of the right femur and the hip joint (coronal section) (from Heuck et al., MRT-Atlas, 2009).

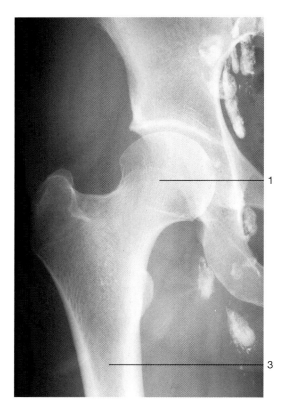

X-ray of the right femur and the hip joint (a.-p. direction).

◁ **Femur of the adult.** Coronal section of the proximal and distal epiphyses displaying the spongy bone and the medullary cavity.

1   Head of the femur
2   Spongy bone
3   Diaphysis of the femur
4   Compact bone
5   Articular cartilage

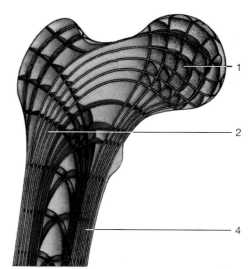

Three-dimensional representation on the trajectorial lines of the femoral head (according to B. Kummer).

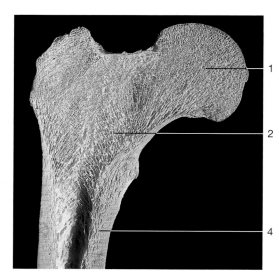

Coronal section through the proximal end of the adult femur showing the characteristic structure of the spongy bone.

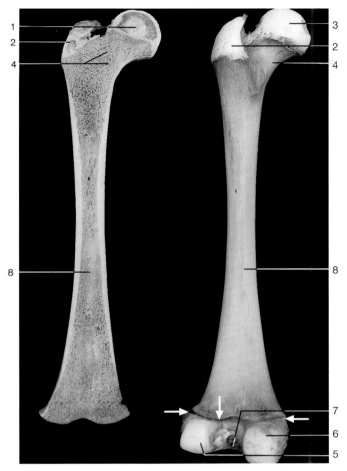

Ossification of the femur (left: coronal section, right: posterior view of the femur). Arrows: distal epiphysis.

The **ossification of the bones** of the limbs starts within the ossification centers of the primary cartilagenous bones. Here, the medullary cavity develops. The ossification process of limb bones is not finished at birth.

◁ 1 Ossification center in the head of the femur
2 Greater trochanter
3 Head of the femur
4 Neck of the femur
5 Lateral condyle
6 Medial condyle
7 Intercondylar notch
8 Diaphysis

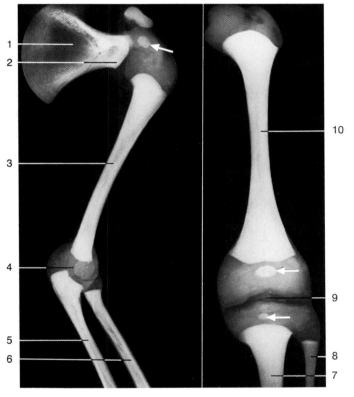

X-ray of the upper and lower limb of a newborn child (left: upper limb, right: lower limb). Arrows: ossification centers.

1 Scapula
2 Shoulder joint
3 Humerus
4 Elbow joint
5 Ulna
6 Radius
7 Tibia
8 Fibula
9 Knee joint
10 Femur

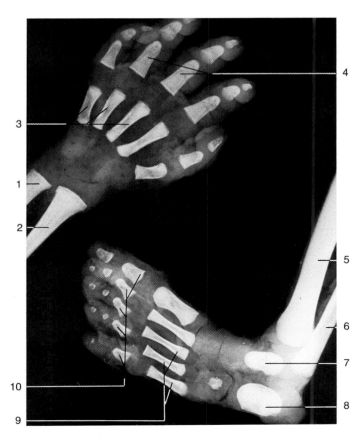

◁ 1 Ulna
2 Radius
3 Metacarpals
4 Phalanges
5 Tibia
6 Fibula
7 Talus
8 Calcaneus
9 Metatarsals
10 Phalanges

X-ray of hand and foot of a newborn.

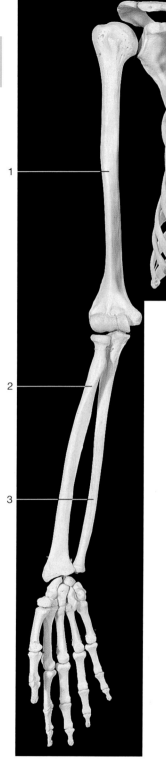

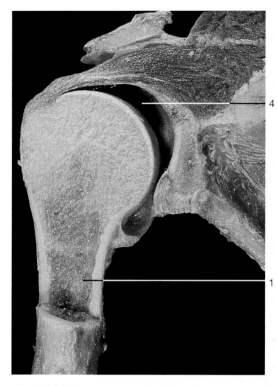

Shoulder joint as an example of a multiaxial ball-and-socket joint (coronal section).

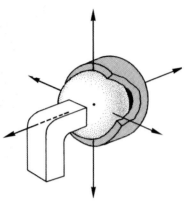

Ball-and-socket joint with its different axes (schematic drawing). Arrows: axes of movement.

1   Humerus
2   Radius
3   Ulna
4   Articular cavity (shoulder joint)
5   Metacarpophalangeal joint
6   Joints of fingers

Skeleton of the right arm and shoulder girdle (anterior aspect).

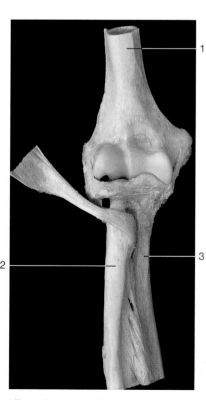

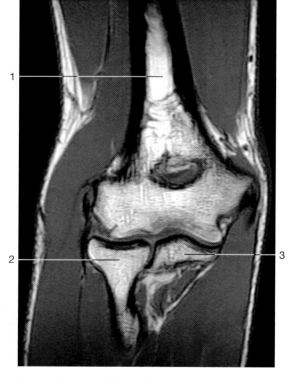

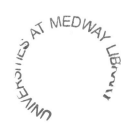

Elbow joint with ligaments as an example of a hinge joint (monaxial humero-ulnar joint) in combination with a pivot joint (monaxial radio-ulnar joint), which allows rotation.

Coronal section of the elbow joint (MRI scan, courtesy of Prof. Heuck, Munich). The possibilities of movement are shown in the schematic drawings on p. 11.

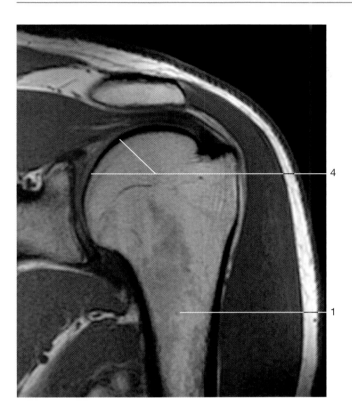

Coronal section of the shoulder joint
(MRI scan, from Heuck et al., MRT-Atlas, 2009).

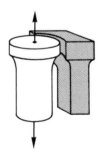

Hinge joint
(e.g. humero-ulnar joint). Left: extension, right: flexion.
Arrows: axes of movement.

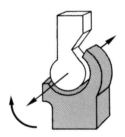

Pivot joint
(e.g. radio-ulnar joint).

Saddle joint
(e.g. carpometacarpal joint of
the thumb).

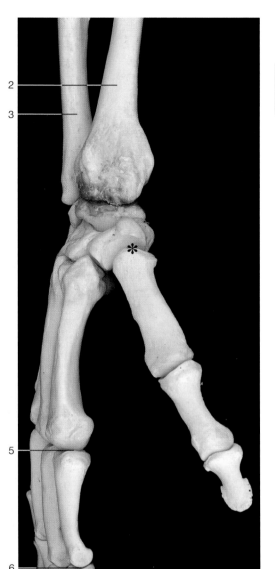

Skeleton of right wrist and hand (medial aspect).
The metacarpophalangeal joints are biaxial, as is
the carpometacarpal joint of the thumb (✻ in the
figure). The joints of the fingers, however, are
monaxial.

Joints exhibit a variety of functions. In
general, mobility becomes reduced in the
direction from proximal to distal. The hip
joint, e.g., is multiaxial; the knee joint is
biaxial, and the joints of toes and fingers are
monaxial.

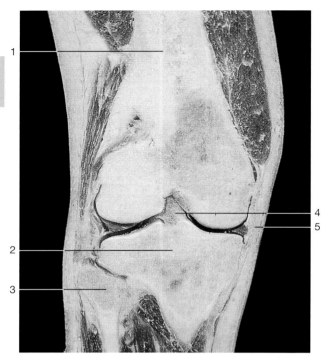

Coronal section through the knee joint (anterior aspect of the right joint in extension).

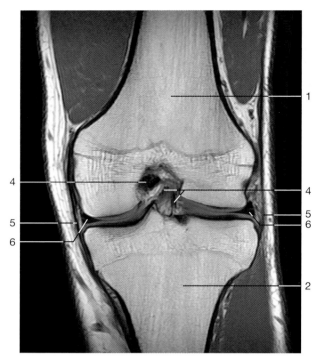

MRI scan of the knee joint (coronal plane) (from Heuck et al., MRT-Atlas, 2009).

1   Femur
2   Tibia
3   Fibula
4   Cruciate ligaments
5   Collateral ligaments
6   Meniscus

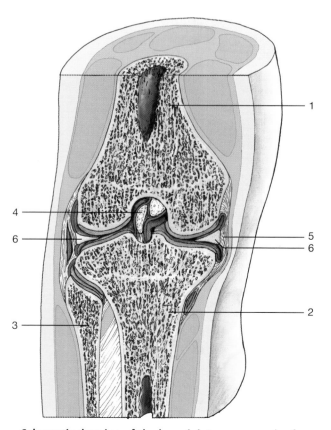

Schematic drawing of the knee joint as an example of a synovial joint, characterized by a joint cavity enclosed by a joint capsule (red) containing synovial fluid. Blue = articular cartilage.

Joints are places of articulation allowing movements between bones. Synovial joints are characterized by a joint cavity enclosed by a joint capsule containing synovial fluid, which is produced by the articular capsule. The kind of movements depends not only on form and structure of the articulating bones but also on ligaments incorporated into the articular capsule. In some synovial joints, fibrocartilagenous articular discs develop, when the articulating surfaces of the bones are incongruous.

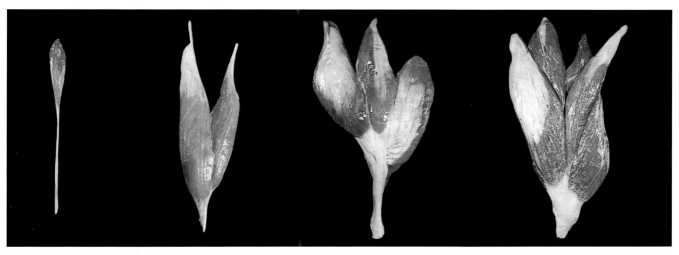

Fusiform
(palmaris longus)

Bicipital
(biceps brachii)

Tricipital (triceps surae,
gastrocnemius, and soleus)

Quadricipital
(quadriceps femoris)

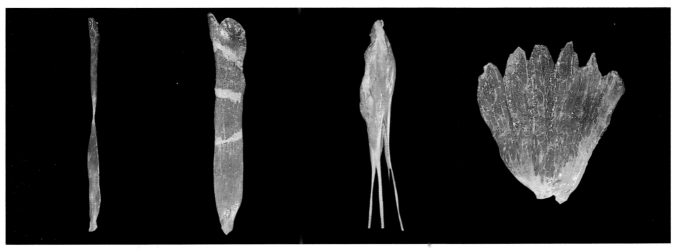

Digastric
(omohyoideus)

Multiventral
(rectus abdominis)

Multicaudal
(flexor digitorum prof.)

Serrated
(serratus anterior)

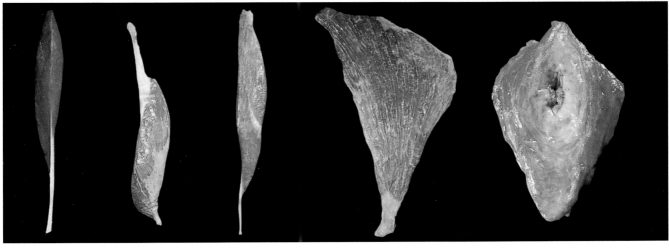

Bipennate
(tibialis anterior)

Unipennate
(semimembranosus)

Semitendinous
(semitendinosus)

Broad, flat muscle
(latissimus dorsi)

Ring-like
(sphincter ani externus)

The human body possesses **a great variety of muscles.** The architecture of the muscles depends on the functional systems in which they are involved, i.e., the kind of movements, the form of the joints with their specific ligaments, etc. The movements themselves vary to a great extent individually.

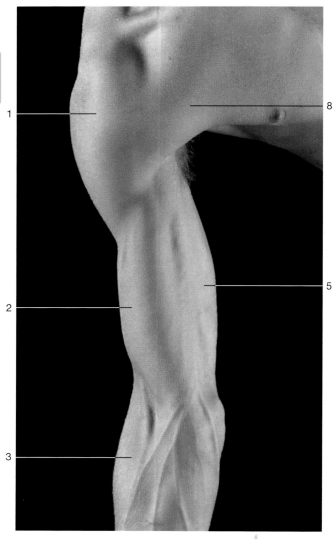

1
8
2
7
5

3

Ventral aspect of the right arm. The biceps muscle appears slightly contracted. In the area of the elbow joint, several subcutaneous veins can be recognized.

1   Deltoid muscle
2   Biceps brachii muscle
3   Brachioradialis muscle
4   Humerus
5   Triceps brachii muscle
6   Elbow joint
7   Brachialis muscle
8   Pectoralis major muscle
9   Radius
10 Ulna

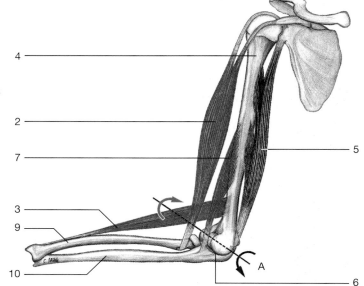

4
2
7
5
3
9
10
A
6

Diagram illustrating the position of the flexor and extensor muscles of the arm and their effect on the elbow joint.
A = axis of humero-ulnar joint; arrows = direction of movements; red = flexion; black = extension.

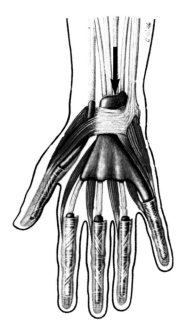

Synovial sheaths of flexor tendons (palmar aspect of right hand, semischematic drawing). **The flexor retinaculum** protects the flexor tendons passing through the carpal tunnel (arrow).

Joints are moved by muscles. The highly differentiated movements are coordinated by special groups of muscles (**synergists**). Their counterparts are called **antagonists**. Movements can only be carried out harmoniously if the contraction of the synergists are supported by a corresponding dilatation of the antagonists. This interaction is controlled by the nervous system. In order to carry out certain directions of movements, often the tendons of muscles have to be directed by ligaments. At those places, the tendons often develop synovial sheaths, e.g., at the wrist joint or at the fingers.

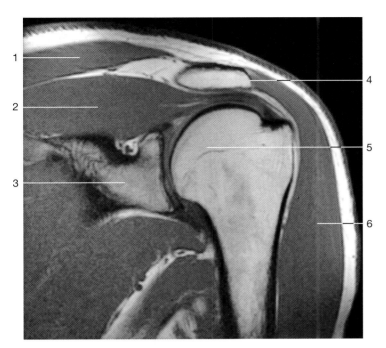

Shoulder joint (MRI scan, coronal section) (from Heuck et al., MRT-Atlas, 2009).

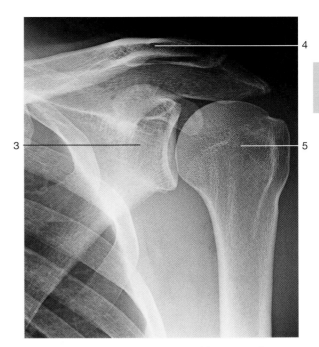

Shoulder joint (X-ray, a.-p. direction) (courtesy of Dr. Holik, Spardorf).

1	Trapezius muscle	6	Deltoid muscle
2	Supraspinatus muscle	7	Cavity of shoulder joint
3	Scapula	8	Articular cartilage
4	Acromion	9	Articular cavity
5	Head of humerus	10	Humerus

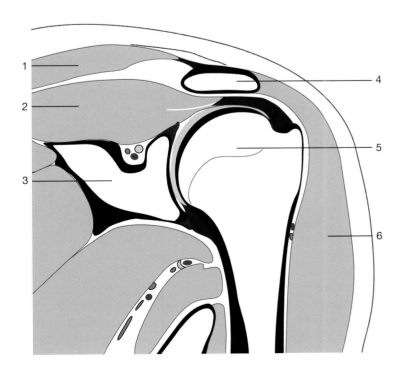

Shoulder joint (schematic drawing of the MRI scan above) (from Heuck et al., MRT-Atlas, 2009).

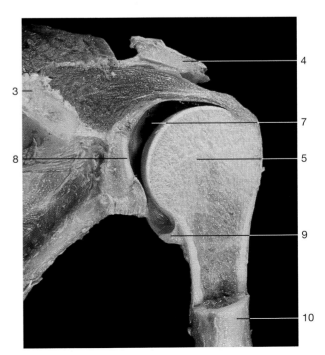

Frontal section of the shoulder joint (compare with the two pictures above).

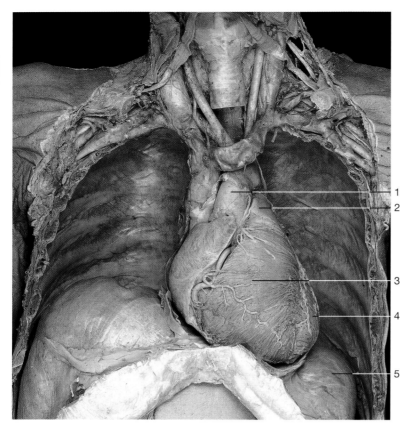

Heart and related vessels in situ (anterior aspect). Anterior thoracic wall, pericardium, and epicardium have been removed. The trachea is divided.

1	Aorta	4	Left heart
2	Pulmonary artery	5	Diaphragm
3	Right heart	6	Abdominal aorta

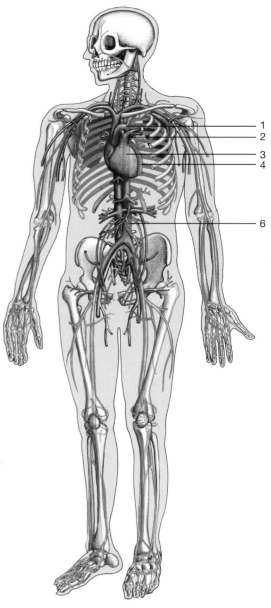

Organization of the circulatory system with the heart in the center. Red = arteries; blue = veins (from Lütjen-Drecoll, Rohen, Innenansichten des menschlichen Körpers, 2010).

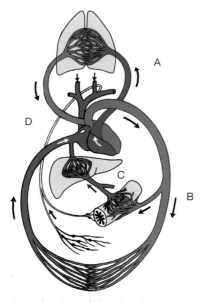

Organization of the circulatory systems in the human body. The center of this system represents the heart. Red = arteries; blue = veins (from Lütjen-Drecoll, Rohen, Innenansichten des menschlichen Körpers, 2010).

A = pulmonary circulation   C = portal circulation
B = systemic circulation   D = lymphatic circulation

The center of the circulatory system is the heart, which is situated in the thoracic cavity and in contact with the diaphragm. In the right ventricle, the venous blood is collected and pumped through the pulmonary artery and into the lung where the blood is oxygenated. The veins of the lung transport the blood to the left ventricle, where it is pumped through the aorta and its branches (arteries) in the human body. Arteries and veins mostly run parallel. The venous blood from the intestine reaches the liver via the portal vein.

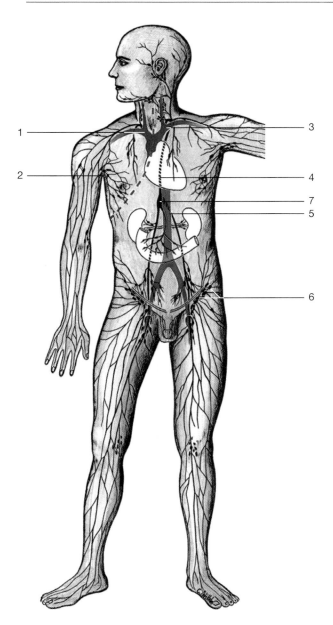

Organization of the lymphatic system.
Course of the main lymphatic vessels and lymph nodes in the body. Dotted red line = border between lymphatic vessels draining toward the right and the left venous angles.

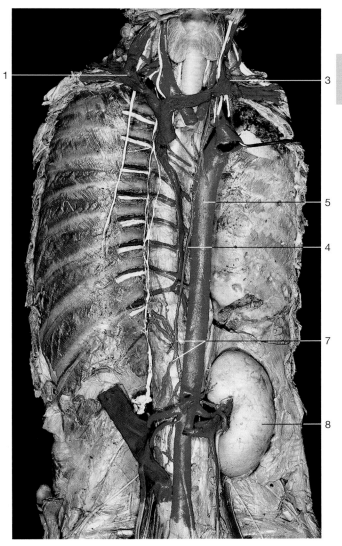

Major lymph vessels of the trunk (green). Blue = veins, red = arteries, white = nerves.

1	Right venous angle	5	Aorta
2	Axillary lymph nodes	6	Inguinal lymph nodes
3	Left venous angle	7	Cisterna chyli
4	Thoracic duct	8	Left kidney

Lymphatic vessels originate in the tissue spaces (lymph capillaries) and unite to form larger vessels (lymphatics). These resemble veins but have a much thinner wall, more valves, and are interrupted by lymph nodes at various intervals. Large groups of lymph nodes are located in the inguinal and axillary regions, deep to the mandible and sternocleidomastoid muscle, and within the root of the mesentery of the intestine. The lymphatic vessels of the right half of the head and neck, the right thorax, and the right upper limb drain toward the right venous angle; those of the rest of the body, toward the left venous angle.

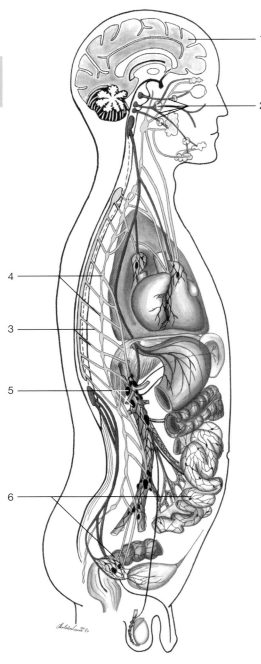

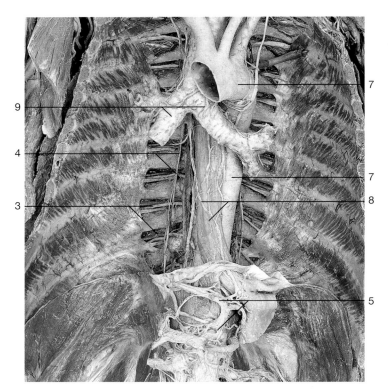

Posterior part of the trunk. The **solar plexus** with its connection to the vagus nerve and the sympathetic trunk has been dissected.

Diagram illustrating the **localization of the three functional portions of the nervous system** (brain, spinal cord and autonomic nervous system). Yellow = sympathetic system; red = parasympathetic system.

1	Cerebrum	6	Nervous plexus of the autonomic system
2	Cranial nerves		
3	Spinal nerves	7	Aorta
4	Sympathetic trunk	8	Vagus nerve and esophagus
5	Solar plexus	9	Bifurcation of trachea

The nervous system can be divided into three functionally distinct parts:
1. The cranial part, which comprises the great sensory organs and the brain.
2. The spinal cord, which shows a segmental structure and serves predominantly as a reflex organ.
3. The autonomic nervous system, which controls the involuntary functions (subconscious control) of organs and tissues. The autonomic part of the nervous system forms many delicate plexuses near or within the organs.

At certain places these plexuses contain aggregations of nerve cells (prevertebral and intramural ganglia).

The spinal nerves leave the spinal cord at regular intervals. The ventral rami of the spinal nerves form the cervical and brachial plexus, which innervates the upper extremity, and the ventral rami of the lumbar and sacral spinal nerves form the lumbosacral plexus, which innervates the pelvis and genital organs and the lower extremity.

2 Head and Neck
2.1 Skull and Muscles of the Head

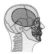

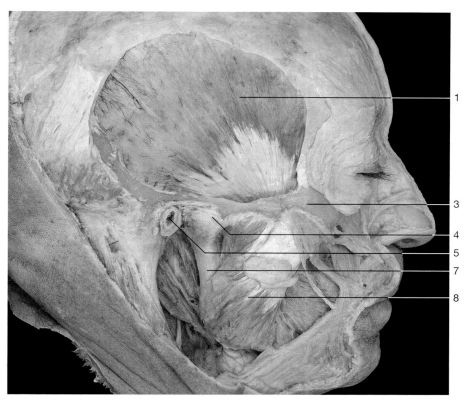

The head contains the brain and the great sensory organs (neurocranium). Anteriorly, the facial bones, the facial muscles, and the muscles of mastication have been developed (viscerocranium). The base of the skull is slightly bent so that the structures of the viscerocranium become located underneath the neurocranium, a specifity of the human head. Therefore mimic movements are possible in the human face.

Muscles of mastication and facial muscles (lateral aspect).
The auricle has been removed.

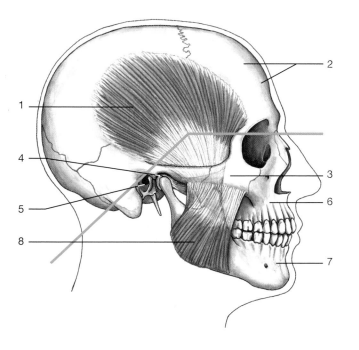

1 Temporalis muscle
2 Frontal bone
3 Zygomatic bone
4 Temporomandibular joint
5 External acoustic meatus
6 Maxilla
7 Mandible
8 Masseter muscle

Lateral aspect of the skull with muscles of mastication
(temporalis and masseter muscles = red).
The base of the skull is bent (grey line).

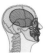

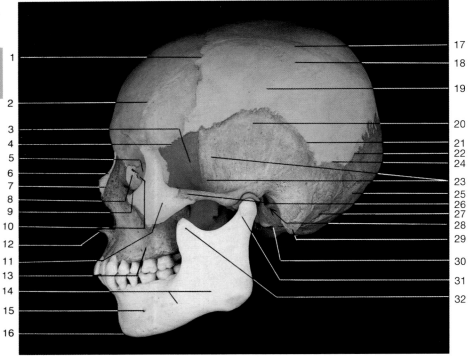

1	Coronal suture
2	Frontal bone
3	Sphenoidal bone
4	Sphenofrontal suture
5	Ethmoidal bone
6	Nasal bone
7	Nasomaxillary suture
8	Lacrimal bone
9	Lacrimomaxillary suture
10	Ethmoidolacrimal suture
11	Zygomatic bone
12	Anterior nasal spine
13	Maxilla
14	Mandible
15	Mental foramen
16	Mental protuberance
17	Superior temporal line
18	Inferior temporal line
19	Parietal bone
20	Temporal bone
21	Squamous suture
22	Lambdoid suture
23	Temporal fossa
24	Parietomastoid suture
25	Occipital bone
26	Zygomatic arch
27	Occipitomastoid suture
28	External acoustic meatus
29	Mastoid process
30	Tympanic portion of temporal bone
31	Condylar process of mandible
32	Coronoid process of mandible

General architecture of the skull (lateral aspect). The different bones are indicated in color (numbers cf. table).

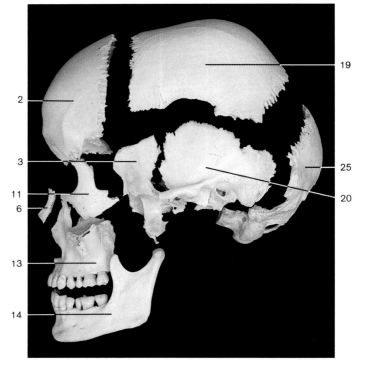

2	Frontal bone (orange)	**Cranial bones**
19	Parietal bone (light yellow)	
3	Greater wing of sphenoidal bone (red)	
25	Squama of occipital bone (blue)	
20	Squama of temporal bone (brown)	
5	Ethmoidal bone (dark green)	**Base of skull**
3	Sphenoidal bone (red)	
	Temporal bone excluding squama (brown)	
30	Tympanic portion of temporal bone (dark brown)	
	Occipital bone excluding squama (blue)	
6	Nasal bone (white)	**Facial bones**
8	Lacrimal bone (light yellow)	
	Inferior nasal concha	
	Vomer	
11	Zygomatic bone (dark yellow)	
	Palatine bone	
13	Maxilla (violet)	
14	Mandible (white)	
	Malleus } within petrous portion of Incus Stapes } temporal bone	**Auditory ossicles**
	Hyoid	

Lateral aspect of the disarticulated skull (palatine bone, lacrimal bone, ethmoidal bone, and vomer are not depicted).

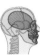

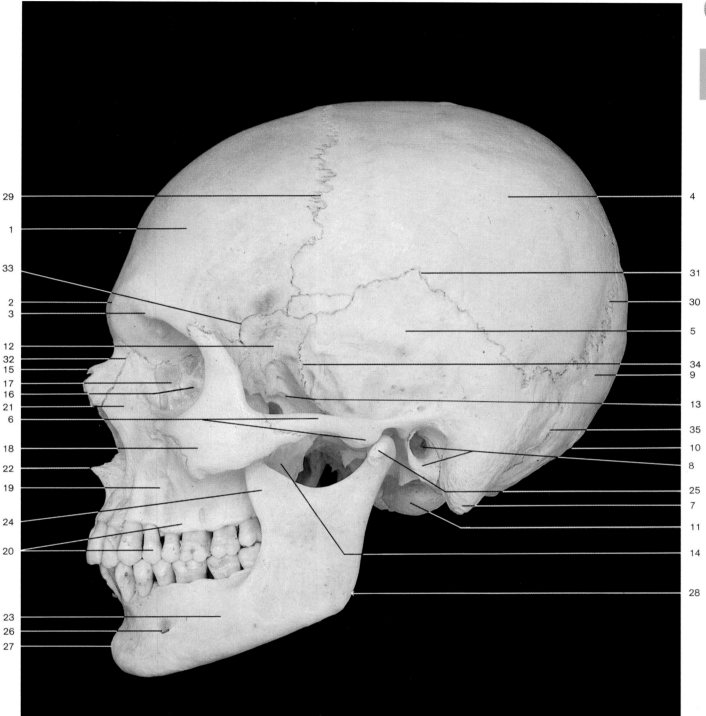

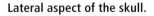

Lateral aspect of the skull.

1   Frontal bone
2   Glabella
3   Supraorbital margin
4   Parietal bone
5   Temporal bone (squamous part)
6   Zygomatic process
    (articular tubercle)
7   Mastoid process
8   Tympanic part (tympanic plate)
    and external acoustic meatus
9   Occipital bone (squamous part)
10 External occipital protuberance
11 Occipital condyle

12 Sphenoidal bone (greater wing)
13 Infratemporal crest of sphenoid
14 Pterygoid process (lateral pterygoid plate)
15 Nasal bone
16 Ethmoidal bone (orbital part)
17 Lacrimal bone
18 Zygomatic bone
19 Maxilla (body)
20 Alveolar process and teeth
21 Frontal process
22 Anterior nasal spine
23 Mandible (body)
24 Coronoid process

25 Condylar process
26 Mental foramen
27 Mental protuberance
28 Angle of the mandible

Sutures
29 Coronal suture
30 Lambdoid suture
31 Squamous suture
32 Nasomaxillary suture
33 Frontosphenoid suture
34 Sphenosquamosal suture
35 Occipitomastoid suture

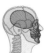

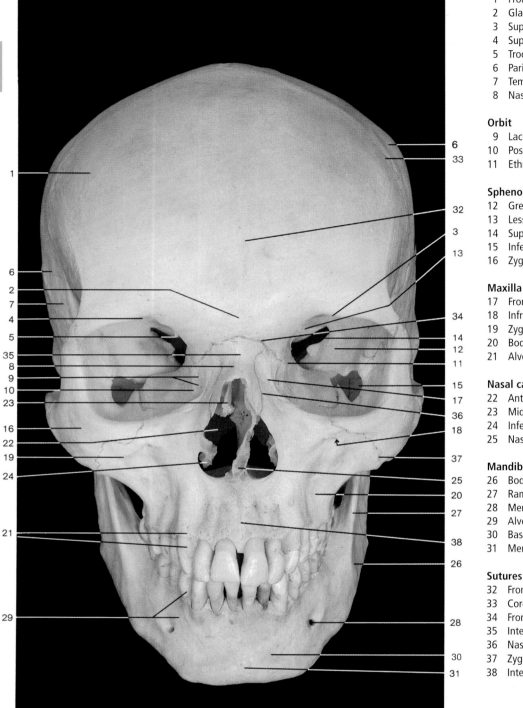

1 Frontal bone
2 Glabella
3 Supra-orbital margin
4 Supra-orbital notch
5 Trochlear spine
6 Parietal bone
7 Temporal bone
8 Nasal bone

Orbit
9 Lacrimal bone
10 Posterior lacrimal crest
11 Ethmoidal bone

Sphenoidal bone
12 Greater wing of sphenoidal bone
13 Lesser wing of sphenoidal bone
14 Superior orbital fissure
15 Inferior orbital fissure
16 Zygomatic bone

Maxilla
17 Frontal process
18 Infra-orbital foramen
19 Zygomatic process
20 Body of maxilla
21 Alveolar process with teeth

Nasal cavity
22 Anterior nasal aperture
23 Middle nasal concha
24 Inferior nasal concha
25 Nasal septum, vomer

Mandible
26 Body of mandible
27 Ramus of mandible
28 Mental foramen
29 Alveolar part with teeth
30 Base of mandible
31 Mental protuberance

Sutures
32 Frontal suture
33 Coronal suture
34 Frontonasal suture
35 Internasal suture
36 Nasomaxillary suture
37 Zygomaticomaxillary suture
38 Intermaxillary suture

Anterior aspect of the skull.

The skull comprises a mosaic of numerous complicated bones that form the cranial cavity protecting the brain (**neurocranium**) and several cavities such as the nasal and oral cavities in the facial region. The neurocranium consists of large bony plates that develop directly from the surrounding sheets of connective tissue (**desmocranium**).

The bones of the skull base are formed out of cartilaginous tissue (**chondrocranium**), which ossifies secondarily. The **visceral skeleton,** which in fish gives rise to the gills, has in higher vertebrates been transformed into the bones of the masticatory and auditory apparatus (maxilla, mandible, auditory ossicles, and hyoid bone).

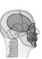

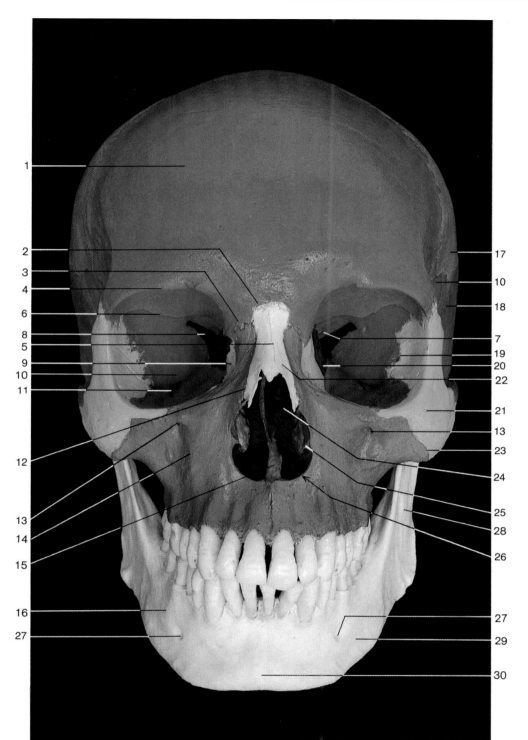

1 Frontal bone
2 Frontonasal suture
3 Frontomaxillary suture
4 Supra-orbital margin
5 Internasal suture
6 Sphenofrontal suture
7 Optic canal in lesser wing
   of sphenoidal bone
8 Superior orbital fissure
9 Lacrimal bone
10 Sphenoidal bone (greater wing)
11 Inferior orbital fissure
12 Nasomaxillary suture
13 Infra-orbital foramen
14 Maxilla
15 Vomer
16 Body of mandible
17 Parietal bone
18 Temporal bone
19 Sphenozygomatic suture
20 Ethmoidal bone
21 Zygomatic bone
22 Nasal bone
23 Zygomaticomaxillary suture
24 Middle nasal concha
25 Inferior nasal concha
26 Anterior nasal aperture
27 Mental foramen
28 Ramus of mandible
29 Base of mandible
30 Mental protuberance

Bones
Brown   = frontal bone
Light green = parietal bone
Dark brown   = temporal bone
Red   = sphenoidal bone
Yellow   = zygomatic bone
Dark green   = ethmoidal bone
Yellow   = lacrimal bone
Orange   = vomer
Violet   = maxilla
White   = nasal bone
White   = mandible

Anterior aspect of the skull (individual bones indicated by color).

The following series of figures are arranged so that the mosaic-like pattern of the skull becomes understandable. It starts with the bones of the **skull base** (sphenoidal and occipital bones) to which the other bones are added step by step. The facial skeleton is built up by the ethmoidal bone to which the palatine bone and maxilla are attached laterally; the small nasal and lacrimal bones fill the remaining spaces. Cartilages remain only in the external part of the nose.

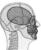

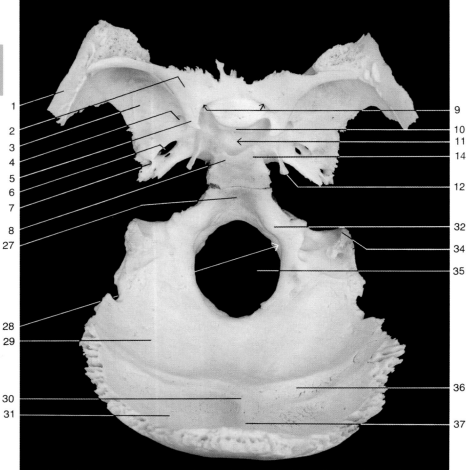

Sphenoidal and occipital bone (from above).

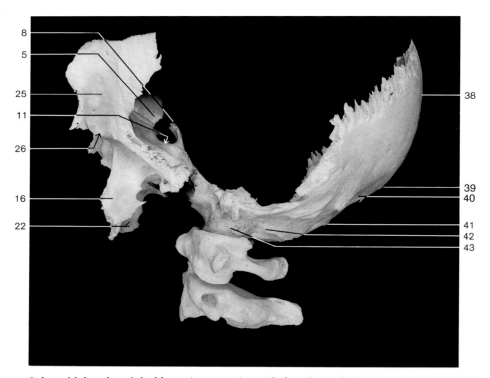

Sphenoidal and occipital bone in connection with the atlas and axis
(1st and 2nd cervical vertebrae) (left lateral view).

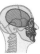

Sphenoidal bone
1   Greater wing
2   Lesser wing
3   Cerebral or superior surface of greater wing
4   Foramen rotundum
5   Anterior clinoid process
6   Foramen ovale
7   Foramen spinosum
8   Dorsum sellae
9   Optic canal
10 Chiasmatic groove (sulcus chiasmatis)
11 Hypophysial fossa (sella turcica)
12 Lingula
13 Opening of sphenoidal sinus
14 Posterior clinoid process
15 Pterygoid canal
16 Lateral pterygoid plate of pterygoid process
17 Pterygoid notch
18 Pterygoid hamulus
19 Orbital surface of greater wing
20 Sphenoidal crest
21 Sphenoidal rostrum
22 Medial pterygoid plate
23 Superior orbital fissure
24 Spine of sphenoid
25 Temporal surface of greater wing
26 Infratemporal crest

Occipital bone
27 Clivus with basilar part of occipital bone
28 Hypoglossal canal
29 Fossa for cerebellar hemisphere
30 Internal occipital protuberance
31 Fossa for cerebral hemisphere
32 Jugular tubercle
33 Condylar canal
34 Jugular process
35 Foramen magnum
36 Groove for transverse sinus
37 Groove for superior sagittal sinus
38 Squamous part of the occipital bone
39 External occipital protuberance
40 Superior nuchal line
41 Inferior nuchal line
42 Condylar fossa
43 Condyle
44 Pharyngeal tubercle
45 External occipital crest

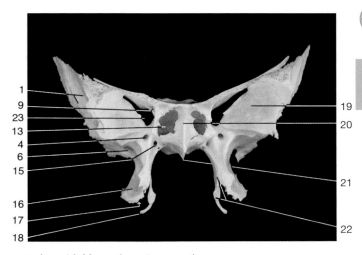

Sphenoidal bone (anterior aspect).

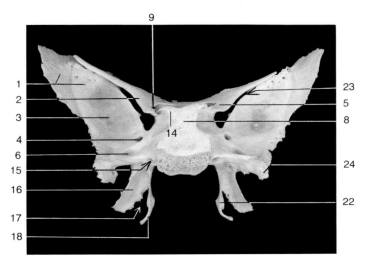

Sphenoidal bone (posterior aspect).

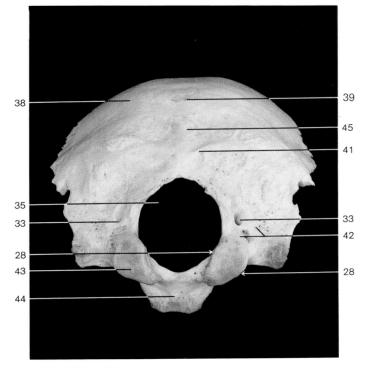

Occipital bone (from below).

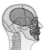

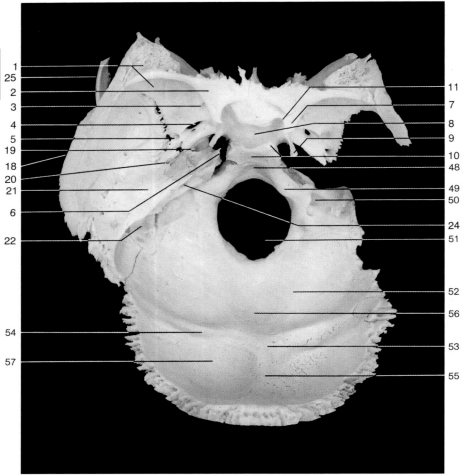

Sphenoidal bone
1   Greater wing
2   Lesser wing
3   Foramen rotundum
4   Foramen ovale
5   Foramen spinosum
6   Foramen lacerum
7   Anterior clinoid process
8   Hypophysial fossa (sella turcica)
9   Lingula
10 Dorsum sellae and posterior clinoid process
11 Optic canal
12 Sphenoidal rostrum
13 Medial pterygoid plate
14 Lateral pterygoid plate
15 Pterygoid hamulus
16 Infratemporal crest
17 Body of the sphenoidal bone

Sphenoidal, occipital, and left temporal bone (from above). Internal aspect of the base of the skull. The left temporal bone has been added to the preceding figure.

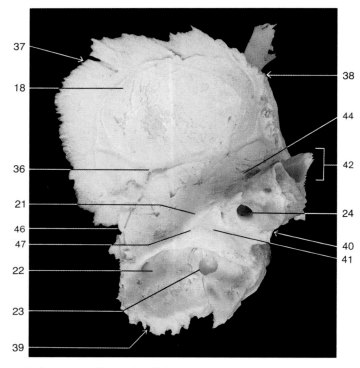

Left temporal bone (medial aspect).

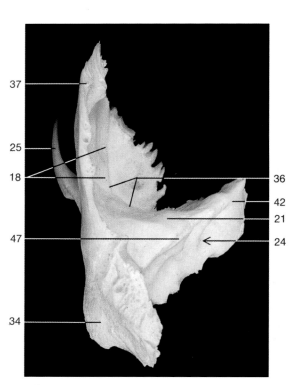

Left temporal bone (from above).

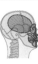

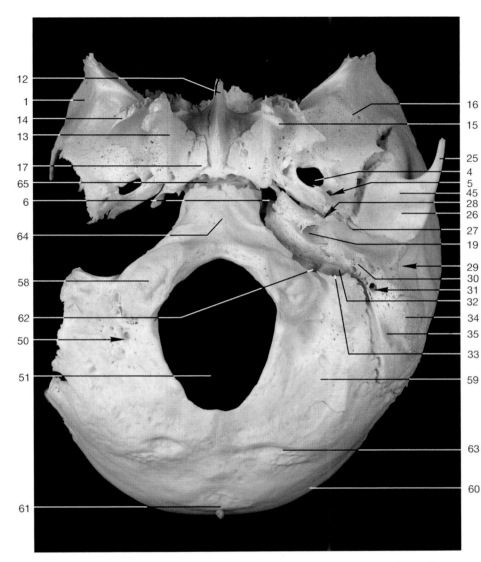

Sphenoidal, occipital, and left temporal bone. Base of the skull (external aspect).

Temporal bone
18 Squamous part
19 Carotid canal
20 Hiatus of facial canal
    (for the greater petrosal nerve)
21 Arcuate eminence
22 Groove for the sigmoid sinus
23 Mastoid foramen
24 Internal acoustic meatus
25 Zygomatic process
26 Mandibular fossa
27 Petrotympanic fissure
28 Canalis musculotubarius
    (bony part of auditory tube)
29 External acoustic meatus
30 Styloid process (remnant only)
31 Stylomastoid foramen
32 Mastoid canaliculus
33 Jugular fossa
34 Mastoid process
35 Mastoid notch
36 Groove for middle
    meningeal vessels
37 Parietal margin
38 Sphenoidal margin
39 Occipital margin
40 Cochlear canaliculus
41 Aqueduct of the vestibule
42 Apex of the petrous part
43 Tympanic part
44 Trigeminal impression
45 Articular tubercle
46 Parietal notch
47 Groove for the superior
    petrosal sinus

Occipital bone
48 Clivus
49 Jugular tubercle
50 Condylar canal
51 Foramen magnum
52 Lower part of squamous
    occipital bone
    (cerebellar fossa)
53 Internal occipital protuberance
54 Groove for the transverse sinus
55 Groove for the superior sagittal sinus
56 Internal occipital crest
57 Upper part of squamous occipital
    bone (cerebral fossa)
58 Condyle
59 Nuchal plane
60 Superior nuchal line
61 External occipital protuberance
62 Jugular foramen
63 Inferior nuchal line
64 Pharyngeal tubercle
65 Spheno-occipital synchondrosis

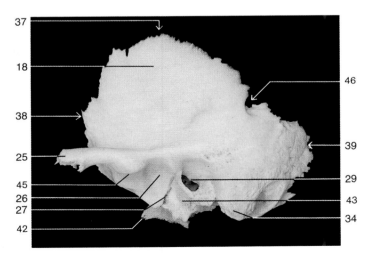

Left temporal bone (lateral aspect).

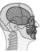

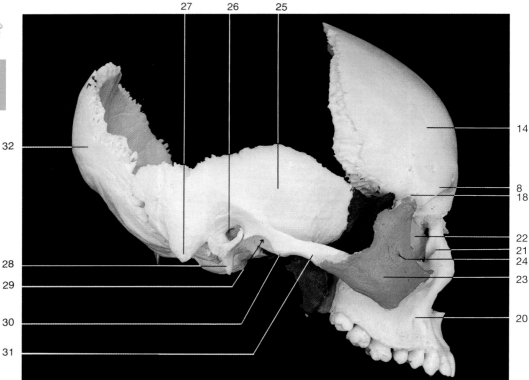

Part of a disarticulated skull (right lateral aspect). The frontal bone and the maxilla are connected with the temporal bone by the zygomatic bone (orange). Sphenoidal bone (black), palatine bone (red), lacrimal bone (yellow).

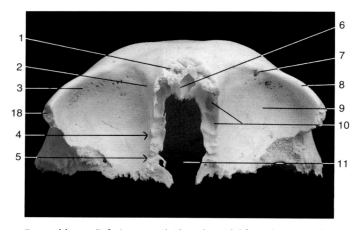

Frontal bone (inferior aspect). The ethmoidal foveolae cover the ethmoidal cavities of the ethmoidal bone.

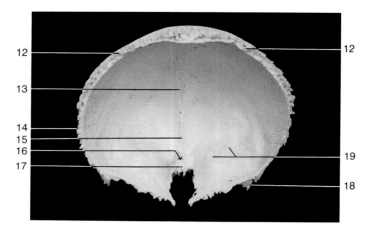

Frontal bone (posterior aspect).

Frontal bone
1 Nasal margin
2 Trochlear fossa
3 Fossa for lacrimal gland
4 Anterior ethmoidal foramen
5 Posterior ethmoidal foramen
6 Nasal spine
7 Supra-orbital notch
8 Supra-orbital margin
9 Orbital plate
10 Roofs of the ethmoidal air cells
11 Ethmoidal notch
12 Parietal margin
13 Groove for superior sagittal sinus
14 Squamous part of frontal bone
15 Frontal crest
16 Foramen cecum
17 Nasal spine
18 Zygomatic process of frontal bone
19 Juga cerebralia

Facial bones
20 Maxilla
21 Frontal process of maxilla
22 Lacrimal bone (yellow)
23 Zygomatic bone (orange)
24 Zygomaticofacial foramen

Temporal bone
25 Squamous part of temporal bone
26 External acoustic meatus
27 Mastoid process
28 Styloid process
29 Mandibular fossa
30 Articular tubercle
31 Zygomatic process

Occipital bone
32 Squamous part of occipital bone

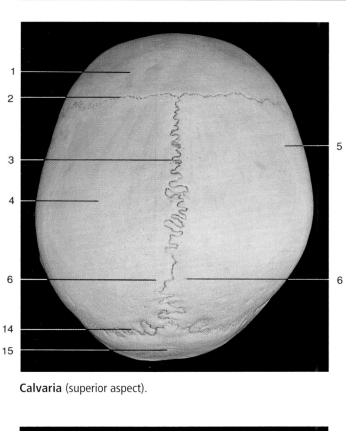

Calvaria (superior aspect).

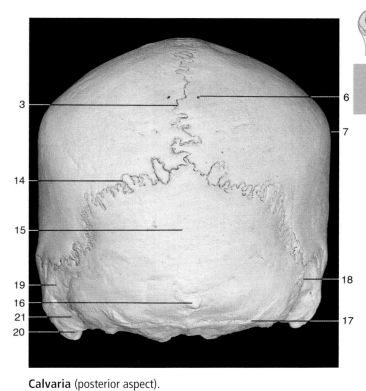

Calvaria (posterior aspect).

Left parietal bone (external aspect).

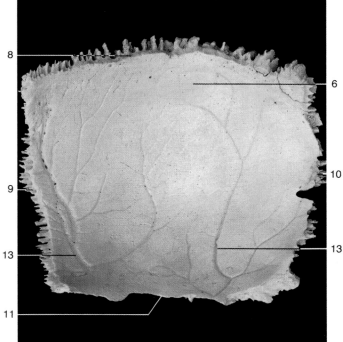

Left parietal bone (internal aspect).

1	Frontal bone	8	Sagittal margin
2	Coronal suture	9	Occipital margin
3	Sagittal suture	10	Frontal margin
4	Parietal bone	11	Squamous margin
5	Superior temporal line	12	Sphenoidal angle
6	Parietal foramen	13	Groove for middle meningeal artery
7	Parietal tuber or eminence	14	Lambdoid suture

15	Occipital bone
16	External occipital protuberance
17	Inferior nuchal line
18	Occipitomastoid suture
19	Temporal bone
20	Mastoid process
21	Mastoid notch

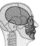

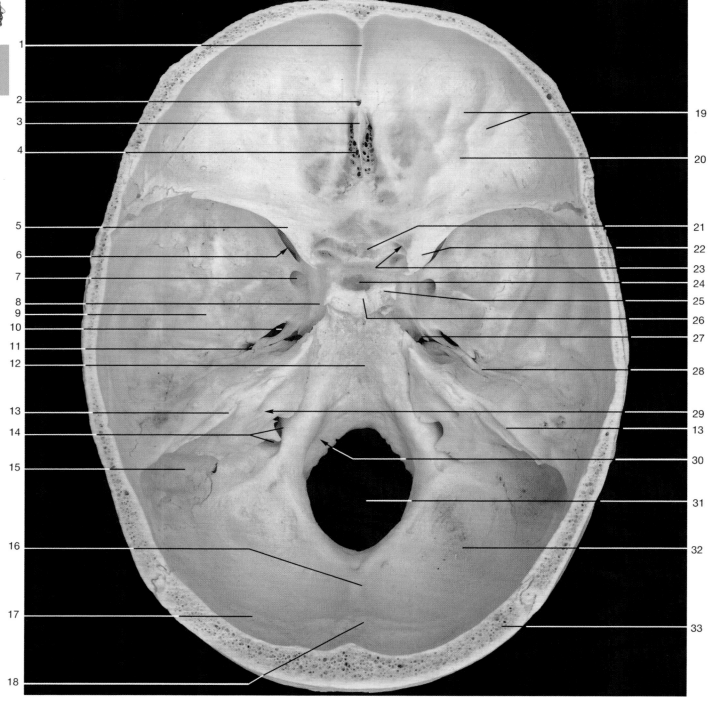

Base of the skull, calvaria removed (internal aspect).

1 Frontal crest	12 Clivus	23 Optic canal
2 Foramen cecum	13 Groove for superior petrosal sinus	24 Sella turcica (hypophysial fossa)
3 Crista galli	14 Jugular foramen	25 Posterior clinoid process
4 Cribriform plate of ethmoidal bone	15 Groove for sigmoid sinus	26 Dorsum sellae
5 Lesser wing of sphenoidal bone	16 Internal occipital crest	27 Foramen lacerum
6 Superior orbital fissure	17 Groove for transverse sinus	28 Groove for greater petrosal nerve
7 Foramen rotundum	18 Internal occipital protuberance	29 Internal acoustic meatus
8 Carotid sulcus	19 Digitate impressions	30 Hypoglossal canal
9 Middle cranial fossa	20 Anterior cranial fossa	31 Foramen magnum
10 Foramen ovale	21 Chiasmatic sulcus	32 Posterior cranial fossa
11 Foramen spinosum	22 Anterior clinoid process	33 Diploe

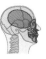

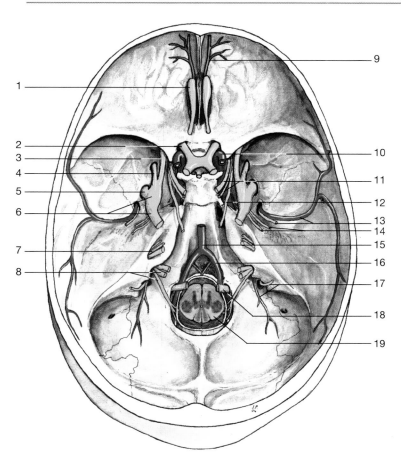

1 Olfactory bulb
2 Optic nerve (n. II)
3 Ophthalmic nerve (n. V₁)
4 Maxillary nerve (n. V₂)
5 Mandibular nerve (n. V₃)
6 Trigeminal nerve (n. V) with trigeminal ganglion
7 Facial nerve (n. VII) and vestibulocochlear nerve (n. VIII)
8 Glossopharyngeal nerve (n. IX), vagus nerve (n. X) and accessory nerve (n. XI)
9 Anterior meningeal artery
10 Internal carotid artery
11 Oculomotor nerve (n. III) and trochlear nerve (n. IV)
12 Abducent nerve (n. VI)
13 Middle meningeal artery and meningeal branch of mandibular nerve
14 Greater and lesser petrosal nerves
15 Basilar artery
16 Vertebral artery
17 Posterior meningeal artery and recurrent meningeal nerve
18 Hypoglossal nerve (n. XII)
19 Medulla oblongata

Base of the skull with cranial nerves and meningeal arteries (internal aspect, schematic drawing).

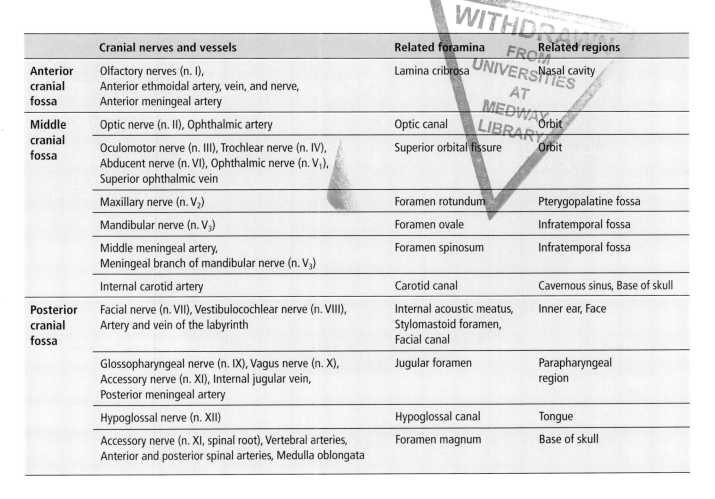

	Cranial nerves and vessels	Related foramina	Related regions
Anterior cranial fossa	Olfactory nerves (n. I), Anterior ethmoidal artery, vein, and nerve, Anterior meningeal artery	Lamina cribrosa	Nasal cavity
Middle cranial fossa	Optic nerve (n. II), Ophthalmic artery	Optic canal	Orbit
	Oculomotor nerve (n. III), Trochlear nerve (n. IV), Abducent nerve (n. VI), Ophthalmic nerve (n. V₁), Superior ophthalmic vein	Superior orbital fissure	Orbit
	Maxillary nerve (n. V₂)	Foramen rotundum	Pterygopalatine fossa
	Mandibular nerve (n. V₃)	Foramen ovale	Infratemporal fossa
	Middle meningeal artery, Meningeal branch of mandibular nerve (n. V₃)	Foramen spinosum	Infratemporal fossa
	Internal carotid artery	Carotid canal	Cavernous sinus, Base of skull
Posterior cranial fossa	Facial nerve (n. VII), Vestibulocochlear nerve (n. VIII), Artery and vein of the labyrinth	Internal acoustic meatus, Stylomastoid foramen, Facial canal	Inner ear, Face
	Glossopharyngeal nerve (n. IX), Vagus nerve (n. X), Accessory nerve (n. XI), Internal jugular vein, Posterior meningeal artery	Jugular foramen	Parapharyngeal region
	Hypoglossal nerve (n. XII)	Hypoglossal canal	Tongue
	Accessory nerve (n. XI, spinal root), Vertebral arteries, Anterior and posterior spinal arteries, Medulla oblongata	Foramen magnum	Base of skull

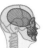

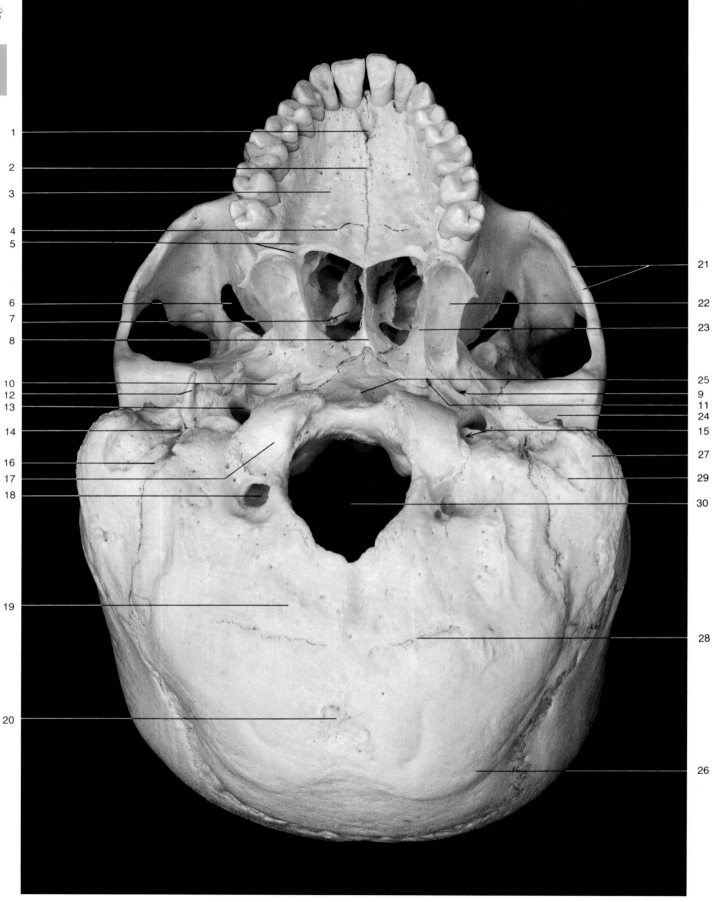

Base of the skull (inferior aspect).

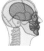

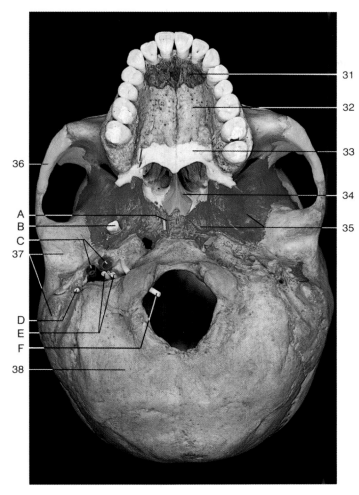

A = **pterygoid canal**
B = **foramen ovale**
C = internal carotid artery within **carotid canal** and internal jugular vein within the venous part of jugular foramen
D = **stylomastoid foramen** (facial nerve)
E = **jugular foramen** (glossopharyngeal, vagus and accessory nerves)
F = **hypoglossal canal** (hypoglossal nerve)

1   Incisive canal
2   Median palatine suture
3   Palatine process of maxilla
4   Palatomaxillary suture
5   Greater and lesser palatine foramina
6   Inferior orbital fissure
7   Middle concha (process of ethmoidal bone)
8   Vomer
9   Foramen ovale
10 Groove for auditory tube
11 Pterygoid canal
12 Styloid process
13 Carotid canal
14 Stylomastoid foramen
15 Jugular foramen
16 Groove for occipital artery
17 Occipital condyle
18 Condylar canal
19 Nuchal plane
20 External occipital protuberance
21 Zygomatic arch
22 Lateral pterygoid plate
23 Medial pterygoid plate
24 Mandibular fossa
25 Pharyngeal tubercle
26 Superior nuchal line
27 Mastoid process
28 Inferior nuchal line
29 Mastoid notch
30 Foramen magnum
31 Incisive bone or premaxilla (dark violet)
32 Maxilla (violet)
33 Palatine bone (white)
34 Vomer (orange)
35 Sphenoidal bone (red)
36 Zygomatic bone (yellow)
37 Temporal bone (brown)
38 Occipital bone (blue)
39 Palatine process of maxilla
40 Vomer
41 Sphenoidal bone
42 Petrous part of temporal bone
43 Basilar part ⎫
44 Lateral part ⎬ of occipital bone
45 Squamous part ⎭
46 Mandible
47 Zygomatic arch
48 Choana
49 Pterygoid process of sphenoidal bone
50 Carotid canal
51 External acoustic meatus (tympanic anulus)
52 Sphenoidal fontanelle
53 Parietal bone
54 Mastoid fontanelle

Base of the skull (from below). The individual bones are indicated by different colors.

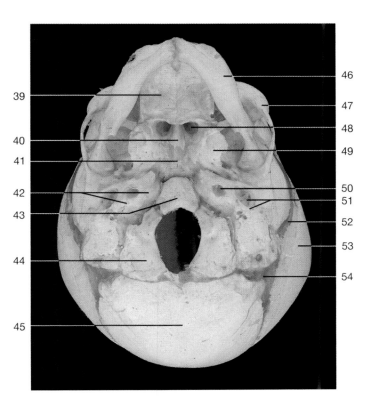

Skull of the newborn (inferior aspect).

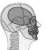

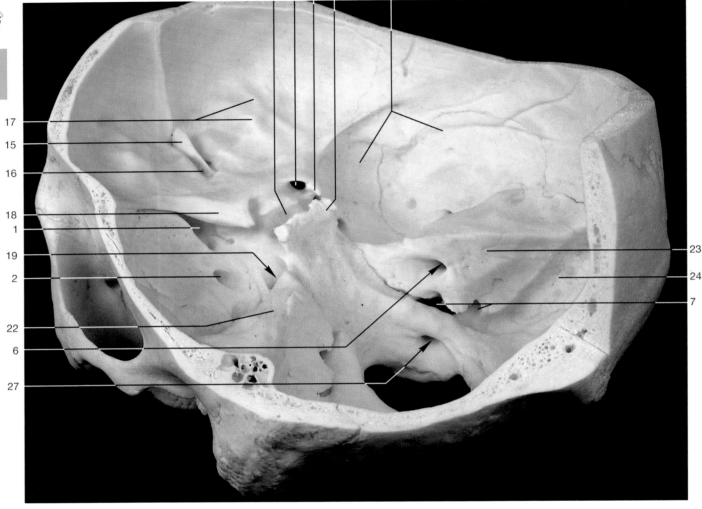

Base of the skull (internal aspect, oblique lateral view from left side).

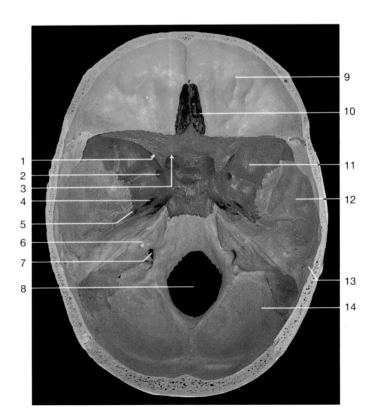

Canals, fissures, and foramina of the base of the skull
1 Superior orbital fissure
2 Foramen rotundum
3 Optic canal
4 Foramen ovale
5 Foramen spinosum
6 Internal acoustic meatus
7 Jugular foramen
8 Foramen magnum

Bones
9   Frontal bone (orange)
10 Ethmoidal bone (dark green)
11 Sphenoidal bone (red)
12 Temporal bone (brown)
13 Parietal bone (yellow)
14 Occipital bone (blue)

Details of bones
15 Crista galli
16 Cribriform plate

17 Digitate impressions (frontal bone)
18 Lesser wing of sphenoidal bone
19 Foramen lacerum
20 Hypophysial fossa (sella turcica)
21 Anterior clinoid process
22 Trigeminal impression
23 Petrous part of temporal bone
24 Groove for sigmoid sinus
25 Dorsum sellae (posterior clinoid process)
26 Greater wing of sphenoidal bone, groove for middle meningeal artery
27 Hypoglossal canal

Base of the skull (internal aspect, superior view). Individual bones indicated by color.

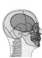

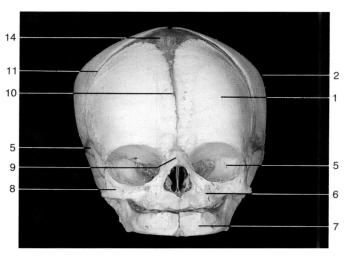

Skull of the newborn (anterior aspect).

Cranial skeleton
1 Frontal tuber or eminence
2 Parietal tuber or eminence
3 Occipital tuber or eminence
4 Squamous part of temporal bone
5 Greater wing of sphenoidal bone

Facial skeleton
6 Maxilla
7 Mandible
8 Zygomatic bone
9 Nasal bone

Sutures and fontanelles
10 Frontal suture
11 Coronal suture
12 Sagittal suture
13 Lambdoid suture
14 Anterior fontanelle
15 Posterior fontanelle
16 Sphenoidal (anterolateral) fontanelle
17 Mastoid (posterolateral) fontanelle

Base of the skull
18 Frontal bone
19 Ethmoidal bone
20 Sphenoidal bone
21 Hypophysial fossa (sella turcica)
22 Dorsum sellae
23 Temporal bone
24 Mastoid (posterolateral) fontanelle
25 Occipital bone

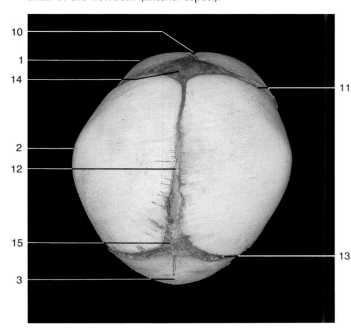

Skull of the newborn (superior aspect). Calvaria.

In the newborn, the facial skeleton, in contrast to the cranial skeleton, appears relatively small. There are no teeth presenting. The bones of the cranium are separated by wide fontanelles.

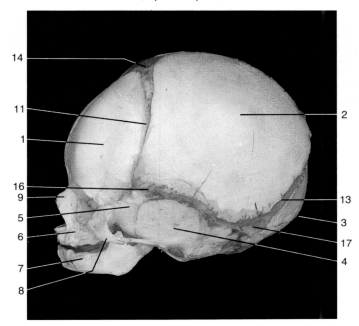

Skull of the newborn (lateral aspect).

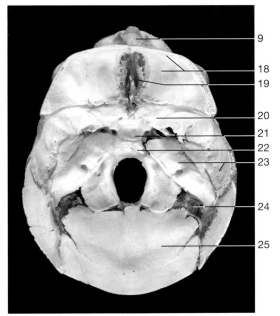

Base of the skull of the newborn (internal aspect).

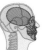

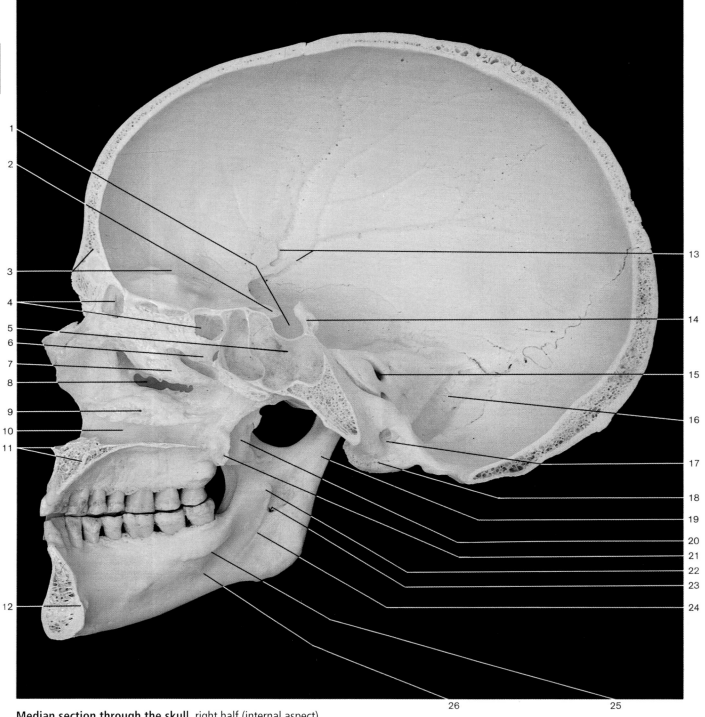

Median section through the skull, right half (internal aspect).

1	Hypophysial fossa (sella turcica)	14	Dorsum sellae
2	Anterior clinoid process	15	Internal acoustic meatus
3	Frontal bone	16	Groove for sigmoid sinus
4	Ethmoidal air cells	17	Hypoglossal canal
5	Sphenoidal sinus	18	Occipital condyle
6	Superior concha	19	Condylar process
7	Middle concha	20	Lateral pterygoid plate ⎫ of pterygoid process
8	Maxillary hiatus	21	Medial pterygoid plate ⎬
9	Inferior concha	22	Lingula of mandible
10	Inferior meatus	23	Mandibular foramen
11	Anterior nasal spine and maxilla	24	Mylohyoid groove
12	Mental spine or genial tubercle	25	Mylohyoid line
13	Groove for middle meningeal artery	26	Submandibular fovea

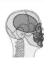

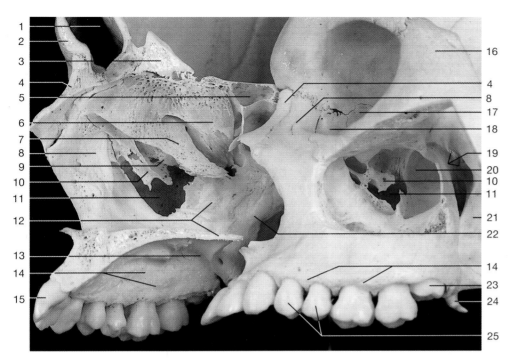

1 Frontal sinus
2 Frontal bone
3 Crista galli
4 Nasal bone
5 Sphenoidal sinus
6 Superior concha ⎱ of ethmoidal
7 Middle concha ⎰ bone
8 Frontal process
   of maxilla
9 Ethmoidal bulla
10 Uncinate process
11 Maxillary hiatus
12 Palatine bone
13 Greater palatine foramen
14 Alveolar process of maxilla
15 Central incisor
16 Zygomatic bone
17 Ethmoidal bone
18 Lacrimal bone
19 Pterygopalatine fossa
20 Maxillary sinus
21 Lateral pterygoid plate
22 Medial pterygoid plate
23 Third molar tooth
24 Pterygoid hamulus
25 Two premolar teeth

Facial part of the skull (viscerocranium), divided in two halves (lateral and medial aspect). Right inferior concha has been removed to show the maxillary hiatus. Left maxillary sinus opened.

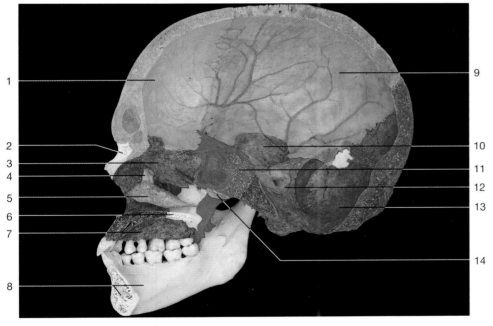

Bones (indicated by colors)
1 Frontal bone (yellow)
2 Nasal bone (white)
3 Ethmoidal bone (dark green)
4 Lacrimal bone (yellow)
5 Inferior nasal concha (pink)
6 Palatine bone (white)
7 Maxilla (violet)
8 Mandible (white)
9 Parietal bone (light green)
10 Temporal bone (brown)
11 Sphenoidal bone (red)
12 Petrous part of temporal
   bone (brown)
13 Occipital bone (blue)
14 Ala of vomer (light brown)

Median section through the skull. The nasal septum has been removed. Bones indicated by colors.

Because of the upright posture that the human developed in the course of evolution, the cranial cavity greatly increased in size, whereas the facial skeleton decreased. As a result, the base of the skull developed an angulation of about 120° between the clivus and the cribriform plate (see drawing on page 19). The hypophysial fossa containing the pituitary gland lies at the angle formed between these two planes.

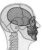

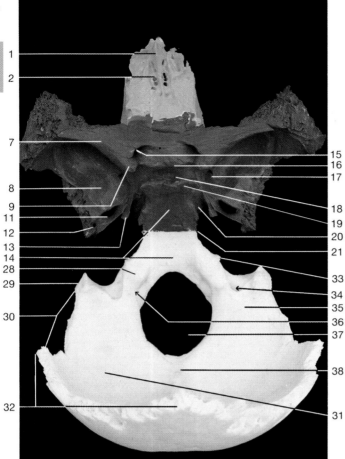

Ethmoidal bone
1 Crista galli
2 Cribriform plate
3 Ethmoidal air cells
4 Middle concha
5 Perpendicular plate (part of nasal septum)
6 Orbital plate

Sphenoidal bone
7 Lesser wing
8 Greater wing
9 Anterior clinoid process
10 Posterior clinoid process
11 Foramen ovale
12 Foramen spinosum
13 Lingula of the sphenoidal bone
14 Clivus
15 Optic canal
16 Tuberculum sellae
17 Foramen rotundum (right side)
18 Hypophysial fossa (sella turcica)
19 Dorsum sellae
20 Carotid sulcus
21 Spheno-occipital synchondrosis
22 Lateral pterygoid plate
23 Greater wing of sphenoidal bone (orbital surface)
24 Greater wing of sphenoidal bone (maxillary surface)
25 Foramen rotundum (left side)
26 Superior orbital fissure
27 Infratemporal crest of the greater wing

Part of the disarticulated base of the skull.
Ethmoidal, sphenoidal, and occipital bones (from above).
Green = sphenoidal bone; yellow = ethmoidal bone.

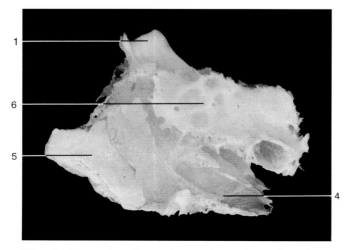

Ethmoidal bone (lateral aspect), posterior portion to the right.

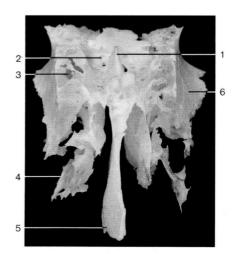

Ethmoidal bone (anterior aspect).

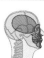

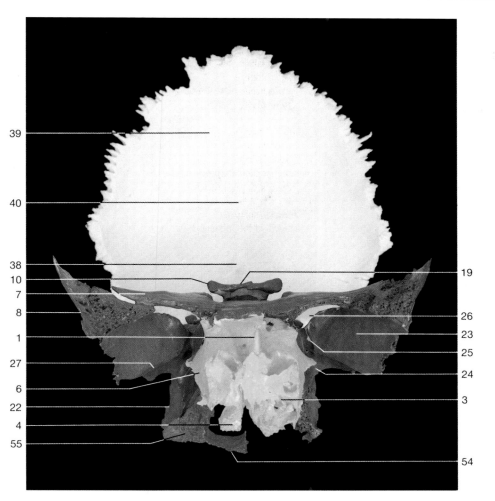

Occipital bone
28 Jugular tubercle
29 Jugular process
30 Mastoid margin
31 Posterior cranial fossa
32 Lambdoid margin
33 Intrajugular process
34 Condylar canal
35 Lateral part of occipital bone
36 Hypoglossal canal
37 Foramen magnum
38 Internal occipital crest
39 Squamous part of occipital bone
40 Internal occipital protuberance

Maxilla
41 Orbital surface
42 Infra-orbital groove
43 Maxillary tuberosity with foramina
44 Frontal process
45 Nasolacrimal groove
46 Infra-orbital margin
47 Anterior nasal spine
48 Zygomatic process
49 Alveolar process

Palatine bone
50 Orbital process
51 Sphenopalatine notch
52 Sphenoidal process
53 Perpendicular plate
54 Horizontal plate
55 Pyramidal process

Disarticulated base of the skull (anterior aspect). Green = sphenoidal bone; yellow = ethmoidal bone; red = palatine bone.

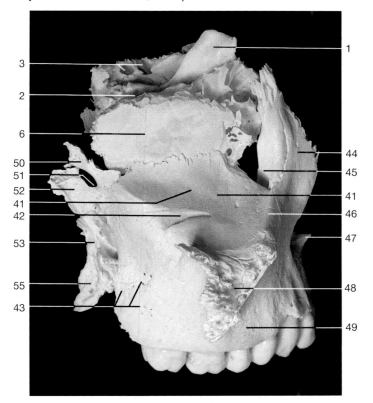

Right maxilla, ethmoidal, and palatine bone (lateral aspect).

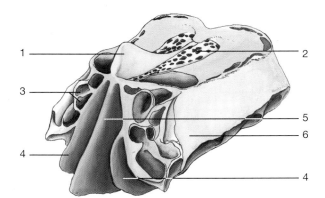

Ethmoidal bone (oblique anterior aspect). (Schematic drawing.)

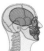

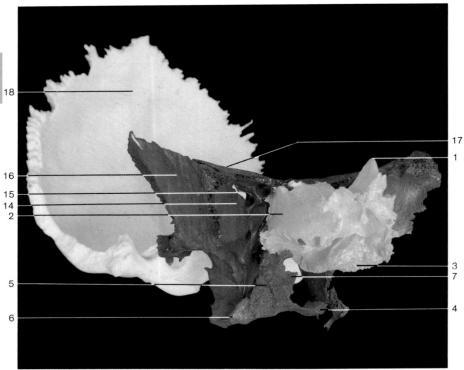

Ethmoidal bone
1 Crista galli
2 Orbital plate
3 Middle concha

Palatine bone
4 Horizontal plate of palatine bone
5 Greater palatine canal
6 Pyramidal process
7 Maxillary process
8 Orbital process
9 Sphenopalatine notch
10 Perpendicular plate of palatine bone
11 Conchal crest
12 Nasal crest
13 Sphenoidal process

Sphenoidal bone
14 Greater wing
15 Superior orbital fissure
16 Greater wing (orbital surface)
17 Lesser wing

Occipital bone
18 Squamous part of occipital bone

Maxilla
19 Maxillary tuberosity
20 Frontal process
21 Orbital surface
22 Infra-orbital margin
23 Infra-orbital groove
24 Zygomatic process
25 Alveolar process

Part of a disarticulated skull base, similar to the preceding figures, but with palatine bone. Green = sphenoidal bone; yellow = ethmoidal bone; red = palatine bone.

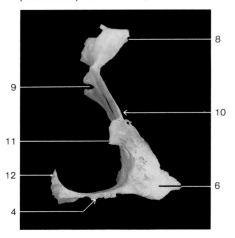

Left palatine bone (medial aspect, posterior aspect to the left).

Left palatine bone (anterior aspect).

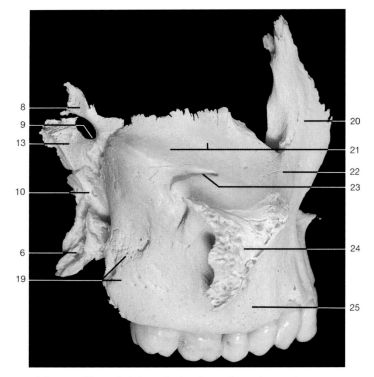

Right maxilla and right palatine bone (lateral aspect).

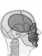

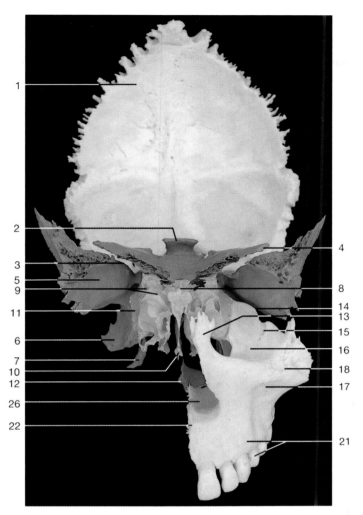

Occipital bone
1 Squamous part

Sphenoidal bone
2 Dorsum sellae
3 Superior orbital fissure
4 Lesser wing
5 Greater wing (orbital surface)
6 Lateral pterygoid plate
7 Medial pterygoid plate

Ethmoidal bone
8 Crista galli
9 Ethmoidal air cells
10 Perpendicular plate
11 Orbital plate

Palatine bone
12 Horizontal plate (nasal crest)

Maxilla
13 Frontal process
14 Inferior orbital fissure
15 Infra-orbital groove
16 Orbital surface
17 Infra-orbital foramen
18 Zygomatic process
19 Anterior lacrimal crest
20 Canine fossa
21 Alveolar process with teeth
22 Anterior nasal spine
23 Juga alveolaria (elevations formed by roots of teeth)
24 Lacrimal groove
25 Maxillary tuberosity with alveolar foramina
26 Palatine process of maxilla

Part of a disarticulated skull.
The left **maxilla** is added to the preceding specimen.

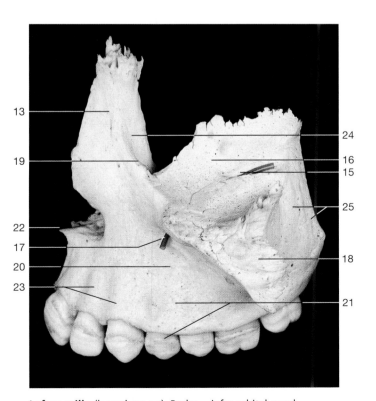

Left maxilla (lateral aspect). Probe = infra-orbital canal.

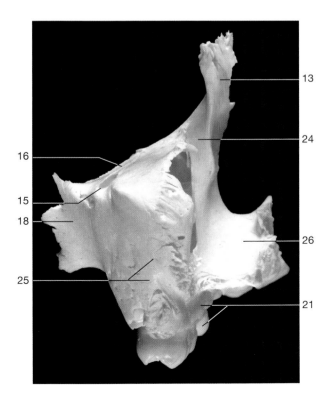

Left maxilla (posterior aspect).

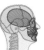

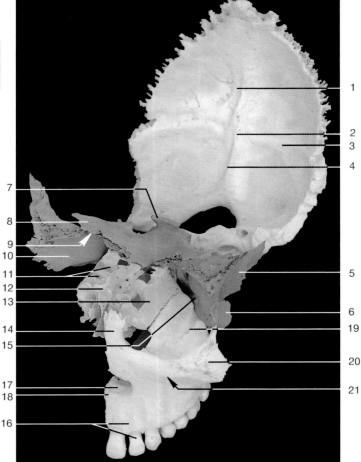

Occipital bone
1 Groove for superior sagittal sinus
2 Internal occipital protuberance
3 Groove for transverse sinus
4 Internal occipital crest

Sphenoidal bone
5 Greater wing (temporal surface)
6 Lateral pterygoid plate
7 Dorsum sellae
8 Lesser wing
9 Superior orbital fissure
10 Greater wing (orbital surface)

Ethmoidal bone
11 Ethmoidal air cells
12 Crista galli
13 Orbital plate

Maxilla
14 Frontal process
15 Inferior orbital fissure
16 Alveolar process with teeth
17 Palatine process
18 Anterior nasal spine
19 Infra-orbital groove
20 Zygomatic process
21 Location of infra-orbital foramen
22 Middle nasal meatus
23 Inferior nasal meatus
24 Maxillary hiatus
   (leading to maxillary sinus)
25 Third molar
26 Lacrimal groove
27 Conchal crest
28 Body of maxilla (nasal surface)
29 Nasal crest
30 Incisive canal

Palatine bone
31 Orbital process
32 Sphenopalatine notch
33 Sphenoidal process
34 Perpendicular plate
35 Conchal crest
36 Horizontal plate
37 Pyramidal process

Frontal bone
38 Squamous part
39 Supra-orbital foramen
40 Frontal notch
41 Frontal spine

Inferior nasal concha
42 Inferior nasal concha
   with maxillary process

Part of a disarticulated base of skull. The mosaic of the facial bones [sphenoidal bone (green), ethmoidal bone (yellow), and palatine bone (red)] is seen from the antero-lateral aspect.

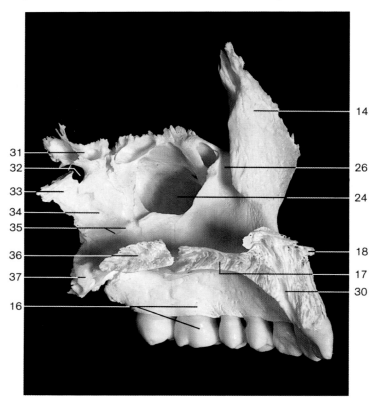

Left maxilla and palatine bone (medial aspect).

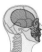

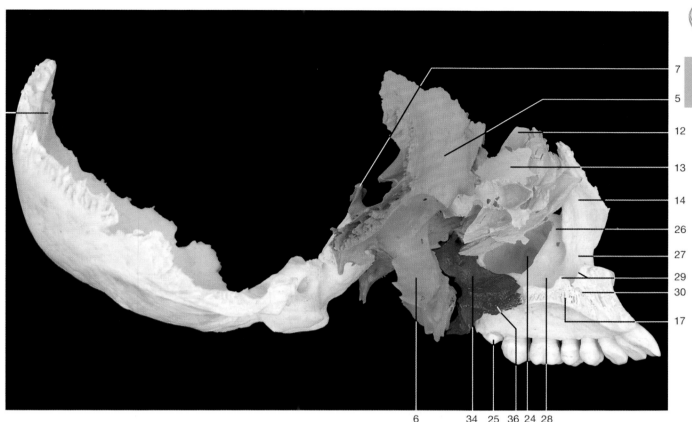

Part of a disarticulated base of skull (medial aspect). Green = sphenoidal bone; yellow = ethmoidal bone; red = palatine bone; natural colored = left maxilla.

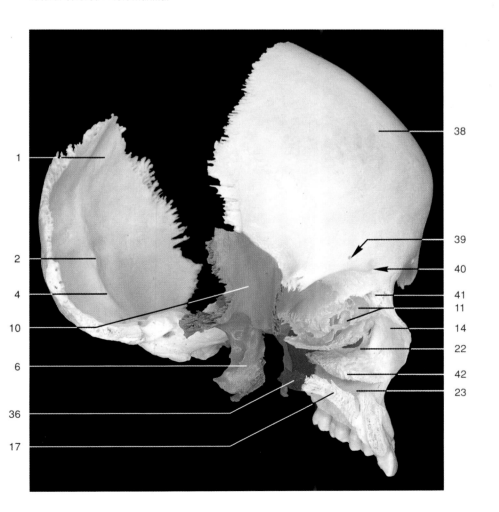

Part of a disarticulated base of skull. The same specimen as shown above but with frontal bone (oblique-lateral aspect).

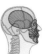

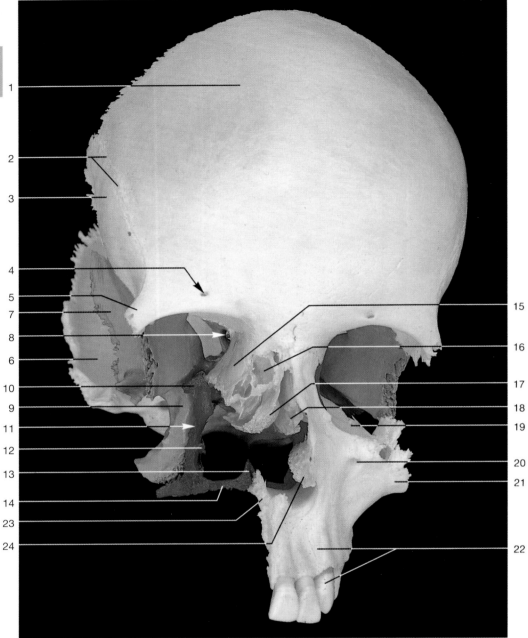

Part of a disarticulated skull showing the connection of the palatine bone (red) and the maxilla with ethmoidal bone (yellow) and sphenoidal bone (green) (anterior aspect).

Frontal bone
1 Squamous part
2 Inferior temporal line
3 Temporal surface
4 Supra-orbital foramen
5 Zygomatic process

Occipital bone
6 Squamous part

Sphenoidal bone
7 Greater wing (temporal surface)
8 Optic canal within the lesser wing
9 Lateral pterygoid plate

Palatine bone
10 Orbital process
11 Perpendicular plate
12 Conchal crest
13 Nasal crest
14 Horizontal plate

Ethmoidal bone
15 Orbital plate
16 Ethmoidal air cell
17 Middle concha
18 Perpendicular plate
(part of bony nasal septum)

Maxilla
19 Infra-orbital groove
20 Infra-orbital foramen
21 Zygomatic process
22 Alveolar process with teeth
23 Palatine process

Left inferior nasal concha
24 Anterior part of
inferior concha

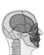

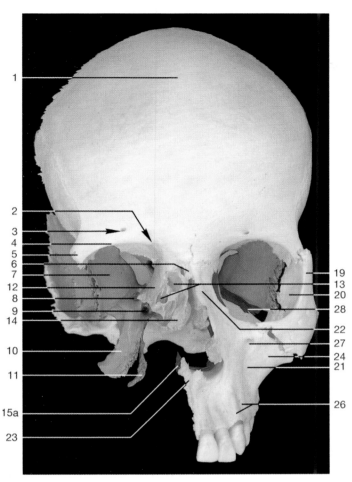

Frontal bone
1   Squamous part
2   Frontal notch
3   Supra-orbital foramen
4   Supra-orbital margin
5   Zygomatic process
6   Frontal spine

Sphenoidal bone
7   Greater wing (orbital surface)
8   Foramen rotundum
9   Pterygoid or Vidian canal
10   Lateral pterygoid plate
11   Medial pterygoid plate

Ethmoidal bone
12   Orbital plate
13   Ethmoidal air cells
14   Middle concha

Palatine bone
15   Horizontal plate
15a Nasal crest
16   Pyramidal process
17   Lesser palatine foramen
18   Greater palatine foramen

Zygomatic bone
19   Frontal process
20   Orbital surface

Maxilla
21   Canine fossa
22   Frontal process
23   Palatine process
24   Zygomatic process
25   Alveolar process and teeth
26   Juga alveolaria
27   Infra-orbital foramen
28   Infra-orbital groove
29   Anterior nasal aperture
30   Anterior nasal spine

Incisive bone
31   Central incisor and incisive bone or premaxilla
32   Incisive fossa

Vomer
33   Ala of the vomer

Sutures and choanae
34   Median palatine suture
35   Transverse palatine suture
36   Choanae

Anterior view of a disarticulated skull showing the connection of the maxilla with the frontal and zygomatic bones. Yellow = ethmoidal bone; red = palatine bone; green = sphenoidal bone.

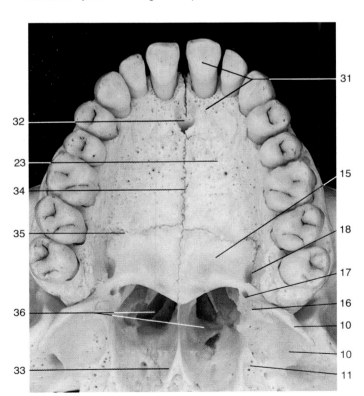

Bony palate and teeth of the maxillae (from below).

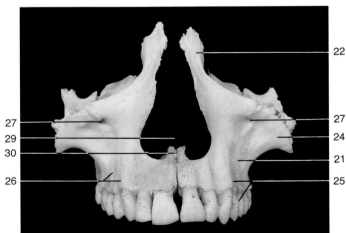

Anterior view of both maxillae forming the anterior bony aperture of the nose.

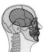

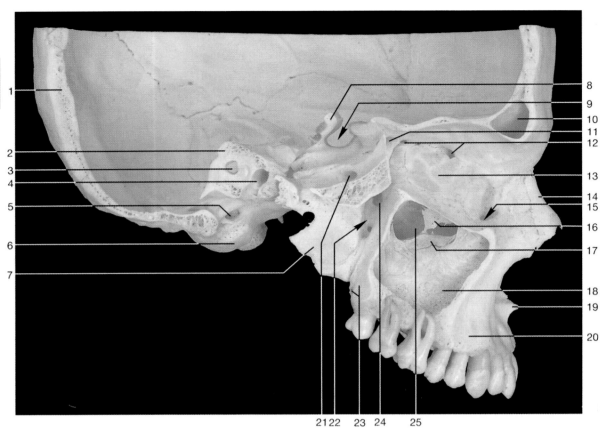

Paramedian section through the skull, right side (lateral aspect). Frontal and maxillary sinuses are opened.

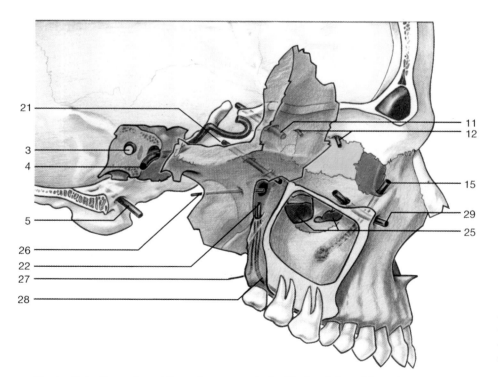

Illustration of canals and foramina connected with the right orbit and pterygopalatine fossa (compare the above figure). The greater wing of sphenoidal bone (green) is shown as being transparent. Brown = temporal bone; yellow = ethmoidal bone; red = lacrimal bone; light red = inferior nasal concha; violet = maxilla; red = palatine bone.

1   Occipital bone
2   Temporal bone (petrous part)
3   Internal acoustic meatus
4   Carotid canal
5   Hypoglossal canal
6   Occipital condyle
7   Lateral plate of pterygoid process
8   Dorsum of sella turcica
9   Sella turcica
10 Frontal sinus
11 Optic canal
12 Posterior and anterior
    ethmoidal foramina
13 Orbital plate of ethmoidal bone
14 Nasal bone
15 Nasolacrimal canal
16 Uncinate process
17 Inferior nasal concha
    (maxillary process)
18 Maxillary sinus
19 Anterior nasal spine
20 Alveolar process of maxilla
21 Foramen rotundum
22 Pterygopalatine fossa
23 Tuberosity of maxilla
    with alveolar foramina
24 Sphenopalatine foramen
25 Maxillary hiatus
26 Pterygoid or Vidian canal
27 Lesser palatine canal
28 Greater palatine canal
29 Infra-orbital canal

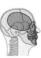

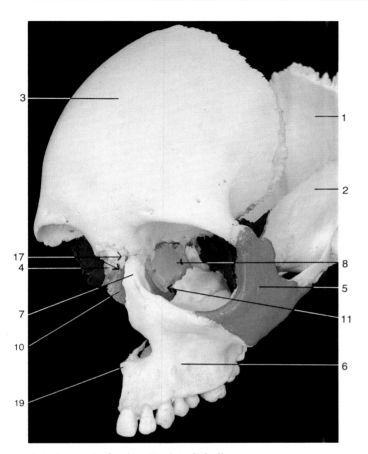

1 Occipital bone
2 Temporal bone
3 Frontal bone
4 Nasal spine of frontal bone
5 Zygomatic bone
6 Maxilla
7 Frontal process of maxilla
8 Ethmoidal bone
9 Orbital plate of ethmoidal bone
10 Perpendicular plate of ethmoidal bone
11 Site of lacrimal bone
12 Lacrimal groove of lacrimal bone
13 Posterior lacrimal crest
14 Fossa for lacrimal sac
15 Lacrimal hamulus
16 Nasolacrimal canal
17 Site of nasal bone
18 Nasal foramina of nasal bone
19 Anterior nasal spine of maxilla
20 Vomer
21 Greater wing of sphenoidal bone
22 Anterior and posterior ethmoidal foramina
23 Optic canal
24 Superior orbital fissure
25 Inferior orbital fissure
26 Infra-orbital groove
27 Infra-orbital foramen

Anterior part of a disarticulated skull.
Orange = zygomatic bone; yellow = ethmoidal bone;
dark green = sphenoidal bone. The arrows indicate the locations
of the lacrimal bone (11) and the nasal bone (17).

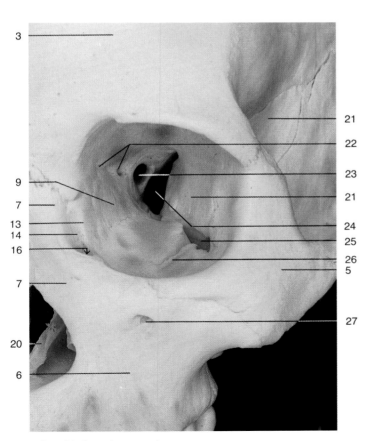

Left orbit (anterior aspect).

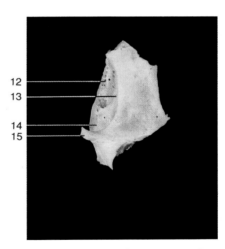

Left lacrimal bone (anterior aspect).

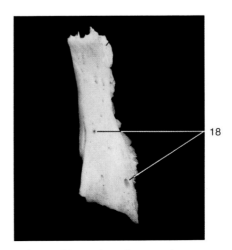

Left nasal bone (anterior aspect).

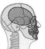

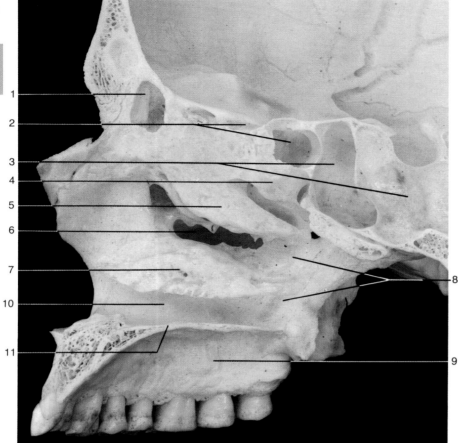

1   Frontal sinus
2   Ethmoidal air cells
3   Sphenoidal sinus
4   Superior nasal concha
5   Middle nasal concha
6   Maxillary hiatus
7   Inferior nasal concha
8   Palatine bone
9   Maxilla
10 Inferior meatus
11 Palatine process of the maxilla

To page 49:

Blue	=	occipital bone
Light green	=	parietal bone
Yellow	=	frontal bone
Dark brown	=	temporal bone
Red	=	sphenoidal bone
Dark green	=	ethmoidal bone
Light blue	=	nasal bone
Pink	=	inferior concha
Orange	=	vomer
Violet	=	maxilla
White	=	palatine bone
White	=	mandible

Lateral wall of the nasal cavity. Median section through the skull.

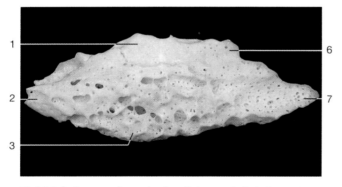

Right inferior nasal concha (medial aspect). Anterior part to the left.

Inferior concha and vomer
1   Ethmoidal process
2   Anterior part of concha
3   Inferior border
4   Ala of vomer
5   Posterior border of nasal septum
6   Lacrimal process
7   Posterior part of concha
8   Maxillary process

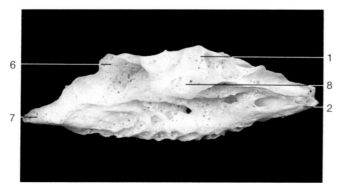

Right inferior nasal concha (lateral aspect). Anterior part to the right.

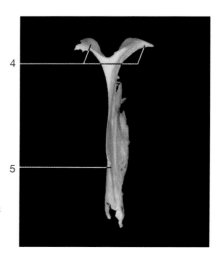

Vomer (posterior aspect).

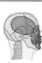

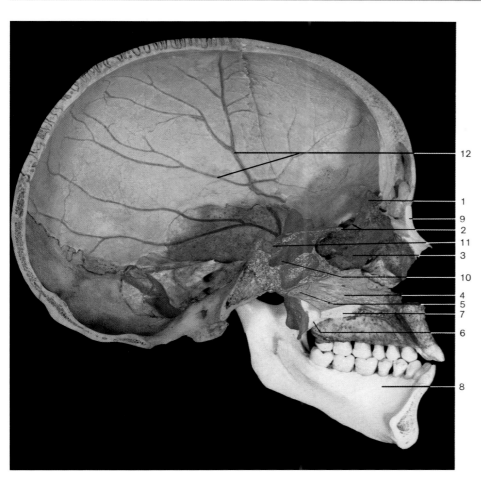

1 Crista galli
2 Cribriform plate
   of ethmoidal bone
3 Perpendicular plate
   of ethmoidal bone
4 Vomer
5 Ala of the vomer
6 Palatine bone
   (perpendicular process)
7 Palatine bone (horizontal plate)
8 Mandible
9 Nasal bone
10 Sphenoidal sinus
11 Hypophysial fossa (sella turcica)
12 Grooves for the middle
   meningeal artery

Cartilages of the nose
13 Lateral nasal cartilage
14 Greater alar cartilage
15 Lesser alar cartilages
16 Septal cartilage
17 Location of nasal bone

Paramedian sagittal section through the skull including the nasal septum.

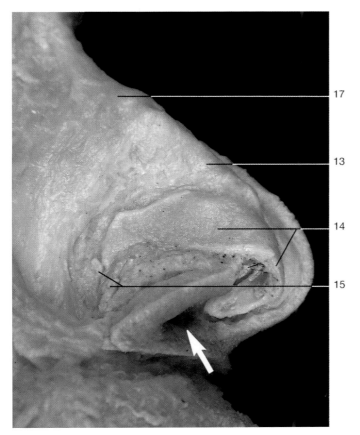

Cartilages of the nose (right anterior aspect). Arrow = nostril, framed by nasal wing.

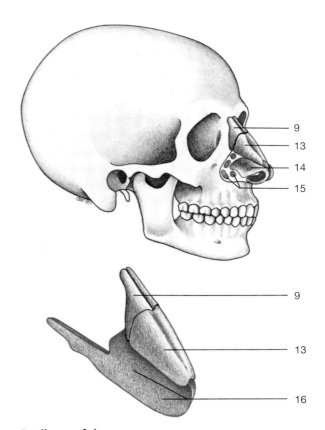

Cartilages of the nose
(schematic diagram of the external nose).

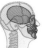

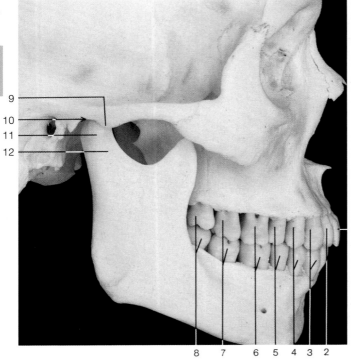

Normal position of teeth. Dentition in centric occlusion (lateral view).

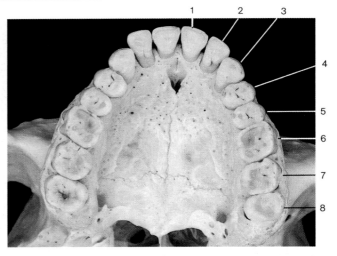

Upper teeth of the adult (inferior aspect).

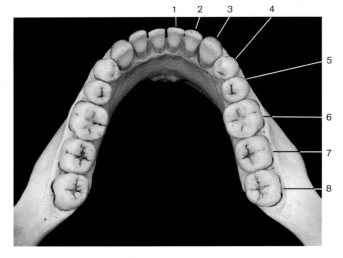

Lower teeth of the adult (superior aspect).

1 Central incisor
2 Lateral incisor
3 Canines
4 First premolars or bicuspids
5 Second premolars or bicuspids
6 First molars
7 Second molars
8 Third molars
9 Articular tubercle
10 Mandibular fossa
11 Head of mandible
12 Condylar process
13 Hard palate and palatine glands
14 Oral cavity
15 Upper molar
16 Oral vestibule
17 Lower molar
18 Platysma muscle
19 Mandible
20 Maxillary sinus
21 Superior longitudinal muscle of tongue
22 Transverse muscle of tongue
23 Buccinator muscle
24 Inferior longitudinal muscle of tongue
25 Sublingual gland
26 Genioglossus muscle

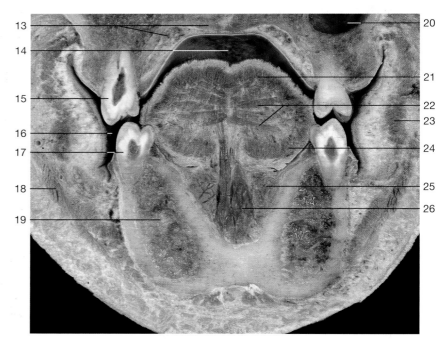

Coronal section through the oral cavity.

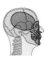

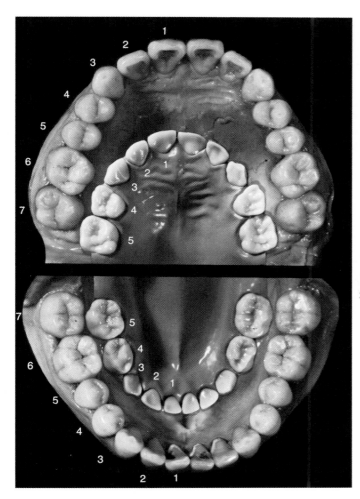

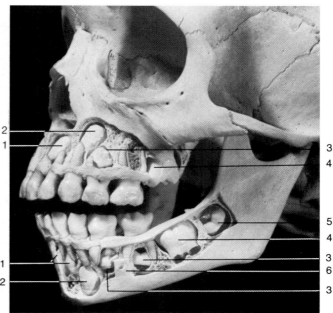

Deciduous teeth in child's skull. The developing crowns of the permanent teeth are displayed in their crypts in the maxilla and mandible.

1   Permanent incisors
2   Permanent cuspid (canine)
3   Premolars
4   First permanent molar
5   Second permanent molar
6   Mental foramen

Comparison of the deciduous and permanent teeth.
Notice that the breadth of the alveolar arch of the child's mandible and maxilla holding the deciduous teeth is nearly the same as the comparable portion in the jaws of the adult. Note the emergence of the third molars. The numbers of the teeth correspond to the numbers in the figure below.

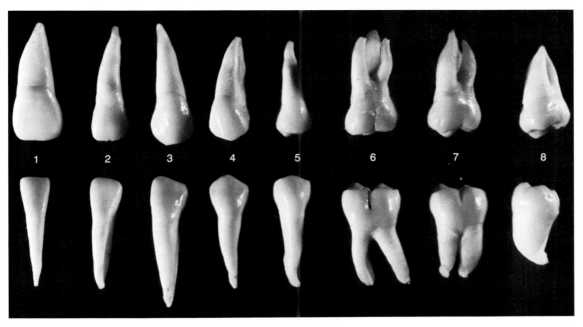

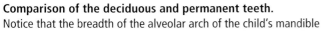

Isolated teeth of the alveolar part of the maxilla (top row) and the mandible (lower row), labial surface of the teeth.

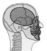

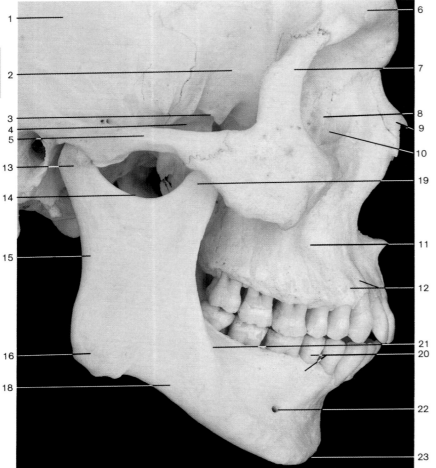

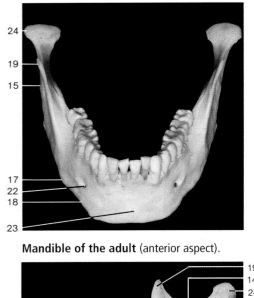

Mandible of the adult (anterior aspect).

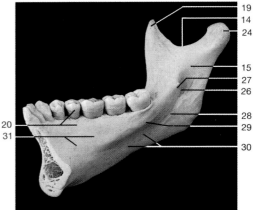

Right half of mandible (medial aspect).

Lateral aspect of the facial bones. Mandible and teeth in the position of occlusion. Upper and lower jaw occluded.

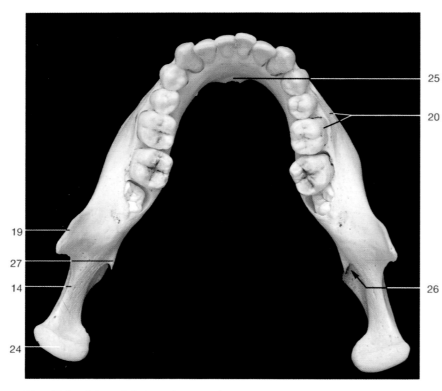

Mandible of the adult (superior aspect).

1   Temporal bone
2   Temporal fossa (greater wing of sphenoidal bone)
3   Infratemporal crest
4   Infratemporal fossa
5   Zygomatic arch
6   Frontal bone
7   Zygomatic bone (frontal process)
8   Lacrimal bone
9   Nasal bone
10 Lacrimal groove
11 Maxilla (canine fossa)
12 Alveolar process of maxilla

Mandible
13 Condylar process
14 Mandibular notch
15 Ramus of the mandible
16 Masseteric tuberosity
17 Angle of the mandible
18 Body of the mandible
19 Coronoid process
20 Alveolar process including teeth
21 Oblique line
22 Mental foramen
23 Mental protuberance
24 Head of the mandible
25 Genial tubercle or mental spine
26 Mandibular foramen (entrance to mandibular canal)
27 Lingula
28 Mylohyoid sulcus
29 Mylohyoid line
30 Submandibular fossa
31 Sublingual fossa

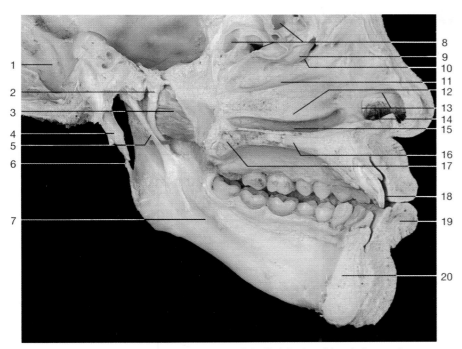

1   Groove for sigmoid sinus
2   Mandibular nerve
3   Lateral pterygoid muscle
4   Styloid process
5   Sphenomandibular ligament
6   Stylomandibular ligament
7   Mylohyoid groove
8   Ethmoidal air cells
9   Ethmoidal bulla
10 Hiatus semilunaris
11 Middle meatus
12 Inferior nasal concha
13 Limen nasi
14 Vestibule with hairs
15 Inferior meatus
16 Hard palate
17 Soft palate
18 Vestibule of oral cavity
19 Lower lip
20 Mandible
21 Calvaria with diploe
22 Sella turcica
23 Internal acoustic meatus
24 Atlanto-occipital articulation
25 Median atlanto-axial articulation
26 Atlas (C₁)
27 Dens of axis (C₂)
28 Spinous process of axis (C₂)
29 Cervical vertebrae (C₃, C₄)
30 Frontal sinus
31 Crista galli
32 Sphenoidal sinus
33 Nasal septum
34 Mandibular foramen
35 Mylohyoid line
36 Bodies of cervical
    vertebrae (C₅, C₆)
37 Articular capsule
38 Lateral ligament
39 Mastoid process
40 Styloid process

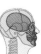

Ligaments of temporomandibular joint. Left half of the head (medial aspect).

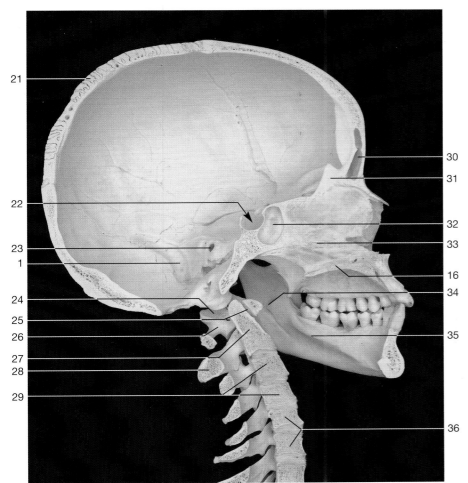

Head and cervical vertebral column (median section through skull and cervical vertebrae, medial aspect).

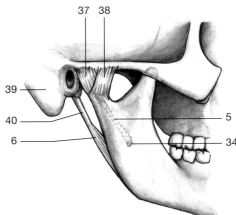

Ligaments related to the temporomandibular joint (schematic drawing).

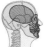

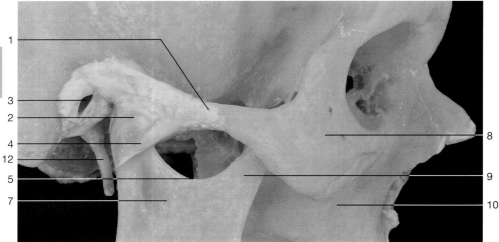

1 Zygomatic arch
2 Articular capsule
3 External acoustic meatus
4 Lateral ligament
5 Mandibular notch
6 Stylomandibular ligament
7 Ramus of the mandible
8 Zygomatic bone
9 Coronoid process
10 Maxilla
11 Articular cartilage of
   condylar process
12 Styloid process
13 Mandibular fossa
14 Articular disc
15 Articular tubercle
16 Lateral pterygoid muscle
17 Condylar process of mandible
18 Temporalis muscle
19 Digastric muscle, posterior belly
20 Masseter muscle
21 Medial pterygoid muscle
22 Parotid duct
23 Buccinator muscle
24 Mandible

Temporomandibular joint with ligaments.

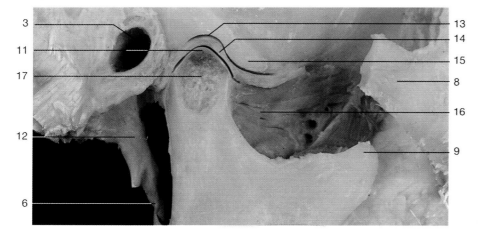

Temporomandibular joint, sagittal section.

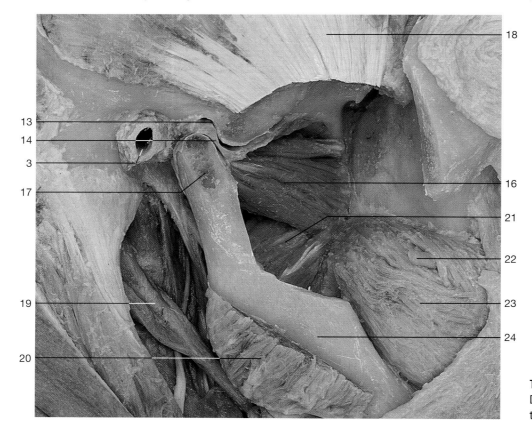

Temporomandibular joint.
Dissection of the articular disc and
the related muscles (lateral aspect).

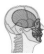

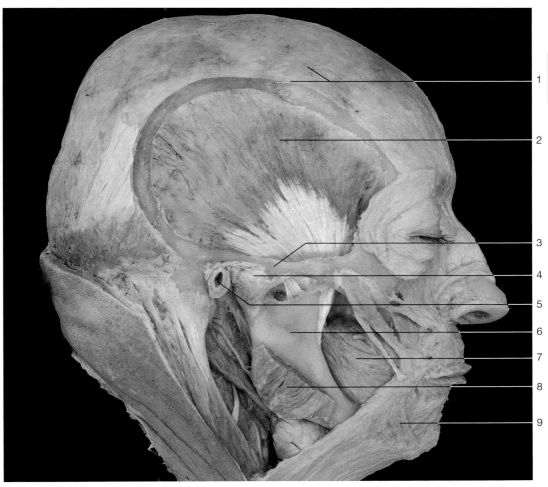

Muscles of mastication and temporomandibular joint. Masseter muscle partly removed.

1   Galea aponeurotica
2   Temporalis muscle
3   Zygomatic arch
4   Temporomandibular joint
5   External acoustic meatus
6   Mandible
7   Buccinator muscle
8   Masseter muscle (cut)
9   Platysma muscle
10 Lateral pterygoid muscle
11 Posterior belly of digastric muscle
12 Stylohyoid muscle
13 Medial pterygoid muscle
14 Anterior belly of digastric muscle
15 Mylohyoid muscle
16 Hyoid bone

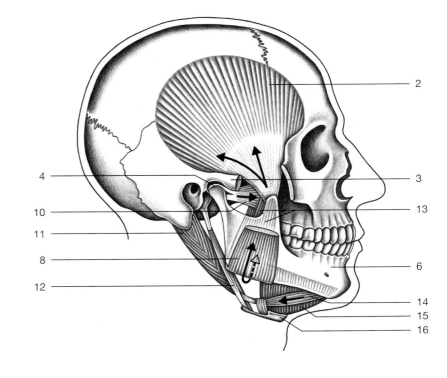

Effect of the masticatory muscles on the temporomandibular joint (arrows).

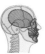

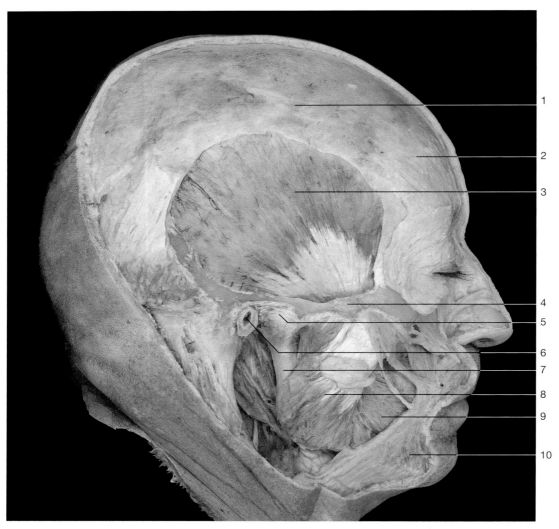

Muscles of mastication. The temporomandibular joint and the masseter and temporalis muscles are shown.

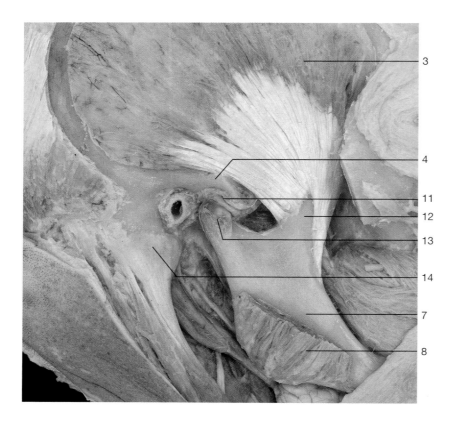

1   Galea aponeurotica
2   Frontal belly of occipitofrontalis muscle
3   Temporalis muscle
4   Zygomatic arch
5   Temporomandibular joint
6   External acoustic meatus
7   Mandible
8   Masseter muscle
9   Buccinator muscle
10 Platysma muscle
11 Articular disc of temporomandibular joint
12 Coronoid process of mandible
13 Condylar process of mandible
14 Mastoid process

Temporalis muscle with insertion at the mandible and the temporomandibular joint. Zygomatic arch and masseter muscle have been partly removed.

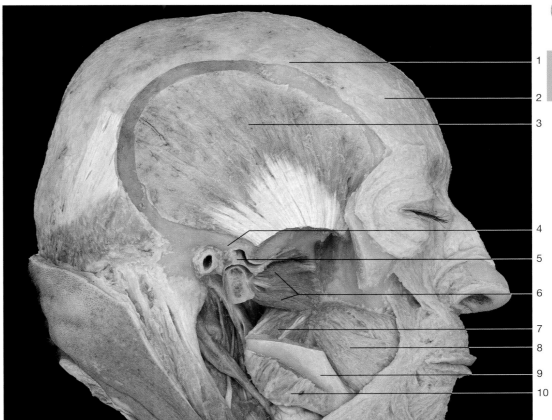

Muscles of mastication. The zygomatic arch and part of the mandible have been removed to reveal the medial and lateral pterygoid muscles.

1	Galea aponeurotica	7	Medial pterygoid muscle
2	Frontal belly of occipitofrontalis muscle	8	Buccinator muscle
3	Temporalis muscle	9	Mandible
4	Zygomatic arch	10	Masseter muscle
5	Articular disc of temporomandibular joint	11	Platysma muscle
6	Lateral pterygoid muscle		

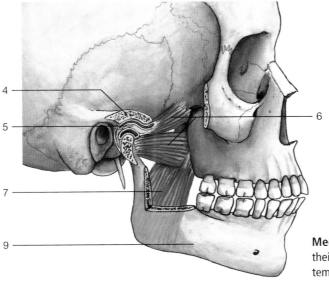

Medial and lateral pterygoid muscles and their connections with the articular disc of the temporomandibular joint (schematic drawing).

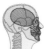

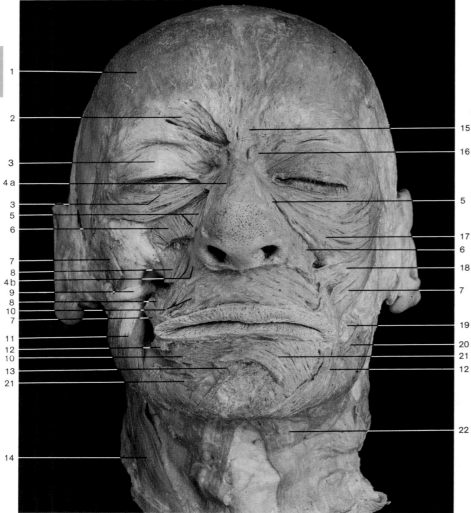

1 Frontal belly of occipitofrontalis muscle
2 Corrugator supercilii muscle
3 Palpebral part of orbicularis oculi muscle
4a Transverse part of nasalis muscle
4b Alar part of nasalis muscle
5 Levator labii superioris alaeque nasi muscle
6 Levator labii superioris muscle
7 Zygomaticus major muscle
8 Levator anguli oris muscle
9 Parotid duct
10 Orbicularis oris muscle
11 Masseter muscle
12 Depressor anguli oris muscle
13 Mentalis muscle
14 Sternocleidomastoid muscle
15 Procerus muscle
16 Depressor supercilii muscle
17 Orbital part of orbicularis oculi muscle
18 Zygomaticus minor muscle
19 Buccinator muscle
20 Risorius muscle
21 Depressor labii inferioris muscle
22 Platysma muscle
23 Galea aponeurotica
24 Temporoparietalis muscle
25 Occipital belly of occipitofrontalis muscle
26 Parotid gland with fascia
27 Temporal fascia
28 Orbicularis oculi muscle
29 Parotid duct and masseter muscle

Facial muscles (anterior aspect). Left side: superficial layer, right side: deeper layer.

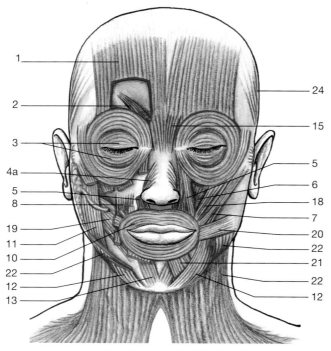

Facial muscles (schematic drawing).
Left side: superficial layer, right side: deeper layer.

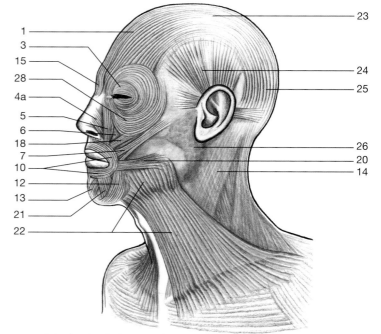

Facial muscles (schematic drawing). Sphincter-like muscles surround the orifices of the head. Radially arranged muscles work as their antagonists.

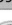

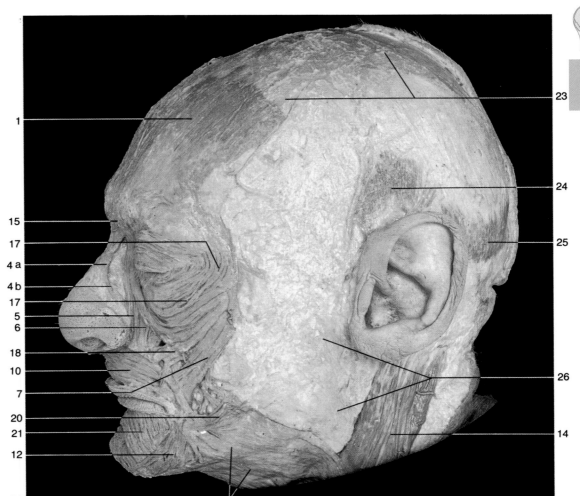

Facial muscles (lateral aspect).

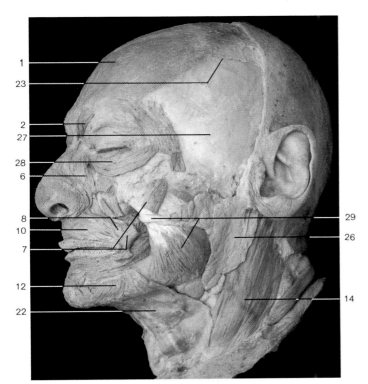

Facial muscles and parotid gland (lateral aspect).

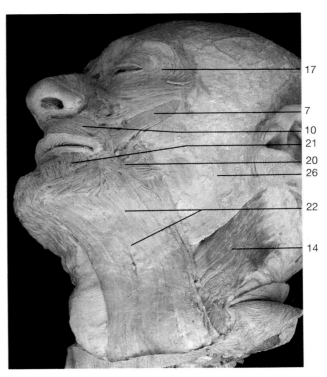

Platysma muscle (oblique lateral aspect). Superficial lamina of cervical fascia partly removed.

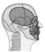

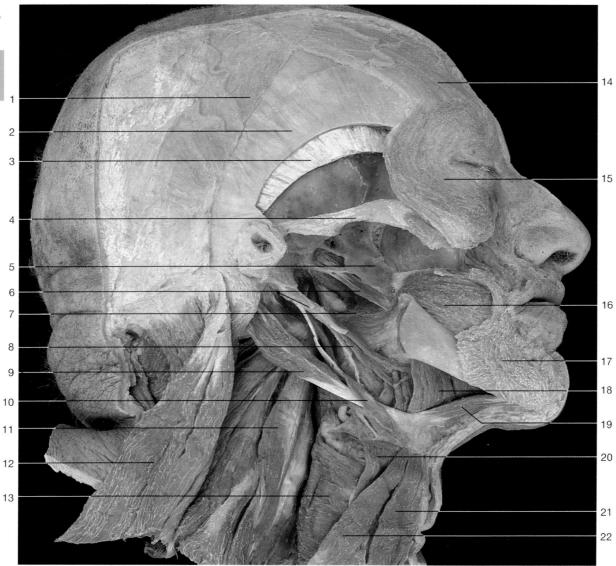

Supra- and infrahyoid muscles and pharynx (lateral aspect). Ramus of mandible, pterygoid muscles, and insertion of temporalis muscle removed.

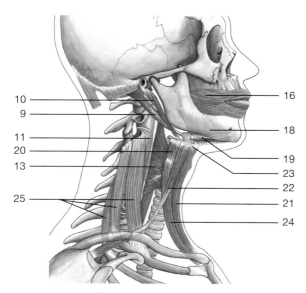

Supra- and infrahyoid muscles (schematic drawing).

1 Galea aponeurotica
2 Temporal fascia
3 Tendon of temporalis muscle
4 Zygomatic arch
5 Lateral pterygoid plate
6 Tensor veli palatini muscle (styloid process)
7 Superior constrictor muscle of pharynx
8 Styloglossus muscle
9 Posterior belly of digastric muscle
10 Stylohyoid muscle
11 Longus capitis muscle
12 Sternocleidomastoid muscle (reflected)
13 Inferior constrictor of pharynx
14 Frontal belly of occipitofrontalis muscle
15 Orbital part of orbicularis oculi muscle
16 Buccinator muscle
17 Depressor anguli oris muscle
18 Mylohyoid muscle
19 Anterior belly of digastric muscle
20 Thyrohyoid muscle
21 Sternohyoid muscle
22 Omohyoid muscle
23 Hyoid bone
24 Sternothyroid muscle
25 Scalenus muscles

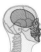

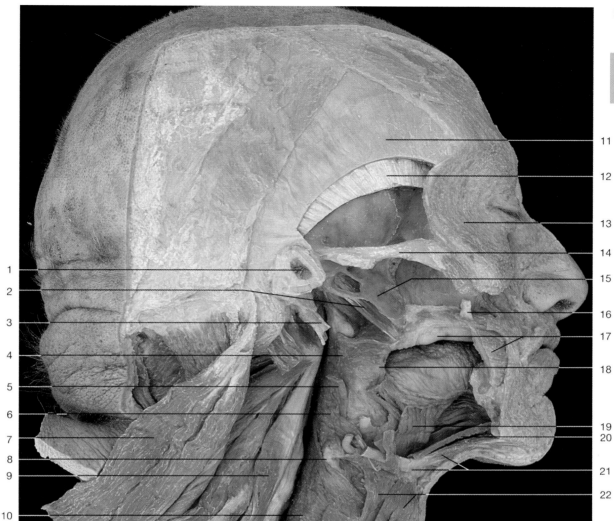

Supra- and infrahyoid muscles and pharynx (lateral aspect). Buccinator muscle removed; oral cavity opened.

1 External acoustic meatus
2 Tensor veli palatini muscle
3 Styloid process
4 Superior constrictor muscle of pharynx
5 Stylopharyngeus muscle (divided)
6 Middle constrictor muscle of pharynx
7 Sternocleidomastoid muscle
8 Greater horn of hyoid bone
9 Longus capitis muscle
10 Inferior constrictor muscle of pharynx
11 Temporal fascia
12 Tendon of temporalis muscle
13 Orbicularis oculi muscle
14 Zygomatic arch
15 Lateral pterygoid plate
16 Parotid duct
17 Gingiva of upper jaw (without teeth),
    buccinator muscle (divided)
18 Pterygomandibular raphe
19 Hyoglossus muscle
20 Mylohyoid muscle
21 Anterior belly of digastric muscle (hyoid bone)
22 Sternohyoid and thyrohyoid muscles
23 Omohyoid muscle

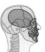

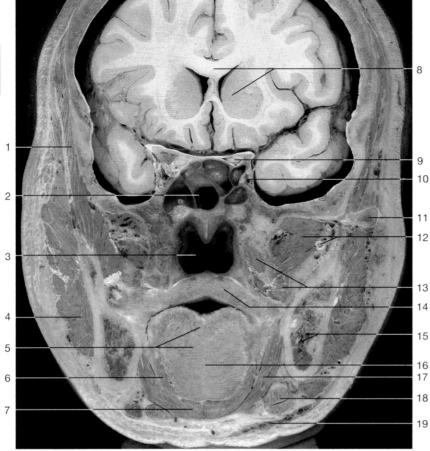

1   Temporalis muscle
2   Sphenoidal sinus
3   Nasopharynx
4   Masseter muscle
5   Superior longitudinal, transverse and vertical muscles of tongue
6   Hyoglossus muscle
7   Geniohyoid muscle
8   Corpus callosum (caudate nucleus)
9   Optic nerve
10 Cavernous sinus
11 Zygomatic arch
12 Cross section of lateral pterygoid muscle and maxillary artery
13 Section of medial pterygoid muscle
14 Soft palate
15 Mandible and inferior alveolar nerve
16 Septum of the tongue
17 Mylohyoid muscle
18 Submandibular gland
19 Platysma muscle
20 Foramen magnum, vertebral artery and spinal cord
21 Internal carotid artery
22 Head of mandible
23 Styloid process
24 Inferior alveolar nerve
25 Lingual nerve and chorda tympani nerve
26 Medial pterygoid muscle
27 Uvula
28 Anterior belly of digastric muscle (cut)
29 Condyle of occipital bone
30 Mastoid process
31 Lateral pterygoid muscle
32 Auditory tube and levator veli palatini muscle
33 Tensor veli palatini muscle

Coronal section through cranial, nasal, and oral cavities at the level of sphenoidal sinus.

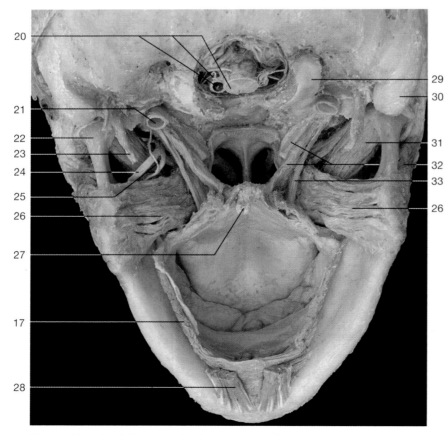

Pterygoid and palatine muscles (posterior aspect).

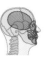

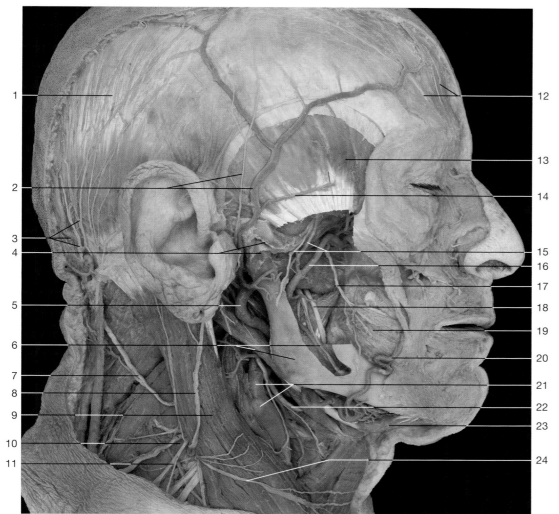

1 Galea aponeurotica
2 Superficial temporal artery and auriculo-temporal nerve
3 Occipital artery and greater occipital nerve (C₂)
4 Temporomandibular joint (opened)
5 External carotid artery
6 Mandible and inferior mandibular artery and nerve
7 Accessory nerve (Var.)
8 Great auricular nerve
9 Sternocleidomastoideus muscle
10 Punctum nervosum
11 Supraclavicular nerves
12 Supra-orbital nerves
13 Temporalis muscle
14 Transverse facial artery
15 Masseteric nerve and deep temporal branch of maxillary artery
16 Maxillary artery
17 Buccal nerve
18 Lingual nerve
19 Buccinator muscle
20 Facial artery
21 External carotid artery and sinus caroticus
22 Hypoglossal nerve
23 Digastric muscle
24 Transverse cervical nerves

Dissection of maxillary artery (lateral aspect). Ramus mandibulae partly removed and canalis mandibulae opened.

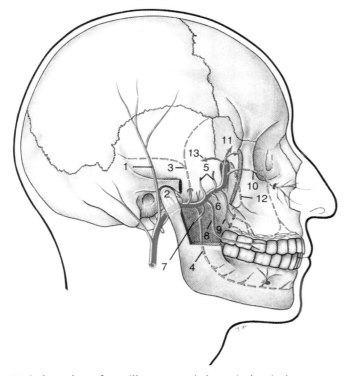

1 Superficial temporal artery

Branches of the first part
2 Deep auricular artery and anterior tympanic artery
3 Middle meningeal artery
4 Inferior alveolar artery

Branches of the second part
5 Deep temporal branches
6 Pterygoid branches
7 Masseteric artery
8 Buccal artery

Branches of the third part
9 Posterior superior alveolar artery
10 Infra-orbital artery
11 Sphenopalatine artery and branches to the nasal cavity
12 Descending palatine artery
13 Artery of the pterygoid canal

Main branches of maxillary artery (schematic drawing).

2.2 Cranial Nerves

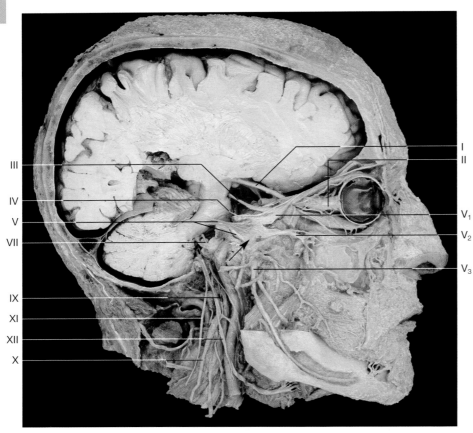

Dissection of the cranial nerves (indicated by I–XII) (lateral aspect). Brain, brain stem, and cerebellum have been partly removed (from Lütjen-Drecoll, Rohen, Innenansichten des menschlichen Körpers, 2010).

The twelve cranial nerves emerge from the brain stem and penetrate the skull at different places. The olfactory nerves (n. I) pass the lamina cribrosa innervating the upper part of the nasal mucous membrane. The optic nerve (n. II) is related to the eye. The external ocular muscles are innervated by the oculomotor, trochlear, and abducent nerves (n. III, n. IV, and n. VI). Facial skin and masticatory muscles are innervated by the trigeminal nerve (n. V) while the facial nerve (n. VII) innervates mainly the mimic musculature. The stato-acoustic organ is related to the vestibulocochlear nerve (n. VIII). The vagus nerve (n. X) is one of the longest cranial nerves, running through the lateral neck region to reach the thoracic and abdominal cavities. It belongs to the parasympathetic part of the autonomic nervous system. The glossopharyngeal (n. IX), accessory (n. XI), and hypoglossal (n. XII) nerves innervate the muscles of the neck, the tongue, and the pharynx. During human evolution, they were incorporated secondarily into the brain cavity.

Cranial nerves

  I = Olfactory nerves
  II = Optic nerve
  III = Oculomotor nerve
  IV = Trochlear nerve
  V = Trigeminal nerve
  VI = Abducent nerve
  VII = Facial nerve
  VIII = Vestibulocochlear nerve
  IX = Glossopharyngeal nerve
  X = Vagus nerve
  XI = Accessory nerve
  XII = Hypoglossal nerve

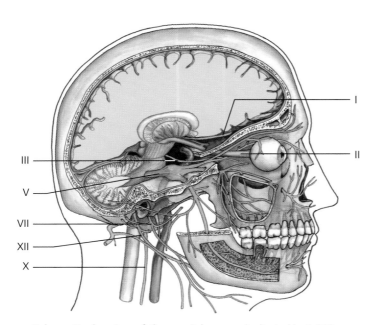

Schematic drawing of the cranial nerves (indicated by I–XII) (lateral aspect).

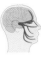

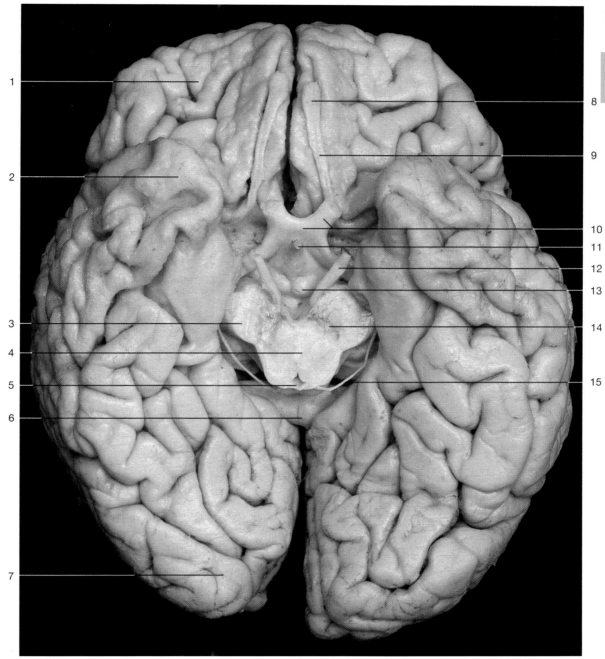

Inferior aspect of the brain with cranial nerves. Midbrain divided.

1	Frontal lobe	9	Olfactory tract
2	Temporal lobe	10	Optic nerve and optic chiasma
3	Pedunculus cerebri	11	Infundibulum
4	Midbrain (divided)	12	Oculomotor nerve (n. III)
5	Cerebral aqueduct	13	Mamillary body
6	Splenium of corpus callosum	14	Substantia nigra
7	Occipital lobe	15	Trochlear nerve (n. IV)
8	Olfactory bulb		

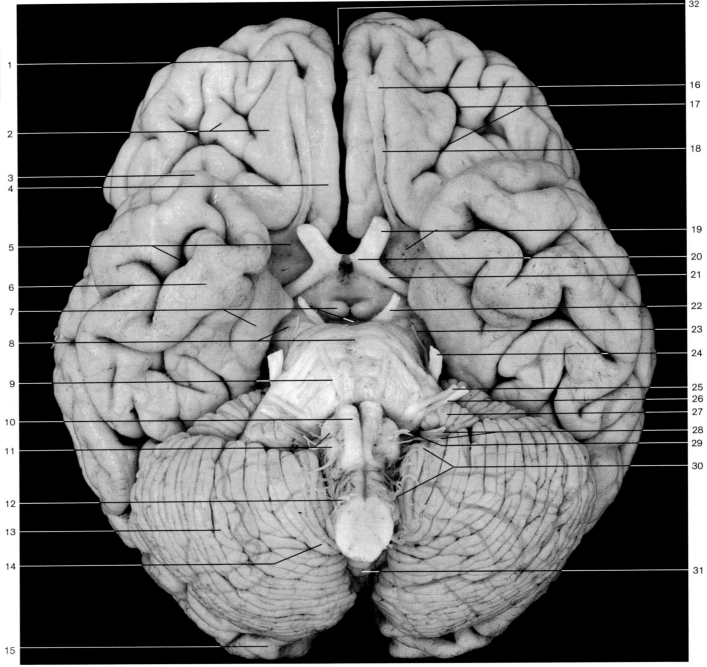

Cranial nerves. Brain (inferior aspect).

1 Olfactory sulcus (termination)	13 Cerebellum	25 Facial nerve (n. VII)
2 Orbital gyri	14 Tonsil of cerebellum	26 Vestibulocochlear nerve (n. VIII)
3 Temporal lobe	15 Occipital lobe (posterior pole)	27 Flocculus of cerebellum
4 Straight gyrus	16 Olfactory bulb	28 Glossopharyngeal nerve (n. IX)
5 Olfactory trigone and inferior temporal sulcus	17 Orbital sulci of frontal lobe	and vagus nerve (n. X)
6 Medial occipitotemporal gyrus	18 Olfactory tract	29 Hypoglossal nerve (n. XII)
7 Parahippocampal gyrus, mamillary body, and	19 Optic nerve (n. II) and anterior	30 Accessory nerve (n. XI)
interpeduncular fossa	perforated substance	31 Vermis of cerebellum
8 Pons and cerebral peduncle	20 Optic chiasma	32 Longitudinal fissure
9 Abducent nerve (n. VI)	21 Optic tract	
10 Pyramid	22 Oculomotor nerve (n. III)	
11 Inferior olive	23 Trochlear nerve (n. IV)	
12 Cervical spinal nerves	24 Trigeminal nerve (n. V)	

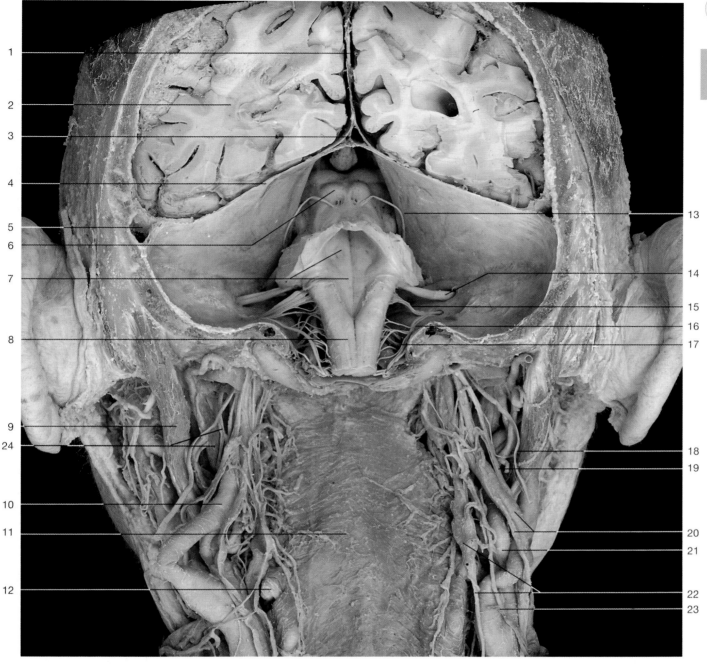

Brain stem and pharynx with cranial nerves (posterior aspect). Cranial cavity opened and cerebellum removed.

1 Falx cerebri
2 Occipital lobe
3 Straight sinus
4 Tentorium cerebelli
5 Transverse sinus
6 Inferior colliculus of midbrain
7 Rhomboid fossa
8 Medulla oblongata
9 Posterior belly of digastric muscle
10 Internal carotid artery
11 Pharynx (middle constrictor muscle)
12 Hyoid bone (greater horn)
13 Trochlear nerve (n. IV)
14 Facial nerve (n. VII) and
    vestibulocochlear nerve (n. VIII)
15 Glossopharyngeal nerve (n. IX)
    and vagus nerve (n. X)
16 Accessory nerve (intracranial portion) (n. XI)
17 Hypoglossal nerve (intracranial portion) (n. XII)
18 Accessory nerve (n. XI)
19 Hypoglossal nerve (n. XII)
20 Vagus nerve (n. X) and internal carotid artery
21 External carotid artery
22 Sympathetic trunk and superior cervical ganglion
23 Ansa cervicalis (superior root of
    hypoglossal nerve)
24 Glossopharyngeal nerve (n. IX) and
    stylopharyngeus muscle

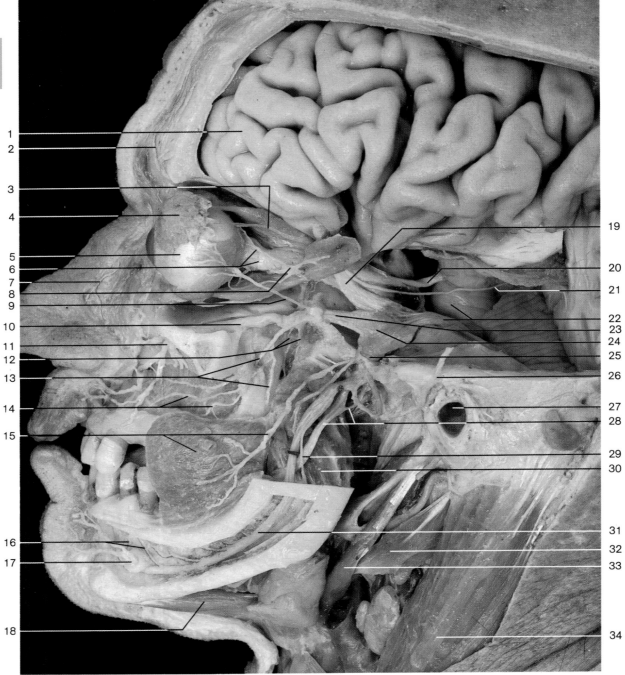

Dissection of the trigeminal nerve in its entirety. Lateral wall of cranial cavity, lateral wall of orbit, zygomatic arch, and ramus of the mandible have been removed and the mandibular canal opened.

1	Frontal lobe of cerebrum	12	Pterygopalatine ganglion and
2	Supra-orbital nerve		pterygopalatine nerves
3	Lacrimal nerve	13	Posterior superior alveolar
4	Lacrimal gland		nerves
5	Eyeball	14	Superior dental plexus
6	Optic nerve and short ciliary nerves	15	Buccinator muscle and buccal nerve
7	External nasal branch of	16	Inferior dental plexus
	anterior ethmoidal nerve	17	Mental foramen and mental nerve
8	Ciliary ganglion	18	Anterior belly of digastric muscle
9	Zygomatic nerve	19	Ophthalmic nerve (n. V₁)
10	Infra-orbital nerve	20	Oculomotor nerve (n. III)
11	Infra-orbital foramen and terminal branches	21	Trochlear nerve (n. IV)
	of infra-orbital nerve	22	Trigeminal nerve and pons

23	Maxillary nerve (n. V₂)
24	Trigeminal ganglion
25	Mandibular nerve (n. V₃)
26	Auriculotemporal nerve
27	External acoustic meatus (divided)
28	Lingual nerve and chorda tympani
29	Mylohyoid nerve
30	Medial pterygoid muscle
31	Inferior alveolar nerve
32	Posterior belly of digastric muscle
33	Stylohyoid muscle
34	Sternocleidomastoid muscle

1 Frontal nerve
2 Lacrimal gland and eyeball
3 Lacrimal nerve
4 Lateral rectus muscle
5 Ciliary ganglion lateral to optic nerve
6 Zygomatic nerve
7 Inferior branch of oculomotor nerve
8 Ophthalmic nerve (n. V$_1$)
9 Maxillary nerve (n. V$_2$)
10 Trigeminal ganglion
11 Mandibular nerve (n. V$_3$)
12 Posterior superior alveolar nerves
13 Tympanic cavity, external acoustic meatus, and tympanic membrane
14 Inferior alveolar nerve
15 Lingual nerve
16 Facial nerve (n. VII)
17 Vagus nerve (n. X)
18 Hypoglossal nerve (n. XII) and superior root of ansa cervicalis
19 External carotid artery
20 Olfactory tract (n. I)
21 Optic nerve (n. II) (intracranial part)
22 Oculomotor nerve (n. III)
23 Abducent nerve (n. VI)
24 Trochlear nerve (n. IV)
25 Trigeminal nerve (n. V)
26 Vestibulocochlear nerve (n. VIII) and facial nerve (n. VII)
27 Glossopharyngeal nerve (n. IX) (leaving brain stem)
28 Rhomboid fossa
29 Vagus nerve (n. X) (leaving brain stem)
30 Hypoglossal nerve (n. XII) (leaving medulla oblongata)
31 Accessory nerve (n. XI) (ascending from foramen magnum)
32 Vertebral artery
33 Spinal ganglion and dura mater of spinal cord
34 Accessory nerve (n. XI)
35 Internal carotid artery
36 Lateral and medial branch of supra-orbital nerve
37 Infratrochlear nerve
38 Infra-orbital nerve
39 Pterygopalatine ganglion and middle superior alveolar nerve
40 Middle superior alveolar nerves (entering superior dental plexus)
41 Buccal nerve
42 Mental nerve and mental foramen
43 Auriculotemporal nerve
44 Otic ganglion (dotted line)
45 Chorda tympani
46 Mylohyoid nerve
47 Submandibular gland
48 Hyoid bone

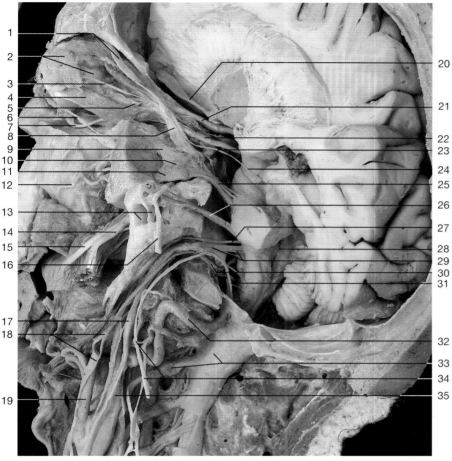

Cranial nerves in connection with the brain stem. Left side (lateral superior aspect). Left half of brain and head partly removed. Notice the location of trigeminal ganglion.

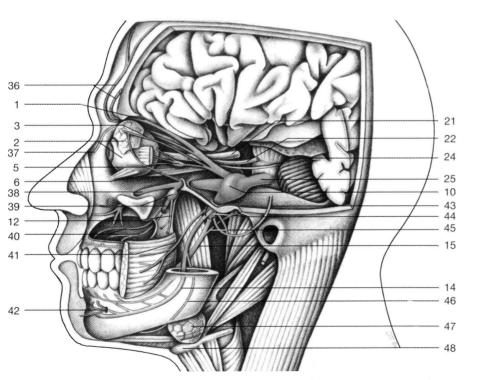

Main branches of trigeminal nerve (schematic drawing of figure on opposite page).

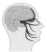

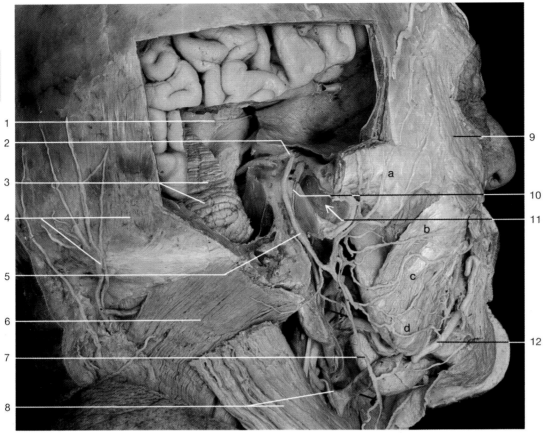

Dissection of facial nerve in its entirety. Cranial cavity fenestrated; temporal lobe partly removed.
Facial canal and tympanic cavity opened, posterior wall of external acoustic meatus removed.
Branches of facial nerve: a = temporal branch; b = zygomatic branches; c = buccal branches;
d = marginal mandibular branch.

1   Trochlear nerve
2   Facial nerve with geniculate ganglion
3   Cerebellum (right hemisphere)
4   Occipital belly of occipitofrontalis muscle
    and greater occipital nerve
5   Facial nerve at stylomastoid foramen
6   Splenius capitis muscle
7   Cervical branch of facial nerve
8   Sternocleidomastoid muscle and
    retromandibular vein
9   Orbicularis oculi muscle
10 Chorda tympani
11 External acoustic meatus
12 Facial artery
13 Mastoid air cells
14 Posterior auricular nerve
15 Nucleus and genu of facial nerve

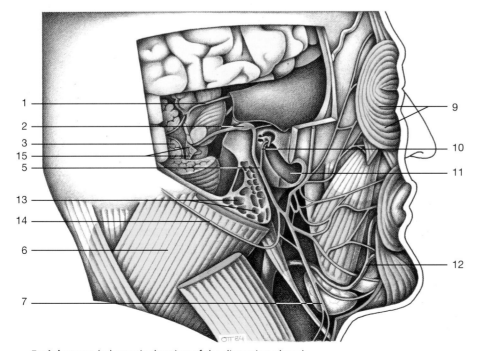

Facial nerve (schematic drawing of the dissection above).

**Cranial nerves in connection with
the brain stem** (oblique-lateral aspect).
Lateral portion of the skull, brain, neck
and facial structures, lateral wall of orbit
and oral cavity have been removed. The
tympanic cavity has been opened.
The mandible has been divided and
the muscles of mastication have been
removed.

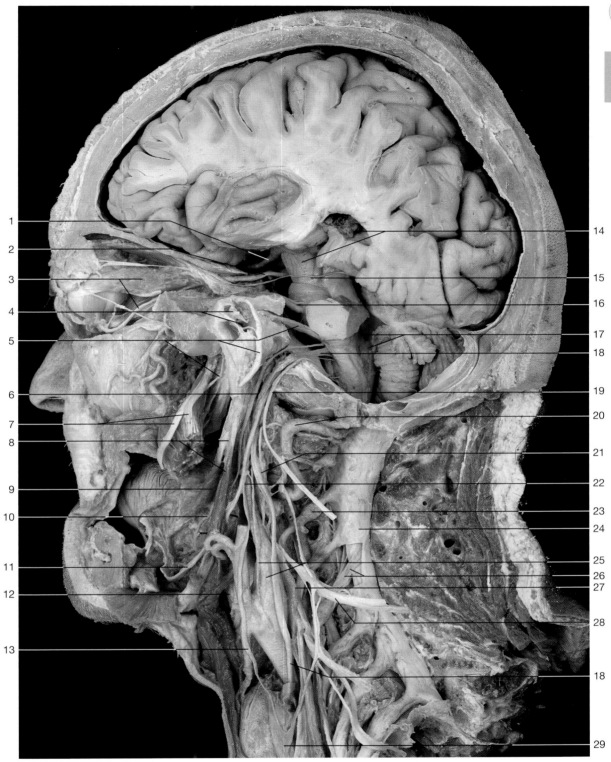

1	Optic tract
2	Oculomotor nerve (n. III)
3	Lateral rectus muscle and inferior branch of oculomotor nerve
4	Malleus and chorda tympani
5	Chorda tympani, facial nerve (n. VII), and vestibulocochlear nerve (n. VIII)
6	Glossopharyngeal nerve (n. XI)
7	Lingual nerve and inferior alveolar nerve
8	Styloid process and stylohyoid muscle
9	Styloglossus muscle
10	Lingual branches of glossopharyngeal nerve
11	Lingual branch of hypoglossal nerve
12	External carotid artery
13	Superior root of ansa cervicalis (branch of hypoglossal nerve, derived from C₁)
14	Lateral ventricle with choroid plexus and cerebral peduncle
15	Trochlear nerve (n. IV)
16	Trigeminal nerve (n. V)
17	Fourth ventricle and rhomboid fossa
18	Vagus nerve (n. X)
19	Accessory nerve (n. XI)
20	Vertebral artery
21	Superior cervical ganglion
22	Hypoglossal nerve (n. XII)
23	Spinal ganglion with dural sheath
24	Dura mater of spinal cord
25	Internal carotid artery and carotid sinus branch of glossopharyngeal nerve
26	Dorsal roots of spinal nerve
27	Sympathetic trunk
28	Branch of cervical plexus (ventral primary ramus of third cervical spinal nerve)
29	Ansa cervicalis

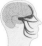
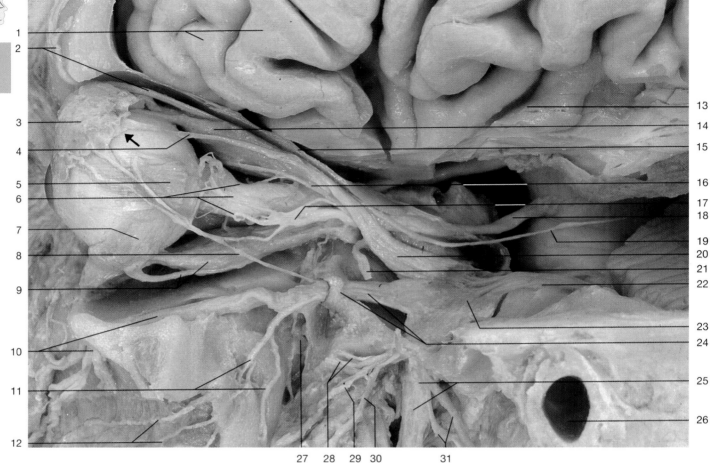

Cranial nerves of the orbit and pterygopalatine fossa. Left orbit (lateral aspect). Note the zygomaticolacrimal anastomosis (arrow).

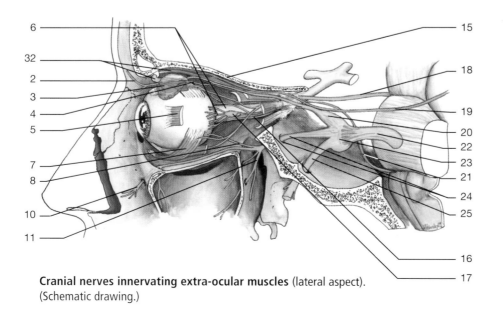

Cranial nerves innervating extra-ocular muscles (lateral aspect). (Schematic drawing.)

1 Frontal lobe
2 Supra-orbital nerve
3 Lacrimal gland
4 Lacrimal nerve
5 Lateral rectus muscle (divided)
6 Optic nerve and short ciliary nerves
7 Inferior oblique muscle
8 Zygomatic nerve
9 Inferior branch of oculomotor nerve and inferior rectus muscle
10 Infra-orbital nerve
11 Posterior superior alveolar nerves
12 Branches of superior alveolar plexus adjacent to mucous membrane of maxillary sinus
13 Central sulcus of insula
14 Superior rectus muscle
15 Periorbita (roof of orbit)
16 Nasociliary nerve
17 Ciliary ganglion
18 Oculomotor nerve (n. III)
19 Trochlear nerve (n. IV)
20 Ophthalmic nerve (n. V_1)
21 Abducent nerve (n. VI) (divided)
22 Trigeminal nerve (n. V)
23 Trigeminal ganglion
24 Maxillary nerve (n. V_2) and foramen rotundum
25 Mandibular nerve (n. V_3)
26 External acoustic meatus
27 Pterygopalatine nerves
28 Deep temporal nerves
29 Buccal nerve
30 Masseteric nerve
31 Auriculotemporal nerve
32 Trochlea and superior oblique muscle

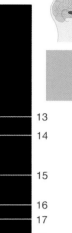

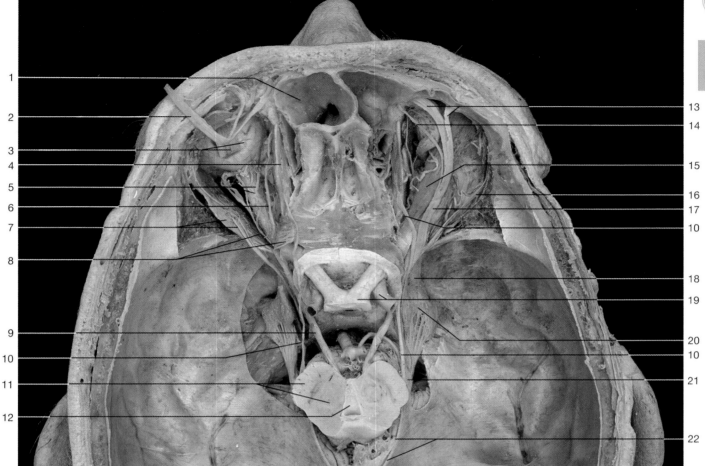

Cranial nerves of the orbit (superior aspect). Right side: superficial layer, left side: middle layer of the orbit (superior rectus muscle and frontal nerve divided and reflected). Tentorium and dura mater partly removed.

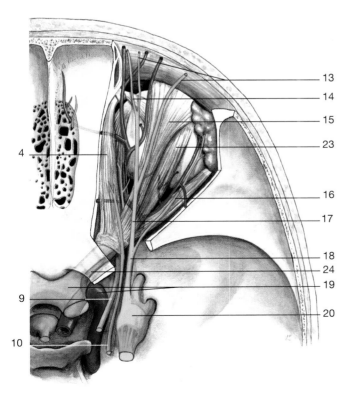

Cranial nerves within the orbit (superior aspect).

1   Frontal sinus (enlarged)
2   Frontal nerve (divided and reflected)
3   Superior rectus muscle (divided) and eyeball
4   Superior oblique muscle
5   Short ciliary nerves and optic nerve (n. II)
6   Nasociliary nerve
7   Abducent nerve (n. VI) and lateral rectus muscle
8   Ciliary ganglion and superior rectus muscle (reflected)
9   Oculomotor nerve (n. III)
10   Trochlear nerve (n. IV)
11   Crus cerebri and midbrain
12   Inferior wall of the third ventricle connected with cerebral aqueduct
13   Lateral and medial branches of supra-orbital nerve
14   Supratrochlear nerve
15   Superior levator palpebrae muscle
16   Lacrimal nerve
17   Frontal nerve
18   Ophthalmic nerve (n. V_1)
19   Optic chiasma and internal carotid artery
20   Trigeminal ganglion
21   Trigeminal nerve (n. V)
22   Tentorial notch
23   Superior rectus muscle
24   Ophthalmic artery

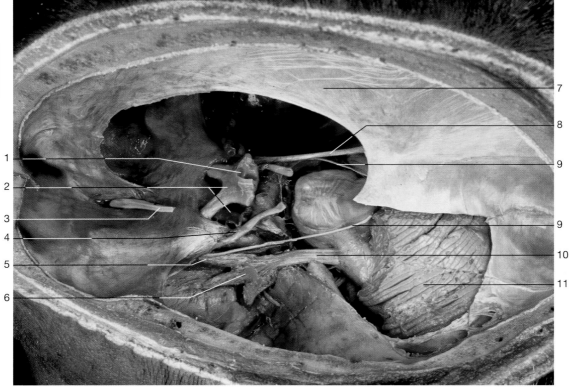

Cranial nerves at the base of the skull. The brain stem was divided and the tentorium fenestrated. Both hemispheres were removed.

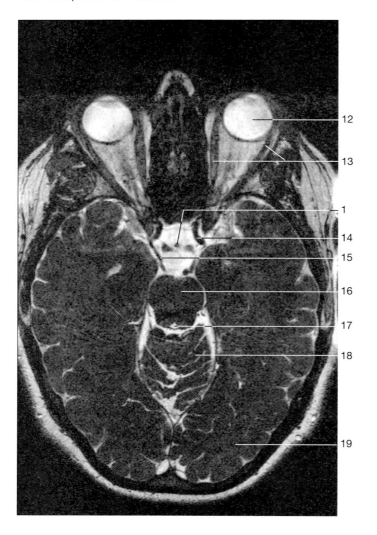

1 Infundibulum
2 Optic chiasma and internal carotid artery
3 Olfactory tract
4 Oculomotor nerve (n. III)
5 Ophthalmic nerve (n. V1)
6 Trigeminal ganglion
7 Falx cerebri
8 Tentorial notch
9 Trochlear nerve (n. IV)
10 Trigeminal nerve (n. V)
11 Cerebellum
12 Eyeball
13 Medial and lateral rectus muscles
14 Internal carotid artery
15 Oculomotor nerve (n. III)
16 Midbrain
17 Cerebral aqueduct
18 Vermis of cerebellum
19 Occipital lobe of the cerebrum
20 Basilar artery

Section through the head at the level of the sella turcica demonstrating cranial nerves (MRI scan, University of Erlangen, Dpt. of Neurosurgery).

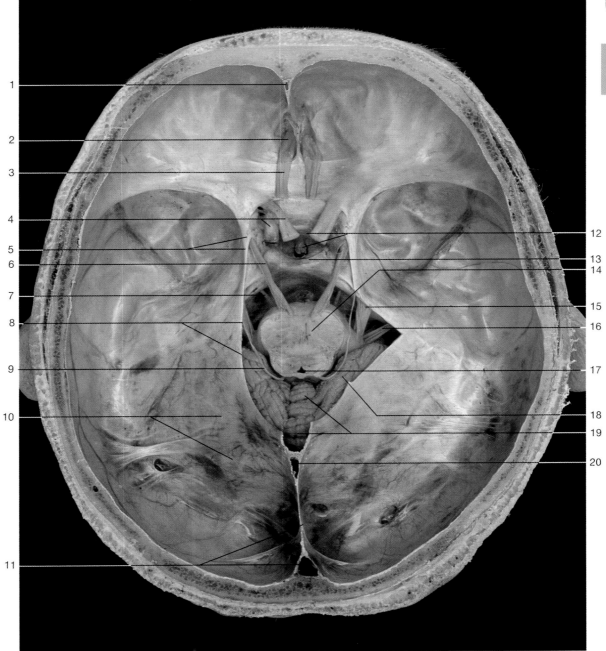

Base of the skull with cranial nerves (internal aspect). Both cerebral hemispheres and upper part of the brain stem removed. Incision on the right tentorium cerebelli to display the cranial nerves of the infratentorial space.

1 Superior sagittal sinus with falx cerebri
2 Olfactory bulb
3 Olfactory tract
4 Optic nerve and internal carotid artery
5 Anterior clinoid process and anterior
   attachment of tentorium cerebelli
6 Oculomotor nerve (n. III)
7 Abducent nerve (n. VI)
8 Tentorial notch (incisura tentorii)
9 Trochlear nerve (n. IV)
10 Tentorium cerebelli
11 Falx cerebri and confluence of sinuses

12 Hypophysial fossa, infundibulum, and
   diaphragma sellae
13 Dorsum sellae
14 Midbrain (divided)
15 Trigeminal nerve (n. V)
16 Facial nerve (n. VII), nervus intermedius, and
   vestibulocochlear nerve (n. VIII)
17 Cerebral aqueduct
18 Right hemisphere of cerebellum
19 Vermis of cerebellum
20 Straight sinus

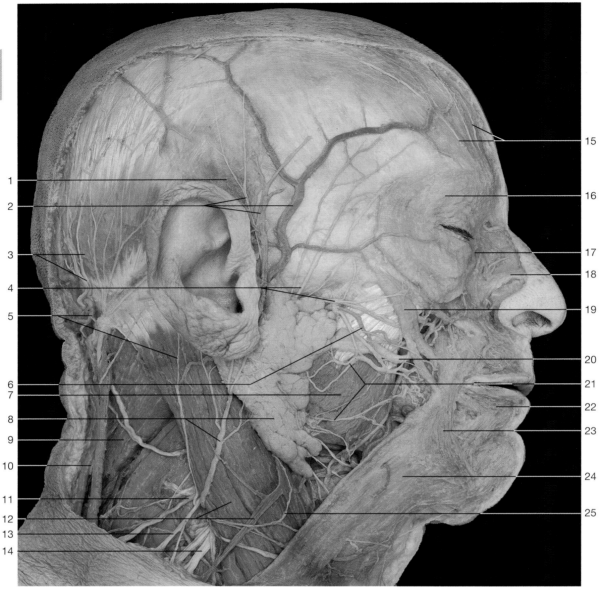

Lateral superficial aspect of the face. Peripheral distribution of facial nerve (n. VII).

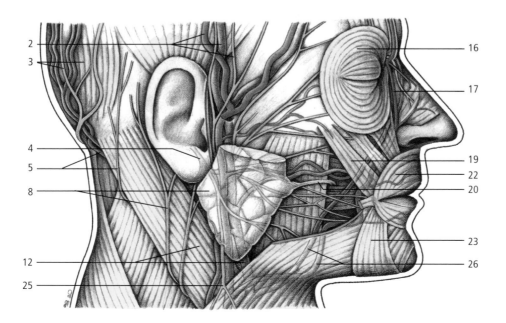

Superficial region of the face. Note the facial plexus within the parotid gland (semischematic drawing).

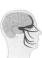

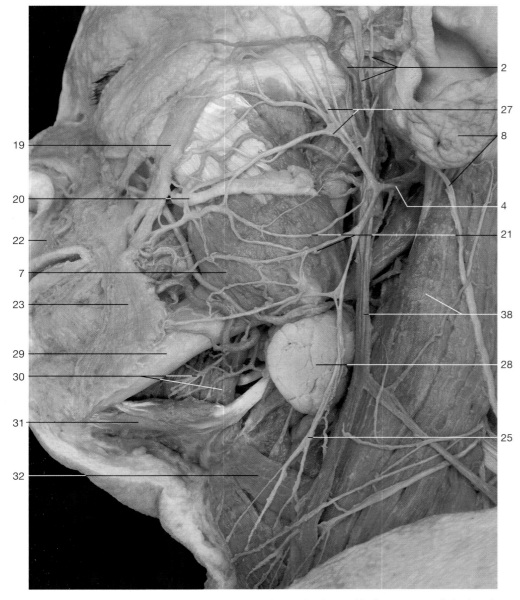

1 Temporoparietalis muscle
2 Superficial temporal artery and vein, and auriculotemporal nerve
3 Occipital belly of occipitofrontalis muscle and greater occipital nerve (C$_2$)
4 Facial nerve (n. VII)
5 Lesser occipital nerve and occipital artery
6 Transverse facial artery
7 Masseter muscle
8 Parotid gland and great auricular nerve
9 Splenius capitis muscle
10 Trapezius muscle
11 Punctum nervosum, point of distribution of cutaneous nerves of cervical plexus
12 Sternocleidomastoid muscle and external jugular vein
13 Supraclavicular nerves
14 Brachial plexus
15 Supra-orbital nerves
16 Orbicularis oculi muscle
17 Angular artery (terminal branch of facial artery)
18 Nasalis muscle
19 Zygomaticus major muscle
20 Parotid duct
21 Zygomatic and buccal branches of facial nerve
22 Orbicularis oris muscle
23 Depressor anguli oris muscle
24 Platysma muscle
25 Cervical branch of facial nerve (anastomosing with transverse cervical nerve of cervical plexus)
26 Facial artery and vein
27 Temporal branches of facial nerve
28 Submandibular gland
29 Mandible
30 Mylohyoideus muscle and nerve
31 Anterior belly of digastric muscle
32 Omohyoid muscle
33 Greater petrosal nerve
34 Geniculate ganglion
35 Chorda tympani
36 Posterior auricular nerve
37 Stylomastoid foramen
38 Sternocleidomastoid muscle and retromandibular vein

Deep dissection of facial nerve. Retromandibular and submandibular regions of the head (lateral aspect). The parotid gland has been removed.

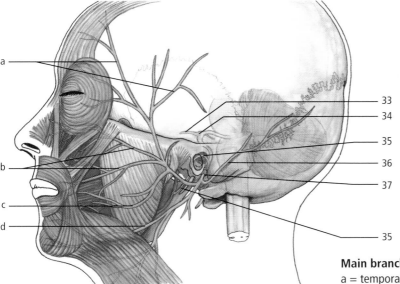

Main branches of facial nerve (schematic drawing).
a = temporal branches; b = zygomatic branches; c = buccal branches; d = marginal mandibular branch.

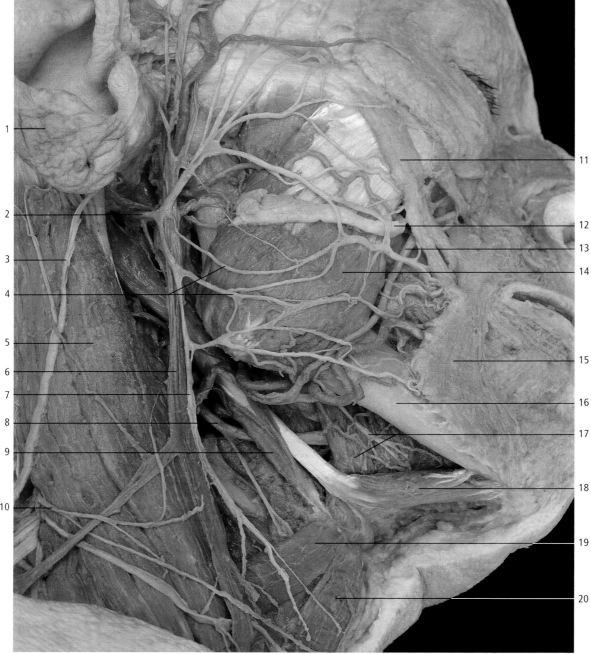

Deep dissection of facial nerve. Retromandibular and submandibular regions of the head (lateral aspect).
The parotid gland and the submandibular gland have been removed. The parotid plexus (4) is formed by anastomosis
of the temporal, zygomatic, buccal, marginal mandibular, and cervical branches of the facial nerve, arising in the
parotid gland.

1	Parotid gland	8	Hypoglossal nerve (n. XII)	15	Depressor anguli oris muscle
2	Facial nerve (n. VII)	9	Stylohyoid muscle	16	Mandible
3	Great auricular nerve	10	Transverse cervical nerve	17	Mylohyoid muscle and nerve
4	Parotid plexus	11	Zygomaticus major muscle	18	Anterior belly of digastric muscle
5	Sternocleidomastoid muscle	12	Parotid duct	19	Omohyoid muscle
6	Retromandibular vein	13	Facial artery	20	Sternohyoid muscle
7	Cervical branch of facial nerve	14	Masseter muscle		

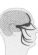

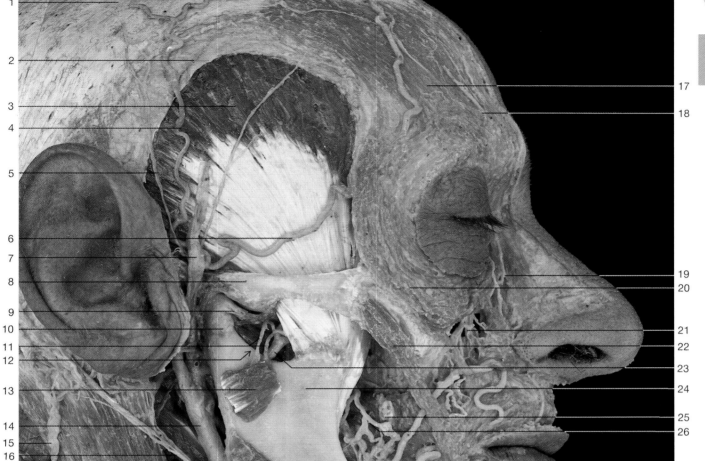

Lateral superficial aspect of the face. Masseter muscle and temporal fascia have been partly removed to display the masseteric artery and nerve.

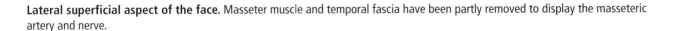

1 Galea aponeurotica	10 Head of mandible	22 Zygomaticus major muscle
2 Temporal fascia	11 Masseteric artery and nerve	23 Maxillary artery
3 Temporalis muscle	12 Mandibular notch	24 Coronoid process
4 Parietal branch of superficial temporal artery	13 Masseter muscle (divided)	25 Parotid duct (divided)
5 Auriculotemporal nerve	14 External carotid artery	26 Buccal nerve
6 Frontal branch of superficial temporal artery	15 Great auricular nerve	27 Facial artery and vein
7 Superficial temporal vein	16 Facial nerve (reflected)	28 Mental nerve
8 Zygomatic arch	17 Frontal belly of occipitofrontalis muscle	29 Mandibular branch of facial nerve
9 Articular disc of temporomandibular joint	18 Medial branch of supra-orbital nerve	30 Cervical branch of facial nerve
	19 Angular artery	31 Transverse cervical nerve (communicating branch with facial nerve) and sternocleidomastoid muscle
	20 Orbicularis oculi muscle	
	21 Infra-orbital nerve	

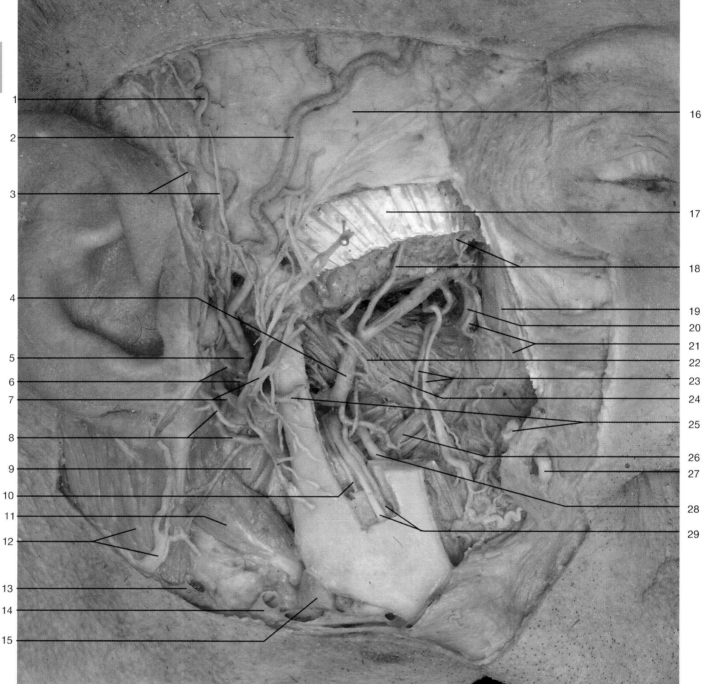

Deep dissection of facial and retromandibular regions. The coronoid process together with the insertions of temporalis muscle have been removed to display the maxillary artery. The upper part of the mandibular canal has been opened.

1 Parietal branch of the superficial temporal artery
2 Frontal branch of the superficial temporal artery
3 Auriculotemporal nerve
4 Maxillary artery
5 Superficial temporal artery
6 Communicating branches between facial and auriculotemporal nerves
7 Facial nerve
8 Posterior auricular artery and anterior auricular branch of superficial temporal artery
9 Internal jugular vein

10 Mylohyoid nerve
11 Posterior belly of digastric muscle
12 Great auricular nerve and sternocleidomastoid muscle
13 External jugular vein
14 Retromandibular vein
15 Submandibular gland
16 Temporal fascia
17 Temporalis tendon
18 Deep temporal arteries
19 Posterior superior alveolar nerve
20 Sphenopalatine artery
21 Posterior superior alveolar arteries

22 Masseteric artery and nerve
23 Buccal nerve and artery
24 Lateral pterygoid
25 Transverse facial artery and parotid duct (divided)
26 Medial pterygoid muscle
27 Facial artery
28 Lingual nerve
29 Inferior alveolar artery and nerve (mandibular canal opened)

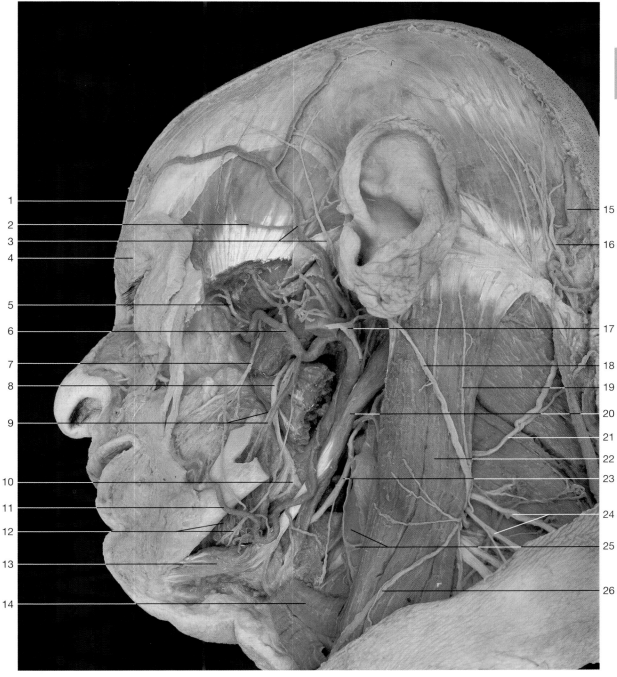

Peripharyngeal and retromandibular regions. The mandible has been partly removed (oblique lateral aspect).

1 Supra-orbital nerve (medial branch)
2 Temporalis muscle
3 Superficial temporal artery and auriculotemporal nerve
4 Orbicularis oculi muscle
5 Anterior deep temporal artery
6 Maxillary artery
7 Buccal nerve
8 Lingual nerve
9 Inferior alveolar nerve and artery

10 Submandibular ganglion
11 Facial artery
12 Mylohyoid muscle and nerve
13 Anterior belly of digastric muscle
14 Omohyoid muscle
15 Occipital artery
16 Greater occipital nerve (C$_2$)
17 Facial nerve (cut) (n. VII)
18 Great auricular nerve
19 Lesser occipital nerve

20 Posterior belly of digastric muscle
21 Accessory nerve (Var.)
22 Sternocleidomastoid muscle
23 Hypoglossus nerve (n. XII)
24 Supraclavicular nerves (lateral and intermedial branches)
25 Internal jugular vein and ansa cervicalis
26 Anterior supraclavicular nerve

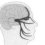

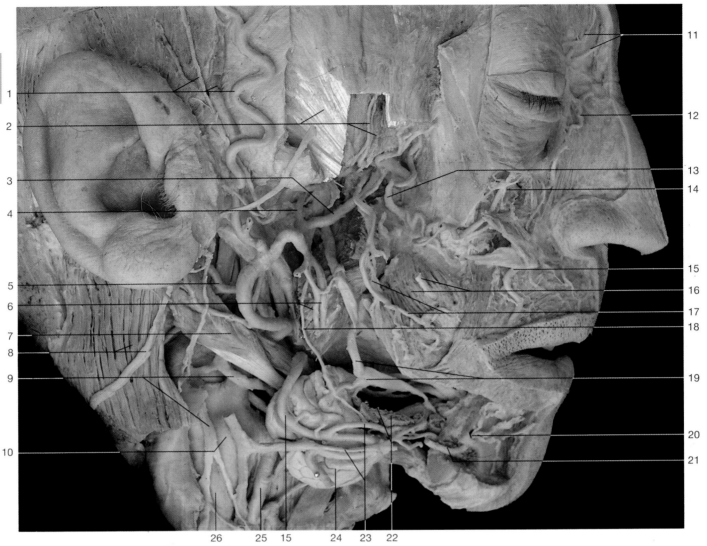

Dissection of deep facial and retromandibular regions after removal of mandible. Pterygoid muscles removed, temporalis muscle fenestrated.

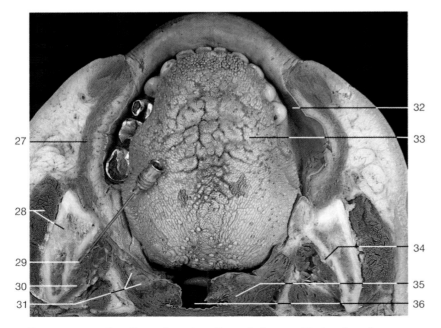

Transverse section through oral cavity and pharynx. The location of inferior alveolar nerve and artery is indicated by a needle.

1 Superficial temporal artery and vein and auriculotemporal nerve
2 Temporalis tendon, deep temporal nerves and artery
3 Maxillary artery
4 Middle meningeal artery
5 Occipital artery
6 Inferior alveolar artery and nerve
7 Posterior belly of digastric muscle
8 Great auricular nerve and sternocleidomastoid muscle
9 Hypoglossal nerve and superior root of ansa cervicalis
10 External carotid artery
11 Supratrochlear nerve and medial branch of supra-orbital artery
12 Angular artery
13 Posterior superior alveolar artery
14 Infra-orbital nerve
15 Facial artery
16 Parotid duct (divided) and buccinator muscle
17 Buccal artery and nerve

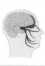

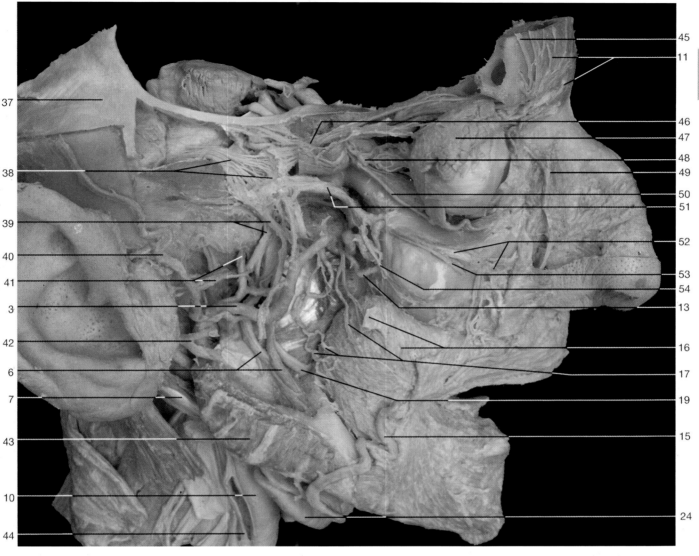

37
38
39
40
41
3
42
6
7
43
10
44

45
11
46
47
48
49
50
51
52
53
54
13
16
17
19
15
24

Para- and retropharyngeal regions. The mandible and the lateral wall of the orbit have been removed. The main branches of the trigeminal nerve and its ganglion are displayed.

18 Mylohyoid nerve
19 Lingual nerve and submandibular ganglion
20 Mental nerve and mental foramen
21 Inferior alveolar nerve
22 Mylohyoid muscle (divided) and hypoglossal nerve
23 Submental artery and vein
24 Submandibular gland
25 Superior thyroid artery
26 Common carotid artery
27 Buccinator muscle
28 Masseter muscle and mandible
29 Entrance of mandibular canal
30 Medial pterygoid muscle
31 Palatine tonsil
32 Oral vestibule
33 Tongue
34 Inferior alveolar nerve, artery, and vein
35 Pharyngeal constrictor muscle

36 Pharynx
37 Tentorium of cerebellum
38 Trigeminal nerve and ganglion
39 Mandibular nerve
40 Superficial temporal artery
41 Auriculotemporal nerve and middle meningeal artery
42 Facial nerve (divided)
43 Masseter muscle
44 Superior root of ansa cervicalis
45 Lateral branch of supra-orbital nerve
46 Ophthalmic nerve
47 Lacrimal gland
48 Ciliary ganglion and short ciliary nerves
49 Angular artery
50 Inferior branch of oculomotor nerve
51 Maxillary nerve
52 Infra-orbital nerve
53 Anterior superior alveolar nerve
54 Posterior superior alveolar nerve

2.3 Brain and Sensory Organs

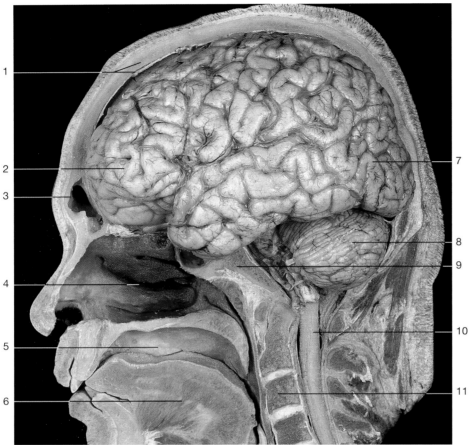

The cranial cavity harbours the brain, the cerebellum, and the brain stem from where the cranial nerves emerge and exit the skull through various openings and fissures. The great sensory organs are located within the orbit (eye), the nasal cavity (olfactory system), and the petrous portion of the temporal bone (vestibulocochlear organ). The brain is enwrapped by the pia mater containing the brain vessels. The dura mater is firmly attached to the skull and provides shelter and stabilization for the brain. Interposed between pia and dura mater lies the arachnoid containing the cerebrospinal fluid.

Dissection of the brain with pia mater and arachnoid in situ. The head is cut in half except for the brain, which is shown in its entirety.

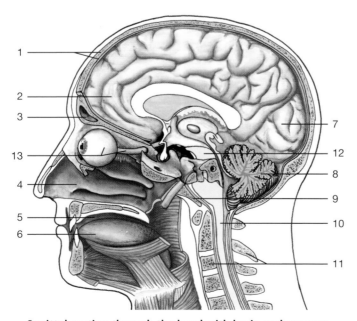

Sagittal section through the head with brain and sensory organs (schematic drawing). The eye with the optic nerve is located within the orbit; the labyrinth organ, within the petrous bone.

1 Vertex of the skull and dura mater
2 Frontal lobe covered by arachnoid and pia mater
3 Frontal sinus
4 Nasal cavity
5 Oral cavity
6 Tongue
7 Occipital lobe
8 Cerebellum
9 Base of skull
10 Spinal cord
11 Vertebral column
12 Brain stem
13 Eye and optic nerve (n. II)

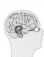

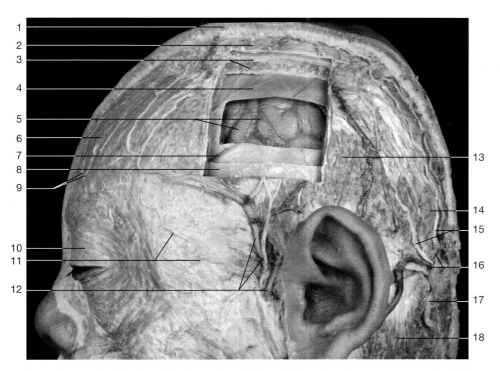

1   Skin
2   Galea aponeurotica
3   Skull diploe
4   Dura mater
5   Arachnoid and pia mater
    with cerebral vessels
6   Frontal belly of occipitofrontalis
    muscle
7   Branch of middle meningeal artery
8   Pericranium (periosteum)
9   Lateral and medial branches of
    supra-orbital nerve
10 Orbicularis oculi muscle
11 Zygomatico-orbital artery
12 Auriculotemporal nerve and
    superficial temporal artery and
    vein
13 Superior auricular muscle
14 Occipital belly of occipitofrontalis
    muscle
15 Occipital nerve
16 Occipital artery and vein
17 Greater occipital nerve
18 Sternocleidomastoid muscle
19 Frontal lobe
20 Chiasmatic cistern
21 Interpeduncular cistern
22 Arachnoid granulations
23 Subarachnoid space
24 Superior sagittal sinus
25 Inferior sagittal sinus
26 Corpus callosum
27 Straight sinus
28 Confluence of sinuses
29 Cerebellum
30 Cerebellomedullar cistern
31 Cerebral cortex

Lateral aspect of the head. Scalp, vertex of the skull, and meninges are demonstrated
by a series of window-like openings.

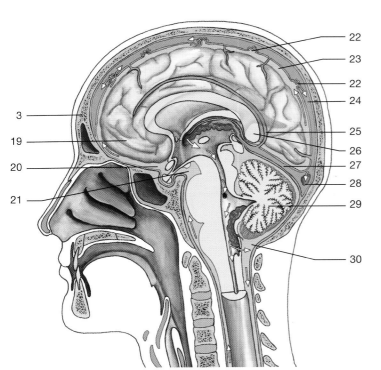

Subarachnoid cisterns of the brain (midsagittal section).
Green = cisterns; blue = dural sinus and ventricles;
red = choroid plexus of third and fourth ventricles; arrows = flow of
cerebrospinal fluid.

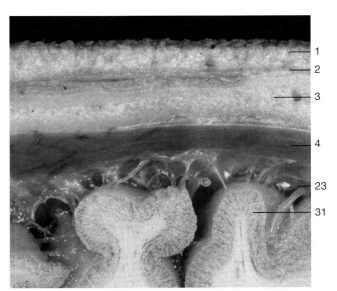

Cross section of the scalp and the meninges.
The subarachnoid space (23) is shown.

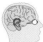

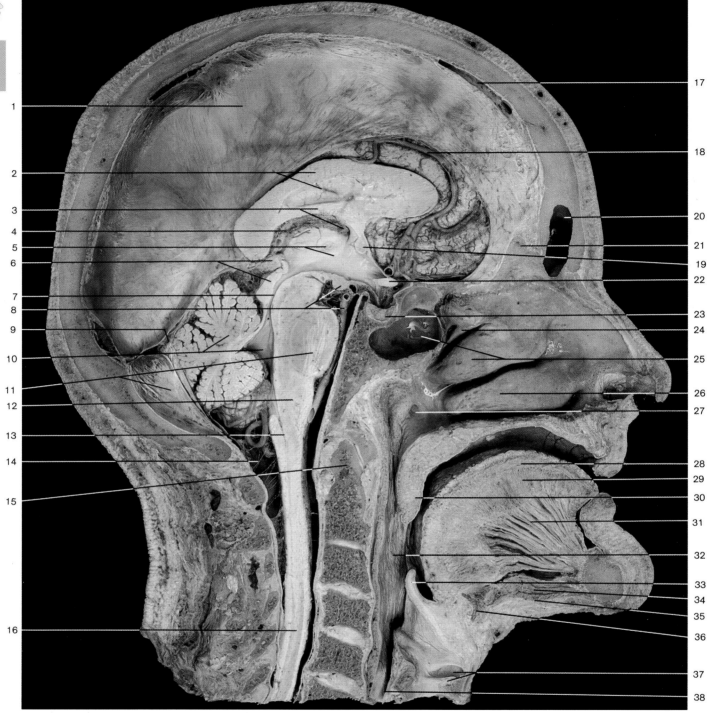

Median sagittal section through the head and neck.

1 Falx cerebri
2 Corpus callosum and septum pellucidum
3 Interventricular foramen and fornix
4 Choroid plexus of third ventricle and internal cerebral vein
5 Third ventricle and interthalamic adhesion
6 Pineal body and colliculi of the midbrain
7 Cerebral aqueduct
8 Mamillary body and basilar artery
9 Straight sinus
10 Fourth ventricle and cerebellum
11 Pons and falx cerebelli
12 Medulla oblongata
13 Central canal

14 Cerebellomedullary cistern
15 Dens of the axis (odontoid process)
16 Spinal cord
17 Superior sagittal sinus
18 Anterior cerebral artery
19 Anterior commissure
20 Frontal sinus
21 Crista galli
22 Optic chiasma
23 Pituitary gland (hypophysis)
24 Superior nasal concha
25 Middle nasal concha and sphenoid sinus
26 Inferior nasal concha

27 Pharyngeal opening of auditory tube
28 Superior longitudinal muscle of tongue
29 Vertical muscle of the tongue
30 Uvula
31 Genioglossus muscle
32 Pharynx
33 Epiglottis
34 Geniohyoid muscle
35 Mylohyoid muscle
36 Hyoid bone
37 Vocal fold and sinus of larynx
38 Esophagus

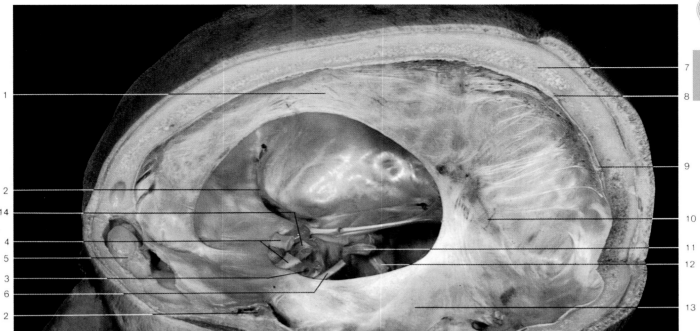

Dura mater and venous sinuses of the dura mater. The brain has been removed (oblique lateral aspect).

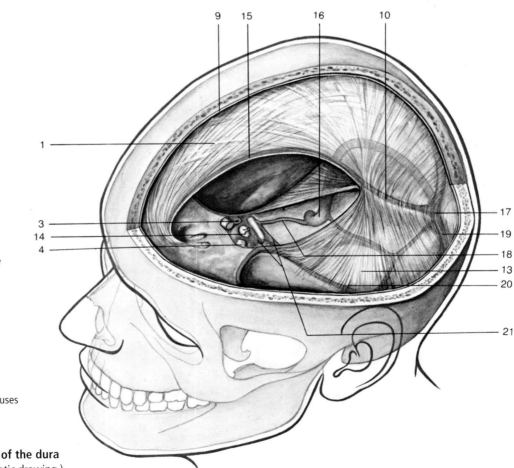

1   Falx cerebri
2   Position of middle meningeal
    artery and vein
3   Internal carotid artery
4   Optic nerve (n. II)
5   Frontal sinus
6   Oculomotor nerve (n. III)
7   Diploe
8   Dura mater
9   Superior sagittal sinus
10 Straight sinus
11 Trigeminal nerve (n. V)
12 Facial and vestibulocochlear nerve
    (n. VII and n. VIII)
13 Tentorium cerebelli
14 Pituitary gland (hypophysis)
15 Inferior sagittal sinus
16 Sigmoid sinus
17 Confluence of sinuses
18 Inferior petrosal sinus
19 Transverse sinus
20 Superior petrosal sinus
21 Cavernous and intercavernous sinuses

Dura mater and venous sinuses of the dura mater (left lateral aspect). (Schematic drawing.)

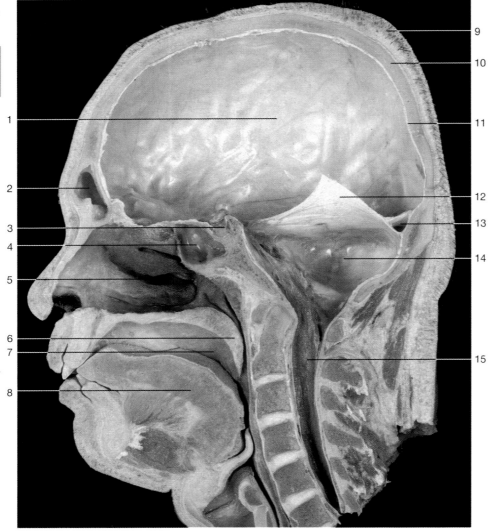

1. Cranial cavity with dura mater (right cerebral hemisphere has been removed)
2. Frontal sinus
3. Hypophysial fossa with pituitary gland
4. Sphenoidal sinus
5. Nasal cavity
6. Soft palate (uvula)
7. Oral cavity
8. Tongue
9. Skin
10. Calvaria
11. Dura mater
12. Tentorium cerebelli
13. Confluence of sinuses
14. Infratentorial space (cerebellum and part of the brain stem have been removed)
15. Vertebral canal
16. Frontal branch of middle meningeal artery and veins
17. Middle meningeal artery
18. Diploe
19. Parietal branch of middle meningeal artery and vein
20. Occipital pole of left hemisphere covered with dura mater

Median section through the head. Demonstration of dura mater covering the cranial cavity. Brain and spinal cord are removed (right half of the head, as seen from medial).

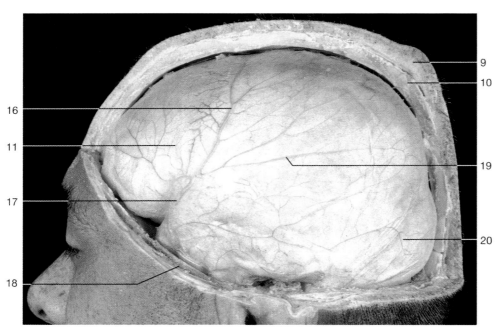

Dissection of dura mater and meningeal vessels. Left half of calvaria removed.

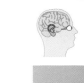

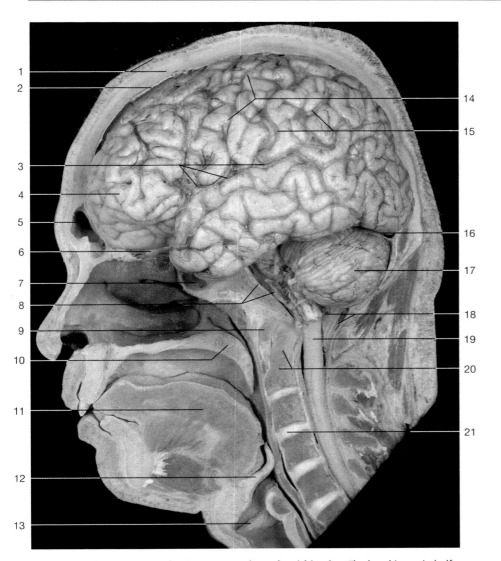

1 Calvaria and skin of the scalp
2 Dura mater (divided)
3 Position of lateral sulcus
4 Frontal lobe covered by arachnoid and pia mater
5 Frontal sinus
6 Olfactory bulb
7 Sphenoidal sinus
8 Dura mater on clivus and basilar artery
9 Atlas (anterior arch, divided)
10 Soft palate
11 Tongue
12 Epiglottis
13 Vocal fold
14 Position of central sulcus
15 Superior cerebral veins
16 Tentorium (divided)
17 Cerebellum
18 Cerebellomedullary cistern
19 Position of foramen magnum and spinal cord
20 Dens of axis
21 Intervertebral disc

Dissection of the brain with pia mater and arachnoid in situ. The head is cut in half except for the brain, which is shown in its entirety.

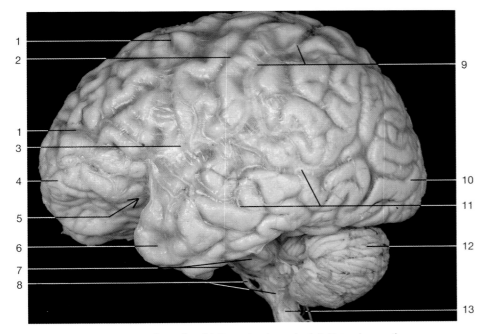

1 Superior cerebral veins
2 Position of central sulcus
3 Position of lateral sulcus and cistern of lateral cerebral fossa
4 Frontal pole
5 Lateral sulcus (arrow)
6 Temporal pole
7 Pons and basilar artery
8 Vertebral arteries
9 Superior anastomotic vein
10 Occipital pole
11 Inferior cerebral veins
12 Hemisphere of cerebellum
13 Medulla oblongata

Brain with pia mater and arachnoid. Frontal pole to the left (lateral aspect).

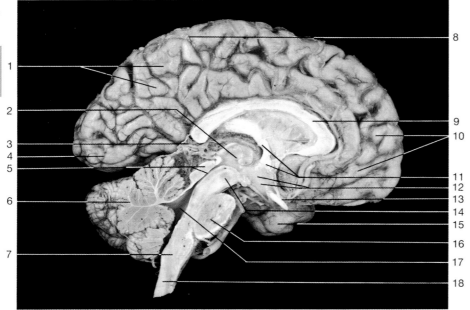

Brain and brain stem, median section. Frontal pole to the right.

1   Parietal lobe
2   Thalamus, third ventricle, and intermediate mass
3   Great cerebral vein
4   Occipital lobe
5   Colliculi of the midbrain and cerebral aqueduct
6   Cerebellum
7   Medulla oblongata
8   Central sulcus
9   Corpus callosum
10 Frontal lobe
11 Fornix and anterior commissure
12 Hypothalamus
13 Optic chiasma
14 Midbrain
15 Temporal lobe
16 Pons
17 Fourth ventricle
18 Spinal cord
19 Inferior concha and nasal cavity
20 Alveolar process of maxilla
21 Tongue
22 Dens of axis
23 Oral part of pharynx
24 Alveolar process of mandible
25 Epiglottis

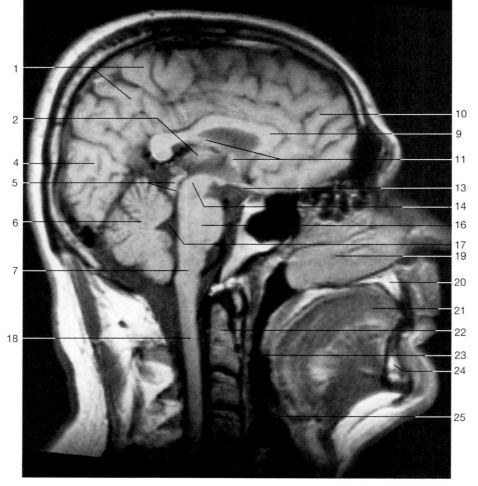

Median section through the head. (MRI scan, cf. section on opposite page.)

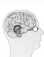

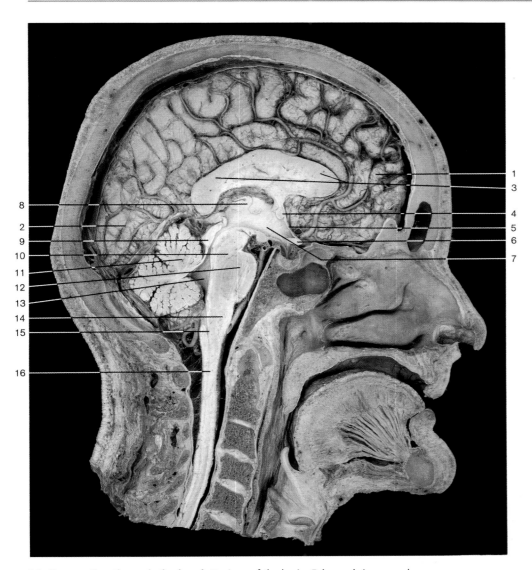

1 Frontal lobe of cerebrum
2 Occipital lobe of cerebrum
3 Corpus callosum
4 Anterior commissure
5 Lamina terminalis
6 Optic chiasma
7 Hypothalamus
8 Thalamus and third
   ventricle
9 Colliculi of the midbrain
10 Midbrain (inferior portion)
11 Cerebellum
12 Pons
13 Fourth ventricle
14 Medulla oblongata
15 Central canal
16 Spinal cord

Median section through the head. Regions of the brain. Falx cerebri removed.

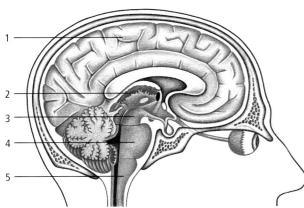

Scheme of brain divisions (cf. table). (Schematic drawing.)
Red = choroidal plexus.

1 Telencephalon (yellow) with lateral ventricles
2 Diencephalon (orange) with third ventricle,
   optic nerve, and retina
3 Mesencephalon (blue) with cerebral aqueduct
4 Metencephalon (green) with fourth ventricle
5 Myelencephalon (yellow-green)

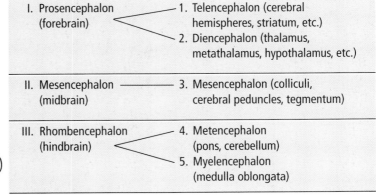

I. Prosencephalon (forebrain)	1. Telencephalon (cerebral hemispheres, striatum, etc.)
	2. Diencephalon (thalamus, metathalamus, hypothalamus, etc.)
II. Mesencephalon (midbrain)	3. Mesencephalon (colliculi, cerebral peduncles, tegmentum)
III. Rhombencephalon (hindbrain)	4. Metencephalon (pons, cerebellum)
	5. Myelencephalon (medulla oblongata)

Main divisions of the brain
I–III = primary brain vesicles; 1–5 = secondary brain vesicles

Diencephalon, midbrain, pons, and medulla oblongata are collectively termed the **brain stem.**

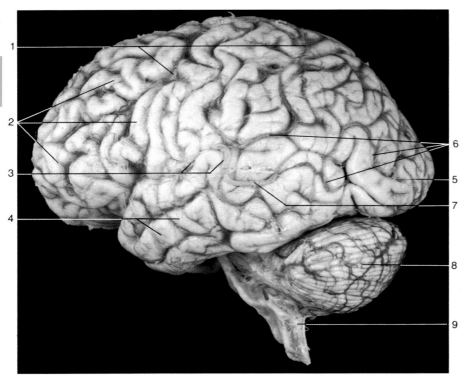

1. Superior cerebral veins and parietal lobe
2. Frontal lobe
3. Superficial middle cerebral vein and cistern of lateral cerebral fossa
4. Temporal lobe
5. Occipital lobe
6. Inferior cerebral veins and transverse occipital sulcus
7. Inferior anastomotic vein
8. Cerebellum
9. Medulla oblongata

Brain with pia mater. Cerebral veins (bluish). In the lateral sulcus the cistern of the lateral fossa is recognizable. Frontal lobe to the left.

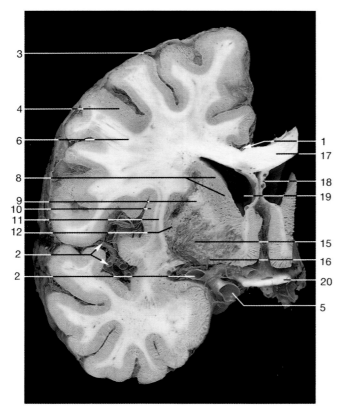

Arteries of the brain. Coronal section. Areas supplied by cortical and central arteries. Dotted lines indicate boundaries of arterial supply areas; arrows = direction of blood flow.

◁ **Coronal section through the right hemisphere,** showing arachnoid, pia mater, and the arterial blood supply (anterior aspect).

1 Anterior cerebral artery	8 Caudate nucleus	15 Pallidostriate artery
2 Middle cerebral arteries	9 Internal capsule	16 Thalamic artery
3 Arachnoid	10 Insular lobe	17 Corpus callosum
4 Cortex	11 Claustrum	18 Septum pellucidum
5 Internal carotid artery	12 Putamen	19 Lateral ventricle
6 Frontal lobe (white matter)	13 Posterior striate branch	20 Optic chiasma
7 Posterior cerebral artery	14 Insular artery	

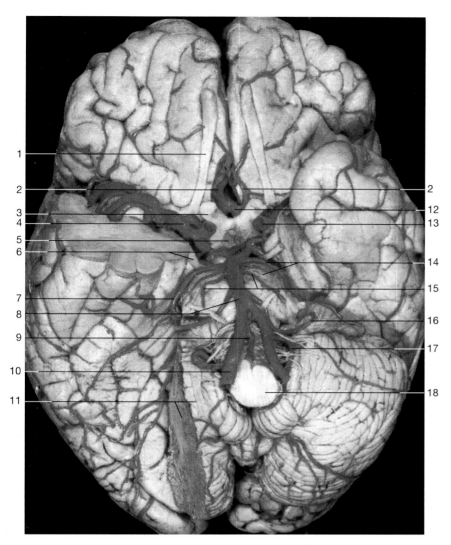

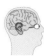

1   Olfactory tract
2   Anterior cerebral artery
3   Optic nerve (n. II)
4   Middle cerebral artery
5   Infundibulum
6   Oculomotor nerve (n. III) and
    posterior communicating
    artery
7   Posterior cerebral artery
8   Basilar artery and abducent
    nerve (n. VI)
9   Anterior spinal artery
10 Vertebral artery
11 Cerebellum
12 Anterior communicating artery
13 Internal carotid artery
14 Superior cerebellar artery
    and pons
15 Labyrinthine arteries
16 Inferior anterior cerebellar
    artery
17 Inferior posterior cerebellar
    artery
18 Medulla oblongata
19 Supratrochlear artery
20 Anterior ciliary arteries
21 Lacrimal artery
22 Posterior ciliary arteries
23 Ophthalmic artery with
    central retinal artery
24 Trigeminal nerve (n. V)
25 Facial nerve (n. VII) and
    vestibulocochlear nerve (n. VIII)
26 Glossopharyngeal nerve (n. IX),
    vagus nerve (n. X), and
    accessory nerve (n. XI)
27 Olfactory bulb
28 Posterior spinal artery

Arteries of the brain (inferior aspect, frontal pole above). Right temporal lobe and
cerebellum partly removed.

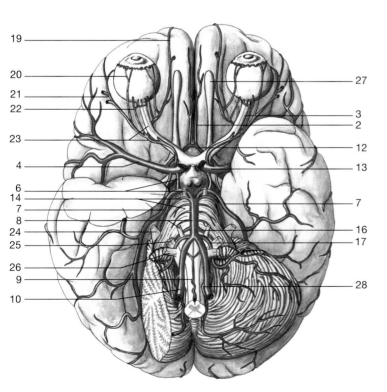

Arteries of the brain (inferior aspect). Right temporal lobe
and cerebellum partly removed. Note the arterial circle of Willis
around the infundibulum.

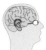

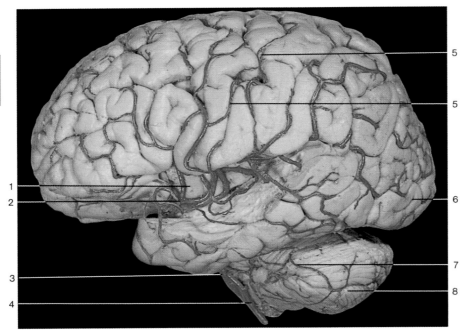

1 Insula
2 Middle cerebral artery (2 branches:
   a Parietal branches,
   b Temporal branches)
3 Basilar artery
4 Vertebral artery
5 Central sulcus
6 Occipital lobe
7 Superior cerebellar artery
8 Cerebellum
9 Anterior cerebral artery
10 Ethmoidal arteries
11 Ophthalmic artery
12 Internal carotid artery
13 Posterior communicating artery
14 Posterior cerebral artery
15 Anterior inferior cerebellar artery
16 Posterior inferior cerebellar artery

Cerebral arteries. Lateral aspect of the left hemisphere. The upper part of the temporal lobe has been removed to display the insula and cerebral arteries.

◁ **Arteries of the brain.**

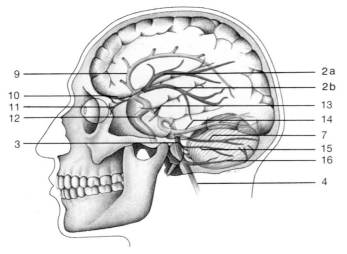

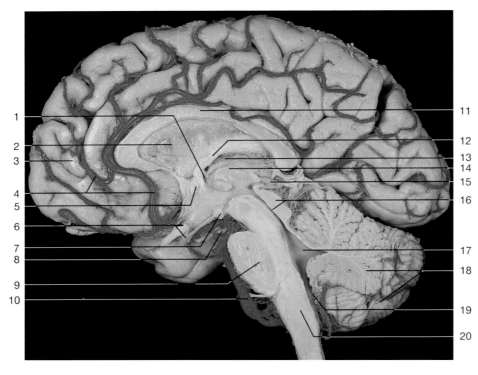

1 Interventricular foramen
2 Septum pellucidum
3 Frontal lobe
4 Anterior cerebral artery
5 Anterior commissure
6 Optic chiasma and infundibulum
7 Mamillary body
8 Oculomotor nerve (n. III)
9 Pons
10 Basilar artery
11 Corpus callosum
12 Fornix
13 Choroid plexus
14 Third ventricle
15 Pineal body
16 Tectum and cerebral aqueduct
17 Fourth ventricle
18 Cerebellum (arbor vitae, vermis)
19 Median aperture of Magendie
20 Medulla oblongata

Median section through the brain and brain stem. Cerebral arteries injected with red resin.

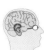

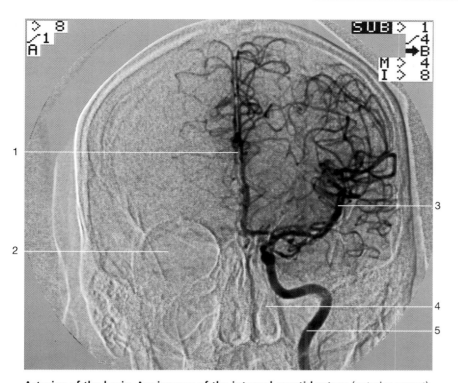

1 Anterior cerebral artery
2 Orbit
3 Middle cerebral artery
4 Nasal cavity
5 Internal carotid artery
6 Arterial circle of Willis
7 Posterior communicating artery
8 Posterior cerebral artery
9 Basilar artery
10 Vertebral artery
11 Subclavian artery
12 Aortic arch
13 Common carotid artery

Arteries of the brain. Angiogram of the internal carotid artery (anterior aspect) (courtesy of Prof. Dr. W. Huk, University of Erlangen-Nürnberg).

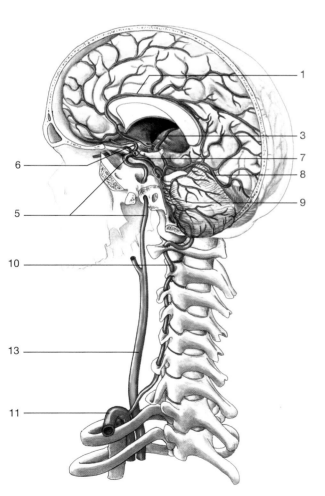

Cerebral arteries (schematic drawing).
Left hemisphere and brain stem have been removed.
Note the arterial circle of Willis around the sella turcica.

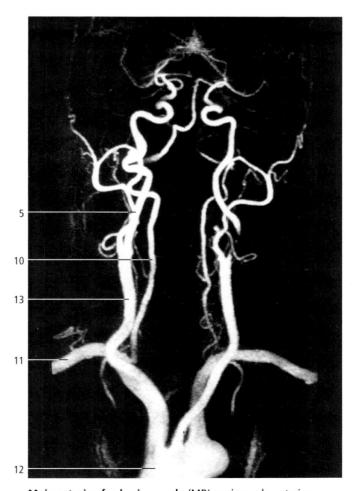

Main arteries for brain supply (MRI angiograph, anterior aspect, courtesy of Prof. Dr. W. Bautz, University of Erlangen-Nürnberg).

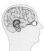

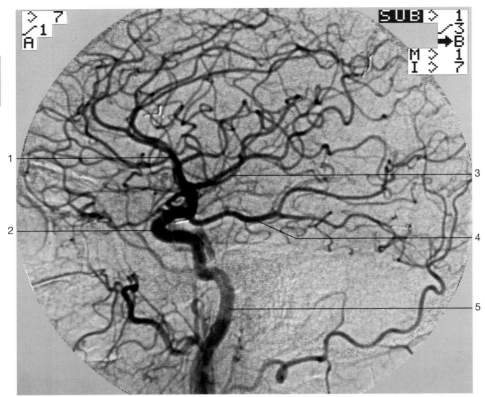

1   Anterior cerebral artery
2   Loop of the internal
    carotid artery
3   Middle cerebral artery
4   Posterior cerebral artery
5   Internal carotid artery
6   Superior cerebellar artery
7   Anterior inferior cerebellar
    artery
8   Posterior inferior cerebellar
    artery
9   Vertebral artery

Arteries of the brain. Angiogram of the internal carotid artery (lateral aspect)
(courtesy of Prof. Dr. W. Huk, University of Erlangen-Nürnberg).

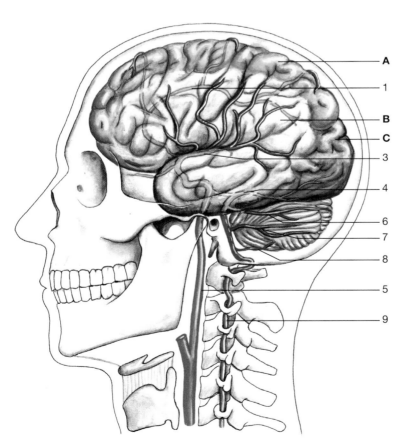

Cerebral arteries. The areas supplied by the main arteries are indicated by
different colors (lateral aspect).

Areas of blood supply of the brain
(cerebellum = light blue).
A = anterior cerebral artery (upper
       and medial parts of the cortex)
       (orange)
B = middle cerebral artery (lateral
       areas of the frontal, parietal, and
       temporal lobes) (white)
C = posterior cerebral artery (occipital
       lobe and inferior parts of the
       temporal lobe) (blue)

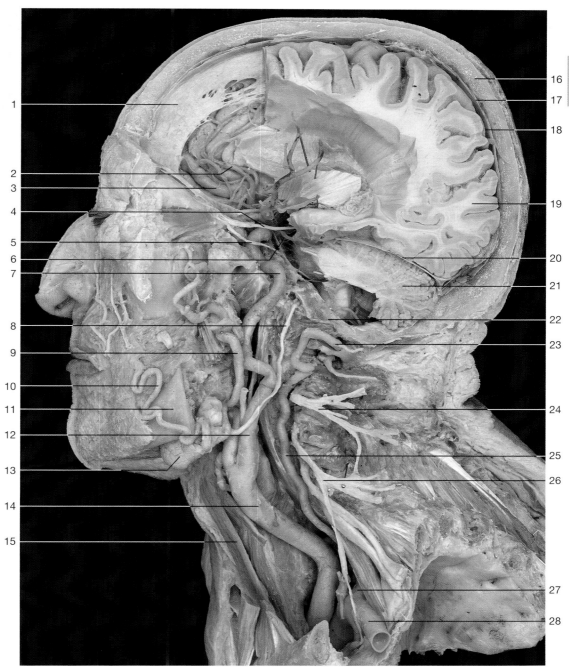

Dissection of the arteries of the brain and head (lateral aspect, superficial layers of facial region and left hemisphere and cerebellum partly removed).

1	Falx cerebri	16	Calvaria
2	Anterior cerebral artery	17	Dura mater
3	Frontal lobe	18	Subarachnoidal space
4	Oculomotor nerve (n. III)	19	Occipital lobe
5	Abducent nerve (n. VI)	20	Tentorium of cerebellum
6	Posterior cerebral artery	21	Cerebellum
7	Internal carotid artery, entering sinus cavernosus	22	Base of skull
8	Hypoglossus nerve (n. XII)	23	Vertebral artery (on the posterior arch of the atlas)
9	Maxillary artery	24	Cervical plexus
10	Facial artery	25	Vertebral artery (removed from the cervical vertebrae)
11	Mandible	26	Brachial plexus
12	External carotid artery	27	Vertebral artery (branching from the subclavian artery)
13	Submandibular gland	28	Subclavian artery
14	Common carotid artery		
15	Sternohyoid muscle		

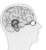

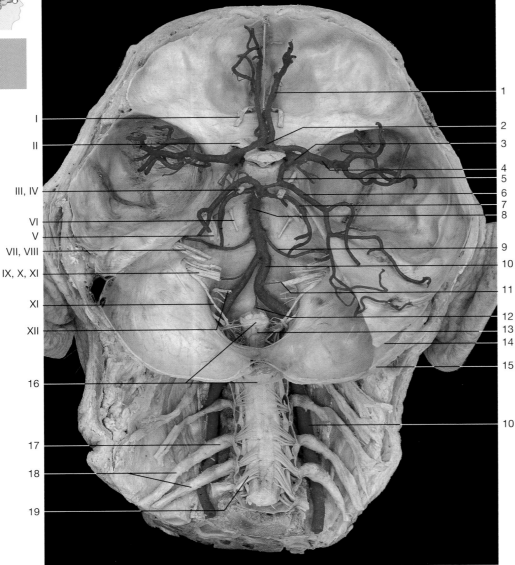

1   Anterior cerebral artery
2   Anterior communicating artery
3   Internal carotid artery
4   Medial cerebral artery
5   Posterior communicating artery
6   Posterior cerebral artery
7   Superior cerebellar artery
8   Basilar artery
9   Anterior inferior cerebellar artery with the artery of the labyrinth
10 Vertebral artery
11 Posterior inferior cerebellar artery
12 Anterior spinal artery
13 Pia mater of spinal cord
14 Tentorium cerebelli
15 Dura mater of the cranial cavity
16 Spinal cord
17 Spinal ganglion
18 Spinal nerves (C_3, C_4)
19 Posterior root filaments (fila radicularia post.)
20 Ophthalmic artery (within the orbit)
21 Internal carotid artery (within carotid canal)
22 Posterior spinal artery

I   Olfactory tract
II   Optic nerve
III   Oculomotor nerve
IV   Trochlear nerve
V   Trigeminal nerve
VI   Abducent nerve
VII   Facial nerve
VIII Vestibulocochlear nerve
IX   Glossopharyngeal nerve
X   Vagus nerve
XI   Accessory nerve
XII   Hypoglossus nerve

Dissection of the arterial circle of the cerebrum at the base of the skull
(from above; calvaria and brain have been removed; arteries are colored in red, cranial nerves [n. I–XII] in yellow).

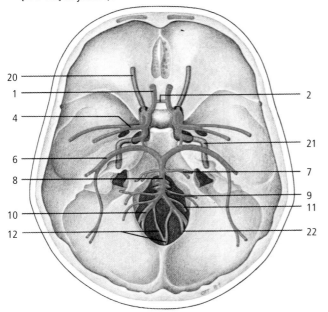

Arterial circle of Willis (superior aspect).
(Schematic drawing.)

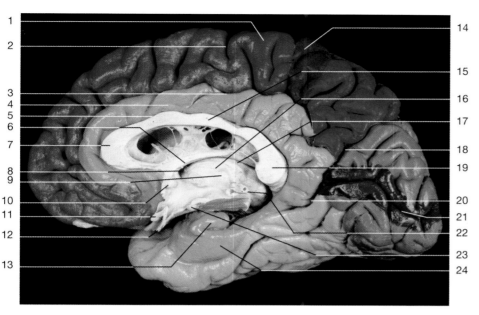

1 Precentral gyrus
2 Precentral sulcus
3 Cingulate sulcus
4 Cingulate gyrus
5 Sulcus of corpus callosum
6 Fornix
7 Genu of corpus callosum
8 Interventricular foramen
9 Intermediate mass
10 Anterior commissure
11 Optic chiasma
12 Infundibulum
13 Uncus hippocampi
14 Postcentral gyrus
15 Body of corpus callosum
16 Third ventricle and thalamus
17 Stria medullaris
18 Parieto-occipital sulcus
19 Splenium of corpus callosum
20 Communication of calcarine and parieto-occipital sulcus
21 Calcarine sulcus
22 Pineal body
23 Mamillary body
24 Parahippocampal gyrus
25 Olfactory bulb
26 Olfactory tract
27 Gyrus rectus
28 Optic nerve
29 Infundibulum and optic chiasma
30 Optic tract
31 Oculomotor nerve
32 Pedunculus cerebri
33 Red nucleus
34 Cerebral aqueduct
35 Corpus callosum
36 Longitudinal fissure
37 Orbital gyri
38 Lateral root of olfactory tract
39 Medial root of olfactory tract
40 Olfactory tubercle and anterior perforated substance
41 Tuber cinereum
42 Interpeduncular fossa
43 Substantia nigra
44 Colliculi of the midbrain
45 Lateral occipitotemporal gyrus
46 Medial occipitotemporal gyrus

Brain, right hemisphere (medial aspect). Frontal pole to the left (midbrain divided, cerebellum and inferior part of brain stem removed).

Red	=	Frontal lobe	Dark blue	=	Postcentral lobe
Blue	=	Parietal lobe	Dark green	=	Calcarine sulcus
Green	=	Occipital lobe	Dark yellow	=	Limbic cortex
Yellow	=	Temporal lobe			(cingulate and
Dark red	=	Precentral lobe			parahippocampal gyri)

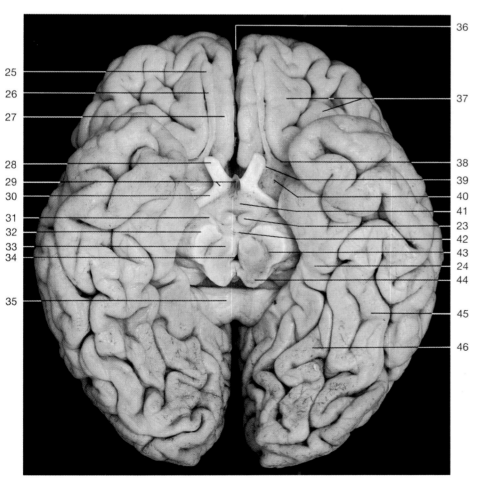

Brain (inferior aspect). Midbrain divided. Cerebellum and inferior part of brain stem removed. Frontal pole at the top.

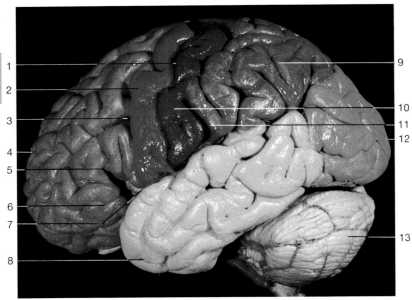

1	Central sulcus
2	Precentral gyrus
3	Precentral sulcus
4	Frontal lobe
5	Anterior ascending ramus of lateral sulcus
6	Anterior horizontal ramus of lateral sulcus
7	Lateral sulcus
8	Temporal lobe
9	Parietal lobe
10	Postcentral gyrus
11	Postcentral sulcus
12	Occipital lobe
13	Cerebellum
14	Superior frontal sulcus
15	Middle frontal gyrus
16	Lunate sulcus
17	Longitudinal fissure
18	Arachnoid granulations

Brain, left hemisphere (lateral aspect). Frontal pole to the left.

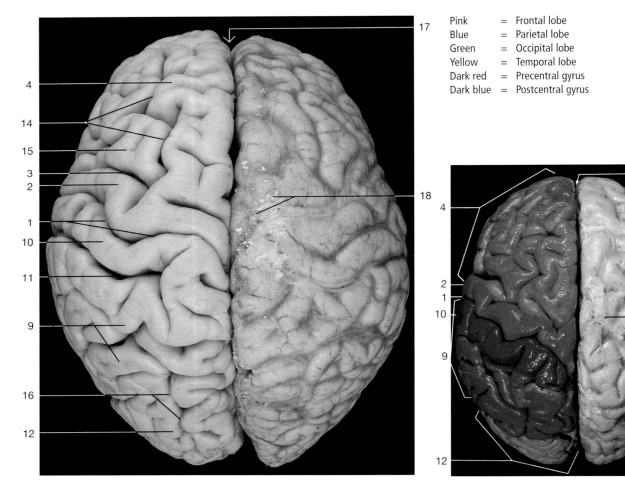

Pink	=	Frontal lobe
Blue	=	Parietal lobe
Green	=	Occipital lobe
Yellow	=	Temporal lobe
Dark red	=	Precentral gyrus
Dark blue	=	Postcentral gyrus

Brain (superior aspect). Right hemisphere with arachnoid and pia mater.

Brain (superior aspect). Lobes of the left hemisphere indicated by color; right hemisphere is covered with arachnoid and pia mater.

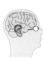

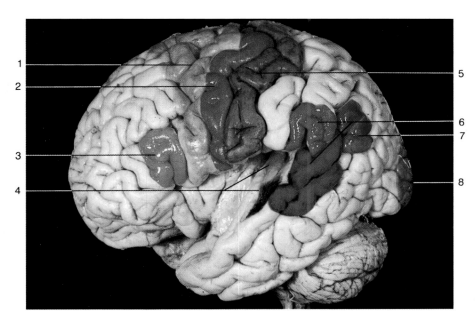

1   Premotor area
2   Somatomotor area
3   Motor speech area of Broca
4   Acoustic area
    (red: high tone, dark green: low tone)
5   Somatosensory area
6   Sensory speech area of Wernicke
7   Reading comprehension area
8   Visuosensory area

Brain, left hemisphere (lateral aspect). **Main cortical areas** are colored.
The lateral sulcus has been opened to display the insula and the inner surface of the
temporal lobe.

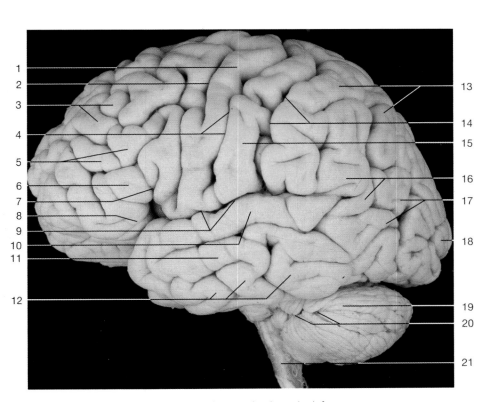

1   Precentral gyrus
2   Precentral sulcus
3   Superior frontal gyrus
4   Central sulcus
5   Middle frontal gyrus
6   Inferior frontal gyrus
7   Ascending ramus } of lateral
8   Horizontal ramus sulcus
9   Posterior ramus
10 Superior temporal gyrus
11 Middle temporal gyrus
12 Inferior temporal gyrus
13 Parietal lobe
14 Postcentral sulcus
15 Postcentral gyrus
16 Supramarginal gyrus
17 Angular gyrus
18 Occipital lobe
19 Cerebellum
20 Horizontal fissure of cerebellum
21 Medulla oblongata

Brain, left hemisphere (lateral aspect). Frontal pole to the left.

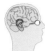

1 Superior cerebellar peduncle
2 Middle cerebellar peduncle
3 Cerebellar tonsil
4 Inferior semilunar lobule
5 Vermis
6 Central lobule of vermis
7 Inferior cerebellar peduncle
8 Superior medullary velum
9 Nodule of vermis
10 Flocculus of cerebellum
11 Biventral lobule
12 Left cerebellar hemisphere
13 Inferior semilunar lobule
14 Biventral lobule
15 Vermis of cerebellum
16 Tuber of vermis
17 Pyramid of vermis
18 Uvula of vermis
19 Tonsil of cerebellum
20 Flocculus of cerebellum
21 Right cerebellar hemisphere
22 Vermis (central lobule)
23 Cerebellar lingula
24 Ala of central lobule
25 Superior cerebellar peduncle
26 Fastigium
27 Fourth ventricle
28 Middle cerebellar peduncle
29 Nodule of vermis
30 Flocculus of cerebellum
31 Cerebellar tonsil
32 Culmen of vermis
33 Declive of vermis
34 Tuber of vermis
35 Inferior semilunar lobule
36 Pyramid of vermis (cut)
37 Uvula of vermis

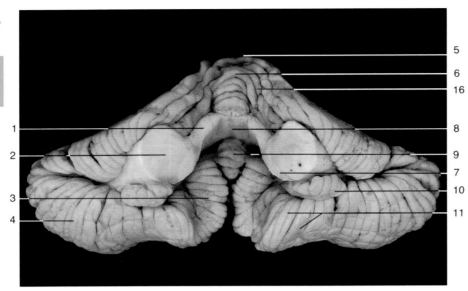

Cerebellum (inferior anterior aspect). The cerebellar peduncles have been severed.

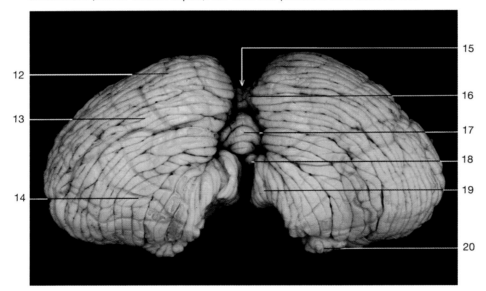

Cerebellum (inferior posterior aspect).

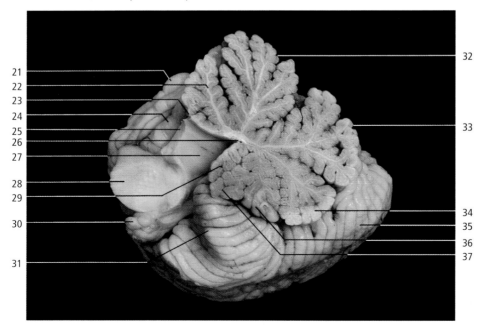

Median section through the cerebellum. Right cerebellar hemisphere and right half of vermis.

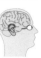

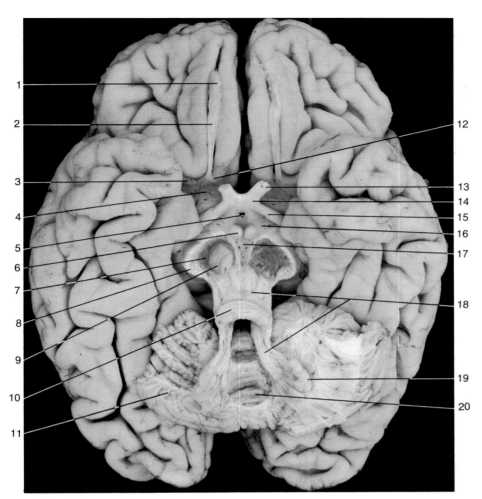

1   Olfactory bulb
2   Olfactory tract
3   Lateral olfactory stria
4   Anterior perforated substance
5   Infundibulum (divided)
6   Mamillary body
7   Substantia nigra
8   Cerebral peduncle (cut)
9   Red nucleus
10 Decussation of superior cerebellar peduncle
11 Cerebellar hemisphere
12 Medial olfactory stria
13 Optic nerve
14 Optic chiasma
15 Optic tract
16 Posterior perforated substance
17 Interpeduncular fossa
18 Superior cerebellar peduncle and cerebellorubral tract
19 Dentate nucleus
20 Vermis of cerebellum
21 Cingulate gyrus
22 Corpus callosum
23 Stria terminalis
24 Septum pellucidum
25 Columna fornicis
26 Cerebral peduncle at midbrain level
27 Pons
28 Inferior olive
29 Medulla oblongata with lateral pyramidal tract
30 Occipital lobe
31 Calcarine sulcus
32 Thalamus
33 Inferior colliculus with brachium
34 Medial lemniscus
35 Superior cerebellar peduncle
36 Inferior cerebellar peduncle
37 Middle cerebellar peduncle
38 Cerebellar hemisphere

Brain and cerebellum (inferior aspect). Parts of the cerebellum have been removed to display the dentate nucleus and the main pathway to the midbrain (cerebellorubral tract).

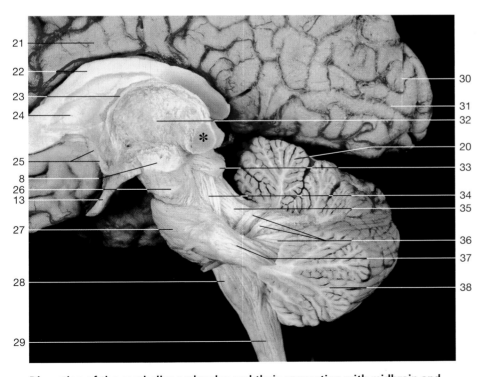

Dissection of the cerebellar peduncles and their connection with midbrain and diencephalon. A small part of pulvinar thalami (✱) has been cut to show inferior brachium.

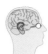

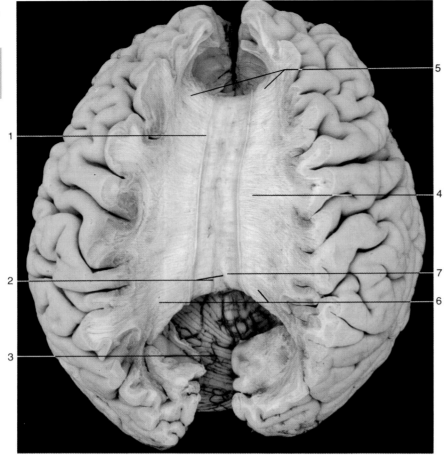

1 Lateral longitudinal stria
   of indusium griseum
2 Medial longitudinal stria
   of indusium griseum
3 Cerebellum
4 Radiating fibers of the corpus callosum
5 Forceps minor of corpus callosum
6 Forceps major of corpus callosum
7 Splenium of corpus callosum

Dissection of the brain I. The fiber system of the corpus callosum has been displayed by removing the cortex lying above it. Frontal pole at the top.

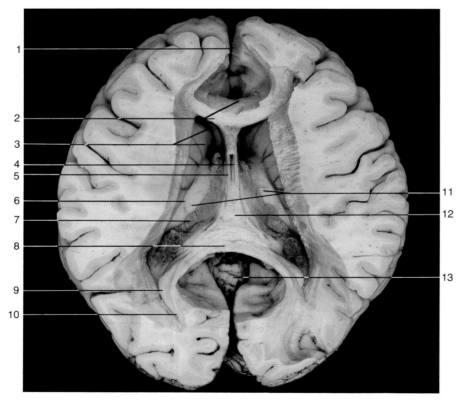

1 Longitudinal cerebral fissure
2 Genu of corpus callosum
3 Head of caudate nucleus and
   anterior horn of lateral ventricle
4 Cavum of septum pellucidum
5 Septum pellucidum
6 Stria terminalis
7 Choroid plexus of lateral ventricle
8 Splenium of corpus callosum
9 Calcar avis
10 Posterior horn of lateral ventricle
11 Thalamus (lamina affixa)
12 Commissure of fornix
13 Vermis of cerebellum

Dissection of the brain II. The lateral ventricles and subcortical nuclei of the brain are dissected. The corpus callosum has been partly removed. Frontal pole at the top.

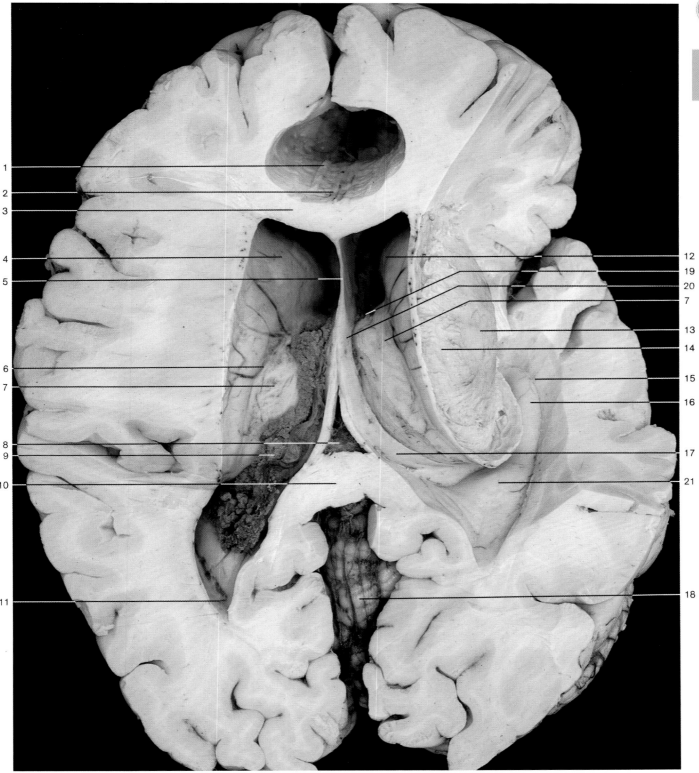
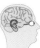

Dissection of the brain III (superior view of lateral ventricle and subcortical nuclei of the brain). Corpus callosum partly removed. At right, the entire lateral ventricle has been opened, the insula with claustrum and the extreme and external capsules have been removed, exposing the lentiform nucleus and the internal capsule.

1   Lateral longitudinal stria
2   Medial longitudinal stria
3   Genu of corpus callosum
4   Head of caudate nucleus
5   Septum pellucidum
6   Stria terminalis
7   Thalamus (lamina affixa)
8   Choroid plexus of third ventricle

9   Choroid plexus of lateral ventricle
10 Splenium of corpus callosum
11 Posterior horn of lateral ventricle
12 Anterior horn of lateral ventricle
    (head of caudate nucleus)
13 Putamen of lentiform nucleus
14 Internal capsule
15 Inferior horn of lateral ventricle

16 Pes hippocampi
17 Crus of fornix
18 Vermis of cerebellum with arachnoid and
    pia mater
19 Interventricular foramen
20 Right column of fornix
21 Collateral eminence

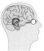

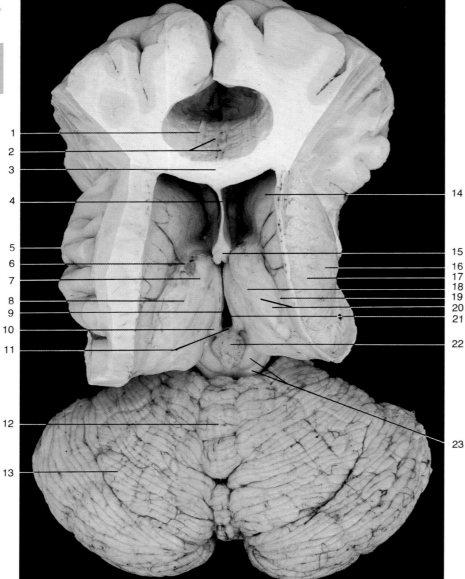

1   Lateral longitudinal stria
2   Medial longitudinal stria
3   Corpus callosum
4   Septum pellucidum
5   Insular gyri
6   Thalamostriate vein
7   Anterior tubercle of thalamus
8   Thalamus
9   Stria medullaris of thalamus
10 Habenular trigone
11 Habenular commissure
12 Vermis of cerebellum
13 Left hemisphere of cerebellum
14 Head of caudate nucleus
15 Columns of fornix
16 Putamen of lentiform nucleus
17 Internal capsule
18 Taenia of choroid plexus
19 Stria terminalis and thalamostriate vein
20 Lamina affixa
21 Third ventricle
22 Pineal body
23 Superior and inferior colliculus of midbrain

Dissection of the brain IVa. Temporal lobe, fornix, and the posterior corpus callosum have been removed (this part of the specimen is depicted below). Frontal pole at top (superior aspect).

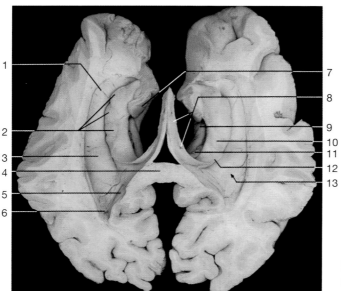

1   Inferior horn of lateral ventricle
2   Hippocampal digitations
3   Collateral eminence
4   Splenium of corpus callosum
5   Calcar avis
6   Posterior horn of lateral ventricle
7   Uncus of parahippocampal gyrus
8   Body and crus of fornix
9   Parahippocampal gyrus
10 Pes hippocampi
11 Dentate gyrus
12 Hippocampal fimbria
13 Lateral ventricle

Dissection of the brain IVb. Depicted is the portion of the brain removed from the specimen above. **Temporal lobe and limbic system** (superior aspect). Columns of fornix are cut.

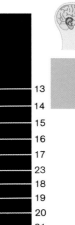

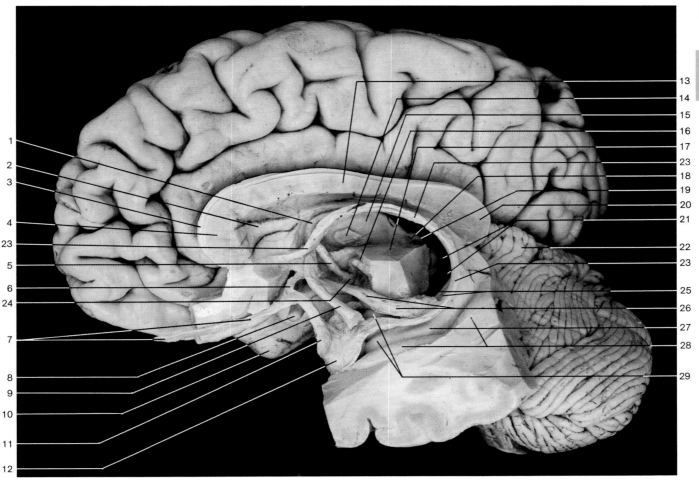

Dissection of the limbic system. Left side, lateral aspect. Corpus callosum has been cut in the median plane. The left thalamus and the left hemisphere have been partly removed.

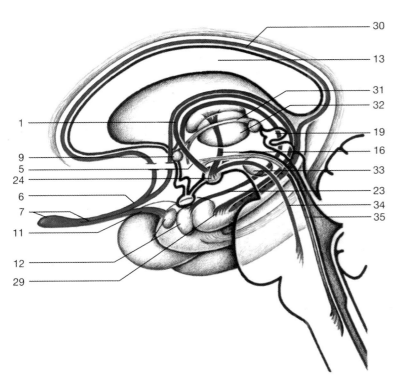

1	Body of fornix	21	Colliculi of midbrain
2	Septum pellucidum	22	Vermis of cerebellum
3	Lateral longitudinal stria	23	Stria terminalis
4	Genu of corpus callosum	24	Mamillary body
5	Column of fornix	25	Fimbria of hippocampus and pes hippocampi
6	Medial olfactory stria		
7	Olfactory bulb and olfactory tract	26	Left optic tract and lateral geniculate body
8	Optic nerve	27	Lateral ventricle and parahippocampal gyrus
9	Anterior commissure (left half)		
10	Right temporal lobe	28	Collateral eminence
11	Lateral olfactory stria	29	Hippocampal digitations
12	Amygdala	30	Supracallosal gyrus (longitudinal stria)
13	Body of corpus callosum		
14	Interthalamic adhesion	31	Stria medullaris of thalamus
15	Third ventricle and right thalamus		
16	Mamillothalamic fasciculus	32	Thalamus
17	Part of the thalamus	33	Red nucleus
18	Habenular commissure	34	Mamillotegmental fasciculus
19	Pineal body		
20	Splenium of corpus callosum	35	Dorsal longitudinal fasciculus (Schütz)

Main pathways of limbic and olfactory system (schematic drawing). Blue = afferent pathways; red = efferent pathways.

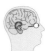

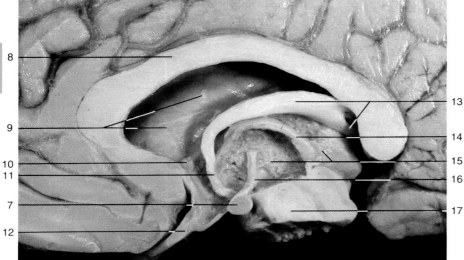

1   Paraventricular nucleus ⎫
2   Pre-optic nucleus   ⎪
3   Ventromedial nucleus   ⎬ Hypothalamic
4   Supra-optic nucleus   ⎪ nuclei
5   Posterior nucleus   ⎪
6   Dorsomedial nucleus   ⎭
7   Mamillary body
8   Corpus callosum
9   Lateral ventricle (showing caudate nucleus)
10   Anterior commissure
11   Column of fornix
12   Optic chiasma
13   Crus of fornix
14   Stria medullaris of thalamus
15   Thalamus and interthalamic adhesion
16   Mamillothalamic fasciculus of Vicq d'Azyr
17   Cerebral peduncle
18   Pineal body
19   Tectum of midbrain
20   Lamina terminalis

Median section through the diencephalon. Medial part of the thalamus and septum pellucidum have been removed to show the fornix and mamillothalamic fasciculus.

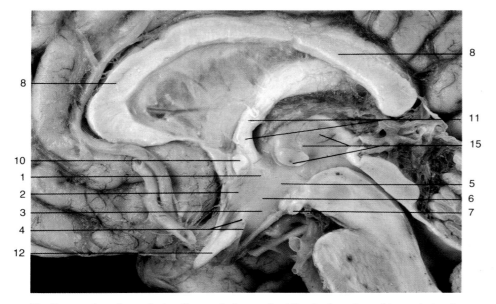

Median section through the diencephalon and midbrain; location of hypothalamic nuclei.

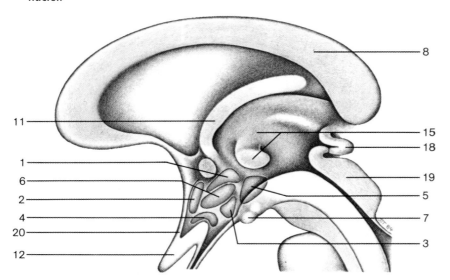

Position of main hypothalamic nuclei (schematic drawing).

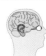

1 Circular sulcus of insula
2 Long gyrus of insula
3 Short gyri of insula
4 Limen insulae
5 Opercula (cut)
  a Frontal operculum
  b Frontoparietal operculum
  c Temporal operculum
6 Corona radiata
7 Lentiform nucleus
8 Anterior commissure
9 Olfactory tract
10 Cerebral arcuate fibers
11 Optic radiation
12 Cerebral peduncle
13 Trigeminal nerve (n. V)
14 Flocculus of cerebellum
15 Pyramidal tract
16 Decussation of pyramidal tract
17 Internal capsule
18 Optic tract
19 Optic nerve (n. II)
20 Infundibulum
21 Temporal lobe (right side)
22 Mamillary bodies
23 Oculomotor nerve (n. III)
24 Transverse fibers of pons

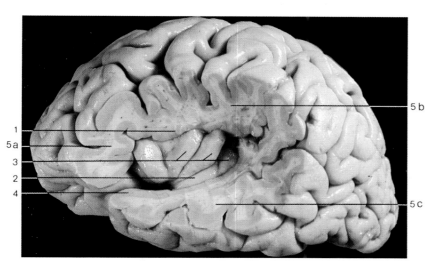

Insula (Reili). The opercula of the frontal, parietal, and temporal lobes have been removed to display the insular gyri. Left hemisphere.

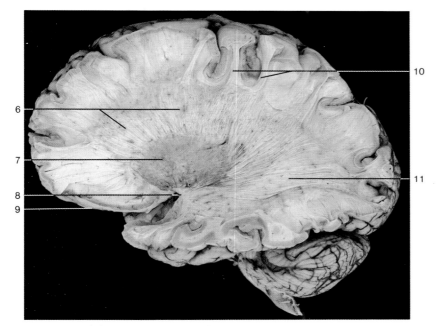

Dissection of the corona radiata, left hemisphere. Frontal pole on the left.

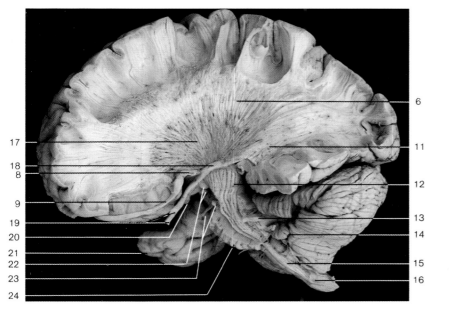

◁ **Corona radiata and internal capsule,** left hemisphere. Lentiform nucleus removed (frontal pole to the left).

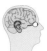

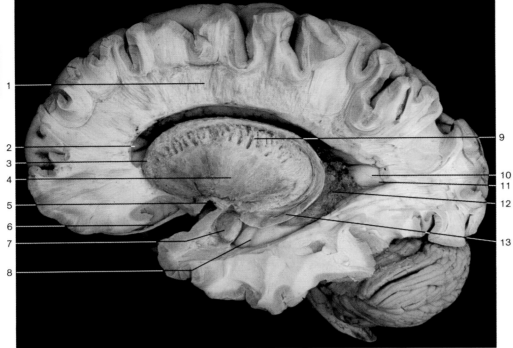

1   Corona radiata
2   Anterior horn of lateral ventricle
3   Head of caudate nucleus
4   Putamen
5   Anterior commissure
6   Olfactory tract
7   Amygdala
8   Hippocampal digitations
9   Internal capsule
10 Calcar avis
11 Posterior horn of lateral ventricle
12 Choroid plexus of lateral ventricle
13 Caudal extremity of caudate nucleus
14 Pulvinar of thalamus
15 Mamillary body
16 Optic tract
17 Anterior commissure
18 Fornix
19 Longitudinal stria
20 Dentate gyrus
21 Hippocampal fimbria
22 Pes hippocampi

Dissection of the subcortical nuclei and internal capsule, left hemisphere (lateral aspect). Frontal pole to the left. The lateral ventricle has been opened, and the insular gyri and claustrum have been removed, revealing the lentiform nucleus and the internal capsule.

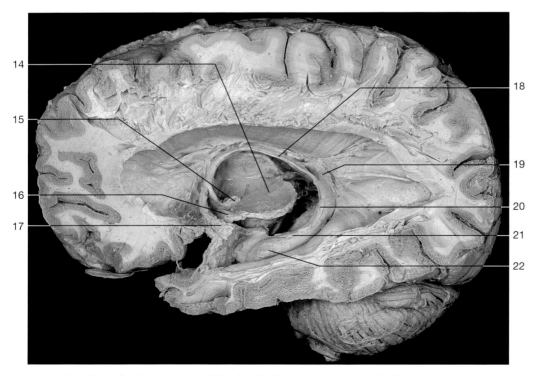

Dissection of the limbic system and the fornix (lateral aspect). Frontal pole to the left.

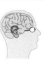

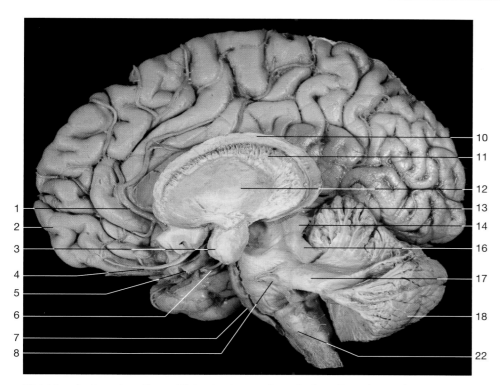

1   Anterior cerebral artery
2   Frontal lobe
3   Amygdala (amygdaloid body)
4   Olfactory tract
5   Internal carotid artery
6   Oculomotor nerve (n. III)
7   Basilar artery
8   Trigeminal nerve (n. V)
9   Hypoglossal nerve (n. XII)
10 Caudate nucleus
11 Internal capsule
12 Lentiform nucleus
13 Caudal extremity of caudate nucleus
14 Inferior colliculus of midbrain
15 Trochlear nerve (n. IV)
16 Superior cerebellar peduncle
17 Middle cerebellar peduncle
18 Cerebellum
19 Facial nerve (n. VII) and vestibulocochlear nerve (n. VIII)
20 Abducent nerve (n. VI)
21 Glossopharyngeal nerve (n. IX), vagus nerve (n. X), and accessory nerve (n. XI)
22 Inferior olive

Right hemisphere together with brain stem and cerebellum (lateral aspect).
The connections of the brain stem with the cerebellum are dissected. The amygdala of the left hemisphere is shown. The corpus callosum has been partly removed.

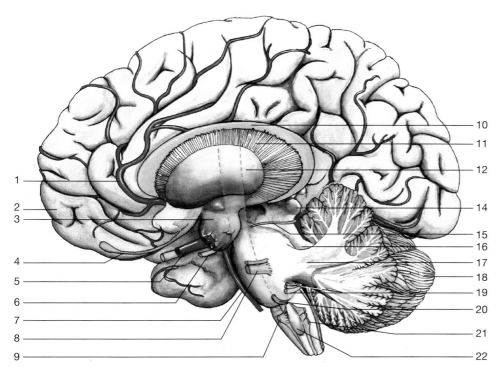

Schematic drawing of the dissected brain shown above (lateral aspect).
The course of the pyramidal tracts is indicated in red. Cranial nerves = yellow.

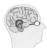

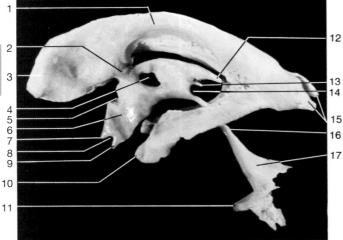

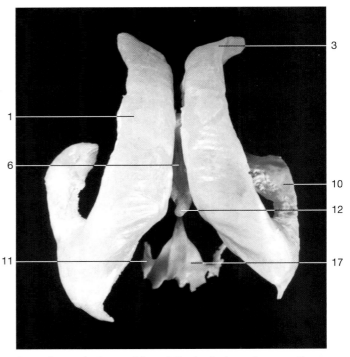

Cast of ventricular cavities of the brain (lateral aspect), frontal pole to the left.

Cast of ventricular cavities of the brain (superior aspect), frontal pole at top.

1   Central part of the lateral ventricle
2   Interventricular foramen of Monro
3   Anterior horn of the lateral ventricle
4   Site of interthalamic adhesion
5   Notch for anterior commissure
6   Third ventricle
7   Optic recess
8   Notch for optic chiasma
9   Infundibular recess
10 Inferior horn of lateral ventricle with indentation of amygdaloid body
11 Lateral recess and lateral aperture of Luschka
12 Suprapineal recess
13 Pineal recess
14 Notch for posterior commissure
15 Posterior horn of lateral ventricle
16 Cerebral aqueduct

17 Fourth ventricle
18 Median aperture of Magendie
19 Cerebellomedullary cistern
20 Superior sagittal sinus
21 Inferior sagittal sinus
22 Intervaginal space of optic nerve
23 Arachnoid granulations of Pacchioni
24 Straight sinus

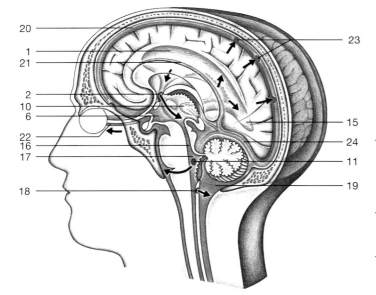

Position of ventricular cavities (schematic drawing). The direction of flow of cerebrospinal fluid is indicated by arrows. Green = right lateral ventricle; red = choroidal plexus with cerebrospinal fluid.

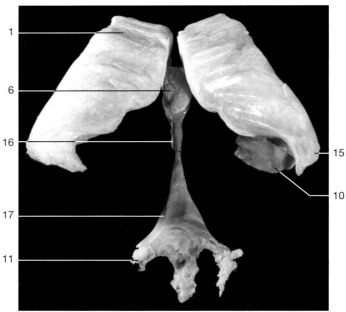

Cast of ventricular cavities of the brain (posterior aspect).

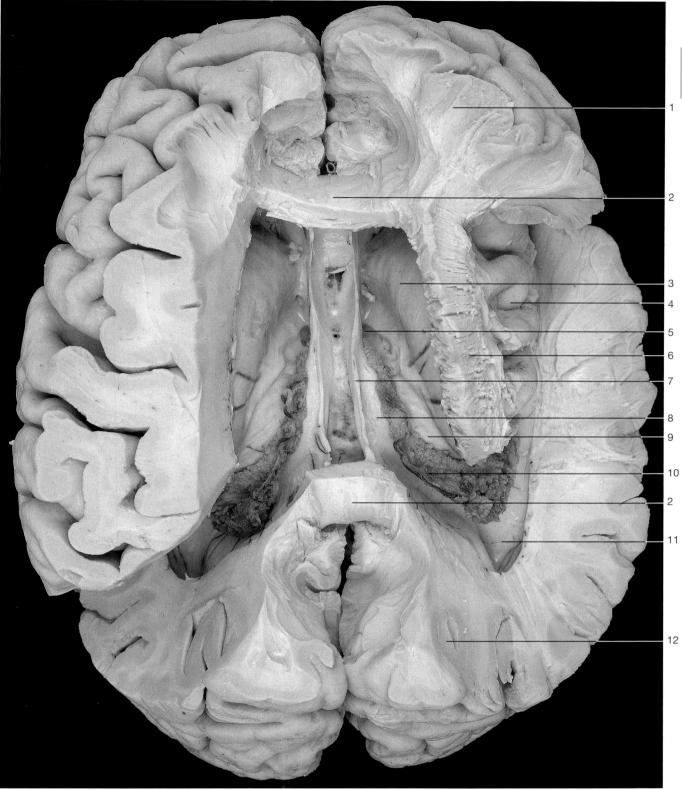

Dissection of the brain (superior view of the lateral ventricle and of the subcortical nuclei of the brain). Corpus callosum partly removed. Fornix and choroid plexus of the left lateral ventricle are shown.

1 Frontal lobe of brain
2 Corpus callosum
3 Caudate nucleus (head)
4 Insular cortex
5 Interventricular foramen
6 Internal capsule

7   Lateral longitudinal stria
8   Body of fornix
9   Thalamus
10 Choroid plexus
11 Lateral ventricle (occipital horn)
12 Occipital lobe of brain

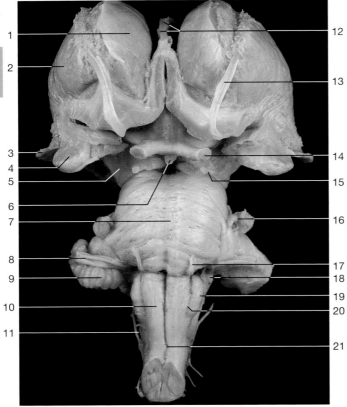

Brain stem (ventral aspect).

1   Caudate nucleus
2   Lentiform nucleus
3   Caudal extremity of caudate nucleus
4   Amygdaloid body
5   Cerebral peduncle
6   Infundibulum
7   Pons
8   Facial nerve (n. VII) and vestibulocochlear nerve (n. VIII)
9   Cerebellar flocculus
10   Medulla oblongata
11   Accessory nerve (n. XI)
12   Fornix and column of fornix
13   Olfactory tract
14   Optic nerve (n. II)
15   Oculomotor nerve (n. III)
16   Trigeminal nerve (n. V)
17   Abducent nerve (n. VI)
18   Glossopharyngeal nerve (n. IX) and vagus nerve (n. X)
19   Inferior olive
20   Hypoglossal nerve (n. XII)
21   Decussation of the pyramids
22   Thalamus
23   Epiphysis
24   Tectum of midbrain (superior and inferior colliculus)
25   Motor nucleus of trigeminal nerve (n. V)
26   Facial nucleus (n. VII)
27   Middle cerebellar peduncle
28   Visceral nucleus of glossopharyngeal and vagus nerves (n. IX and n. X), salivatory nucleus
29   Vestibular nucleus (n. VIII)
30   Ambiguus nucleus (n. IX, n. X, n. XI)
31   Spinal nucleus of accessory nerve (n. XI)
32   Motor nucleus of oculomotor nerve (n. III)
33   Trochlear nucleus and nerve (n. IV)
34   Sensory nucleus of trigeminal nerve (n. V)
35   Abducent nucleus (n. VI)
36   Hypoglossal nucleus (n. XII)

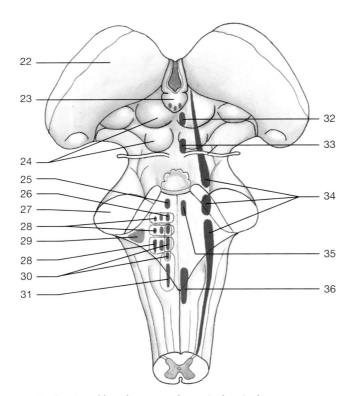

Brain stem (dorsal aspect, schematic drawing).
Location of cranial nerve nuclei.

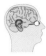

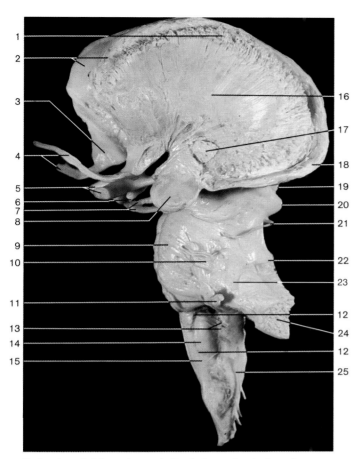

Brain stem (left lateral aspect). Cerebellar peduncles have been severed, cerebellum and cerebral cortex have been removed.

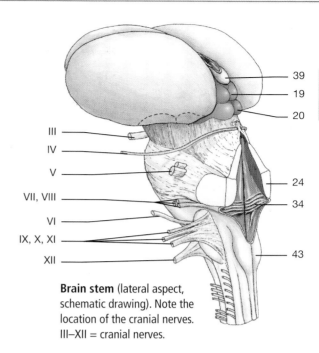

Brain stem (lateral aspect, schematic drawing). Note the location of the cranial nerves. III–XII = cranial nerves.

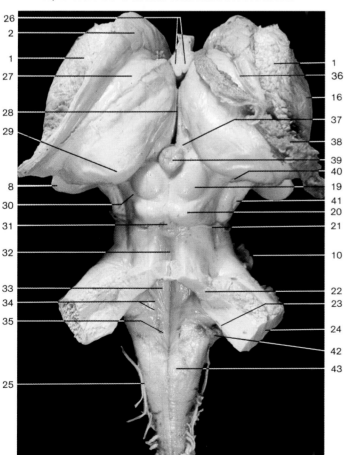

Brain stem (dorsal aspect). Cerebellum removed.

1   Internal capsule
2   Head of the caudate nucleus
3   Olfactory trigone
4   Olfactory tracts
5   Optic nerves (n. II)
6   Infundibulum
7   Oculomotor nerve (n. III)
8   Amygdaloid body
9   Pons
10 Trigeminal nerve (n. V)
11 Facial and vestibulocochlear nerves (n. VII, n. VIII)
12 Hypoglossal nerve (n. XII)
13 Glossopharyngeal and vagus nerves (n. IX, n. X)
14 Inferior olive
15 Medulla oblongata
16 Lentiform nucleus
17 Anterior commissure
18 Tail of caudate nucleus
19 Superior colliculus
20 Inferior colliculus
21 Trochlear nerve (n. IV)
22 Superior cerebellar peduncle
23 Inferior cerebellar peduncle
24 Middle cerebellar peduncle
25 Accessory nerve (n. XI)
26 Columns of fornix (divided)
27 Lamina affixa
28 Third ventricle
29 Pulvinar of thalamus
30 Inferior brachium
31 Frenulum veli
32 Superior medullary velum
33 Facial colliculus
34 Striae medullares and rhomboid fossa
35 Hypoglossal trigone
36 Stria terminalis and thalamostriate vein
37 Habenular trigone
38 Choroid plexus of lateral ventricle
39 Pineal body
40 Medial geniculate body
41 Cerebral peduncle
42 Choroid plexus of fourth ventricle
43 Clava

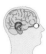

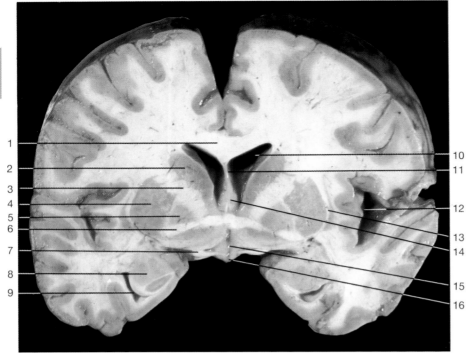

Coronal section through the brain at the level of the anterior commissure. Section 1.

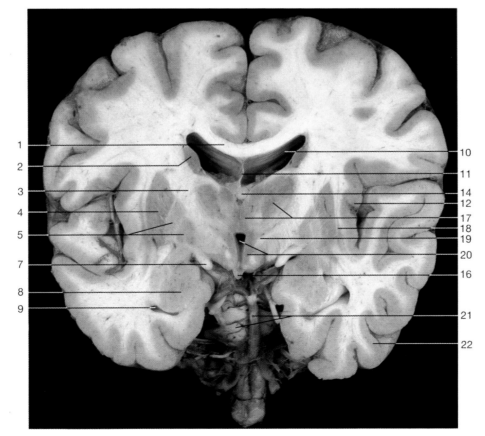

Coronal section through the brain at the level of the third ventricle and the interthalamic adhesion. Section 2.

1   Corpus callosum
2   Head of caudate nucleus
3   Internal capsule
4   Putamen
5   Globus pallidus
6   Anterior commissure
7   Optic tract
8   Amygdaloid body
9   Inferior horn of lateral ventricle
10   Lateral ventricle
11   Septum pellucidum
12   Lobus insularis (insula)
13   External capsule
14   Column of fornix
15   Optic recess
16   Infundibulum
17   Thalamus
18   Claustrum
19   Lenticular ansa
20   Third ventricle and hypothalamus
21   Basilar artery and pons
22   Cortex of temporal lobe
23   Inferior colliculus
24   Superior colliculus
25   Cerebral aqueduct
26   Red nucleus
27   Substantia nigra
28   Cerebral peduncle
29   Trochlear nerve (n. IV)
30   Gray matter
31   Nucleus of oculomotor nerve
32   Fibers of oculomotor nerve (n. III)
33   Vermis of cerebellum
34   Fourth ventricle
35   Reticular formation
36   Pons and transverse pontine fibers
37   Emboliform nucleus
38   Dentate nucleus
39   Middle cerebellar peduncle
40   Choroid plexus
41   Hypoglossal nucleus at rhomboid fossa
42   Medial longitudinal fasciculus
43   Trigeminal nerve (n. V.)
44   Inferior olivary nucleus
45   Corticospinal fibers and arcuate fibers
46   Fourth ventricle with choroid plexus
47   Vestibular nuclei
48   Nucleus and tractus solitarius
49   Inferior cerebellar peduncle
      (restiform body)
50   Reticular formation
51   Medial lemniscus
52   Cuneate nucleus of Burdach
53   Central canal
54   Pyramidal tract
55   Flocculus of cerebellum
56   Cerebellar hemisphere with pia mater
57   "Arbor vitae" of cerebellum
58   Nucleus gracilis of Goll
59   Lateral recess of choroid plexus
      of fourth ventricle
60   Posterior inferior cerebellar artery
61   Choroid plexus of lateral ventricle

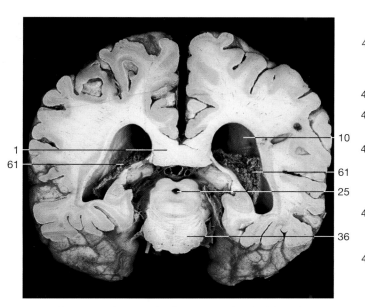

Coronal section through the brain at the level of the inferior colliculus (posterior aspect). Section 3.

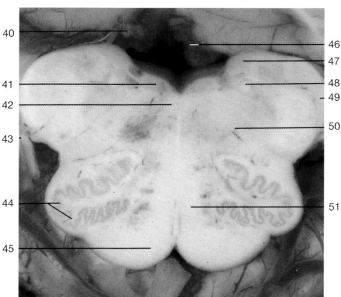

Cross section of the rhombencephalon at the level of the olive (inferior aspect). Section 6.

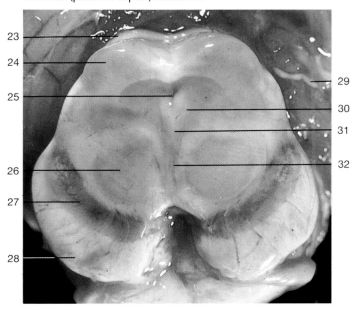

Cross section of the midbrain (mesencephalon) at the level of the superior colliculus (superior aspect). Section 4.

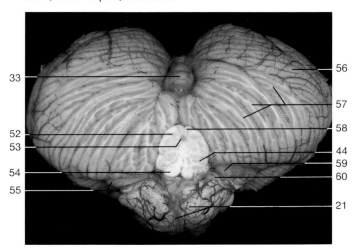

Cross section through medulla oblongata and cerebellum (inferior aspect). Section 7.

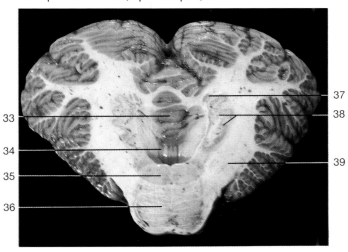

Cross section through the rhombencephalon at the level of the pons (inferior aspect). Section 5.

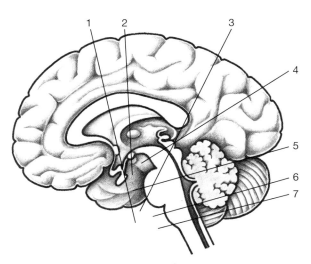

Right half of the brain. Levels of the sections are indicated.

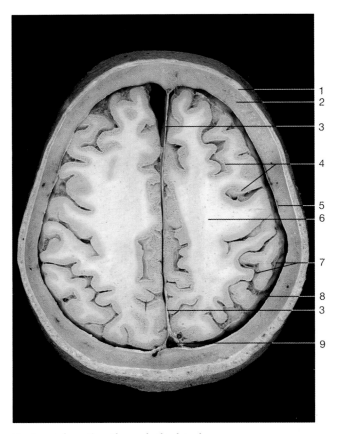

Horizontal section through the head.
Section 1.

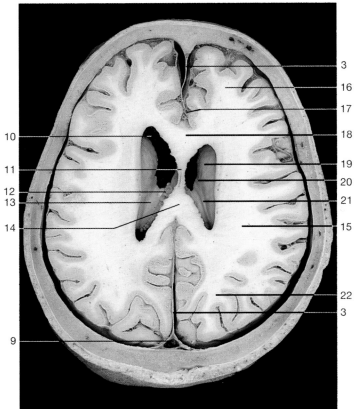

Horizontal section through the head.
Section 2.

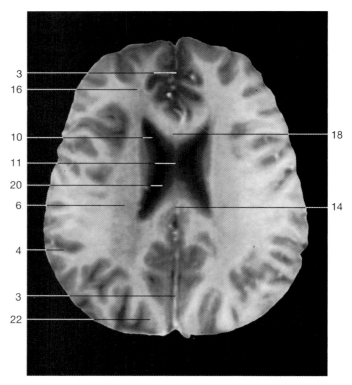

MRI scan of the human head at the level of section 2.

1 Skin of scalp
2 Calvaria (diploe of the skull)
3 Falx cerebri
4 Gray matter of brain (cortex)
5 Dura mater
6 White matter of brain
7 Arachnoid and pia mater with vessels
8 Subdural space (slightly expanded due to shrinkage of the brain)
9 Superior sagittal sinus
10 Anterior horn of lateral ventricle
11 Septum pellucidum
12 Choroid plexus
13 Thalamus
14 Splenium of corpus callosum
15 Parietal lobe
16 Frontal lobe
17 Anterior cerebral artery
18 Genu of corpus callosum
19 Caudate nucleus
20 Central part of lateral ventricle
21 Stria terminalis
22 Occipital lobe

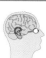

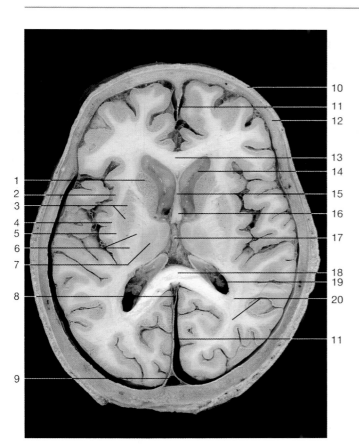

1   Caudate nucleus
2   Lobus insularis (insula)
3   Lentiform nucleus
4   Claustrum
5   External capsule
6   Internal capsule
7   Thalamus
8   Inferior sagittal sinus
9   Superior sagittal sinus
10 Skin of scalp
11 Falx cerebri
12 Calvaria (diploe of skull)
13 Genu of corpus callosum
14 Anterior horn of lateral ventricle
15 Septum pellucidum
16 Column of fornix
17 Choroid plexus of third ventricle
18 Splenium of corpus callosum
19 Entrance to inferior horn of lateral ventricle with
     choroid plexus
20 Optic radiation
21 Third ventricle

Horizontal section through the head at the level of third ventricle of internal capsule and neighboring nuclei.
Section 3.

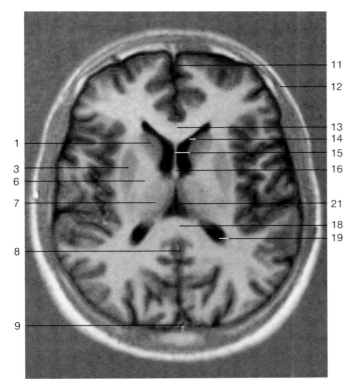

MRI scan at the corresponding level to the above figure.
Section 3.

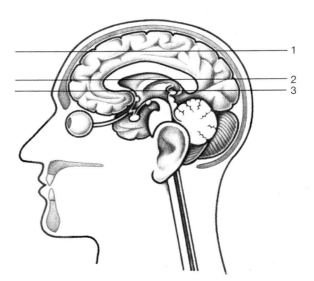

Sagittal section through the head.
Levels of the horizontal sections are indicated.

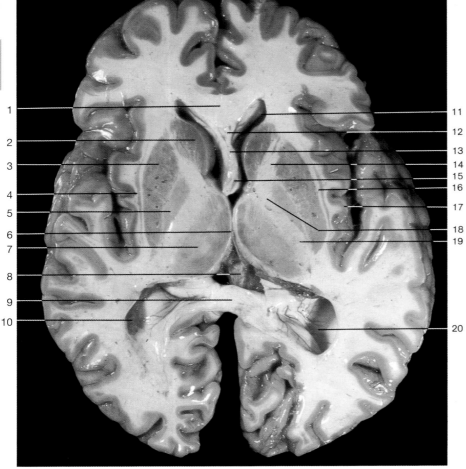

1   Genu of corpus callosum
2   Head of caudate nucleus
3   Putamen
4   Claustrum
5   Globus pallidus
6   Third ventricle
7   Thalamus
8   Pineal body
9   Splenium of corpus callosum
10 Choroid plexus of the lateral ventricle
11 Anterior horn of lateral ventricle
12 Cavity of septum pellucidum
13 Septum pellucidum
14 Anterior limb of internal capsule
15 Column of fornix
16 External capsule
17 Lobus insularis (insula)
18 Genu of internal capsule
19 Posterior limb of internal capsule
20 Posterior horn of lateral ventricle
21 Anterior commissure
22 Optic radiation
23 Falx cerebri
24 Maxillary sinus
25 Position of auditory tube
26 Tympanic cavity
27 External acoustic meatus
28 Medulla oblongata
29 Fourth ventricle
30 Cerebellum (left hemisphere)
31 Temporomandibular joint
32 Tympanic membrane
33 Base of cochlea
34 Mastoid air cells
35 Sigmoid sinus
36 Vermis of cerebellum
37 Intermediate mass

Horizontal section through the brain, showing the subcortical nuclei and internal capsule. Section 1.

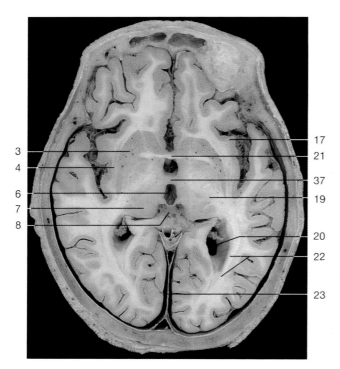

Horizontal section through the head. Section 2.

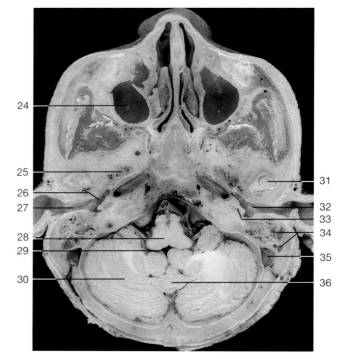

Horizontal section through the head. Section 4.

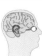

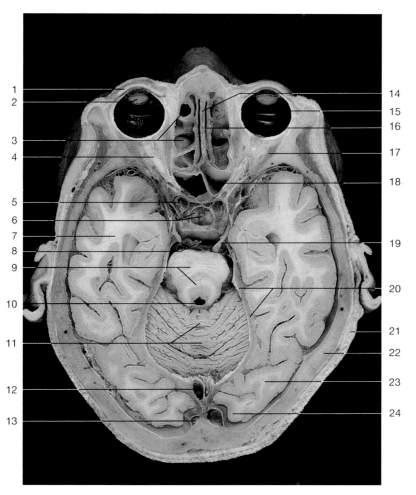

1   Upper lid (tarsal plate)
2   Lens
3   Ethmoidal sinus
4   Optic nerve (n. II)
5   Internal carotid artery
6   Infundibulum and pituitary gland
7   Temporal lobe
8   Basilar artery
9   Pons (cross section of brain stem)
10 Cerebral aqueduct (beginning of fourth ventricle)
11 Vermis of cerebellum
12 Straight sinus
13 Transverse sinus
14 Nasal septum
15 Eyeball (sclera)
16 Nasal cavity
17 Lateral rectus muscle
18 Sphenoidal sinus
19 Oculomotor nerve (n. III)
20 Tentorium of cerebellum
21 Skin of scalp
22 Calvaria
23 Occipital lobe
24 Striate cortex (visual cortex)

Horizontal section through the head. Section 3.

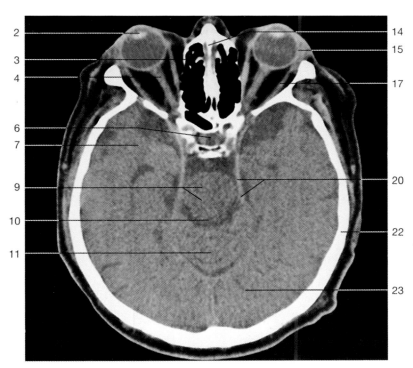

Horizontal section through the head. (CT scan.) Section 3.

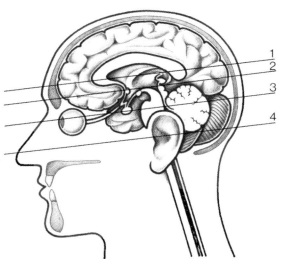

Sagittal section through the head.
Levels of the horizontal sections are indicated.

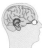

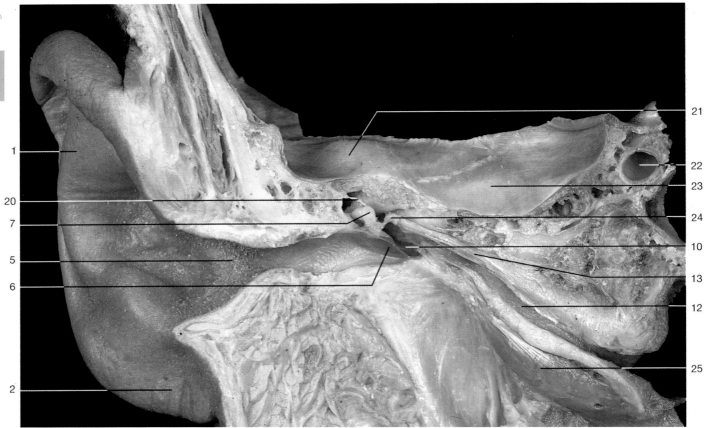

Longitudinal section through the right temporal bone. The outer and middle ear and auditory ossicles and tube are shown (anterior aspect).

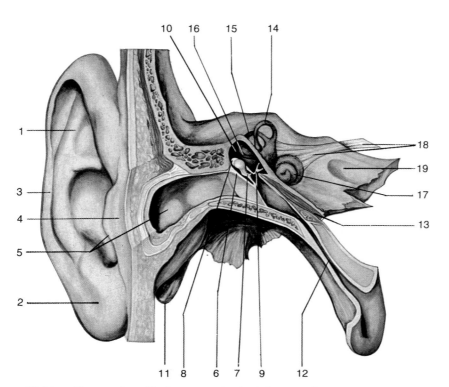

Right auditory and vestibular apparatus (anterior aspect). (Schematic drawing.)

Outer ear
1 Auricle
2 Lobule of auricle
3 Helix
4 Tragus
5 External acoustic meatus

Middle ear
6 Tympanic membrane
7 Malleus
8 Incus
9 Stapes
10 Tympanic cavity
11 Mastoid process
12 Auditory tube
13 Tensor tympani muscle

Inner ear
14 Anterior semicircular duct
15 Posterior semicircular duct
16 Lateral semicircular duct
17 Cochlea
18 Vestibulocochlear nerve
19 Petrous part of the temporal bone

Additional structures
20 Superior ligament of malleus
21 Arcuate eminence
22 Internal carotid artery
23 Anterior surface of pyramid with dura mater
24 Stapes
25 Levator veli palatini muscle

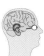

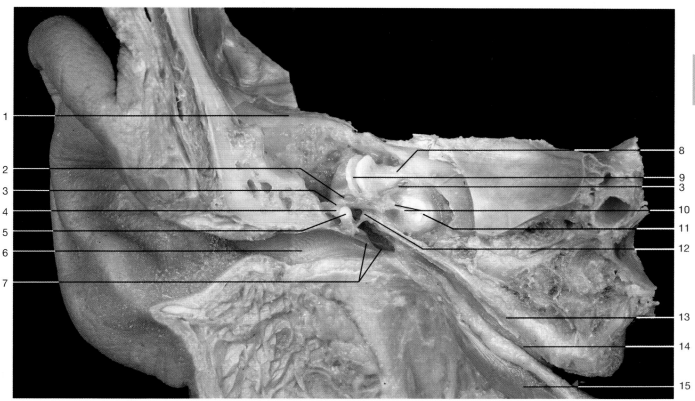

Longitudinal section through the right outer, middle, and inner ear. The cochlea and semicircular canals have been further dissected (anterior aspect).

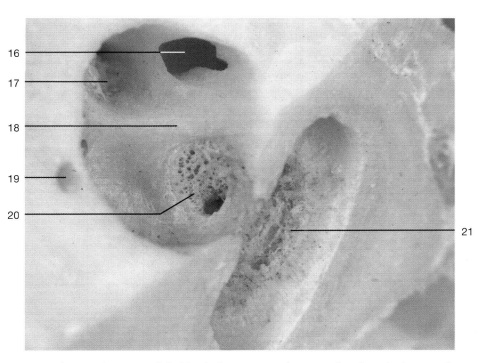

Internal acoustic meatus, left side. The bone was partly removed to show the bottom of the meatus.

1 Roof of tympanic cavity
2 Lateral osseous semicircular canal
3 Facial nerve
4 Incus
5 Malleus
6 External acoustic meatus
7 Tympanic cavity and tympanic membrane
8 Vestibulocochlear nerve
9 Anterior osseous semicircular canal
10 Geniculate ganglion and greater petrosal nerve
11 Cochlea
12 Stapes
13 Tensor tympani muscle
14 Auditory tube
15 Levator veli palatini muscle
16 Area of facial nerve
17 Superior vestibular area
18 Transverse crest
19 Foramen singulare
20 Foraminous spiral tract (outlet of cochlear part of vestibulocochlear nerve)
21 Base of cochlea

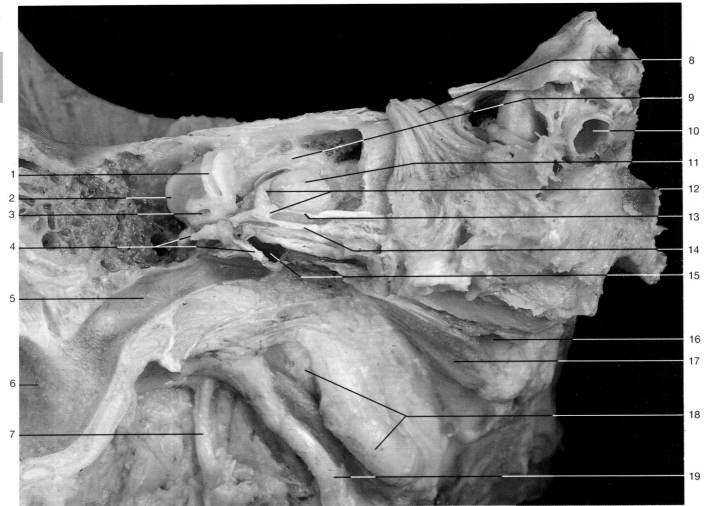

Longitudinal section through the outer, middle, and inner ear. Deeper dissection to display facial nerve and lesser and greater petrosal nerves (anterior aspect).

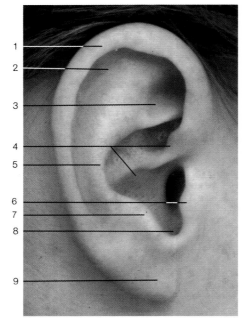

Right auricle (lateral aspect).

◁
1 Helix
2 Scaphoid fossa
3 Triangular fossa
4 Concha
5 Antihelix
6 Tragus
7 Antitragus
8 Intertragic notch
9 Lobule

△
1 Anterior osseous semicircular canal (opened)
2 Posterior osseous semicircular canal
3 Lateral osseous semicircular canal (opened)
4 Facial nerve and chorda tympani
5 External acoustic meatus
6 Auricle
7 Facial nerve
8 Trigeminal nerve
9 Bony base of internal acoustic meatus
10 Internal carotid artery within cavernous sinus
11 Cochlea
12 Facial nerve with geniculate ganglion
13 Greater petrosal nerve
14 Lesser petrosal nerve
15 Tympanic cavity
16 Auditory tube
17 Levator veli palatini muscle
18 Internal carotid artery and internal jugular vein
19 Styloid process

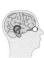

1 Anterior semicircular canal (red)
2 Posterior semicircular canal (yellow)
3 Lateral or horizontal semicircular canal (green)
4 Fenestra vestibuli
5 Fenestra cochleae
6 Tympanic cavity
7 Mastoid process
8 Petrotympanic fissure (red probe: chorda tympani)
9 Lateral pterygoid plate
10 Mastoid air cells
11 Facial canal (blue)
12 Foramen ovale
13 Carotid canal (red)
14 Tympanic ring
15 Petromastoid part of temporal bone
16 Squamous part of temporal bone
17 Squamomastoid suture
18 Zygomatic process of temporal bone
19 Incisure of tympanic ring
20 Promontory
21 Apex of cochlea (cupula)
22 Spiral canal of cochlea at base of cochlea
23 Epitympanic recess
24 Auditory ossicles and tympanic cavity
25 Hypotympanic recess
26 Canaliculus chordae tympani (green probe)
27 Mastoid process
28 Canaliculus for stapedius nerve (red)
29 Cochlea
30 Canaliculus mastoideus (red probe)

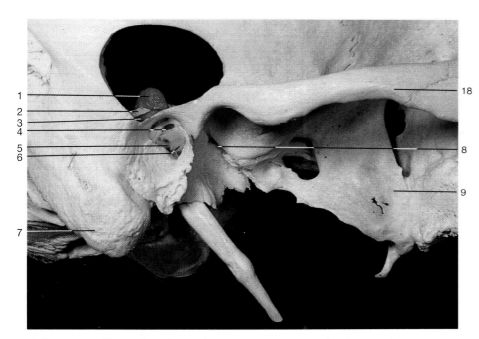

Right temporal bone (lateral aspect). Petrosquamous portion has been partly removed to display the semicircular canals.

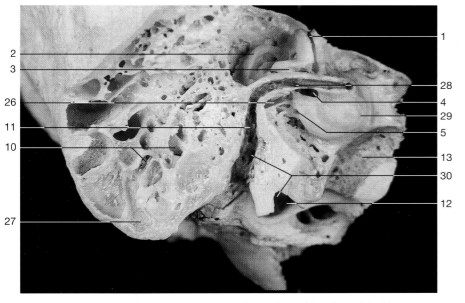

Right temporal bone (lateral aspect). Mastoid air cells and facial canal had been opened. The three semicircular canals were dissected.

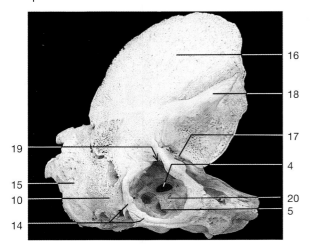

Right temporal bone of the newborn (lateral aspect).

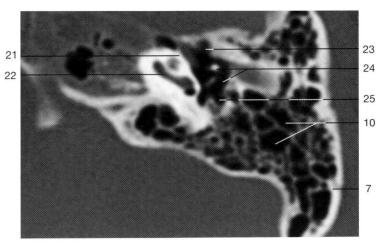

Frontal section through petrous part. (CT scan.)

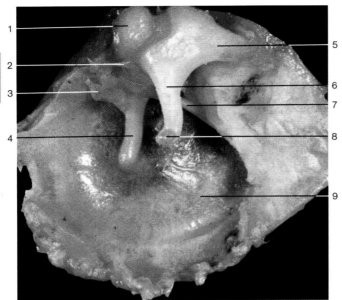

1   Head of malleus
2   Anterior ligament of malleus
3   Tendon of tensor tympani muscle
4   Handle of malleus
5   Short crus of incus
6   Long crus of incus
7   Chorda tympani
8   Lenticular process
9   Tympanic membrane

Tympanic membrane with malleus and incus (internal aspect; right side).

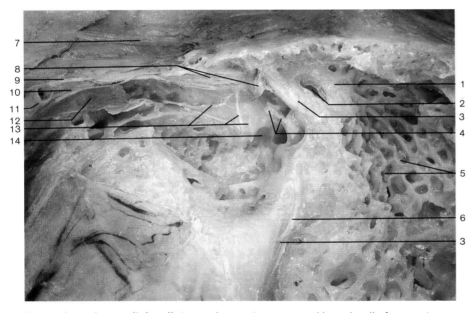

1   Tympanic antrum
2   Lateral semicircular canal (opened)
3   Facial canal
4   Stapes with tendon of stapedius
5   Mastoid air cells
6   Chorda tympani (intracranial part)
7   Greater petrosal nerve
8   Tensor tympani muscle (processus cochleariformis)
9   Lesser petrosal nerve
10 Anterior tympanic artery
11 Middle meningeal artery
12 Auditory tube
13 Promontory with tympanic plexus
14 Fenestra cochleae

Tympanic cavity, medial wall. External acoustic meatus and lateral wall of tympanic cavity together with incus. Malleus and tympanic membrane have been removed; mastoid air cells are opened (left side).

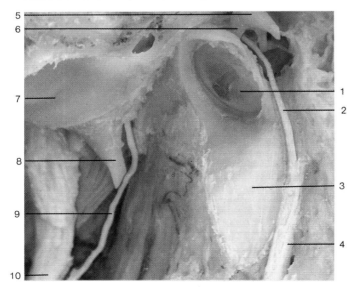

1   Tympanic membrane
2   Chorda tympani (intracranial part)
3   Floor of the external acoustic meatus
4   Facial nerve and facial canal
5   Incus
6   Head of malleus
7   Mandibular fossa
8   Spine of sphenoid
9   Chorda tympani (extracranial part)
10 Styloid process

Tympanic membrane (lateral aspect). External acoustic meatus and facial canal have been opened to expose the chorda tympani (magn. ~1.5×) (left side).

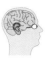

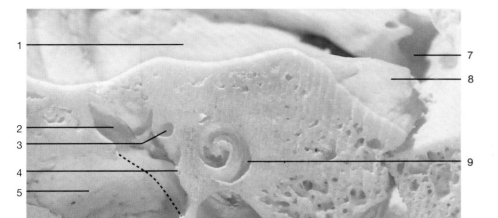

Frontal section through the petrous part of the left temporal bone at the level of the cochlea (posterior aspect). Position of tympanic membrane indicated by dotted line.

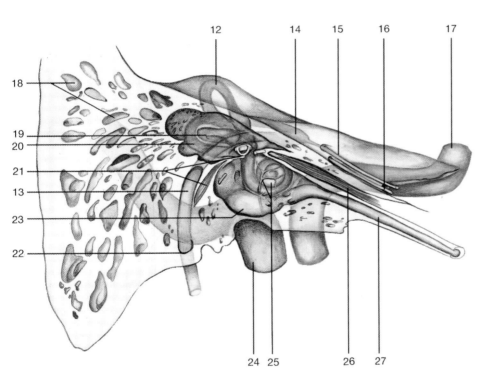

Medial wall of tympanic cavity and its relation to neighboring structures of the inner ear, facial nerve, and blood vessels (schematic drawing). Frontal section through the right temporal bone (anterior aspect).

1 Anterior surface of the pyramid	10 Carotid canal	20 Posterior semicircular duct
2 Mastoid antrum	11 Pterygoid process	21 Stapes with stapedius muscle
3 Lateral semicircular canal	12 Anterior semicircular duct	22 Stylomastoid foramen
4 Cochleariform process	13 Facial nerve	23 Inferior recess of tympanic cavity
5 External acoustic meatus	14 Geniculate ganglion	(hypotympanon)
6 Jugular fossa	15 Greater petrosal nerve	24 Internal jugular vein
7 Foramen lacerum	16 Lesser petrosal nerve	25 Promontory with tympanic plexus
8 Apex of petrous part	17 Internal carotid artery	(position of cochlea)
9 Position of cochlea (modiolus with	18 Mastoid air cells	26 Tensor muscle of tympanum
crista spiralis ossea)	19 Lateral semicircular duct	27 Auditory tube

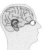

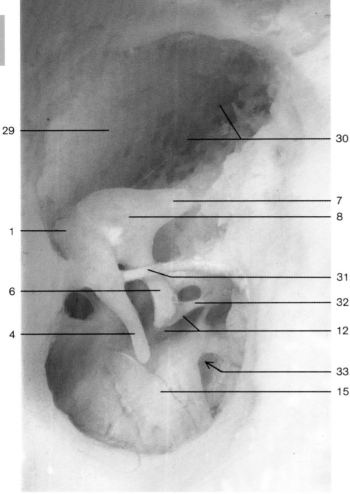

Tympanic cavity with malleus, incus, and stapes, left side (lateral aspect). Tympanic membrane removed, mastoid antrum opened.

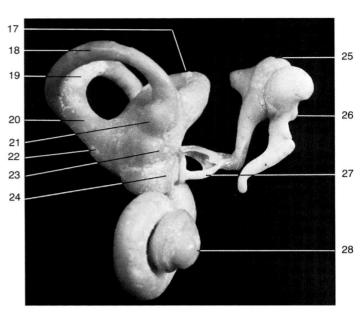

Chain of auditory ossicles in connection with the inner ear, left side (antero-lateral aspect).

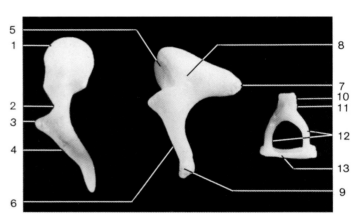

Auditory ossicles (isolated).

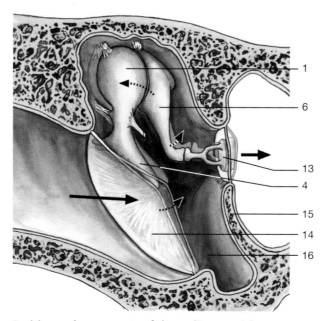

Position and movements of the auditory ossicles (schematic drawing).

Malleus
1 Head
2 Neck
3 Lateral process
4 Handle

Incus
5 Articular facet for malleus
6 Long crus
7 Short crus
8 Body
9 Lenticular process

Stapes
10 Head
11 Neck
12 Anterior and posterior crura
13 Base

Walls of tympanic cavity
14 Tympanic membrane
15 Promontory
16 Hypotympanic recess of tympanic cavity

Internal ear (labyrinth)
17 Lateral semicircular duct
18 Anterior semicircular duct
19 Posterior semicircular duct
20 Common crus
21 Ampulla
22 Beginning of endolymphatic duct
23 Utricular prominence
24 Saccular prominence
25 Incus
26 Malleus
27 Stapes
28 Cochlea

Tympanic cavity
29 Epitympanic recess
30 Mastoid antrum
31 Chorda tympani
32 Tendon of stapedius muscle
33 Round window (fenestra cochleae)

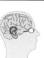

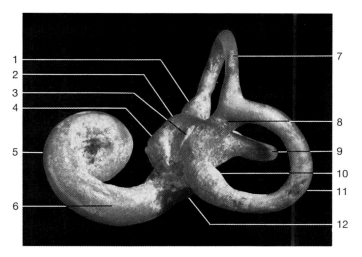

Cast of the right labyrinth (postero-medial aspect).

1   Ampulla (anterior
    semicircular canal)
2   Elliptical recess
3   Aqueduct of the vestibule
4   Spherical recess
5   Cochlea
6   Base of cochlea
7   Anterior semicircular canal
8   Crus commune or common
    limb
9   Lateral semicircular canal
10 Posterior bony ampulla
11 Posterior semicircular canal
    (posterior canal)
12 Fenestra cochleae
13 Bony ampulla
14 Fenestra vestibuli
15 Cupula of cochlea
16 External acoustic meatus
17 Mastoid air cells
18 Tympanic cavity and
    fenestra cochleae (probe)
19 External acoustic meatus
20 Facial canal
21 Base of cochlea and
    musculotubal canal
22 Malleus and incus
23 Stapes
24 Tympanic membrane
25 Tympanic cavity
26 Aqueduct of cochlea
27 Endolymphatic sac
28 Endolymphatic duct
29 Macula of utricle
30 Macula of saccule

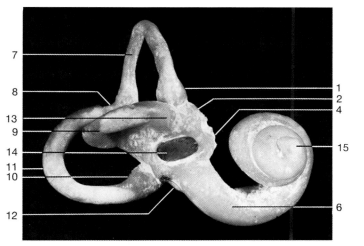

Cast of the right labyrinth (lateral aspect).

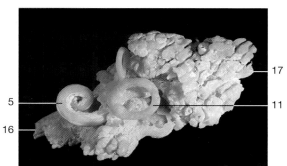

Cast of the labyrinth and mastoid cells.
Life size (posterior aspect).

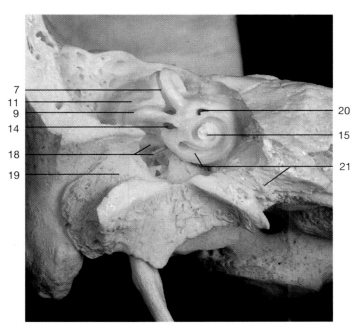

Dissection of bony labyrinth in situ. Semicircular canals and
cochlear duct opened.

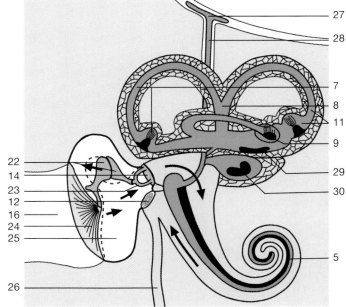

Auditory and vestibular apparatus. Arrows = direction of sound
waves; blue = perilymphatic ducts (schematic drawing; from
Lütjen-Drecoll, Rohen, Innenansichten des menschlichen Körpers,
2010).

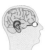

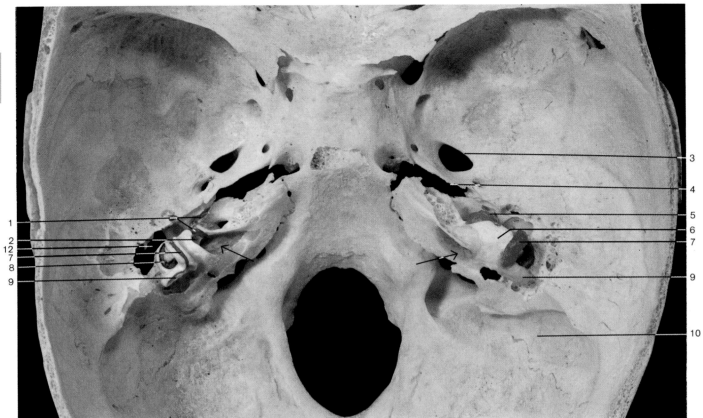

Bony labyrinth, petrous part of the temporal bone (from above). At left: semicircular canals opened; at right: closed. Arrows: internal acoustic meatus.

1 Facial canal and semicanal of auditory tube
2 Superior vestibular area
3 Foramen ovale
4 Foramen lacerum
5 Cochlea
6 Vestibule
7 Anterior semicircular canal
8 Lateral semicircular canal

9 Posterior semicircular canal
10 Groove for sigmoid sinus
11 Sigmoid sinus
12 Tympanic cavity
13 Auditory tube
14 Mastoid air cells
15 Facial and vestibulocochlear nerves
16 Temporal fossa

17 Fenestra vestibuli
18 Promontory
19 Zygomatic process
20 Fenestra cochleae
21 Mastoid process

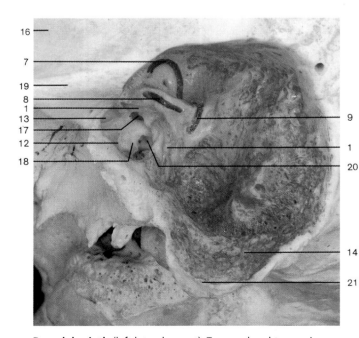

Bony labyrinth (left lateral aspect). Temporal and tympanic bone partly removed, semicircular canals opened.

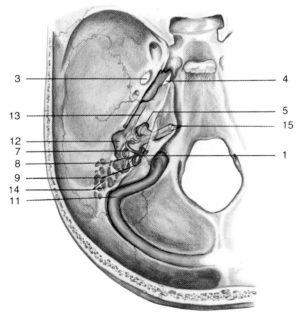

Internal ear. Diagram showing the position of the membranous labyrinth and the tympanic cavity.

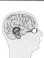

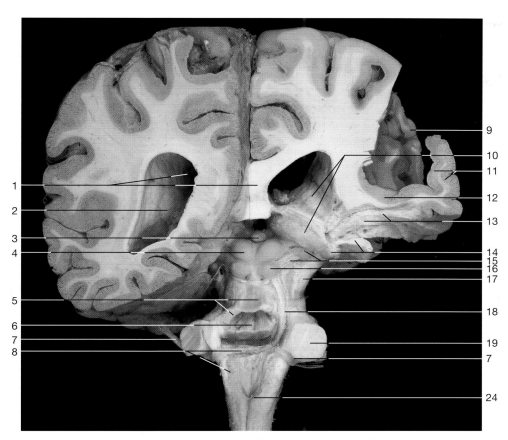

1   Left lateral ventricle and corpus callosum
2   Thalamus
3   Pineal gland (epiphysis)
4   Superior colliculus
5   Superior medullary velum and superior cerebellar peduncle
6   Rhomboid fossa
7   Vestibulocochlear nerve (n. VIII)
8   Dorsal acoustic striae and inferior cerebellar peduncle
9   Insular lobe
10 Caudate nucleus and thalamus
11 Temporal lobe (superior temporal gyrus) (area of acoustic centers)
12 Transverse temporal gyri of Heschl (area of primary acoustic centers)
13 Acoustic radiation of internal capsule
14 Lateral geniculate body and optic radiation (cut)
15 Medial geniculate body and brachium of inferior colliculus
16 Inferior colliculus
17 Cerebral peduncle
18 Lateral lemniscus
19 Middle cerebellar peduncle
20 Dorsal (posterior) cochlear nucleus
21 Ventral (anterior) cochlear nucleus
22 Inferior olive with olivo-cochlear tract of Rasmussen (red)
23 Ganglion spirale
24 Obex
25 Frontal lobe
26 Temporal lobe
27 Middle temporal gyrus (area of tertiary acoustic centers)
28 Trapezoid body

Dissection of the brain stem showing the auditory pathway. Cerebellum and posterior part of the two hemispheres have been removed (dorsal aspect).

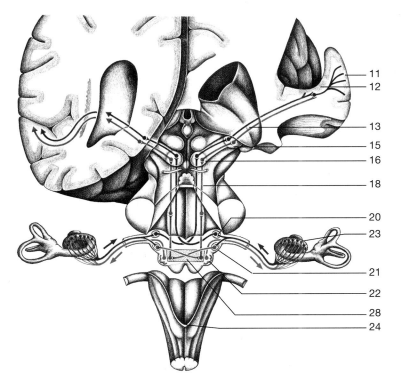

Auditory pathway (schematic drawing, compare with figure above). Red = descending (efferent) pathway (olivocochlear tract of Rasmussen); green and blue = ascending (afferent) pathways.

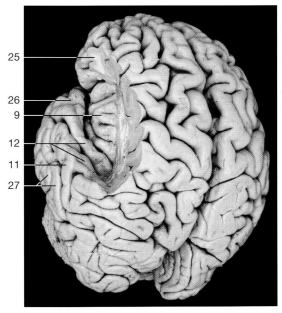

Auditory areas in the left hemisphere (supero-lateral aspect). Parts of the frontal and parietal lobes have been removed.

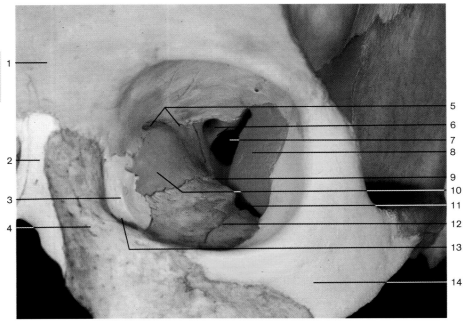

1 Frontal bone
2 Nasal bone
3 Lacrimal bone
4 Maxilla (frontal process)
5 Ethmoidal foramina
6 Lesser wing of sphenoid bone and optic canal
7 Superior orbital fissure
8 Greater wing of sphenoid bone
9 Orbital process of palatine bone
10 Orbital plate of ethmoid bone
11 Inferior orbital fissure
12 Infra-orbital sulcus
13 Nasolacrimal canal
14 Zygomatic bone
15 Frontal sinus
16 Superior rectus muscle
17 Orbital fatty tissue
18 Optic nerve
19 Sclera
20 Inferior rectus muscle
21 Periorbita and maxilla
22 Maxillary sinus
23 Levator palpebrae superioris muscle
24 Superior conjunctival fornix
25 Superior tarsal plate
26 Inferior tarsal plate
27 Inferior conjunctival fornix
28 Inferior oblique muscle
29 Lateral rectus muscle
30 Medial rectus muscle
31 Superior oblique muscle
32 Nasal septum
33 Middle nasal concha
34 Inferior nasal concha
35 Tenon's space
36 Ophthalmic artery
37 Cornea
38 Lens

Bones of the left orbit (indicated by different colors).

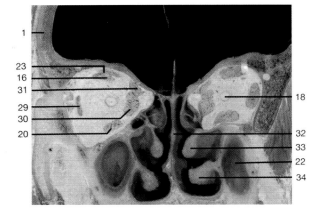

Frontal section through the posterior part of the orbit.

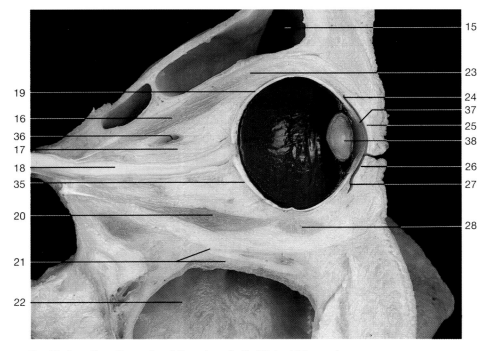

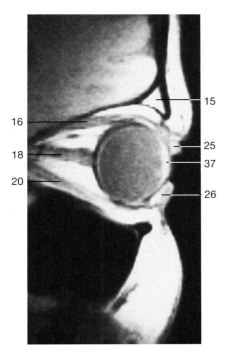

Sagittal section through orbit and eyeball. (Right: MRI scan.)

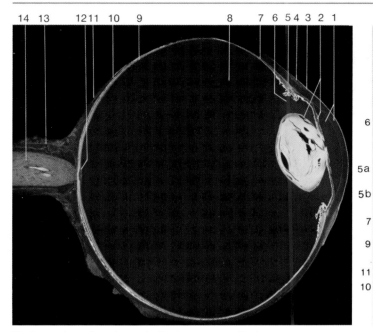

Horizontal section through the human eye (2×).

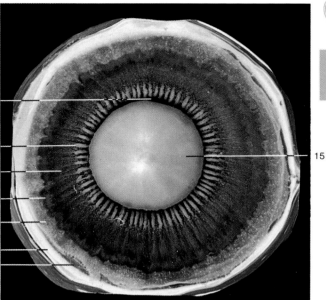

Anterior segment of the eyeball (posterior aspect). The opacity of the lens is an artifact.

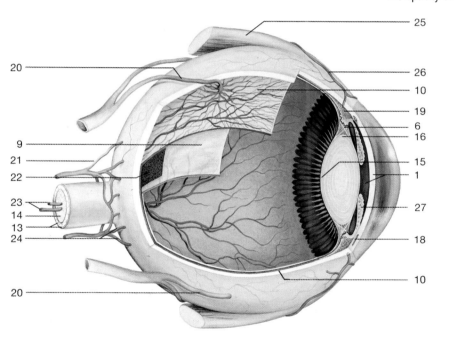

◁

Organization of the eyeball.
Demonstration of vascular tunic of bulb (schematic drawing).

1 Cornea and anterior chamber
2 Iris and lens
3 Transitional zone between corneal and conjunctival epithelium
4 Conjunctiva of the eyeball
5 Ciliary body
   a Ciliary processes (pars plicata)
   b Ciliary ring (pars plana)
6 Zonular fibers
7 Ora serrata
8 Vitreous body
9 Retina
10 Choroid
11 Sclera
12 Optic disc
13 Dura mater and subarachnoid space
14 Optic nerve (n. II)
15 Lens (posterior pole)
16 Equator of lens
17 Lens (anterior pole)
18 Canal of Schlemm
19 Ciliary muscle
20 Vena vorticosa
21 Long posterior ciliary artery
22 Retinal pigmented epithelium
23 Central retinal artery and vein
24 Short posterior ciliary arteries
25 External ocular muscle
26 Anterior ciliary artery
27 Iris

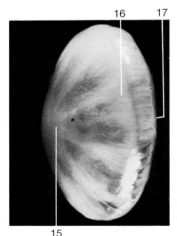

Lens (equatorial aspect), anterior pole to the right.

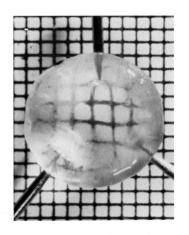

Lens (frontal aspect). Note the magnification effect.

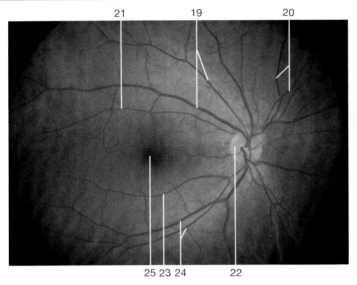

Fundus of a normal right eye (courtesy of Prof. Okamura, Univ. Eye Dept., Kumamoto, Japan). Notice, the arteries are smaller and lighter than the veins.

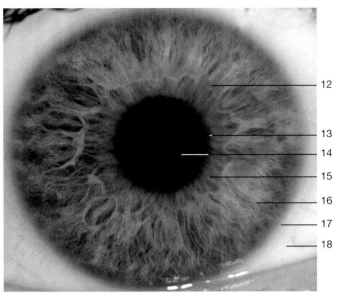

Anterior segment of the human eye (courtesy of Prof. Naumann, Eye Dept., University of Erlangen, Germany). Note the colored iris (16) and the location of the lens behind the iris (14).

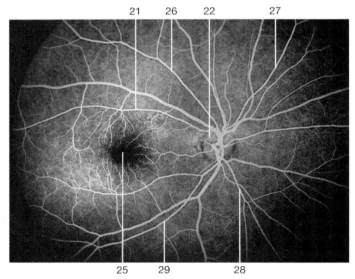

Fluorescent angiography of the right eye; retinal vessels. The same eye as above (courtesy of Prof. Okamura, Univ. Eye Dept., Kumamoto, Japan).

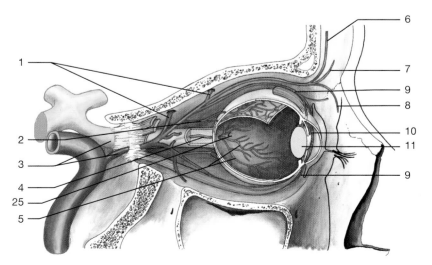

Diagram of the ophthalmic artery and its branches.

1   Posterior and anterior ethmoidal arteries
2   Long and short posterior ciliary arteries
3   Optic nerve and ophthalmic artery
4   Central retinal artery
5   Retinal arteries
6   Supratrochlear artery
7   Supra-orbital artery
8   Dorsal nasal artery
9   Anterior ciliary artery
10   Iridial arteries
11   Lens
12   Iridial fold
13   Pupillary margin of iris
14   Anterior pole of lens
15   Lesser circle of iris
16   Greater circle of iris
17   Margin of cornea or limbus
18   Sclera
19   Superior temporal artery and vein of retina
20   Superior nasal artery and vein of retina
21   Superior macular artery
22   Optic disc
23   Inferior macular artery
24   Inferior temporal artery and vein
25   Fovea centralis and macula lutea
26   Superior temporal artery ⎫
27   Superior nasal artery   ⎬ of retina
28   Inferior nasal artery   ⎪
29   Inferior temporal artery ⎭

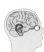

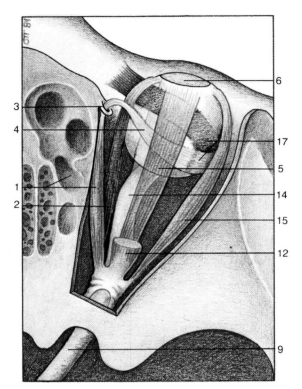

Schematic diagram of the extra-ocular muscles. Right orbit (from above). Levator palpebrae superioris muscle has been severed.

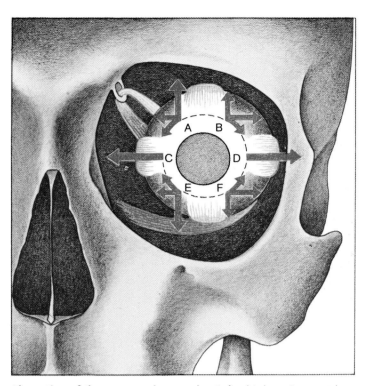

The action of the extra-ocular muscles. Left orbit (anterior aspect).

A = Superior rectus muscle
B = Inferior oblique muscle
C = Medial rectus muscle

D = Lateral rectus muscle
E = Inferior rectus muscle
F = Superior oblique muscle

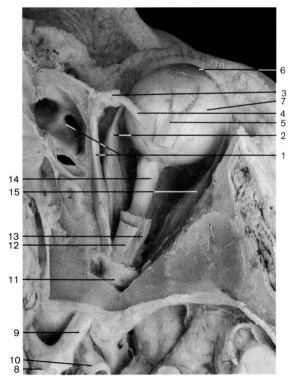

Right orbit with eyeball and extra-ocular muscles (from above). The roof of the orbit has been removed, the superior rectus muscle and the levator palpebrae superioris muscle have been severed.

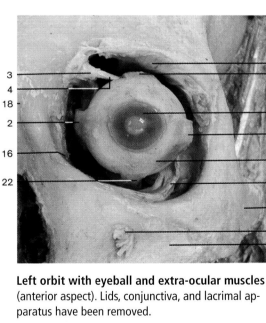

Left orbit with eyeball and extra-ocular muscles (anterior aspect). Lids, conjunctiva, and lacrimal apparatus have been removed.

1 Superior oblique muscle and ethmoid air cells
2 Medial rectus muscle
3 Trochlea
4 Tendon of superior oblique muscle
5 Superior rectus muscle
6 Cornea
7 Eyeball
8 Optic chiasma
9 Optic nerve (intracranial part)
10 Internal carotid artery
11 Common annular tendon
12 Levator palpebrae superioris muscle
13 Superior rectus muscle
14 Optic nerve (extracranial part)
15 Lateral rectus muscle
16 Nasolacrimal duct
17 Inferior oblique muscle
18 Nasal bone
19 Maxilla
20 Infra-orbital foramen and nerves
21 Zygomatic bone
22 Inferior rectus muscle

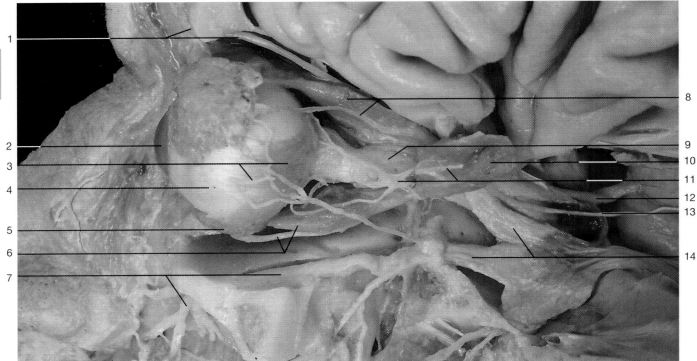

Extra-ocular muscles and their nerves (lateral aspect of left eye). Lateral rectus divided and reflected.

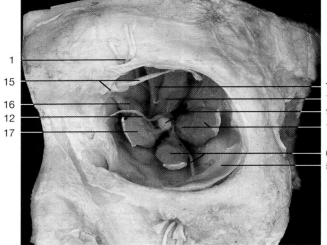

Left orbit with extra-ocular muscles (anterior aspect). Eyeball removed.

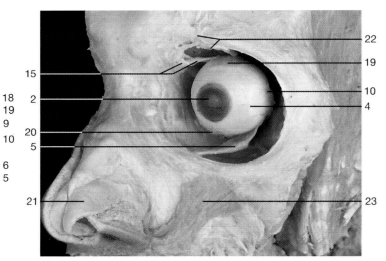

Extra-ocular eye muscles (antero-lateral aspect).

1   Supra-orbital nerve
2   Cornea
3   Insertion of lateral rectus muscle
4   Eyeball (sclera)
5   Inferior oblique muscle
6   Inferior rectus muscle and inferior branch of oculomotor nerve
7   Infra-orbital nerve
8   Superior rectus muscle and lacrimal nerve
9   Optic nerve
10 Lateral rectus muscle
11 Ciliary ganglion and abducens nerve (n. VI)

12 Oculomotor nerve (n. III)
13 Trochlear nerve (n. IV)
14 Ophthalmic nerve (n. V$_1$) and maxillary nerve (n. V$_2$)
15 Trochlea and tendon of superior oblique muscle
16 Superior oblique muscle
17 Medial rectus muscle
18 Levator palpebrae superioris muscle
19 Superior rectus muscle
20 Inferior rectus muscle
21 Greater alar cartilage
22 Supra-orbital nerve and levator palpebrae superioris muscle
23 Levator labii superioris muscle

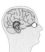

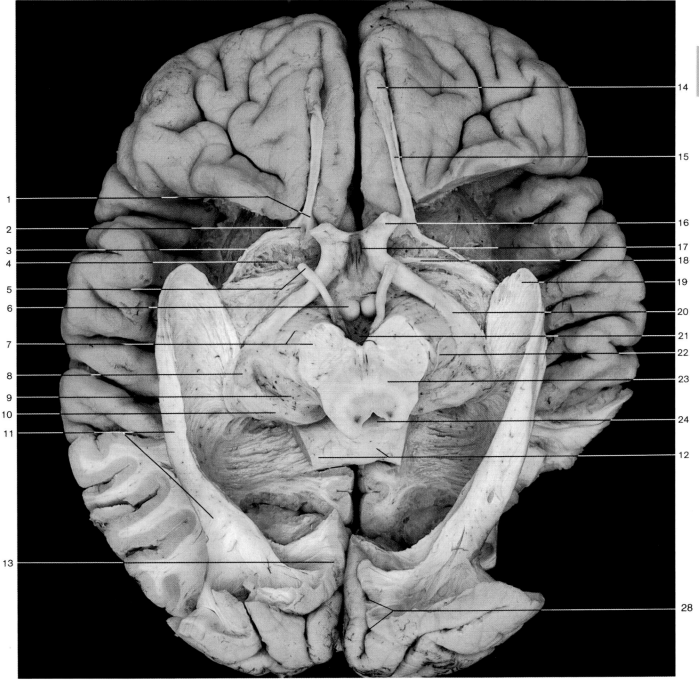

Dissection of the visual pathway (inferior aspect). Frontal pole at top, midbrain divided.

1 Medial olfactory stria	15 Olfactory tract
2 Olfactory trigone	16 Optic nerve (n. II)
3 Lateral olfactory stria	17 Infundibulum
4 Anterior perforated substance	18 Anterior commissure
5 Oculomotor nerve (n. III)	19 Genu of optic radiation
6 Mamillary body	20 Optic tract
7 Cerebral peduncle	21 Interpeduncular fossa and
8 Lateral geniculate body	posterior perforated substance
9 Medial geniculate body	22 Trochlear nerve (n. IV)
10 Pulvinar of thalamus	23 Substantia nigra
11 Optic radiation	24 Cerebral aqueduct
12 Splenium of the corpus	25 Visual cortex
callosum (commissural fibers)	26 Line of Gennari
13 Cuneus	27 Gyrus of striate cortex
14 Olfactory bulb	28 Calcarine sulcus

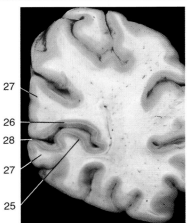

Frontal section of the striate cortex at the level of the striate area in the occipital lobe.

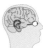

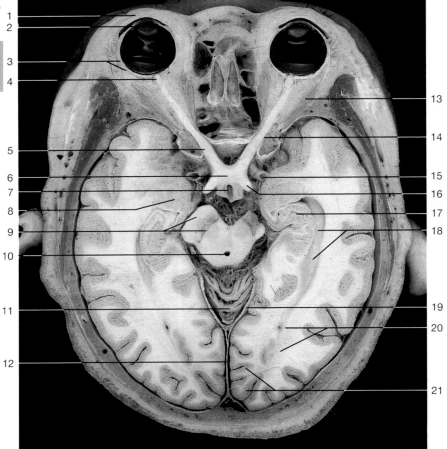

1 Upper lid
2 Cornea
3 Eyeball (sclera, retina)
4 Head of optic nerve
5 Optic nerve
6 Optic chiasma
7 Infundibular recess of hypothalamus
8 Amygdaloid body
9 Substantia nigra and crus cerebri
10 Cerebral aqueduct
11 Vermis of cerebellum
12 Falx cerebri
13 Lateral rectus muscle
14 Optic canal
15 Internal carotid artery
16 Optic tract
17 Hippocampus
18 Inferior horn of lateral ventricle
19 Tentorium cerebelli
20 Optic radiation of Gratiolet
21 Visual cortex (area calcarina, striate cortex)
22 Lens
23 Eyeball
24 Ethmoidal cells
25 Optic nerve with dura sheath
26 Cerebral peduncle
27 Aqueduct of mesencephalon
28 Vermis of cerebellum

Horizontal section through the head at the level of optic chiasma and striate cortex (superior aspect). Note the relationship of hypothalamic infundibulum to optic chiasma.

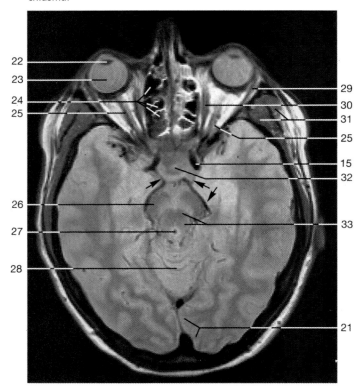

Horizontal section through the human head
(MRI scan, courtesy of Prof. W. J. Huk, Erlangen, Germany).
Arrows = branches of arterial circle of Willis.

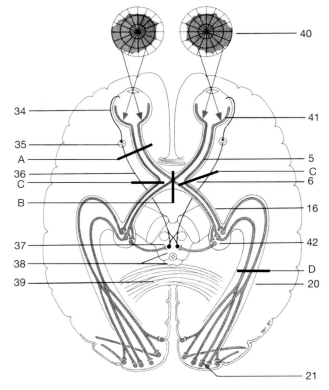

Diagram of the visual pathway and path of the light reflex.

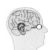

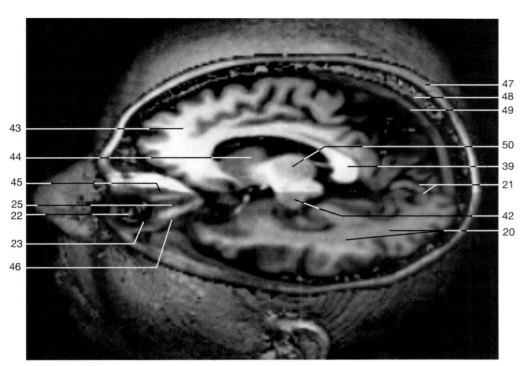

29 Lateral rectus muscle
30 Medial rectus muscle
31 Temporalis muscle
32 Hypophysis (pituitary gland)
33 Midbrain
34 Ciliary nerves (long and short)
35 Ciliary ganglion
36 Oculomotor nerve
37 Accessory oculomotor nucleus
38 Colliculi of midbrain
39 Corpus callosum
40 Visual field
41 Retina
42 Lateral geniculate body
43 Frontal lobe
44 Caudate nucleus
45 Medial rectus muscle
46 Lateral rectus muscle
47 Skin
48 Diploe (skull)
49 Dura mater
50 Thalamus
51 Anterior cerebral artery
52 Caudate nucleus
53 Frontal sinus
54 Internal capsule
55 Lentiform nucleus (putamen)
56 Hippocampus
57 Temporal lobe of left hemisphere

3-D reconstruction of the human visual system (MRI scan flash 40°, courtesy of Prof. Huk, University of Erlangen, Germany).

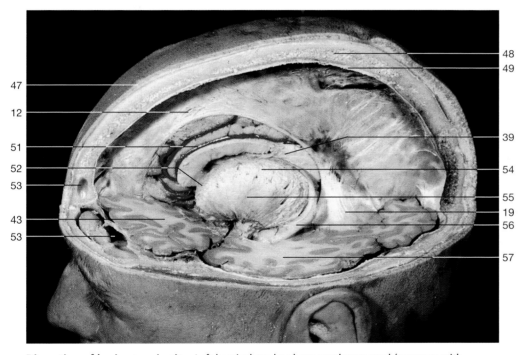

Dissection of brain stem in situ. Left hemisphere has been partly removed (compare with MRI scan above).

In **binocular vision** the visual field (40) is projected upon portions of both retinae (blue and red in the drawing). In the chiasma the fibers from the two retinal portions are combined to form the left optic tract. The fibers of the two eyes remain separated from each other throughout the entire visual pathway up to their final termination in the calcarine cortex (21). **Injuries on the optic pathway** produce visual defects whose nature depends on the location of the injury. Destruction of one optic nerve (A) produces **blindness in the corresponding eye** with loss of pupillary light reflex. If **lesions of the chiasma** destroy the crossing fibers of the nasal portions of the retina (B), both temporal fields of vision are lost **(bitemporal hemianopsia)**. If both lateral angles of the chiasma are compressed (C), the nondecussating fibers from the temporal retinae are affected, resulting in loss of nasal visual fields **(binasal hemianopsia)**. Lesions posterior to the chiasma (D) (i.e., optic tract, lateral geniculate body, optic radiation, or visual cortex) result in a loss of the entire opposite field of vision **(homonymous hemianopsia)**.

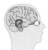

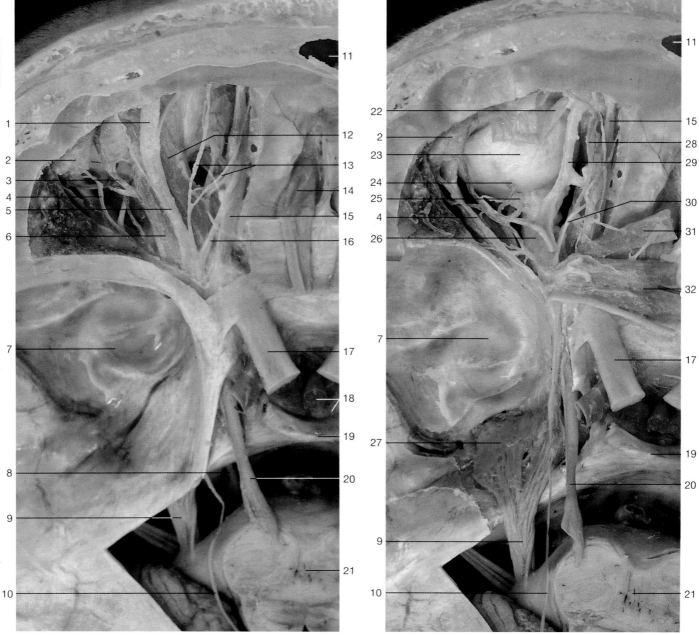

Superficial layer of the left orbit (superior aspect). The roof of the orbit and a portion of the left tentorium have been removed.

Middle layer of the left orbit (superior aspect). The roof of the orbit has been removed and the superior extra-ocular muscles have been divided and reflected.

1	Lateral branch of frontal nerve	10	Trochlear nerve (intracranial part) (n. IV)
2	Lacrimal gland	11	Frontal sinus
3	Lacrimal vein	12	Levator palpebrae superioris muscle
4	Lacrimal nerve	13	Branches of supratrochlear nerve
5	Frontal nerve	14	Olfactory bulb
6	Superior rectus	15	Superior oblique muscle
7	Middle cranial fossa	16	Trochlear nerve (intra-orbital part) (n. IV)
8	Abducent nerve (n. VI)	17	Optic nerve (intracranial part)
9	Trigeminal nerve (n. V)	18	Pituitary gland and infundibulum

19	Dorsum sellae
20	Oculomotor nerve (n. III)
21	Midbrain
22	Tendon of superior oblique muscle
23	Eyeball
24	Vena vorticosa
25	Short ciliary nerves
26	Optic nerve (extracranial part)
27	Trigeminal ganglion

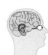

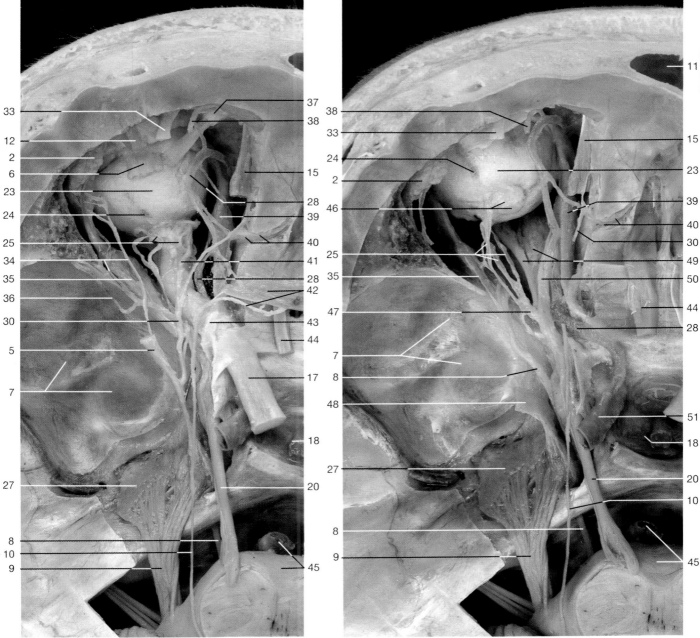

Middle layer of the left orbit (superior aspect). The roof of the orbit and the superior extra-ocular muscles have been removed.

Deeper layer of the left orbit (superior aspect). The optic nerve has now been removed.

28	Ophthalmic artery	37	Trochlea	45	Basilar artery and pons
29	Superior ophthalmic vein	38	Medial branch of supra-orbital nerve	46	Optic nerve (external sheath of optic nerve, divided)
30	Nasociliary nerve	39	Medial rectus muscle		
31	Levator palpebrae superioris muscle (reflected)	40	Anterior ethmoidal artery and nerve	47	Ciliary ganglion
		41	Long ciliary nerve	48	Ophthalmic nerve (divided, reflected)
32	Superior rectus muscle (reflected)	42	Superior oblique muscle and trochlear nerve	49	Inferior branch of oculomotor nerve and inferior rectus muscle
33	Lateral branch of supra-orbital nerve				
34	Lacrimal nerve and artery	43	Common tendinous ring	50	Superior branch of oculomotor nerve
35	Lateral rectus muscle	44	Olfactory tract	51	Internal carotid artery
36	Meningolacrimal artery (anastomosing with middle meningeal artery)				

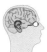

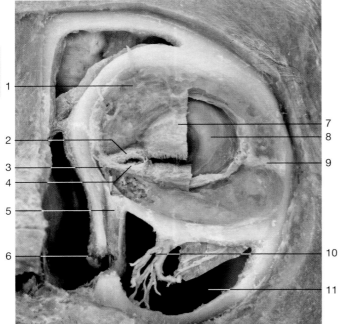

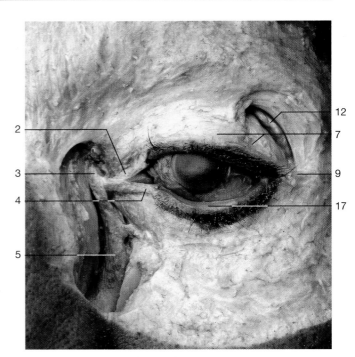

Lids and lacrimal apparatus of the left eye. Parts of the eyelids have been removed to reveal the underlying eyeball. The maxillary sinus has been opened.

Lacrimal apparatus of the left eye.

1	Orbicularis oculi muscle	10	Infra-orbital artery and nerve
2	Superior lacrimal canaliculus	11	Maxillary sinus
3	Lacrimal sac	12	Lacrimal gland
4	Inferior lacrimal canaliculus	13	Medial palpebral ligament
5	Nasolacrimal duct	14	Aponeurosis of levator palpebrae superioris muscle
6	Inferior nasal concha	15	Palpebral portion of the orbicularis oculi muscle
7	Upper eyelid	16	Infra-orbital foramen
8	Eyeball	17	Palpebral conjunctiva of lower lid
9	Lateral palpebral ligament		

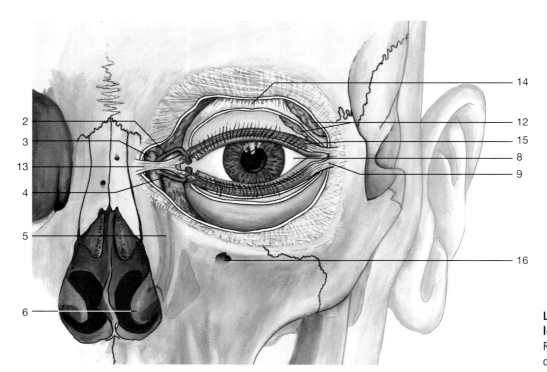

Lacrimal apparatus of the left eye (schematic drawing). Red = Palpebral portion of the orbicularis oculi muscle.

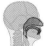

2.4 Oral and Nasal Cavities

During evolution, the oral and nasal cavities of the human head were situated upon each other, so the human face developed in the frontal plane. The **nasal cavities** are separated by the nasal septum. They contain three conchae, where openings to the ethmoidal and maxillary sinus are located. Posteriorly the two nasal cavities open into the nasopharynx through the choanae.

The **oral cavity** is separated from the nasal cavity by the palate. When the mouth is closed, the oral cavity is fully occupied by the tongue, which is characterized by its high mobility, necessary for the development of speech and song. Specific lymphatic organs (tonsils) are located at the entrance of the nasopharynx in both the nasal and oval cavities to protect the digestive tract from infection. The respiratory and digestory tracts cross each other within the nasopharynx, the most important requirement for the development of speech.

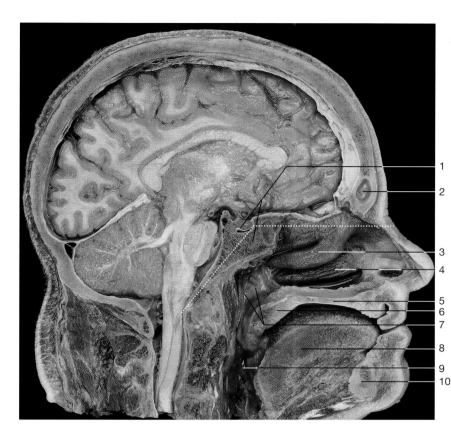

Median sagittal section through the head. The palate separates nasal and oral cavities. The base of the skull forms an angle of about 150° at the sella turcica (dotted line).

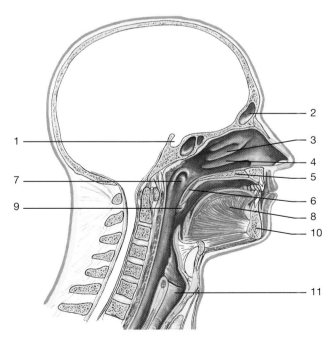

Median sagittal section through the head (schematic drawing). The tongue has been disposed to show the connection of the oral cavity with the pharynx and the position of the palatine tonsil.

1   Hypophysis within hypophysial fossa
2   Frontal sinus
3   Middle nasal concha
4   Inferior nasal concha
5   Hard palate
6   Soft palate
7   Pharynx with auditory tube
8   Tongue
9   Pharynx with palatine tonsil
10 Mandible
11 Larynx

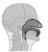

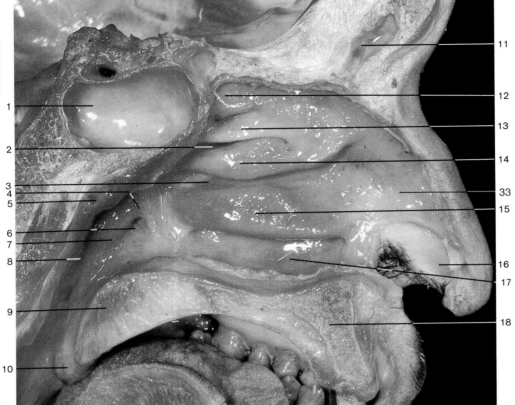

1	Sphenoidal sinus
2	Superior meatus
3	Middle meatus
4	Tubal elevation
5	Pharyngeal tonsil
6	Pharyngeal orifice of auditory tube
7	Salpingopharyngeal fold
8	Pharyngeal recess
9	Soft palate
10	Uvula
11	Frontal sinus
12	Spheno-ethmoidal recess
13	Superior nasal concha
14	Middle nasal concha
15	Inferior nasal concha
16	Vestibule
17	Inferior meatus
18	Hard palate
19	Grooves for the middle meningeal artery and parietal bone (yellow)
20	Maxillary hiatus
21	Perpendicular process of palatine bone
22	Openings of ethmoidal air cells
23	Opening of frontal sinus
24	Medial pterygoid plate (red)
25	Horizontal plate of palatine process
26	Ethmoidal air cells
27	Maxillary sinus
28	Nasal septum
29	Pterygoid hamulus
30	Nasal bone (white)
31	Frontal process of maxilla (violet)
32	Palatine process of maxilla (violet)
33	Nasal atrium

Lateral wall of the nasal cavity. Septum removed.

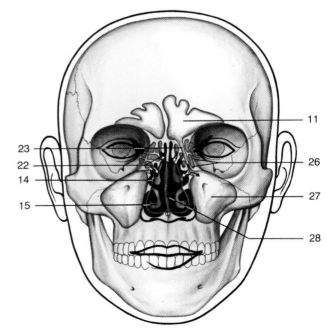

Bones of left nasal cavity (medial aspect).

Schematic diagram showing the position of paranasal sinuses. Openings indicated by arrows.

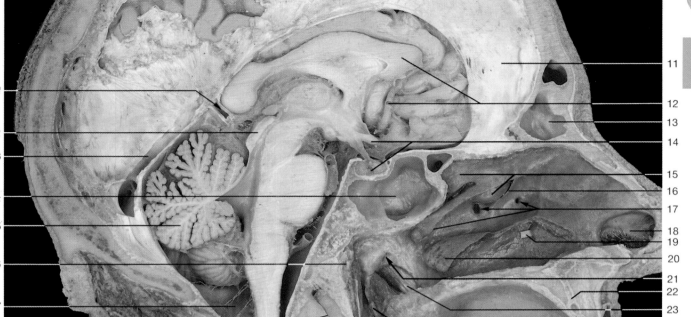

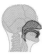

Median section through the head with nasal and oral cavities. The middle and inferior nasal conchae have been partly removed to show the openings of paranasal sinuses.

1 Great cerebral vein (Galen's vein)
2 Tectum of midbrain
3 Straight sinus
4 Sphenoidal sinus
5 Cerebellum
6 Pharyngeal tonsil
7 Cerebellomedullary cistern
8 Median atlanto-axial joint
9 Spinal cord
10 Oral part of pharynx
11 Falx cerebri
12 Corpus callosum and anterior cerebral artery
13 Frontal sinus
14 Optic chiasm and pituitary gland
15 Superior nasal concha and ethmoidal bulla
16 Semilunar hiatus
17 Accessory openings to maxillary sinus and cut edge of middle nasal concha
18 Vestibule
19 Opening of nasolacrimal duct
20 Inferior nasal concha (cut)
21 Opening of auditory tube
22 Incisive canal
23 Levator veli palatini muscle
24 Salpingopharyngeal fold
25 Lingual nerve and submandibular ganglion
26 Submandibular duct
27 Nasofrontal duct
28 Nasolacrimal duct
29 Spheno-ethmoidal recess (of Rosenmüller)
30 Salpingopalatine fold

Lateral wall of nasal cavity. Openings indicated by red arrows (schematic drawing).

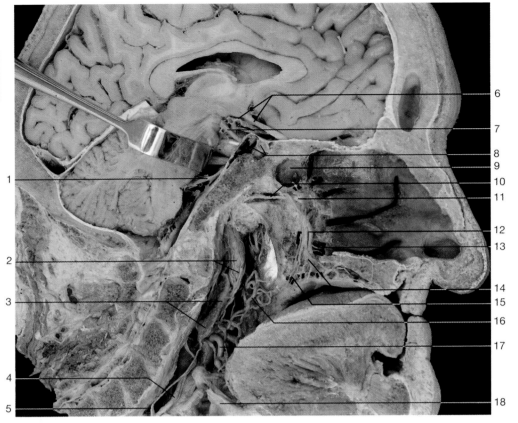

1   Facial nerve
2   Internal carotid artery and internal carotid plexus
3   Superior cervical ganglion
4   Vagus nerve
5   Sympathetic trunk
6   Optic nerve and ophthalmic artery
7   Oculomotor nerve
8   Internal carotid artery and cavernous sinus
9   Sphenoidal sinus
10   Nerve of the pterygoid canal
11   Pterygopalatine ganglion
12   Descending palatine artery
13   Lateral inferior posterior nasal branches and lateral posterior nasal and septal arteries
14   Greater palatine nerves and artery
15   Lesser palatine nerves and arteries
16   Branches of ascending pharyngeal artery
17   Lingual artery
18   Epiglottis
19   Anterior ethmoidal artery
20   Olfactory bulb
21   Olfactory tract
22   Nasopalatine nerve
23   Choanae
24   Frontal sinus
25   Crista galli
26   Anterior ethmoidal artery and nerve, and nasal branch of anterior ethmoidal artery
27   Nasal septum
28   Septal artery
29   Crest of nasal septum
30   Hard palate
31   Tentorium cerebelli
32   Trochlear nerve
33   Trigeminal nerve with motor root
34   Internal carotid plexus
35   Lingual nerve with chorda tympani
36   Medial pterygoid muscle and medial pterygoid plate
37   Inferior alveolar nerve
38   Sympathetic trunk
39   Oculomotor nerve
40   Palatine nerves
41   Tongue
42   Trigeminal ganglion
43   Trigeminal nerve (n. V)
44   Facial nerve (n. VII)
45   Geniculate ganglion
46   Stylomastoid foramen
47   Medial pterygoid muscle

Nerves of the lateral wall of nasal cavity. Sagittal section through the head. Mucous membranes partly removed, pterygoid canal opened.

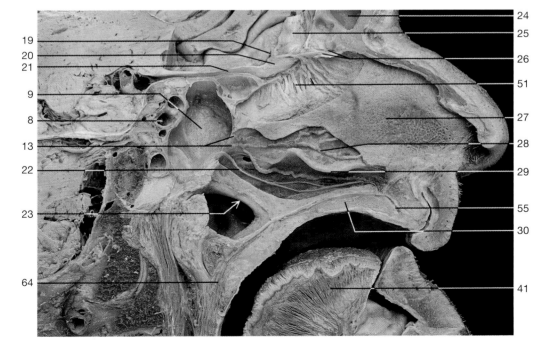

Nasal septum. Dissection of nerves and vessels.

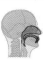

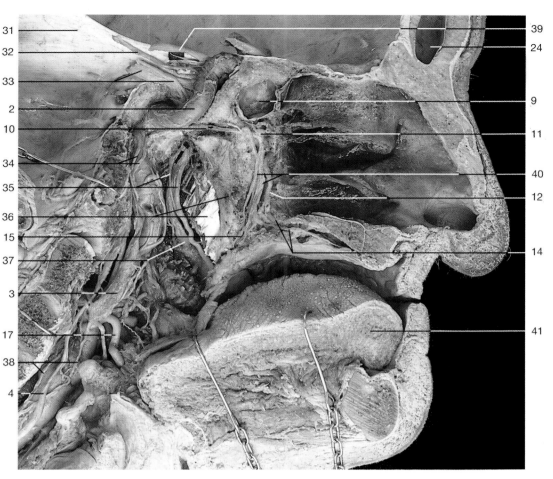

48 Greater petrosal nerve
49 Maxillary nerve
50 Olfactory bulb
51 Olfactory nerves
52 Internal nasal branches of anterior ethmoidal nerve
53 Lateral superior posterior nasal branches
54 Lateral inferior posterior nasal branches
55 Incisive canal with nasopalatine nerve
56 Greater palatine nerve
57 Deep petrosal nerve
58 Mandibular nerve
59 Nasal cavity and inferior nasal concha
60 Opening of auditory tube
61 Tensor veli palatini muscle
62 Levator veli palatini muscle
63 Pharyngeal recess in the nasopharynx
64 Uvula
65 Palatoglossal arch
66 Tonsillar branch of ascending palatine artery
67 Palatine tonsil
68 Palatopharyngeal arch

Nerves of the lateral wall of nasal cavity. Carotid canal opened, mucous membranes of pharynx and nasal cavity partly removed.

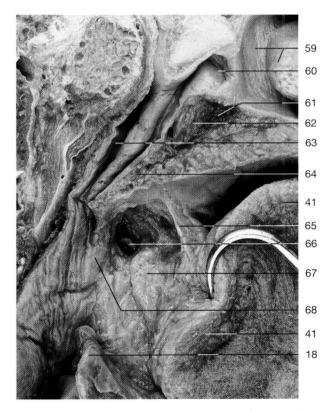

Dissection of palatine tonsil located in the lateral wall of the nasopharynx (left side). Root of tongue reflected.

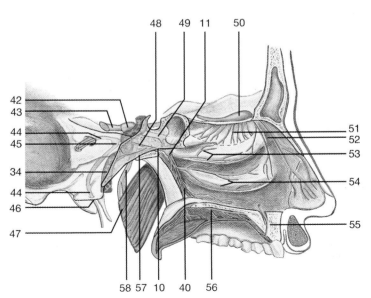

Nerves of the lateral wall of nasal cavity. Body of sphenoid bone appears transparent (schematic drawing).

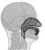

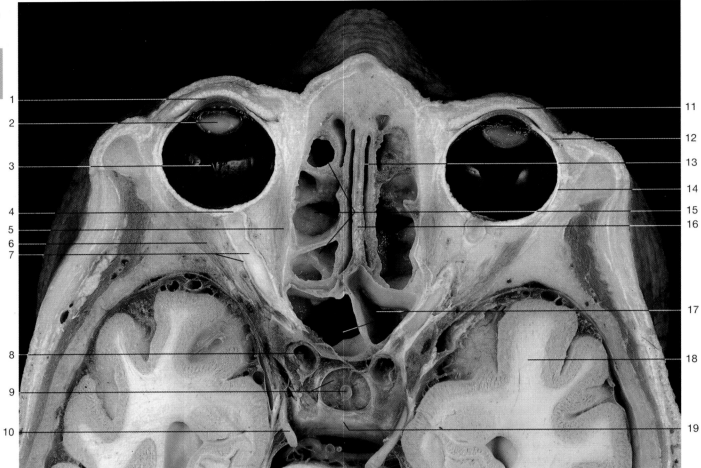

Horizontal section through the nasal cavity, the orbits, and temporal lobes of the brain at the level of pituitary gland.

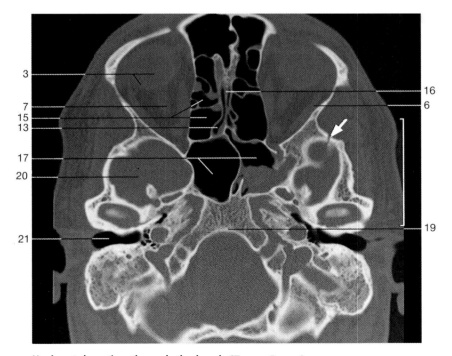

Horizontal section through the head. CT scan. Bar = 2 cm.
Arrow: fracture.

1 Cornea
2 Lens
3 Vitreous body (eyeball)
4 Head of optic nerve
5 Medial rectus muscle
6 Lateral rectus muscle
7 Optic nerve with dural sheath
8 Internal carotid artery
9 Pituitary gland and infundibulum
10 Oculomotor nerve
11 Superior tarsal plate of eyelid
12 Fornix of conjunctiva
13 Nasal cavity
14 Sclera
15 Ethmoidal sinus
16 Nasal septum
17 Sphenoidal sinus
18 Temporal lobe
19 Clivus
20 Middle cranial fossa
21 External acoustic meatus
22 Superior sagittal sinus
23 Falx cerebri
24 Superior rectus and levator
    palpebrae superioris muscles
25 Eyeball and lacrimal gland
26 Inferior rectus and inferior oblique muscles
27 Zygomatic bone
28 Maxillary sinus
29 Inferior nasal concha
30 Hard palate

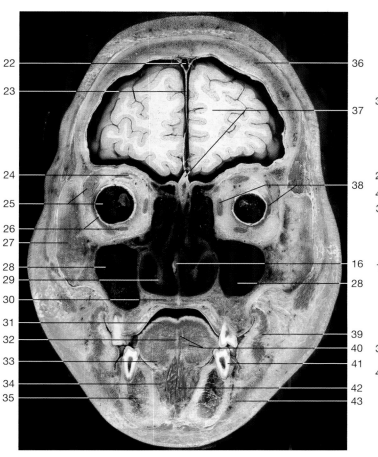

22
23
36
37
24
25
38
26
27
28 16
29 28
30
31
32 39
33 40
41
34 42
35 43

Coronal section through the head at the level of the second premolar of the mandible.

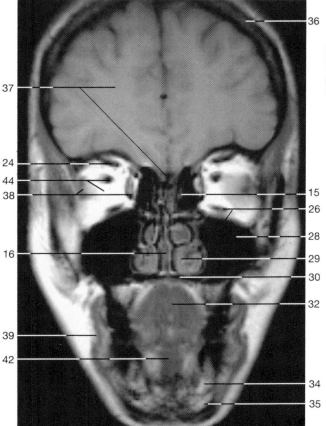

36
37
24
44 15
38 26
28
16 29
30
32
39
42
34
35

Coronal section through the head (MRI scan, courtesy of Prof. Heuck, Munich, Germany). Note the situation of the head cavities.

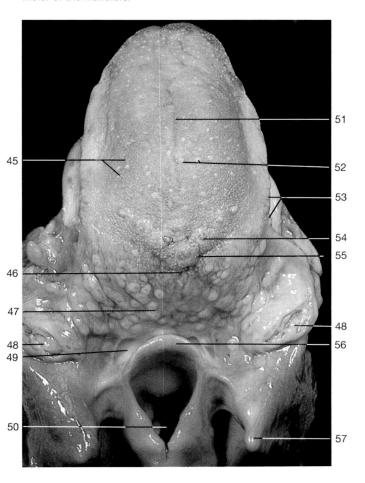

45
46
47
48
49
50

51
52
53
54
55
48
56
57

31   Superior longitudinal muscle of tongue
32   Lingual septum
33   Inferior longitudinal muscle of tongue
34   Sublingual gland
35   Mandible
36   Calvaria
37   Frontal lobe of brain and crista galli
38   Lateral and medial rectus muscles
39   Buccinator muscle
40   Vertical and transverse muscles of tongue
41   Second premolar of mandible
42   Genioglossus muscle
43   Platysma muscle
44   Orbit and optic nerve
45   Filiform papillae
46   Foramen cecum
47   Root of tongue (lingual tonsil)
48   Palatine tonsil
49   Vallecula of epiglottis
50   Vestibule of larynx
51   Median sulcus of tongue
52   Fungiform papillae
53   Foliate papillae
54   Circumvallate papilla
55   Sulcus terminalis
56   Epiglottis
57   Greater cornu of hyoid bone

◁ **Dorsal surface of the tongue and laryngeal inlet.**

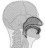

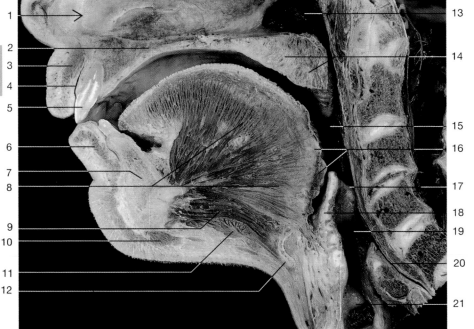

1	Nasal cavity
2	Hard palate
3	Upper lip and orbicularis oris muscle
4	Vestibule of oral cavity
5	First incisor
6	Lower lip and orbicularis oris muscle
7	Mandible
8	Genioglossus muscle
9	Geniohyoid muscle
10	Anterior belly of diagastric muscle
11	Mylohyoid muscle
12	Hyoid bone
13	Nasopharynx
14	Soft palate and uvula
15	Oropharynx
16	Root of tongue and lingual tonsil
17	Laryngopharynx
18	Epiglottis
19	Ary-epiglottic fold
20	Laryngopharynx continuous with esophagus
21	Larynx

Median sagittal section through the oral cavity and pharynx.

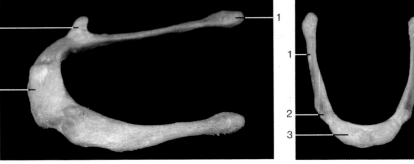

1	Greater cornu	
2	Lesser cornu	} of hyoid bone
3	Body	

Hyoid bone (oblique lateral aspect).   **Hyoid bone** (anterior aspect).

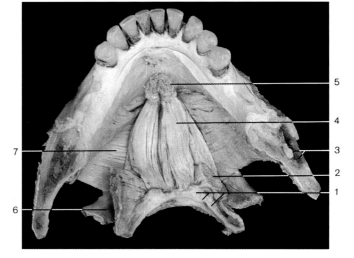

Muscles of the floor of the oral cavity (superior aspect).

1   Lesser cornu and body of hyoid bone
2   Hyoglossus muscle (divided)
3   Ramus of mandible and inferior alveolar nerve
4   Geniohyoid muscle
5   Genioglossus muscle (divided)
6   Stylohyoid muscle (divided)

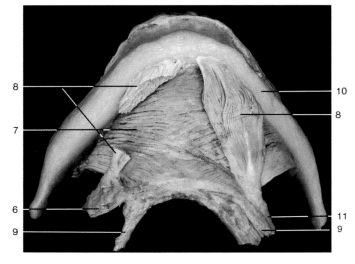

Oral diaphragm, muscles (inferior aspect). Cut on the base.

7   Mylohyoid muscle
8   Anterior belly of digastric muscle
9   Hyoid bone
10 Mandible
11 Intermediate tendon of digastric muscle

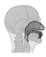

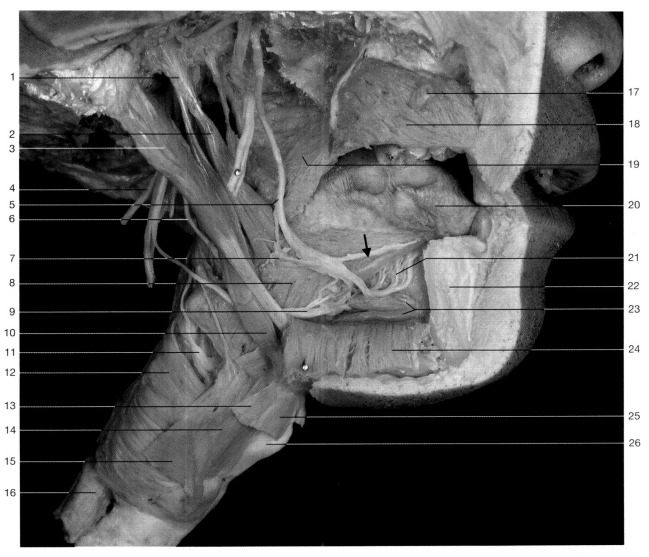

Parapharyngeal and sublingual regions. Innervation of the tongue. Lateral part of face and mandible removed, oral cavity opened. Arrow: submandibular duct.

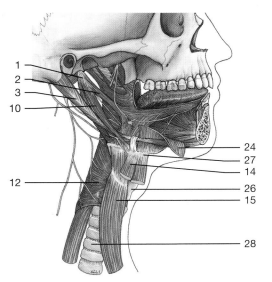

Supra- and infrahyoid muscles and pharynx (schematic drawing).

1 Styloid process
2 Styloglossus muscle
3 Digastric muscle (posterior belly)
4 Vagus nerve (n. X)
5 Lingual nerve (n. V₃)
6 Glossopharyngeal nerve (n. IX)
7 Submandibular ganglion
8 Hyoglossus muscle
9 Hypoglossal nerve (n. XII)
10 Stylohyoid muscle
11 Internal branch of superior laryngeal nerve (branch of vagus nerve, not visible)
12 Middle constrictor muscle of pharynx
13 Omohyoid muscle (divided)

14 Thyrohyoid muscle
15 Sternothyroid muscle
16 Esophagus
17 Parotid duct (divided)
18 Buccinator
19 Superior constrictor muscle of pharynx
20 Tongue
21 Terminal branches of lingual nerve
22 Mandible (divided)
23 Genioglossus and geniohyoid muscles
24 Mylohyoid muscle (divided and reflected)
25 Sternohyoid muscle (divided)
26 Thyroid cartilage
27 Hyoid bone
28 Trachea

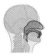

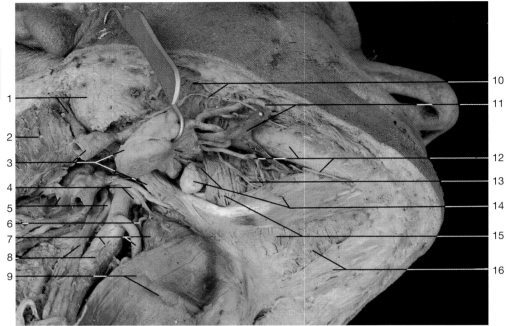

1   Parotid gland and
    retromandibular vein
2   Sternocleidomastoid muscle
3   Retromandibular vein,
    submandibular gland, and
    stylohyoid muscle
4   Hypoglossal nerve and lingual
    artery
5   Vagus nerve and internal
    jugular vein
6   Superior laryngeal artery
7   External carotid artery,
    thyrohyoid muscle, and
    superior thyroid artery
8   Common carotid artery and
    superior root of ansa cervicalis
9   Omohyoid and sternohyoid
    muscles
10 Masseter muscle and marginal
    mandibular branch of facial
    nerve
11 Facial artery and vein
12 Mandible and submental
    artery and vein
13 Mylohyoid nerve
14 Submandibular duct, sublingual
    gland, and anterior belly of
    digastric muscle
15 Mylohyoid muscle
16 Mylohyoid muscle and anterior
    belly of left digastric muscle
17 Hyoglossus muscle and lingual
    artery
18 Lingual nerve
19 Hypoglossal nerve
20 Geniohyoid muscle
21 Anterior belly of right digastric
    muscle
22 Submandibular gland and duct

Submandibular triangle, superficial dissection. Right side (inferior aspect). Submandibular gland has been reflected.

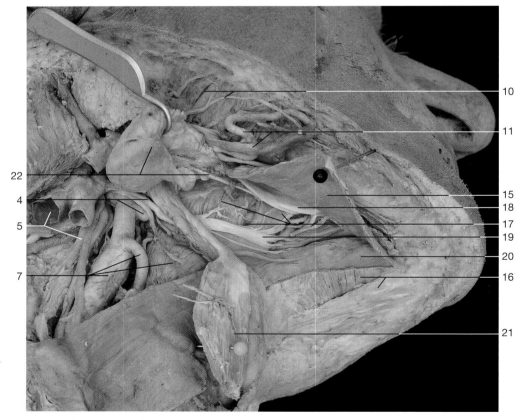

Submandibular triangle, deep dissection. Right side (inferior aspect). Mylohyoid muscle has been severed and reflected to display the lingual and hypoglossal nerves.

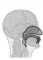

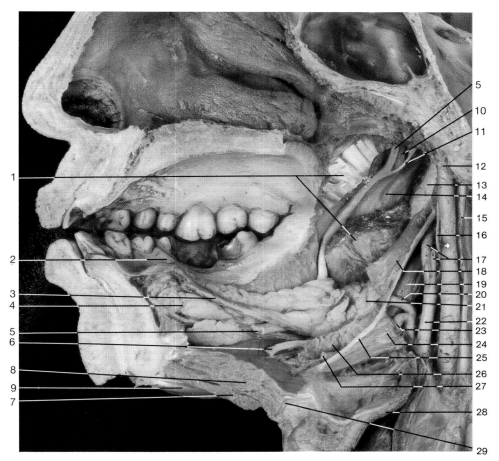

1   Medial pterygoid muscle
2   Sublingual papilla
3   Submandibular duct
4   Sublingual gland
5   Lingual nerve
6   Hypoglossal nerve
7   Mylohyoid muscle
8   Geniohyoid muscle
9   Anterior belly of digastric muscle
10 Inferior alveolar nerve
11 Chorda tympani
12 Internal carotid artery
13 Parotid gland
14 Sphenomandibular ligament
15 Vagus nerve
16 Glossopharyngeal nerve
17 Superficial temporal artery and ascending pharyngeal artery
18 Styloglossus muscle
19 Posterior belly of digastric muscle
20 Facial artery
21 Submandibular gland
22 External carotid artery
23 Lingual artery
24 Middle pharyngeal constrictor muscle
25 Stylohyoid ligament
26 Hyoglossus muscle
27 Deep lingual artery
28 Epiglottis
29 Hyoid bone
30 Buccinator muscle
31 Tongue
32 Mandible (divided)
33 Parotid duct
34 Masseter muscle
35 Right and left sublingual papillae

Oral cavity (internal aspect). Tongue and pharyngeal wall removed.

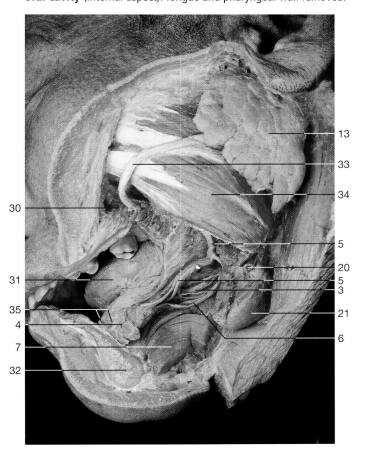

Dissection of major salivary glands. Left mandible and buccinator muscle partly removed to view the oral cavity (infero-lateral aspect).

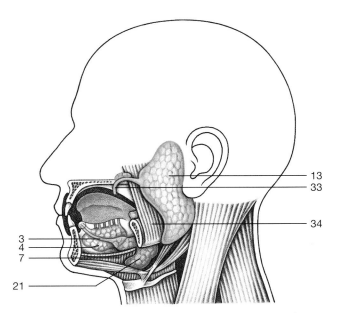

Location of the major salivary glands in relation to the oral cavity.

2.5 Neck and Organs of the Neck

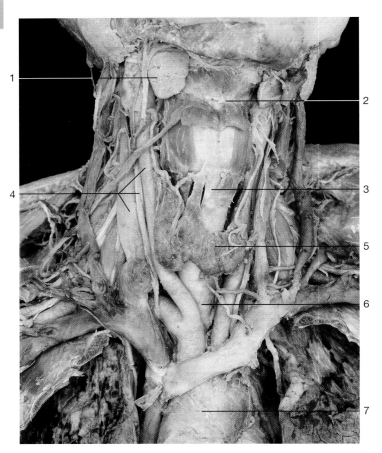

Regional anatomy of the neck (anterior aspect). The anteriorly located muscles and the thoracic wall have been removed.

The anterior aspect of the neck contains the trachea and larynx, which are connected to the nasal cavity via the pharynx. Behind the trachea lies the esophagus, which is connected to the oral cavity, again via the pharynx.

The thyroid gland is located anterior to the trachea, whereas the carotid artery and jugular vein together with the vagus nerve are situated laterally, conjoining the head with the thoracic organs and upper limb.

Underneath the sternocleidomastoid muscle, the cervical portion of the spinal nerves forms the cervical and brachial nervous plexuses that give rise to the innervations of neck and upper limb respectively.

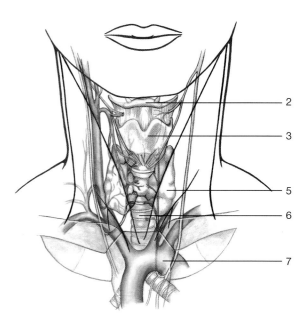

1   Submandibular gland
2   Hyoid bone
3   Larynx (thyroid cartilage)
4   Nerves and vessels of the neck
    (carotid artery, internal jugular vein, and vagus nerve)
5   Thyroid gland
6   Trachea
7   Aortic arch

Organs of the neck (anterior aspect, schematic drawing). The main arterial trunks are indicated in red.

1 Nasal septum
2 Uvula
3 Genioglossus muscle
4 Mandible
5 Geniohyoid muscle
6 Mylohyoid muscle
7 Hyoid bone
8 Thyroid cartilage
9 Manubrium sterni
10 Sphenoidal sinus
11 Nasopharynx
12 Oropharynx
13 Epiglottis
14 Laryngopharynx
15 Arytenoid muscle
16 Vocal fold
17 Cricoid cartilage
18 Trachea
19 Left brachiocephalic vein
20 Thymus
21 Esophagus

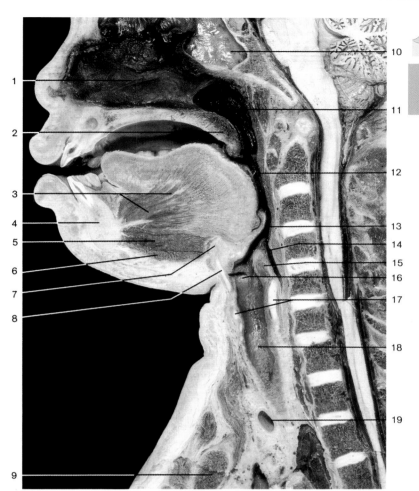

Median section through adult head and neck. Note the low position of the adult larynx when compared with that of the neonate (cf. with the figure below).

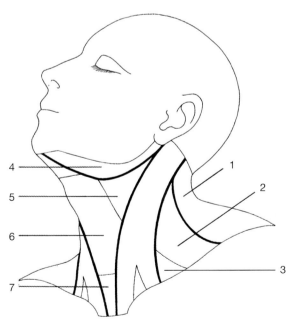

Regions and triangles of the neck (schematic drawing).

1 Posterior cervical region
2 Lateral cervical region
3 Supraclavicular triangle
4 Submandibular triangle
5 Carotid triangle
6 Anterior cervical region
7 Jugular fossa

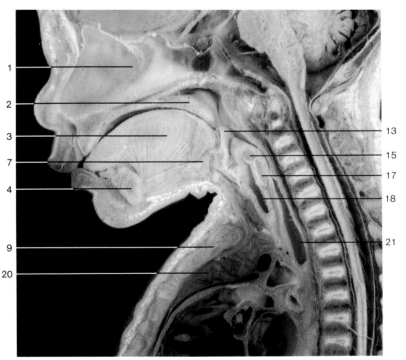

Median section through neonate head and neck. Note the high position of the larynx permitting the epiglottis to nearly reach the uvula (cf. with the figure above).

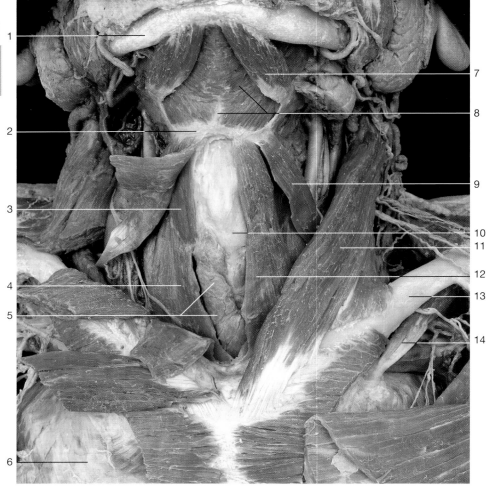

1	Mandible
2	Hyoid bone
3	Thyrohyoid muscle
4	Sternothyroid muscle
5	Thyroid gland
6	Second rib
7	Anterior belly of digastric muscle
8	Mylohyoid muscle (and mylohyoid raphe)
9	Omohyoid muscle
10	Thyroid cartilage
11	Sternocleidomastoid muscle
12	Sternohyoid muscle
13	Clavicle
14	Subclavius muscle
15	Posterior belly of digastric muscle
16	Stylohyoid muscle
17	Scalenus muscles
18	Trapezius muscle
19	First rib
20	Scapula
21	Trachea
22	Manubrium sterni

Muscles of the neck (anterior aspect). Sternocleidomastoid and sternohyoid muscles on the right have been divided and reflected.

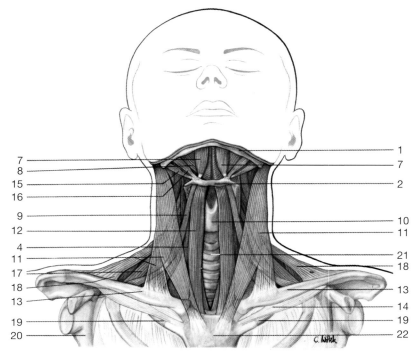

Muscles of the neck (anterior aspect, schematic drawing).

The muscles of the neck are complex and highly sophisticated. There are two major groups of muscles to be distinguished according to their functional aspects. One group is constituted by muscles connecting head to the hyoid bone and the larynx. The second category of muscles links the head and the ribcage.

The sternocleidomastoid muscle represents the border between the anterior and posterior cervical triangle.

1 Sternohyoid and thyrohyoid muscles
2 Larynx
3 Cricoid cartilage
4 Internal jugular vein, common carotid artery, and vagus nerve
5 Esophagus
6 Body of cervical vertebra
7 Vertebral artery
8 Spinal cord
9 Scalenus posterior muscle
10 Deep muscles of the neck
11 Trapezius muscle
12 Omohyoid muscle
13 Thyroid gland
14 Sternocleidomastoid muscle
15 Longus colli and longus capitis muscles
16 Cervical spinal nerve
17 Vertebral artery and vein, and foramen transversarium
18 Ventral and dorsal root of cervical spinal nerve
19 Trachea
20 Sympathetic trunk
21 Anterior tubercle of transverse process and origin of scalenus anterior and medius muscles
22 Superior facet of articular process
23 Spinous process

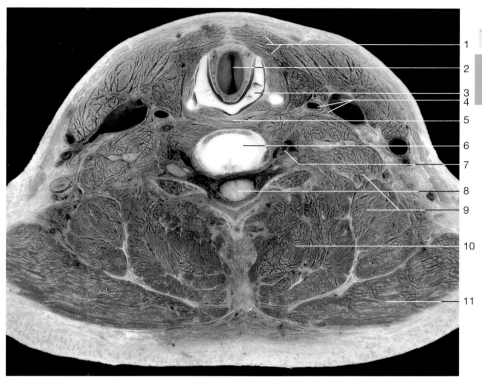

Axial section of the neck at the level of the intervertebral disc between the 5th and 6th cervical vertebra (inferior aspect).

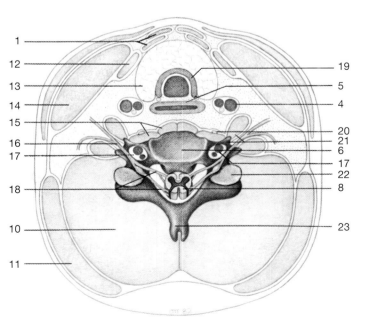

Organization of the neck (axial section at the level of the thyroid gland; schematic drawing).

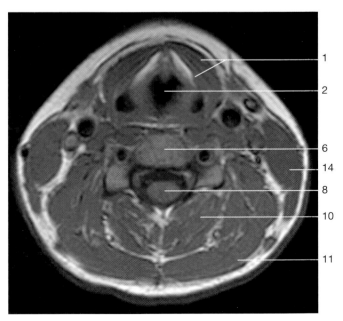

Axial section of the neck at the level of the 4th cervical vertebra (MRI scan; from Heuck et al., MRT-Atlas, 2009).

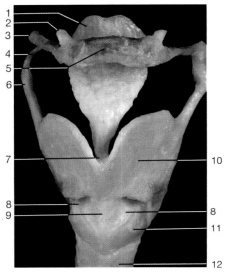

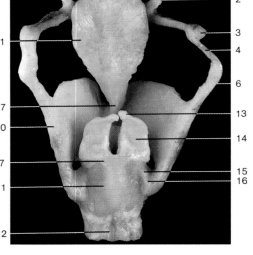

1 Epiglottis
2 Lesser cornu of hyoid bone
3 Greater cornu of hyoid bone
4 Lateral thyrohyoid ligament
5 Body of hyoid bone
6 Superior cornu of thyroid cartilage
7 Thyro-epiglottic ligament
8 Conus elasticus
9 Cricothyroid ligament
10 Thyroid cartilage
11 Cricoid cartilage
12 Trachea
13 Corniculate cartilage
14 Arytenoid cartilage
15 Posterior crico-arytenoid ligament
16 Cricothyroid joint
17 Crico-arytenoid joint

Cartilages of the larynx and the hyoid bone (anterior aspect).

Cartilages of the larynx and the hyoid bone (posterior aspect).

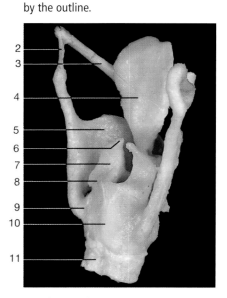

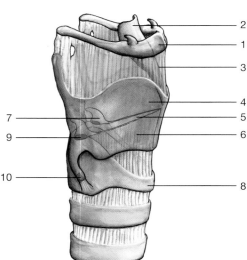

1 Hyoid bone
2 Epiglottis
3 Thyrohyoid membrane
4 Thyroid cartilage
5 Vocal ligament
6 Conus elasticus
7 Arytenoid cartilage
8 Cricoid cartilage
9 Crico-arytenoid joint
10 Cricothyroid joint
11 Tracheal cartilages
12 Corniculate cartilage
13 Muscular process of arytenoid cartilage
14 Vocal process of arytenoid cartilage
15 Lamina of cricoid cartilage
16 Arch of cricoid cartilage

Cartilages of the larynx (anterior aspect). Thyroid cartilage is indicated by the outline.

Cartilages and ligaments of the larynx (lateral aspect).

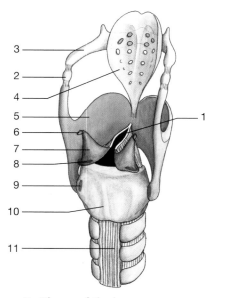

1 Vocal ligament
2 Lateral thyrohyoid ligament
3 Greater cornu of hyoid bone
4 Epiglottis
5 Thyroid cartilage
6 Corniculate cartilage
7 Arytenoid cartilage
8 Crico-arytenoid joint
9 Cricothyroid joint
10 Cricoid cartilage
11 Trachea

Cartilages of the larynx (oblique-posterior aspect).

Cartilages of the larynx (oblique-posterior aspect).

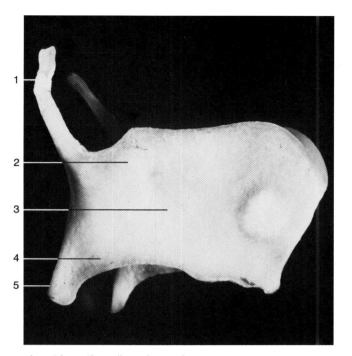

Thyroid cartilage (lateral aspect).

1 Superior cornu
2 Superior thyroid tubercle
3 Lamina of thyroid cartilage

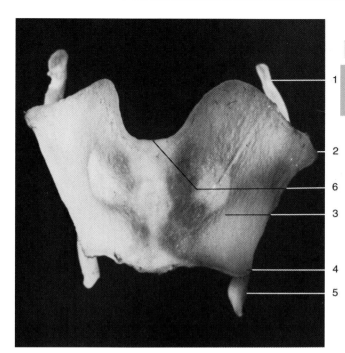

Thyroid cartilage (anterior aspect).

4 Inferior thyroid tubercle
5 Inferior cornu
6 Superior thyroid notch

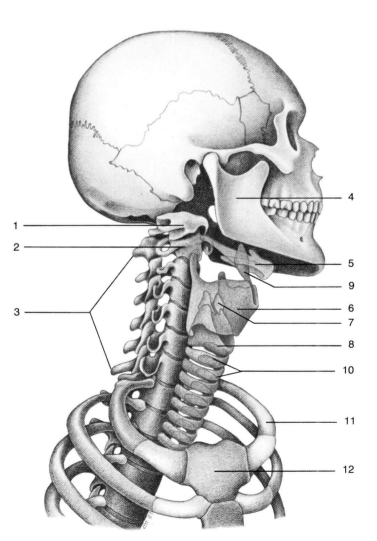

1 Atlas
2 Axis
3 Cervical vertebrae (C$_2$–C$_7$)
4 Mandible
5 Hyoid bone
6 Thyroid cartilage
7 Arytenoid cartilage
8 Cricoid cartilage
9 Epiglottis
10 Tracheal cartilages
11 First rib
12 Manubrium sterni

Position of the larynx in the neck (oblique-lateral aspect).
(Schematic drawing.)

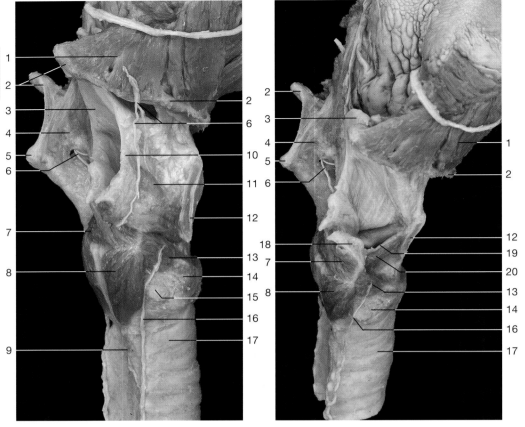

Laryngeal muscles (lateral aspect).
Thyroid cartilage (12) and thyro-arytenoid
muscle have been partly removed.

Laryngeal muscles (lateral aspect).
Half of the thyroid cartilage (12) has been
removed. Dissection of the vocal ligament (19).

1   Hyoglossus muscle
2   Hyoid bone
3   Epiglottis
4   Thyrohyoid membrane
5   Superior cornu of thyroid
    cartilage
6   Superior laryngeal nerve
7   Transverse arytenoid
    muscle
8   Posterior crico-arytenoid
    muscle
9   Transverse muscle of
    trachea
10 Ary-epiglottic fold
11 Thyro-epiglottic muscle
12 Thyroid cartilage
13 Lateral crico-arytenoid
    muscle
14 Cricoid cartilage
15 Articular facet for thyroid
    cartilage
16 Inferior laryngeal nerve
    (branch of recurrent nerve)
17 Trachea
18 Arytenoid cartilage
19 Vocal ligament
20 Vocalis muscle (part of
    thyro-arytenoid muscle)
21 Thyrohyoideus muscle
22 Cricothyroideus muscle
23 Root of tongue
24 Cuneiform tubercle
25 Corniculate tubercle
26 Ary-epiglottic muscle

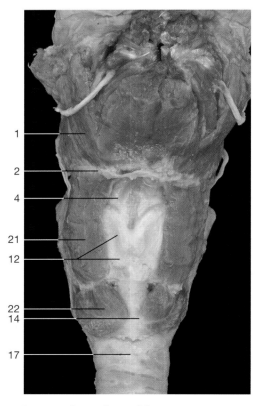

Laryngeal muscles and larynx
(anterior aspect).

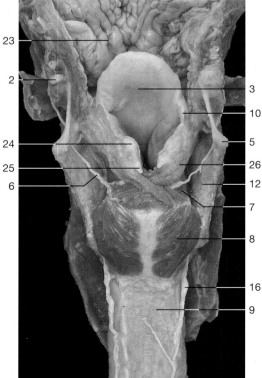

Laryngeal muscles and larynx
(posterior aspect).

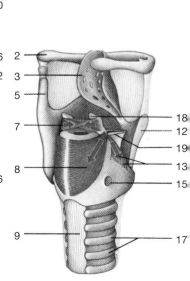

**Action of internal muscles of
the larynx** (schematic drawing).

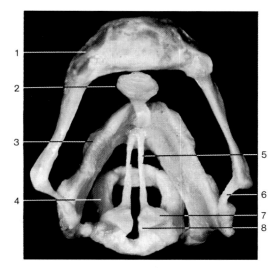

Laryngeal cartilages (superior aspect).

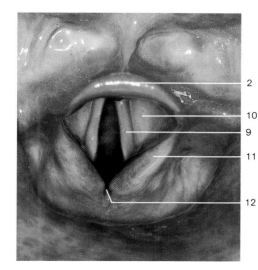

Glottis in vivo (superior aspect).

1   Hyoid bone
2   Epiglottis
3   Thyroid cartilage
4   Cricoid cartilage
5   Vocal ligament
6   Thyrohyoid ligament
7   Arytenoid cartilage
8   Corniculate cartilage
9   Vocal fold
10 Vestibular fold
11 Ary-epiglottic fold
12 Interarytenoid notch
13 Mandible
14 Anterior belly of
    digastric muscle
15 Mylohyoid muscle
16 Pyramidal lobe of
    thyroid gland
17 Sternohyoid and
    sternothyroid muscles
18 Common carotid
    artery
19 Internal jugular vein
20 Rima glottidis
21 Sternocleidomastoid
    muscle
22 Transverse arytenoid
    muscle
23 Pharynx and inferior
    constrictor muscle
24 Ventricle of larynx
25 Vocalis muscle
26 Trachea
27 Superior cornu of
    thyroid cartilage
28 Root of tongue
    (lingual tonsil)
29 Piriform recess
30 Vocalis muscle
31 Lateral crico-arytenoid
    muscle
32 Thyroid gland

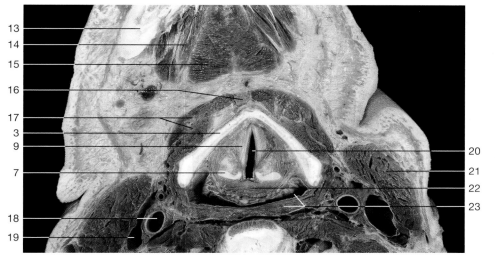

Horizontal section through the larynx at the level of the vocal folds (superior aspect).

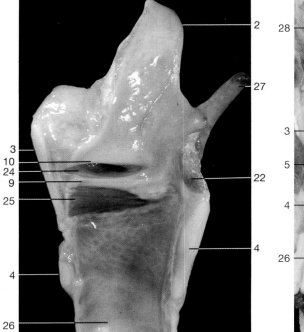

Sagittal section through the larynx.

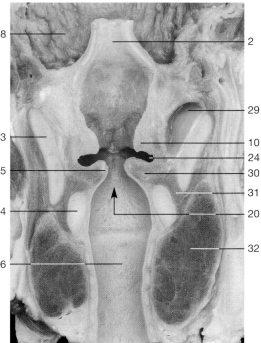

Coronal section through larynx and trachea.

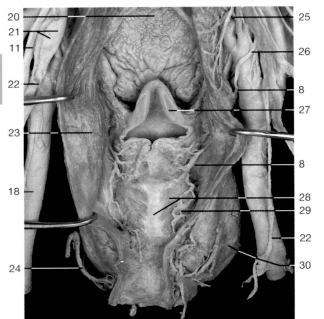

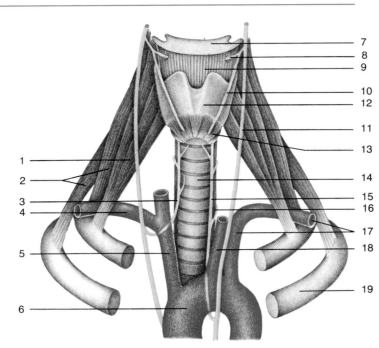

Larynx and its innervation (posterior aspect).
Dissection of superior and inferior laryngeal nerves.
Pharynx has been opened.

Innervation of the larynx (schematic drawing).

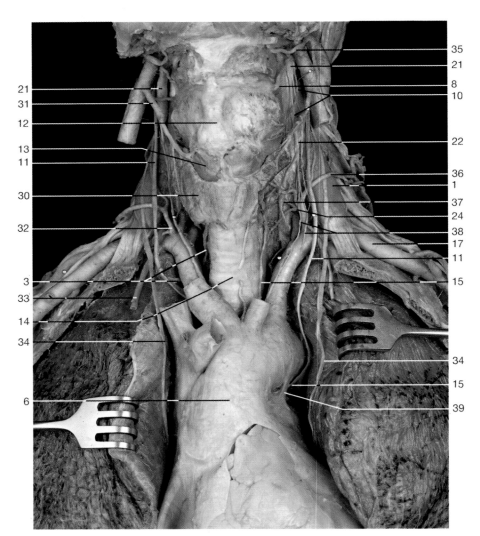

Larynx and thoracic organs (anterior aspect). Dissection of vagus and recurrent laryngeal nerves.

1 Scalenus anterior muscle
2 Scalenus medius and posterior muscles
3 Right recurrent laryngeal nerve
4 Right subclavian artery
5 Brachiocephalic trunk
6 Aortic arch
7 Hyoid bone
8 Internal branch of superior laryngeal nerve
9 Thyrohyoid membrane
10 External branch of superior laryngeal nerve
11 Vagus nerve
12 Thyroid cartilage
13 Cricothyroid muscle
14 Trachea
15 Left recurrent laryngeal nerve
16 Esophagus
17 Left subclavian artery
18 Left common carotid artery
19 Second rib
20 Tongue
21 Superior cervical ganglion
22 Sympathetic trunk
23 Inferior constrictor muscle of pharynx
24 Inferior thyroid artery
25 Glossopharyngeal nerve
26 Superior laryngeal nerve
27 Epiglottis
28 Posterior crico-arytenoid muscle and cricoid cartilage
29 Inferior laryngeal branch of recurrent laryngeal nerve
30 Thyroid gland
31 Superior thyroid artery
32 Thyrocervical trunk
33 Internal thoracic artery
34 Phrenic nerve
35 Hypoglossal nerve
36 Transverse cervical artery
37 Middle cervical ganglion
38 Middle cervical cardiac nerves (branches of sympathetic trunk)
39 Ligamentum arteriosum

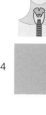

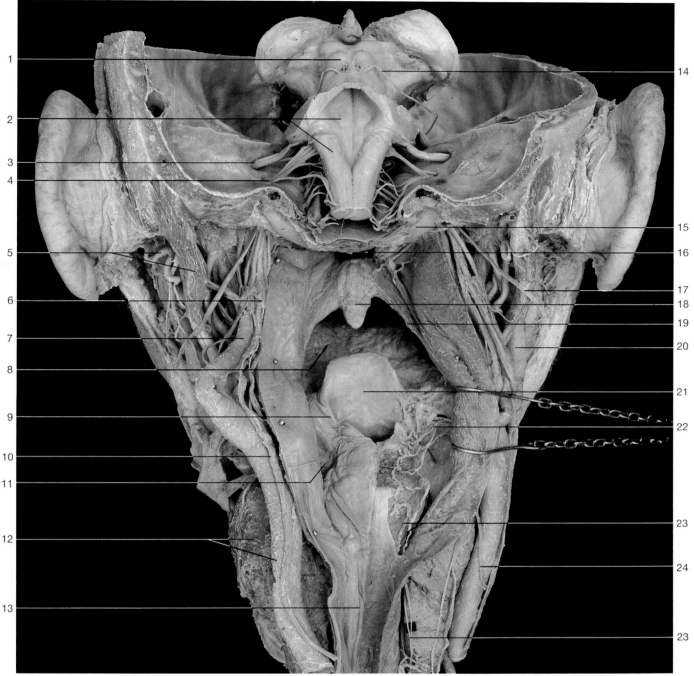

Larynx and oral cavity (posterior aspect). Mucous membrane on the right half of pharynx has been removed.

1 Midbrain (inferior colliculus)	9 Ary-epiglottic fold	18 Uvula and soft palate
2 Rhomboid fossa and medulla oblongata	10 Vagus nerve	19 Palatopharyngeus muscle
3 Vestibulocochlear and facial nerve	11 Piriform recess	20 External carotid artery
4 Glossopharyngeal, vagus, and accessory nerves	12 Thyroid gland and common carotid artery	21 Epiglottis
5 Occipital artery and posterior belly of digastric muscle	13 Esophagus	22 Internal branch of superior laryngeal nerve
6 Superior cervical ganglion	14 Trochlear nerve	23 Inferior laryngeal nerve
7 Internal carotid artery	15 Occipital condyle	24 Ansa cervicalis
8 Oral cavity (tongue)	16 Nasal cavity (choana)	
	17 Accessory nerve	

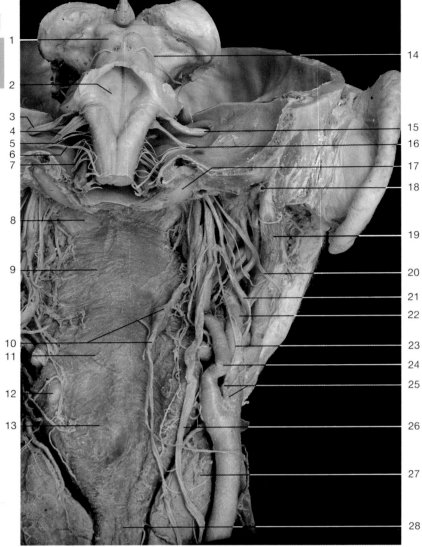

1   Inferior colliculus of midbrain
2   Facial colliculus in floor of rhomboid fossa
3   Vestibulocochlear and facial nerves
4   Glossopharyngeal nerve
5   Vagus nerve
6   Accessory nerve
7   Hypoglossal nerve
8   Pharyngobasilar fascia
9   Superior constrictor muscle of pharynx
10 Sympathetic trunk and superior cervical
    ganglion (medially displaced)
11 Middle constrictor muscle of pharynx
12 Greater cornu of hyoid bone
13 Inferior constrictor muscle of pharynx
14 Trochlear nerve
15 Internal acoustic meatus with facial and
    vestibulocochlear nerves
16 Jugular foramen with glossopharyngeal,
    vagus, and assessory nerves
17 Occipital condyle
18 Occipital artery
19 Posterior belly of digastric muscle
20 Accessory nerve (extracranial part)
21 Hypoglossal nerve (extracranial part)
22 External carotid artery
23 Carotid sinus nerve
24 Internal carotid artery
25 Carotid sinus and carotid body
26 Vagus nerve
27 Thyroid gland
28 Esophagus
29 Choanae
30 Medial pterygoid plate
31 Foramen lacerum
32 Pharyngeal tubercle
33 Hard palate
34 Greater and lesser palatine foramen
35 Pterygoid hamulus
36 Lateral pterygoid plate
37 Pterygoid canal
38 Foramen ovale
39 Mandibular fossa
40 Carotid canal
41 Styloid process and stylomastoid
    foramen

Pharynx and parapharyngeal nerves in connection with brain stem
(posterior aspect).

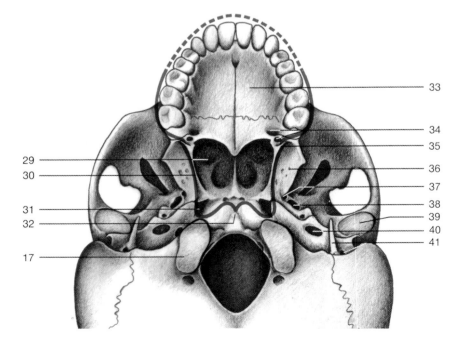

Inferior aspect of the skull.
Red line = outline of superior constrictor muscle
in continuation with buccinator muscle and
orbicularis oris muscle (semischematic drawing).

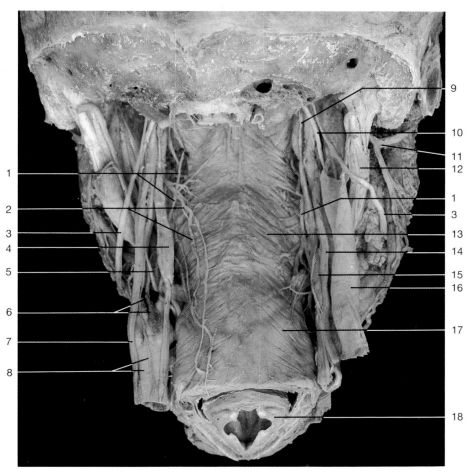

Parapharyngeal nerves and vessels. Dorsal aspect of the pharynx.

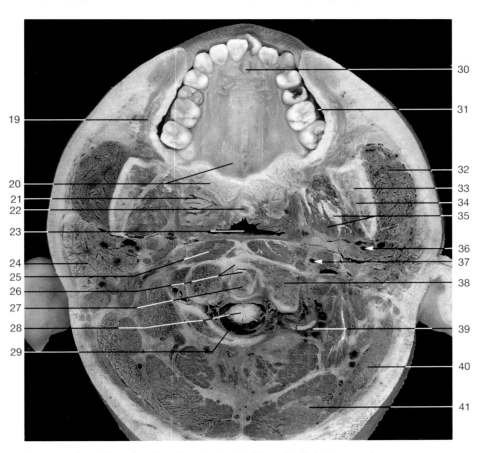

Cross section of head and neck at the level of the atlas (inferior aspect).

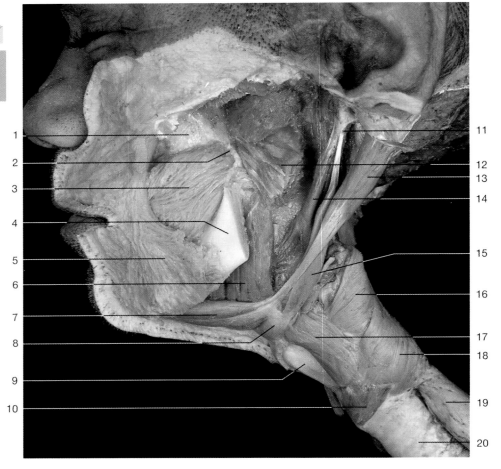

1	Maxilla
2	Pterygomandibular raphe
3	Buccinator muscle
4	Mandible (divided)
5	Depressor anguli oris muscle
6	Mylohyoid muscle
7	Anterior belly of digastric muscle
8	Hyoid bone
9	Thyroid cartilage
10	Cricothyroid muscle
11	Styloid process
12	Medial pterygoid muscle (divided)
13	Posterior belly of digastric muscle
14	Styloglossus muscle
15	Stylohyoid muscle
16	Thyropharyngeal part of inferior constrictor muscle of pharynx
17	Thyrohyoid muscle
18	Cricopharyngeal part of inferior constrictor muscle of pharynx
19	Esophagus
20	Trachea
21	First molar of maxilla
22	Tongue
23	Inferior longitudinal muscle of tongue
24	Genioglossus muscle
25	Superior constrictor muscle of pharynx
26	Hypoglossal nerve
27	Hyoglossus muscle
28	Superior laryngeal nerve and superior laryngeal artery

Dissection of pharynx, supra-, and infrahyoid muscles. Mandible partly removed (lateral aspect).

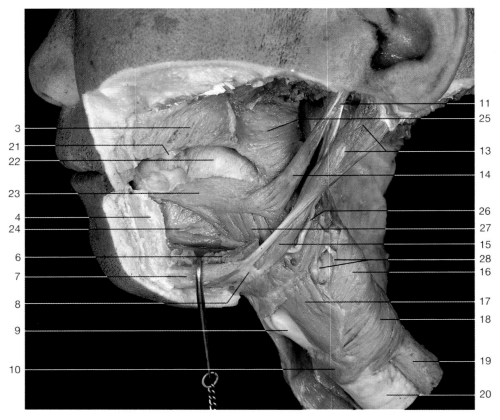

Dissection of pharynx, supra-, and infrahyoid muscles. Oral cavity opened (lateral aspect).

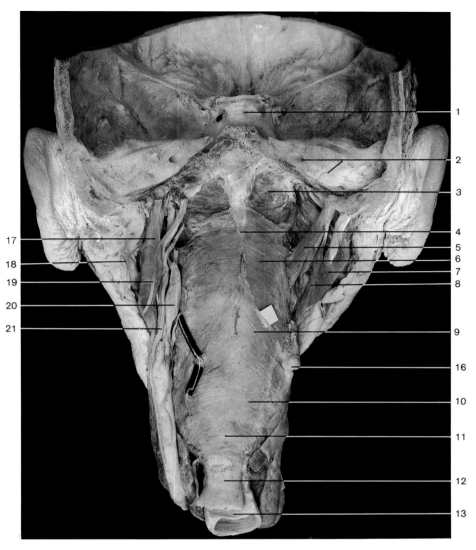

1   Sella turcica
2   Internal acoustic meatus and petrous part of temporal bone
3   Pharyngobasilar fascia
4   Fibrous raphe of pharynx
5   Stylopharyngeal muscle
6   Superior constrictor muscle of pharynx
7   Posterior belly of digastric muscle
8   Stylohyoid muscle
9   Middle constrictor muscle of pharynx
10 Inferior constrictor muscle of pharynx
11 Muscle-free area (Killian's triangle)
12 Esophagus
13 Trachea
14 Thyroid and parathyroid glands
15 Medial pterygoid muscle
16 Greater horn of hyoid bone
17 Internal jugular vein
18 Parotid gland
19 Accessory nerve
20 Superior cervical ganglion of sympathetic trunk
21 Vagus nerve
22 Laimer's triangle (area prone to developing diverticula)
23 Orbicularis oculi muscle
24 Nasalis muscle
25 Levator labii superioris and levator labii alaeque nasi muscles
26 Levator anguli oris muscle
27 Orbicularis oris muscle
28 Buccinator muscle
29 Depressor labii inferioris muscle
30 Hyoglossus muscle
31 Thyrohyoid muscle
32 Thyroid cartilage
33 Cricothyroid muscle
34 Pterygomandibular raphe
35 Tensor veli palatini muscle
36 Levator veli palatini muscle
37 Depressor anguli oris muscle
38 Mentalis muscle
39 Styloglossus muscle

Muscles of the pharynx (posterior aspect).

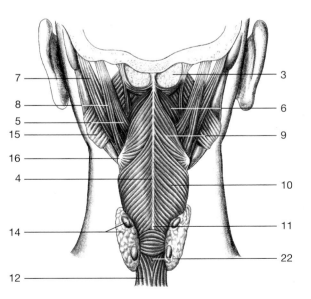

Muscles of the pharynx (posterior aspect). (Schematic drawing.)

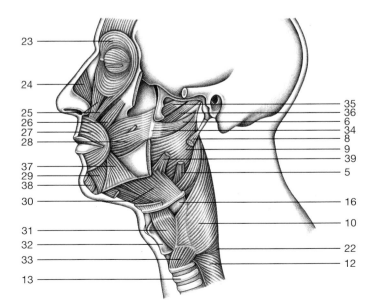

Muscles of the pharynx (lateral aspect). (Schematic drawing.)

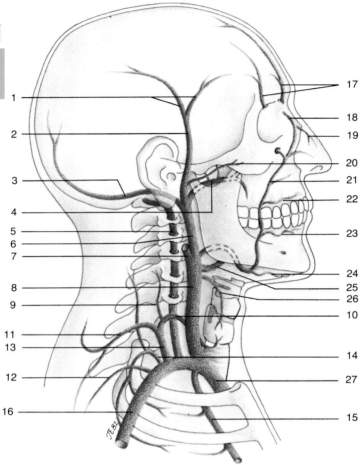

1   Frontal and parietal branches of superficial
    temporal artery
2   Superficial temporal artery
3   Occipital artery
4   Maxillary artery
5   Vertebral artery
6   External carotid artery
7   Internal carotid artery
8   Common carotid artery (divided)
9   Ascending cervical artery
10 Inferior thyroid artery
11 Transverse cervical artery with two branches
    (superficial cervical artery and descending
    scapular artery)
12 Suprascapular artery
13 Thyrocervical trunk
14 Costocervical trunk with two branches
    (deep cervical artery and superior intercostal artery)
15 Internal thoracic artery
16 Axillary artery
17 Supra-orbital and supratrochlear arteries
18 Angular artery
19 Dorsal nasal artery
20 Transverse facial artery
21 Facial artery
22 Superior labial artery
23 Inferior labial artery
24 Submental artery
25 Lingual artery
26 Superior thyroid artery
27 Brachiocephalic trunk

Arteries of head and neck. Diagram of the main branches
of external carotid and subclavian arteries.

▷   **To page 169:**

1   Galea aponeurotica
2   Frontal branch ⎱ of superficial
3   Parietal branch ⎰ temporal artery
4   Superior auricular muscle
5   Superficial temporal artery and vein
6   Middle temporal artery
7   Auriculotemporal nerve
8   Branches of facial nerve
9   Facial nerve
10 External carotid artery within the
    retromandibular fossa
11 Posterior belly of digastric muscle
12 Sternocleidomastoid artery
13 Sympathetic trunk and superior cervical ganglion
14 Sternocleidomastoid muscle (divided and reflected)
15 Clavicle (divided)
16 Transverse cervical artery
17 Ascending cervical artery and phrenic nerve
18 Scalenus anterior muscle
19 Suprascapular artery

20 Dorsal scapular artery
21 Brachial plexus and axillary artery
22 Thoraco-acromial artery
23 Lateral thoracic artery
24 Median nerve (displaced) and
    pectoralis minor muscle (reflected)
25 Frontal belly of occipitofrontalis muscle
26 Orbital part of orbicularis oculi muscle
27 Angular artery and vein
28 Facial artery
29 Superior labial artery
30 Zygomaticus major muscle
31 Inferior labial artery
32 Parotid duct
33 Buccal fat pad
34 Maxillary artery
35 Masseter muscle
36 Facial artery and mandible
37 Submental artery
38 Anterior belly of digastric muscle

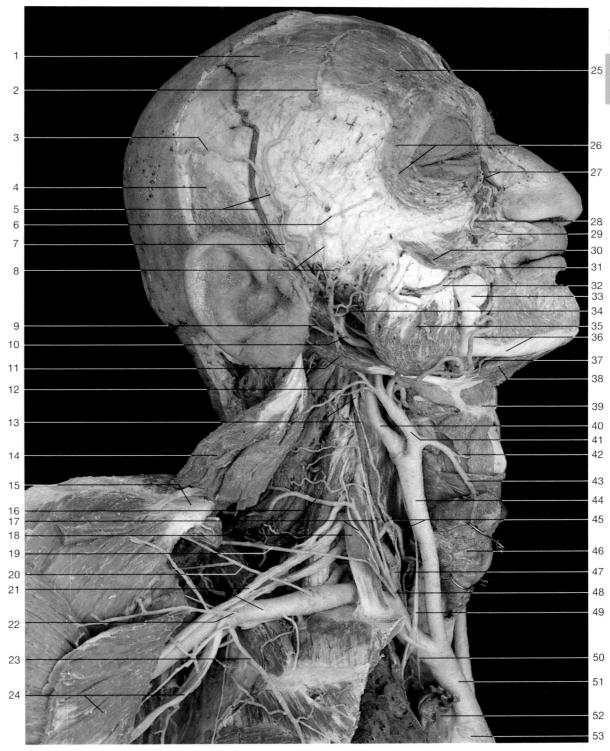

Main branches of head and neck arteries (lateral aspect). Anterior thoracic wall and clavicle partly removed; pectoralis muscles have been reflected to display the subclavian and axillary arteries.

39 Hyoid bone
40 Internal carotid artery
41 External carotid artery
42 Superior laryngeal artery
43 Superior thyroid artery
44 Common carotid artery
45 Thyroid ansa of sympathetic
   trunk and inferior thyroid artery

46 Thyroid gland (right lobe)
47 Vertebral artery
48 Thyrocervical trunk
49 Vagus nerve
50 Ansa subclavia of sympathetic trunk
51 Brachiocephalic trunk
52 Superior vena cava (divided)
53 Aortic arch

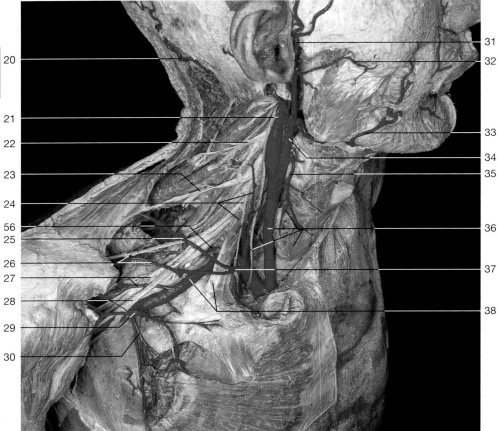

Arteries of head and neck (antero-lateral aspect). Clavicle, sternocleidomastoid muscle, and veins have been partly removed; the arteries have been colored.

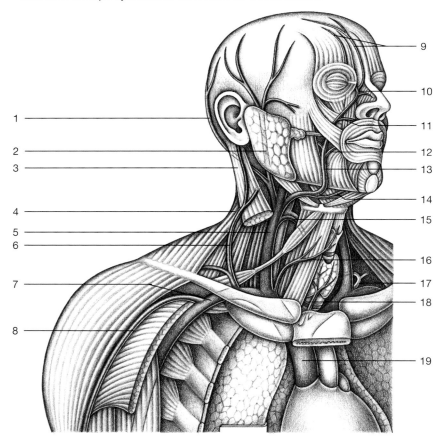

Veins of head and neck. Sternocleidomastoid muscle and anterior thoracic wall partly removed. Note the venous connection with the superior vena cava.

1 Occipital vein
2 Superficial temporal vein
3 Sternocleidomastoid muscle
4 Trapezius muscle
5 Internal jugular vein
6 External jugular vein
7 Subclavian vein
8 Cephalic vein
9 Supra-orbital veins
10 Angular vein
11 Superior labial vein
12 Inferior labial vein
13 Facial vein
14 Submental vein
15 Superior thyroid vein
16 Anterior jugular vein
17 Thoracic duct
18 Inferior thyroid vein
19 Superior vena cava
20 Occipital branch of occipital artery
21 Internal carotid artery
22 Cervical plexus
23 Supraclavicular nerve
24 Phrenic nerve and ascending cervical artery on scalenus anterior muscle
25 Superficial cervical artery
26 Suprascapular artery and nerve
27 Brachial plexus and anterior circumflex humeral artery
28 Lateral cord of brachial plexus
29 Thoraco-acromial artery
30 Lateral thoracic artery
31 Superficial temporal artery
32 Transverse facial artery
33 Facial artery
34 External carotid artery
35 Superior thyroid artery
36 Common carotid artery, vagus nerve, and thyroid gland
37 Thyrocervical trunk
38 Subclavian artery and scalenus anterior muscle
39 Parotid gland and facial nerve
40 Great auricular nerve
41 External jugular vein
42 Brachial plexus
43 Cephalic vein in deltopectoral groove
44 Axillary vein and artery
45 Right brachiocephalic vein
46 Superior vena cava
47 Right lung (reflected)
48 Superficial temporal artery and vein
49 Facial artery and vein
50 Cervical branch of facial nerve and submandibular gland
51 Internal jugular vein, common carotid artery, and omohyoid muscle
52 Anterior jugular vein and thyroid gland
53 Jugular venous arch
54 Left brachiocephalic vein
55 Pericardium of heart (location of right atrium)
56 Transverse cervical artery

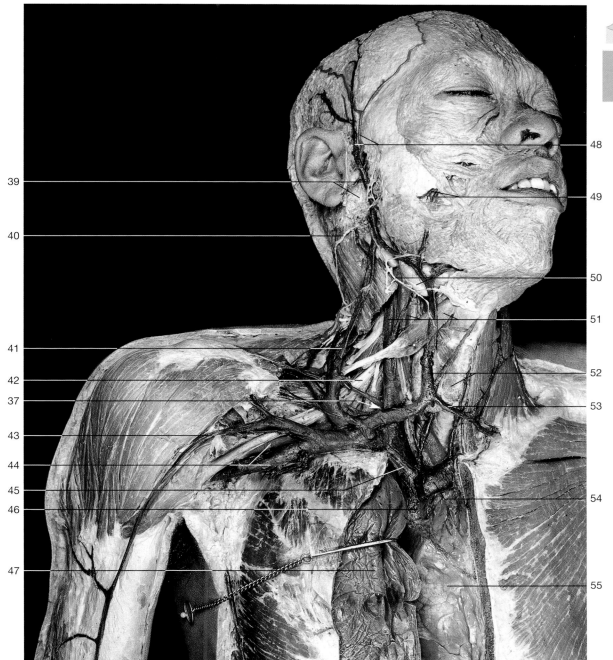

Veins of head and neck (anterior aspect). Part of the thoracic wall, clavicle, and sternocleidomastoid muscle have been removed. Veins are colored blue; arteries, red.

The **internal jugular vein** is the continuation of the sigmoid sinus, which drains most of the venous blood from the brain together with the external cerebrospinal fluid. By joining the subclavian vein, it forms the right brachiocephalic vein, which continues on the right side directly into the superior vena cava. The common way to introduce the lead from a pacemaker device into the heart is by way of the cephalic vein. On the left side, the thoracic duct joins the internal jugular vein at the point where the subclavian vein and the internal jugular vein form the left brachiocephalic vein. Note that the subclavian vein lies in front of the scalenus anterior muscle, whereas the subclavian artery and the brachial plexus lie posterior to that muscle. The **cephalic vein** joins the axillary vein by passing into the deltopectoral triangle. **The subclavian vein** is strongly fixed to the first rib, so it can be punctured with a needle at that point (underneath the sternal end of the clavicle) to introduce a catheter (subclavian line).

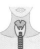

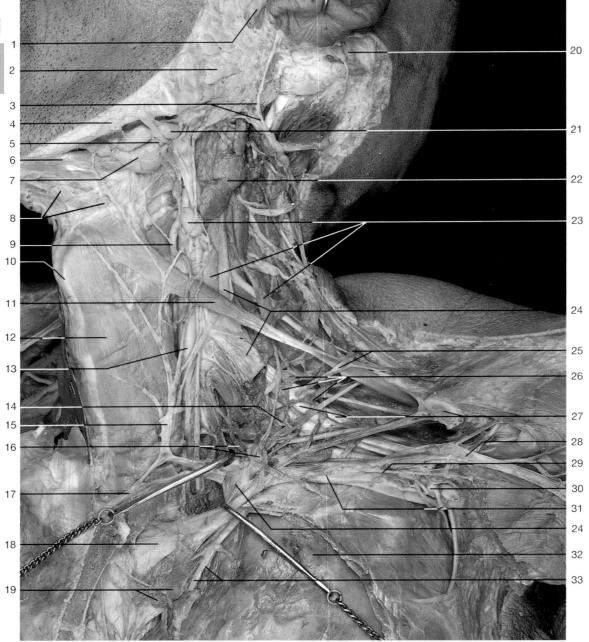

Lymph nodes and lymph vessels of the neck, left side oblique (oblique-lateral aspect). The sternocleidomastoid muscle and the left half of the thoracic wall have been removed. Lower part of the internal jugular vein has been cut and laterally displaced to show the thoracic duct.

1	Superficial parotid lymph node	13	Common carotid artery	24	Internal jugular vein
2	Parotid gland	14	Supraclavicular lymph nodes	25	External jugular vein
3	Great auricular nerve	15	Anterior jugular vein	26	Jugulo-omohyoid lymph nodes
4	Mandible	16	Thoracic duct and internal jugular vein	27	Brachial plexus
5	Facial vein	17	Jugular venous arch	28	Cephalic vein
6	Anterior belly of digastric muscle	18	Left brachiocephalic vein	29	Subclavian trunk
7	Submandibular gland	19	Superior mediastinal lymph nodes	30	Infraclavicular lymph nodes
8	Submental lymph nodes	20	Retro-auricular lymph nodes	31	Subclavian vein
9	Superior thyroid artery	21	Submandibular nodes	32	Lung
10	Thyroid cartilage	22	Superficial cervical lymph nodes	33	Internal thoracic artery and vein
11	Omohyoid muscle	23	Jugulodigastric lymph nodes and jugular trunk		
12	Sternohyoid muscle				

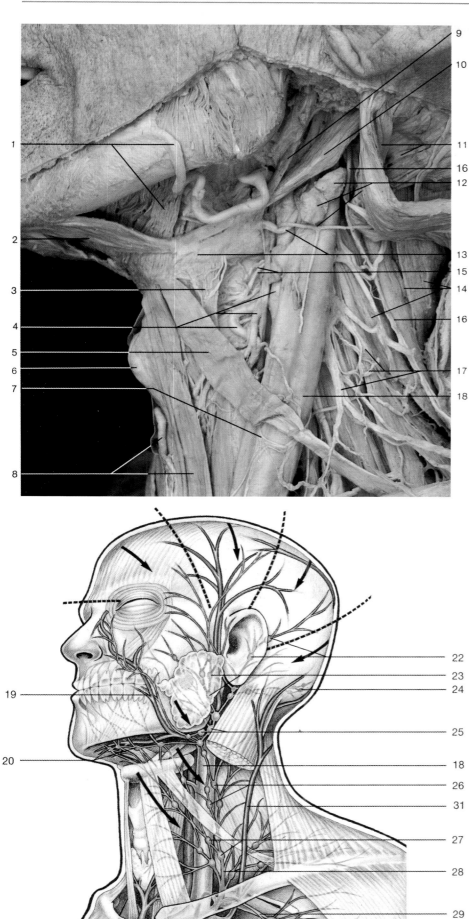

Carotid triangle, left side (lateral aspect). Sternocleidomastoid muscle reflected.

1   Mylohyoid muscle and facial artery
2   Anterior belly of digastric muscle
3   Thyrohyoid
4   External carotid artery,
    superior thyroid artery, and vein
5   Omohyoid muscle
6   Thyroid cartilage
7   Ansa cervicalis
8   Sternohyoid muscle and superior
    thyroid artery
9   Stylohyoid muscle
10 Posterior belly of digastric muscle
11 Sternocleidomastoid muscle (reflected)
12 Superior cervical lymph nodes and
    sternocleidomastoid artery
13 Hyoid bone and hypoglossal nerve
    (n. XII)
14 Splenius capitis and levator
    scapulae muscles
15 Superior laryngeal artery and
    internal branch of superior
    laryngeal nerve
16 Accessory nerve
17 Cervical plexus
18 Internal jugular vein
19 Facial vein
20 Submental nodes
21 Thoracic duct
22 Retro-auricular nodes
23 Parotid nodes
24 Occipital nodes
25 Submandibular nodes
26 Jugulodigastric nodes   } deep cervical
27 Jugulo-omohyoid nodes   } nodes
28 Jugular trunk
29 Subclavian trunk
30 Infraclavicular nodes
31 External jugular vein

Lymph nodes and veins of head and neck. Dotted lines = border between irrigation areas; arrows: direction of lymph flow.

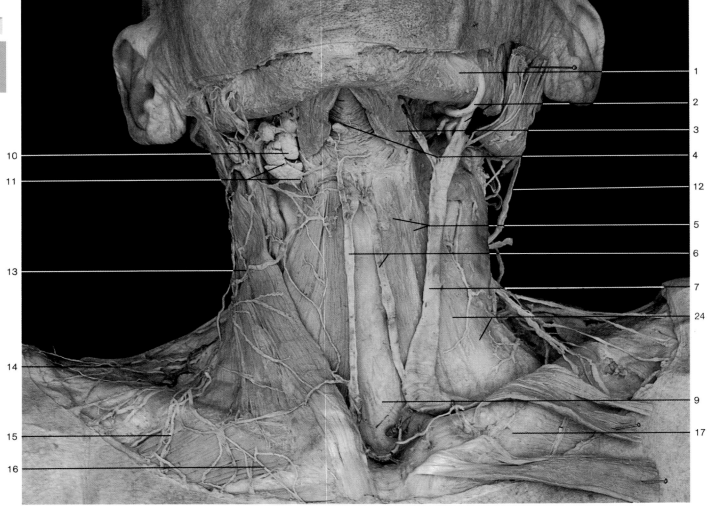

Anterior region of the neck. The superficial fascia has been removed.

1	Mandible
2	Facial artery and vein
3	Anterior belly of digastric muscle
4	Mylohyoid muscle
5	Infrahyoid muscles (sternohyoid, sternothyroid, and omohyoid muscles)
6	Anterior jugular veins
7	External jugular vein
8	Sternocleidomastoid muscle
9	Thyroid gland
10	Submandibular gland
11	Cervical branch of facial nerve
12	Great auricular nerve
13	Transverse cervical nerves
14	Lateral supraclavicular nerves
15	Middle supraclavicular nerves
16	Medial supraclavicular nerves

Cutaneous branches of cervical plexus (12, 13, 14, 15, 16)

17	Clavicle
18	Platysma muscle
19	Prevertebral lamina of cervical fascia, covering longus colli muscle
20	Vertebral artery and vein
21	Scalenus muscles
22	Trapezius muscle
23	Superficial lamina of cervical fascia
24	Pretracheal lamina of cervical fascia
25	Prevertebral lamina of cervical fascia
26	Carotid sheath with common carotid artery, internal jugular vein, and vagus nerve
27	Cervical part of sympathetic trunk
28	Carotid sheath

◁ **Cross section of the neck** at the level of the thyroid gland. Notice the position of the three laminae of cervical fascia (23, 24, 25).

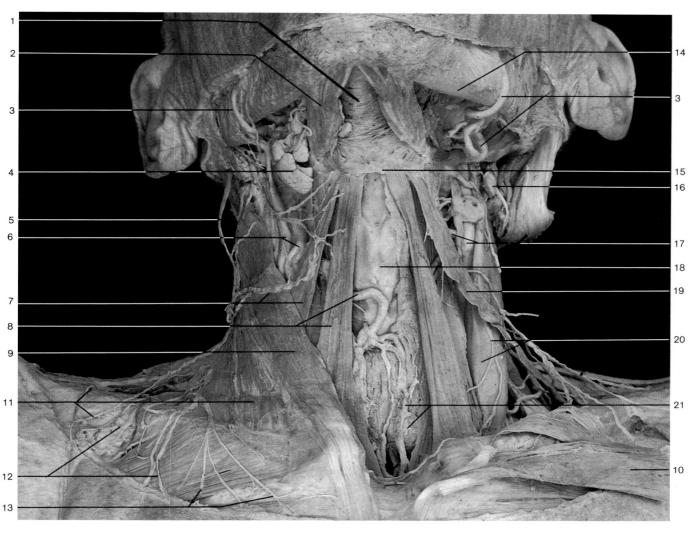

Anterior region of the neck with anterior triangle. The pretracheal lamina of cervical fascia and left sternocleidomastoid muscle have been removed.

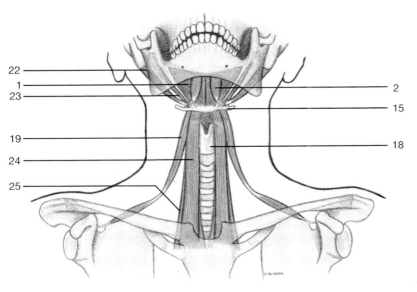

Supra- and infrahyoid muscles (schematic drawing).

1 Mylohyoid muscle
2 Anterior belly of digastric muscle
3 Facial artery
4 Submandibular gland
5 Great auricular nerve
6 Internal jugular vein and common carotid artery
7 Transverse cervical nerve and omohyoid muscle
8 Sternohyoid muscle and superior thyroid artery
9 Sternocleidomastoid muscle (sternal head)
10 Left sternocleidomastoid muscle (reflected)
11 Sternocleidomastoid muscle (clavicular head) and lateral supraclavicular nerves
12 Middle supraclavicular nerves
13 Medial supraclavicular nerves
14 Mandible
15 Hyoid bone
16 Superficial cervical lymph nodes
17 Left superior thyroid artery and external carotid artery
18 Thyroid cartilage
19 Omohyoid muscle (superior belly)
20 Internal jugular vein and branches of ansa cervicalis
21 Thyroid gland and unpaired inferior thyroid vein
22 Posterior belly of digastric muscle
23 Stylohyoid muscle
24 Sternohyoid muscle
25 Sternothyroid muscle

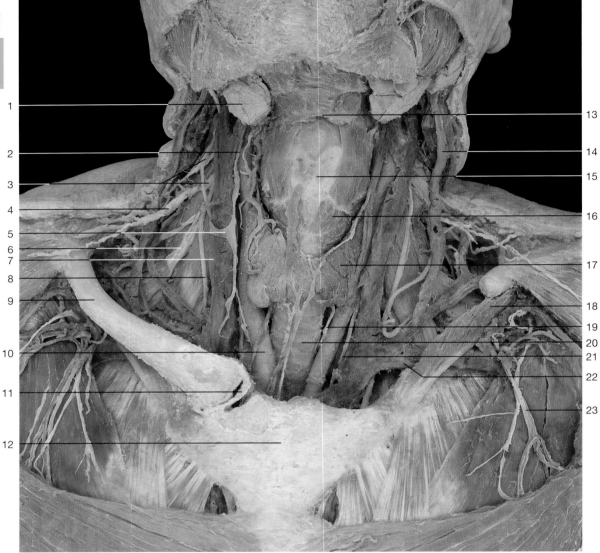

Anterior region of the neck. Sternocleidomastoid muscles and left clavicle have been removed. Thyroid gland in relation to trachea, larynx, and vessels of the neck is shown.

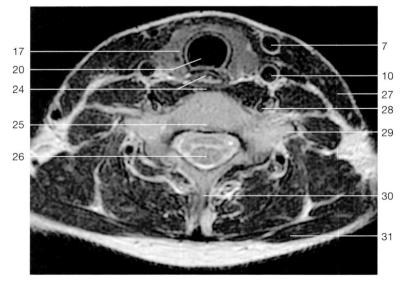

Cross section of the neck at the level of the thyroid gland (MRI scan, courtesy of Prof. Heuck, Munich).

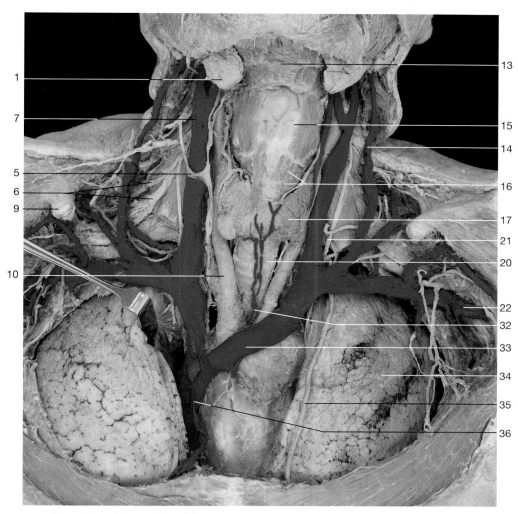

1   Submandibular gland
2   Cervical branch of facial nerve (n. VII)
3   Cervical plexus
4   Middle supraclavicular nerves
5   Ansa cervicalis
6   Brachial plexus
7   Internal jugular vein
8   Phrenic nerve
9   Clavicle
10 Common carotid artery
11 Sternoclavicular articulation with articular disc
12 Manubrium of sternum
13 Hyoid bone
14 External jugular vein
15 Thyroid cartilage
16 Cricothyroid muscle
17 Thyroid gland
18 Subclavius muscle
19 Recurrent laryngeal nerve
20 Trachea
21 Vagus nerve (n. X)
22 Subclavian vein
23 Middle pectoral nerve
24 Esophagus
25 Body of cervical vertebra
26 Spinal cord
27 Sternocleidomastoid muscle
28 Vertebral artery
29 Transverse process of cervical vertebra
30 Spinous process of cervical vertebra
31 Trapezius muscle
32 Inferior thyroid vein
33 Left brachiocephalic vein
34 Superior lobe of left lung
35 Internal thoracic artery
36 Superior vena cava
37 Superior thyroid artery
38 Inferior thyroid artery
39 Thyrocervical trunk
40 Subclavian artery
41 Aortic arch

Anterior region of the neck and thoracic cavity. Both clavicles, sternum, and ribs have been removed. Main veins are colored in blue.

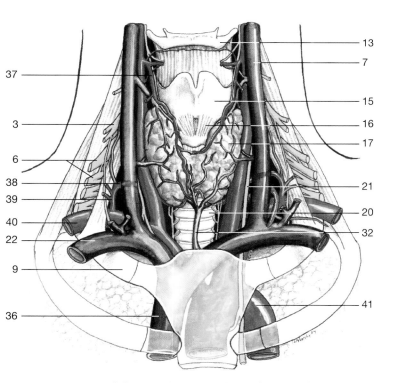

Anterior region of the neck (schematic drawing). Regional anatomy of the thyroid gland with related blood vessels.

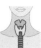

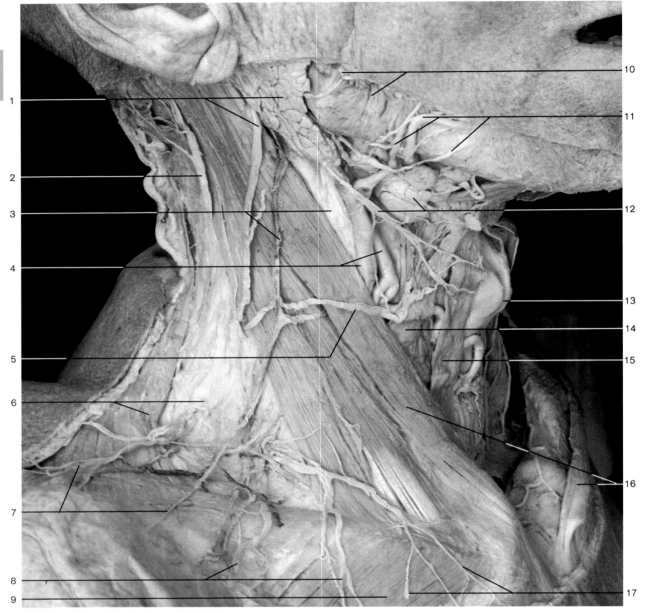

Lateral region of the neck with posterior and carotid triangles. Superficial dissection.

1 Parotid gland and great auricular nerve
2 Lesser occipital nerve
3 Internal and external jugular veins
4 Retromandibular vein and external carotid artery
5 Transverse cervical nerve with communicating branch to cervical branch of facial nerve
6 Trapezius muscle and superficial lamina of cervical fascia
7 Lateral supraclavicular nerves
8 Middle supraclavicular nerves
9 Pectoralis major muscle
10 Buccal branch of facial nerve and masseter muscle

11 Facial artery and vein and mandibular branch of facial nerve
12 Cervical branch of facial nerve and submandibular gland
13 Thyroid cartilage
14 Omohyoid muscle
15 Sternohyoid muscle
16 Sternocleidomastoid muscle
17 Medial supraclavicular nerves
18 Mandibular branch of facial nerve
19 Cervical branch of facial nerve with communicating branch to transverse cervical nerve

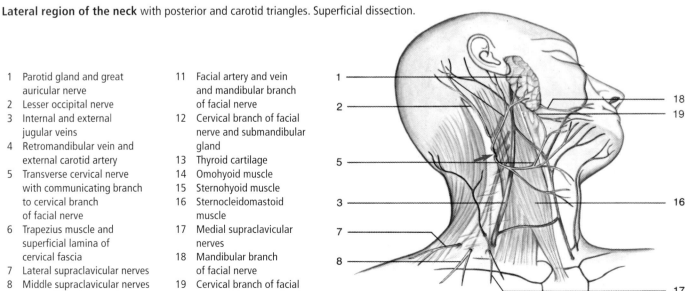

Cutaneous branches of cervical plexus. Erb's point is indicated by an arrowhead (schematic drawing).

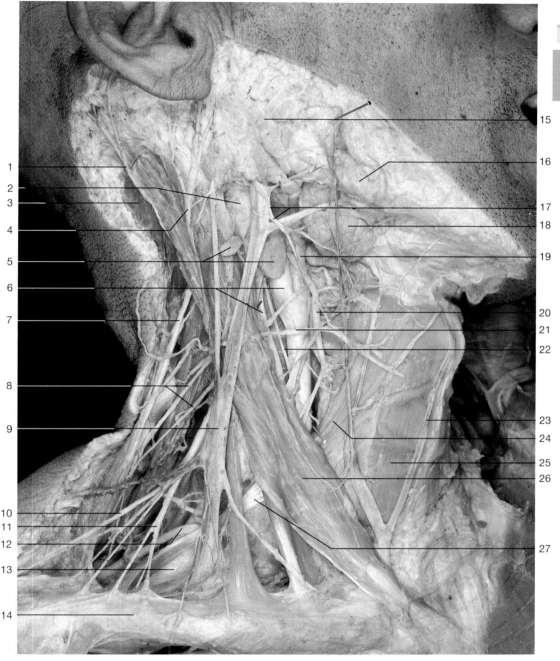

Lateral region of the neck with posterior and carotid triangles. Superficial dissection. The superficial lamina of cervical fascia has been removed to display the cutaneous branches of the cervical plexus and subcutaneous veins.

1 Lesser occipital nerve	15 Parotid gland
2 Internal jugular vein	16 Mandible
3 Splenius capitis muscle	17 Cervical branch of facial nerve
4 Great auricular nerve	18 Submandibular gland
5 Submandibular nodes	19 External carotid artery
6 Internal carotid artery and vagus nerve	20 Superior thyroid artery
7 Accessory nerve	21 Transverse cervical nerve
8 Muscular branches of cervical plexus	22 Superior root of ansa cervicalis
9 External jugular vein	23 Anterior jugular vein
10 Posterior supraclavicular nerves	24 Omohyoid muscle
11 Middle supraclavicular nerves	25 Sternohyoid muscle
12 Suprascapular artery	26 Sternocleidomastoid muscle
13 Pretracheal lamina of fascia of neck	27 Intermediate tendon of omohyoid muscle
14 Clavicle	

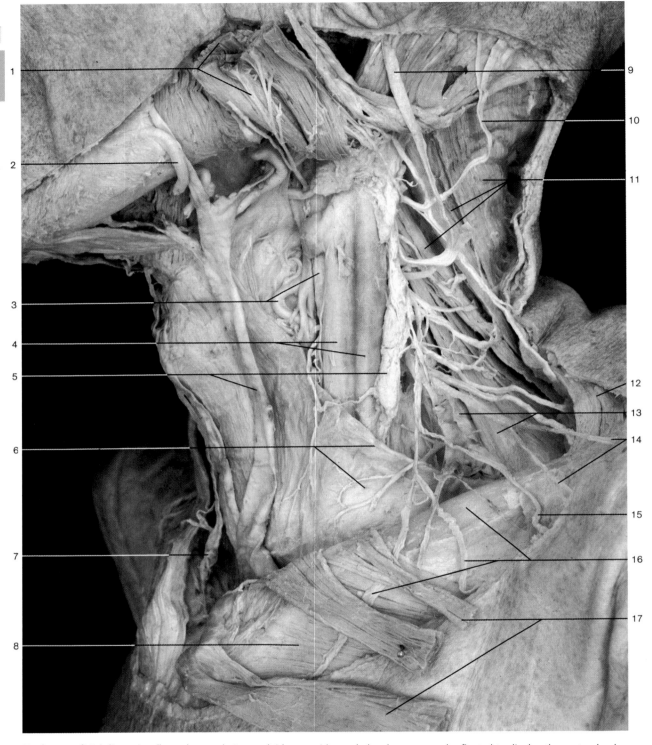

Neck, superficial dissection (lateral aspect). Sternocleidomastoid muscle has been cut and reflected to display the pretracheal lamina of the cervical fascia.

1 Sternocleidomastoid muscle (reflected) and branch of accessory nerve
2 Facial artery
3 External carotid artery and superior thyroid artery
4 Internal jugular vein
5 Deep cervical lymph nodes and external jugular vein
6 Omohyoid muscle and pretracheal lamina of cervical fascia
7 Anterior jugular vein
8 Pectoralis major muscle

9 Great auricular nerve
10 Lesser occipital nerve
11 Splenius capitis and levator scapulae muscles
12 Trapezius muscle
13 Scalenus medius muscle and brachial plexus
14 Posterior supraclavicular nerves
15 Middle supraclavicular nerve
16 Clavicle and anterior supraclavicular nerves
17 Sternocleidomastoid muscle (reflected)

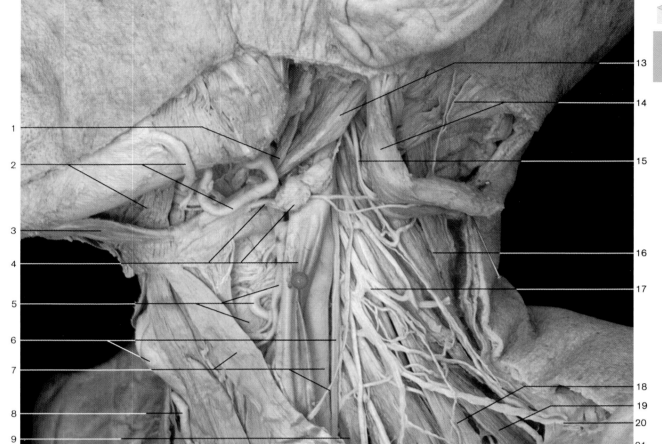

Neck, deep dissection (lateral aspect). The internal jugular vein has been reflected to expose the carotid artery and vagus nerve.

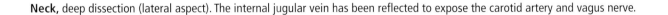

1 Stylohyoid muscle	13 Posterior belly of digastric muscle
2 Facial artery and mylohyoid muscle	14 Sternocleidomastoid muscle and lesser occipital nerve
3 Anterior belly of digastric muscle	15 Accessory nerve
4 Internal jugular vein, hypoglossal nerve, and superficial cervical lymph nodes	16 Splenius capitis muscle
5 Superior thyroid artery and vein and inferior pharyngeal constrictor muscle	17 Cervical plexus
6 Thyroid cartilage and vagus nerve	18 Scalenus posterior muscle
7 Ansa cervicalis, omohyoid muscle, and common carotid artery	19 Levator scapulae muscle
8 Right superior thyroid artery	20 Posterior supraclavicular nerves
9 Scalenus anterior muscle	21 Phrenic nerve
10 Sternothyroid muscle and inferior thyroid artery	22 Middle supraclavicular nerve
11 Muscular branches of ansa cervicalis to the infrahyoid muscles	23 Brachial plexus
12 Inferior thyroid vein	24 Anterior supraclavicular nerves
	25 Sternocleidomastoid muscle

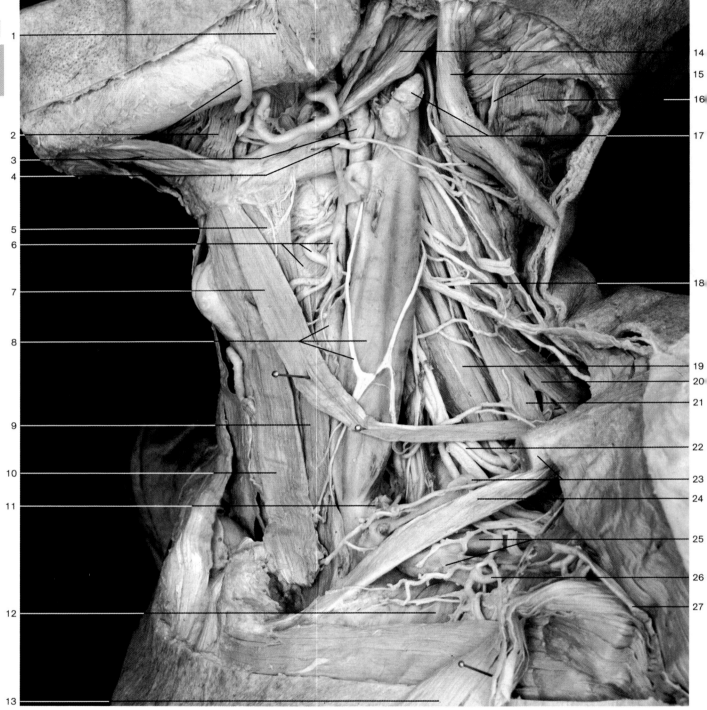

Neck, deeper dissection (lateral aspect). **Ansa cervicalis.** The cervical fascia and the clavicle are partly removed. Ansa cervicalis and infrahyoid muscles are displayed.

1 Masseter muscle	9 Sternothyroid muscle	18 Cervical plexus
2 Mylohyoid muscle and facial artery	10 Sternohyoid muscle	19 Scalenus medius muscle
3 External carotid artery and anterior belly of digastric muscle	11 Thoracic duct	20 Levator scapulae muscle
4 Hypoglossal nerve	12 Pectoralis minor muscle	21 Scalenus posterior muscle
5 Thyrohyoid muscle	13 Pectoralis major muscle	22 Brachial plexus
6 Superior thyroid artery and vein and inferior pharyngeal constrictor muscle	14 Posterior belly of digastric muscle	23 Transverse cervical artery and clavicle
7 Omohyoid muscle (superior belly)	15 Sternocleidomastoid muscle and lesser occipital nerve	24 Subclavius muscle
8 Ansa cervicalis, thyroid gland, and internal jugular vein	16 Splenius capitis muscle	25 Subclavian artery and vein
	17 Superficial cervical lymph nodes and accessory nerve	26 Thoraco-acromial artery
		27 Cephalic vein

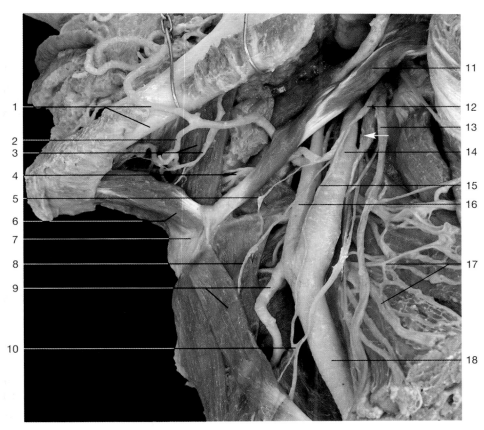

1   Facial artery and mandible
2   Submental artery
3   Mylohyoid muscle and nerve
4   Hypoglossal nerve
    (lingual branches)
5   Thyrohyoid branch of hypoglossal
    nerve (n. XII)
6   Anterior belly of digastric muscle
7   Hyoid bone
8   Omohyoid branch of hypoglossal
    nerve (n. XII)
9   Omohyoid muscle and superior
    thyroid artery
10 Ansa cervicalis
11 Posterior belly of digastric muscle
12 Hypoglossal nerve (n. XII)
13 Vagus nerve (n. X)
14 Internal carotid artery
15 Superior root of ansa cervicalis
16 External carotid artery
17 Cervical plexus
18 Common carotid artery
19 Facial artery and vein
20 Omohyoid muscle
21 Internal jugular vein
22 Sternohyoid and sternothyroid
    muscles
23 Clavicle
24 Superficial temporal artery and vein
25 Occipital artery
26 Spinal nerves (C$_3$ and C$_4$)
27 Spinal processes of cervical
    vertebrae (C$_4$ and C$_5$)
28 Scapula

Neck with submandibular region (lateral aspect). **Hypoglossal nerve** (n. XII). Mandible slightly elevated. Arrow = superior cervical ganglion.

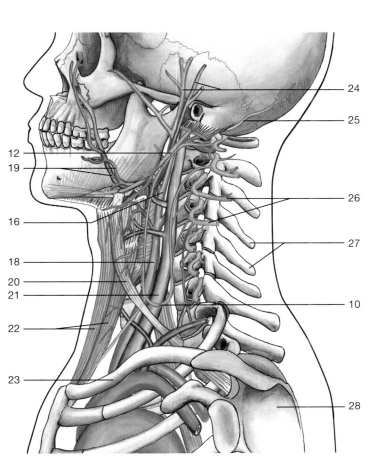

Nerves and vessels of the neck (lateral aspect).
The ansa cervicalis with connection to the spinal nerves is depicted.

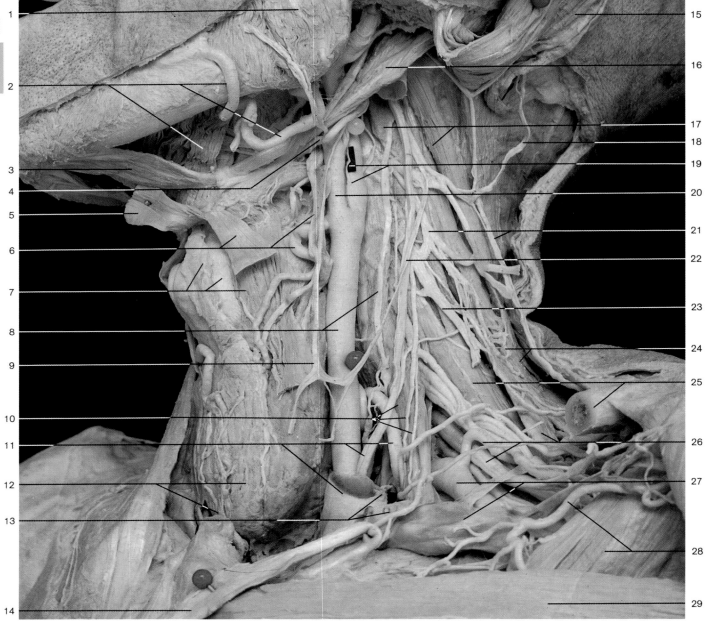

Neck, deeper dissection (lateral aspect). Clavicle partly removed to show the slit between the scalenus muscles. Internal jugular vein removed.

1	Masseter muscle
2	Mylohyoid muscle and facial artery
3	Anterior belly of digastric muscle
4	Hypoglossal nerve
5	Sternohyoid muscle
6	Omohyoid muscle, superior thyroid artery and vein
7	Sternothyroid muscle, thyroid cartilage, and pyramidal lobe of thyroid gland
8	Common carotid artery and sympathetic trunk
9	Ansa cervicalis
10	Phrenic nerve, ascending cervical artery, and anterior scalenus muscle
11	Inferior thyroid artery, vagus nerve, and internal jugular vein (cut)
12	Thyroid gland and unpaired inferior thyroid venous plexus
13	Thoracic duct and left subclavian trunk
14	Subclavius muscle (reflected)
15	Sternocleidomastoid muscle (reflected)
16	Posterior belly of digastric muscle
17	Superior cervical ganglion and splenius muscle
18	Lesser occipital nerve
19	Internal carotid artery and branch of the glossopharyngeal nerve to the carotid body
20	External carotid artery
21	Cervical plexus and accessory nerve
22	Inferior root of ansa cervicalis
23	Supraclavicular nerve
24	Levator scapulae muscle
25	Scalenus medius muscle and clavicle
26	Transverse cervical artery, brachial plexus, and scalenus posterior muscle
27	Subclavian artery and vein
28	Thoraco-acromial artery and pectoralis minor muscle
29	Pectoralis major muscle

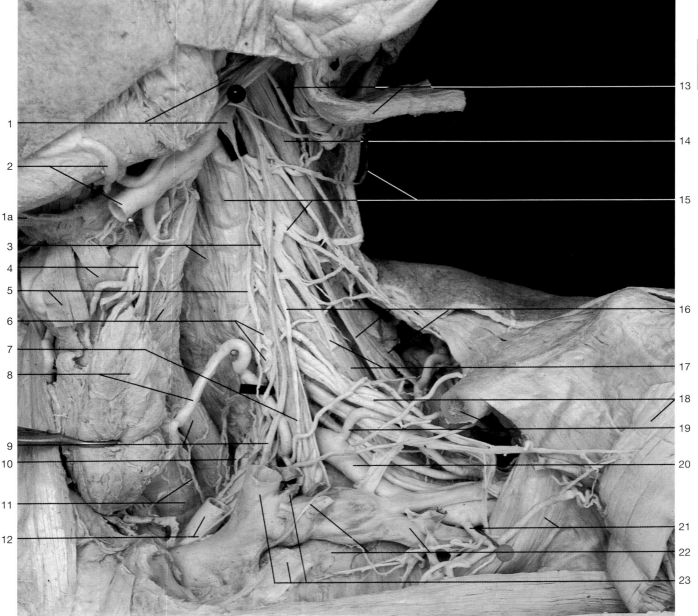

Neck, deepest dissection (antero-lateral aspect). Thyroid gland reflected to expose the esophagus and the recurrent laryngeal nerve.

1 Superior cervical ganglion of sympathetic trunk and posterior belly of digastric muscle
1a Anterior belly of digastric muscle
2 Facial artery and common carotid artery (reflected anteriorly)
3 Ascending cervical artery and longus colli muscle
4 Omohyoid muscle and superior thyroid artery
5 Sympathetic trunk and sternohyoid muscle
6 Middle cervical ganglion and inferior pharyngeal constrictor muscle
7 Scalenus anterior muscle and phrenic nerve
8 Thyroid gland and inferior thyroid artery
9 Vagus nerve and esophagus
10 Stellate ganglion
11 Recurrent laryngeal nerve and trachea

12 Common carotid artery and cervical cardiac branch of vagus nerve
13 Sternocleidomastoid muscle and accessory nerve
14 Splenius capitis muscle
15 Lesser occipital nerve, longus capitis muscle, and cervical plexus
16 Phrenic nerve, scalenus posterior muscle, and levator scapulae muscle
17 Supraclavicular nerves and scalenus medius muscle
18 Brachial plexus and pectoralis major muscle (clavicular head)
19 Transverse cervical artery and clavicle
20 Subclavian artery
21 Thoraco-acromial artery and pectoralis minor muscle
22 First rib, accessory phrenic nerve, and subclavian vein
23 Internal jugular vein, thoracic duct, and subclavius muscle

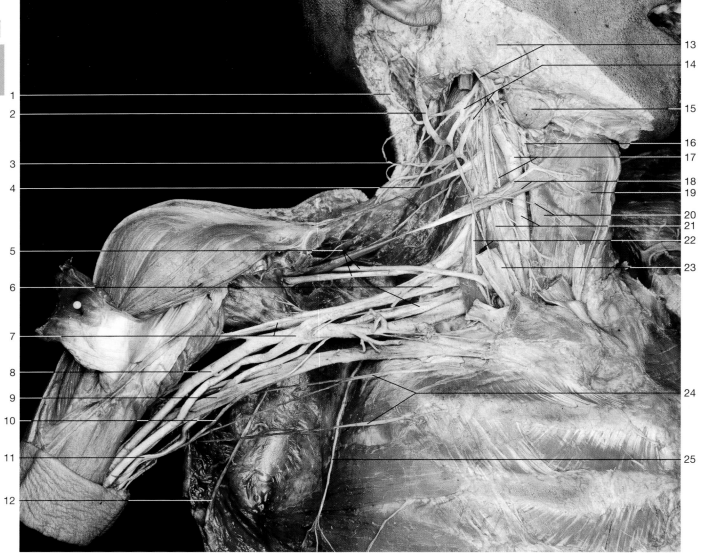

Neck and arm, deepest dissection (antero-lateral aspect). **Cervical and brachial plexuses** and their relation to the blood vessels are shown. Note the location and content of scalene triangle. Sternocleidomastoid muscle and clavicle have been removed; the internal jugular vein was divided to display the roots of cervical and brachial plexuses.

1 Lesser occipital nerve
2 Great auricular nerve
3 Cutaneous branches of cervical plexus
4 Supraclavicular nerve
5 Suprascapular nerve and artery
6 Brachial plexus
7 Median nerve (with two roots) and musculocutaneous nerve
8 Axillary artery
9 Axillary vein
10 Medial brachial cutaneous nerve
11 Ulnar nerve
12 Thoracodorsal nerve
13 Parotid gland and facial nerve (cervical branch)
14 Cervical plexus

15 Submandibular gland
16 Superior thyroid artery
17 Common carotid artery dividing in internal and external carotid artery and superior root of ansa cervicalis
18 Omohyoid muscle and cervical branch of facial nerve joining the transverse cervical nerve (C_2, C_3)
19 Sternohyoid muscle
20 Transverse cervical nerve and sternothyroid muscle
21 Common carotid artery and vagus nerve
22 Phrenic nerve and scalenus anterior muscle
23 Internal jugular vein
24 Intercostobrachial nerves
25 Long thoracic nerve

3 Trunk

The anterior abdominal and thoracic walls reveal a segmental structure. The ribs are connected by intercostal muscles forming defined skeleto-motoric and neuro-vascular segments.

At the abdominal wall, the segments form great flat muscles, that end anteriorly in strong sheet-like aponeuroses. The aponeurosis interlace at the linea alba with their counterparts from the opposite side to form the tough tendinous sheath of the rectus muscle. Movements of the abdominal wall also support the process of respiration functionally related to the diaphragm.

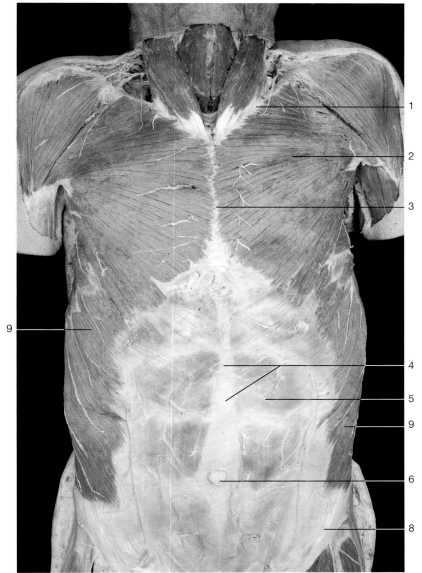

Anterior thoracic and abdominal walls with superficial musculature.
The fascia of pectoralis major muscle and the abdominal wall have been removed; the anterior layer of the sheath of the rectus abdominis muscle is displayed.

1 Clavicle
2 Pectoralis major muscle
3 Sternum
4 Linea alba
5 Anterior layer of rectus sheath
6 Umbilicus
7 Internal abdominal oblique muscle
8 Inguinal ligament
9 External abdominal oblique muscle

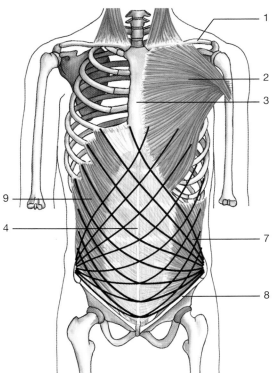

Organization of the thoracic and abdominal walls.
The architecture of tendon fibers of the two abdominal oblique muscles in the rectus sheath is shown.

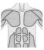

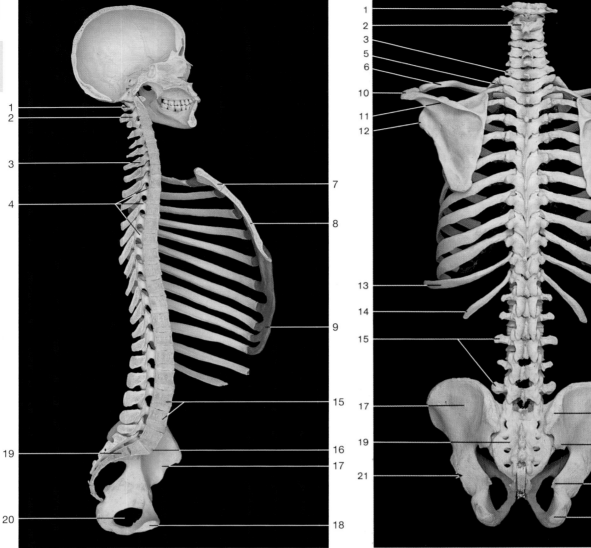

Median sagittal section through the vertebral column, head, and thorax of the adult.

Skeleton of the trunk, vertebral column, thorax, and pelvis (posterior aspect).

1	Atlas	14	Twelfth rib
2	Axis	15	Lumbar vertebrae
3	Seventh cervical vertebra (vertebra prominens)	16	Sacral promontory
4	Vertebral canal	17	Hip bone
5	First rib	18	Pubic symphysis
6	Clavicle	19	Sacrum
7	Manubrium sterni	20	Obturator foramen
8	Body of sternum	21	Acetabulum
9	Costal arch	22	Scapula with coracoid process
10	Acromion	23	Posterior superior iliac spine
11	Spine of scapula	24	Posterior inferior iliac spine
12	Glenoid cavity (lateral angle of scapula)	25	Ischial spine
13	Eleventh rib	26	Ischial tuberosity

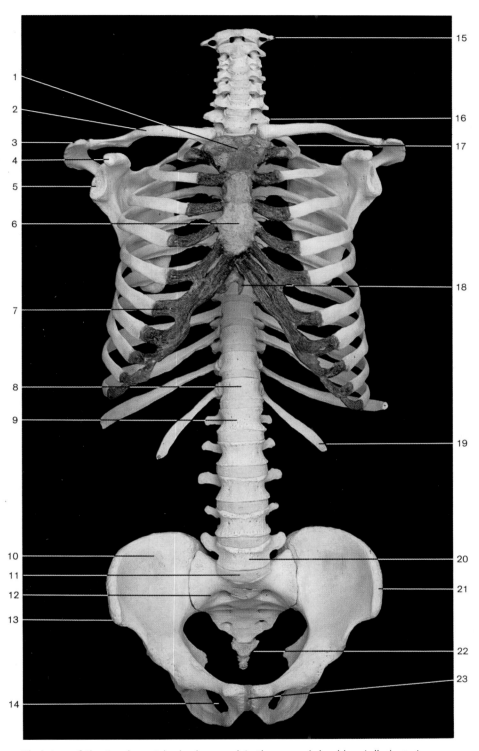

Skeleton of the trunk, vertebral column, pelvis, thorax, and shoulder girdle (anterior aspect).

1   Manubrium sterni
2   Clavicle
3   Acromion
4   Coracoid process
5   Glenoid cavity
6   Body of sternum
7   Costal cartilage
8   Body of the twelfth thoracic vertebra
9   Body of the first lumbar vertebra
10 Hip bone
11 Sacral promontory
12 Sacrum

13 Anterior superior iliac spine
14 Obturator foramen
15 Atlas
16 Seventh cervical vertebra
17 First rib
18 Xiphoid process
19 Twelfth rib
20 Body of the fifth lumbar vertebra
21 Iliac crest
22 Coccyx
23 Pubic symphysis

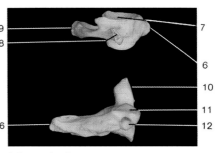

Atlas and axis.

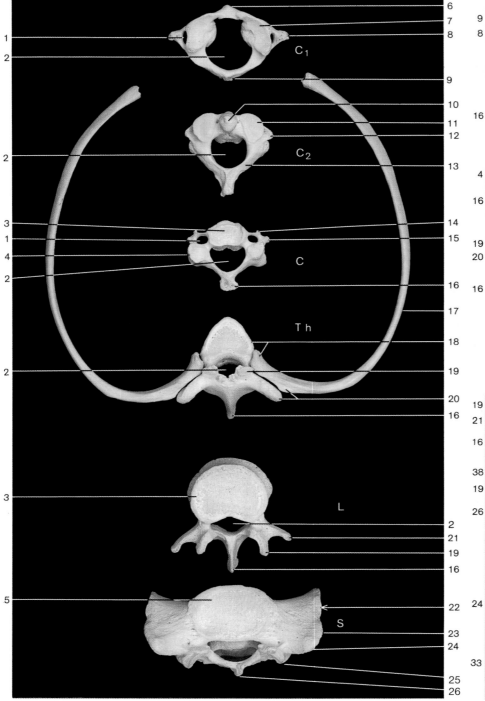

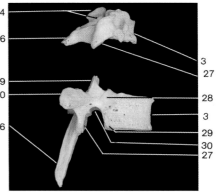

Typical cervical and thoracic vertebrae.

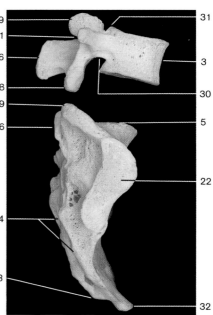

Representative vertebrae from each region of the vertebral column (superior aspect). From top to bottom: atlas (C₁), axis (C₂), cervical vertebra (C), thoracic vertebra (Th), lumbar vertebra (L), and sacrum (S).

Typical lumbar vertebra and sacrum.

Representative vertebrae from each region of the vertebral column (lateral aspect, ventral surface on the right).

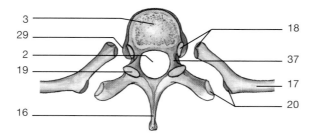

General organization of ribs and vertebrae (schematic drawing).

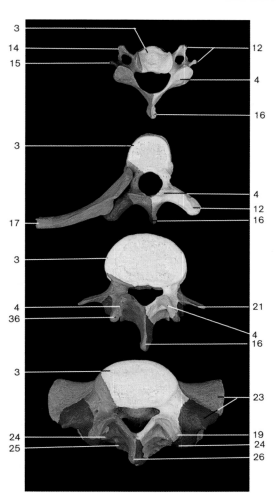

General characteristics of the vertebrae.
Typical cervical, thoracic, and lumbar vertebrae and sacrum.

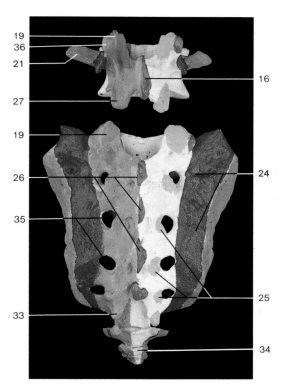

General characteristics of lumbar vertebrae and sacrum (posterior aspect).

Green = ribs or homologous processes
Red   = muscular processes
         (transverse and spinous processes)
Orange = laminae and articular processes
Yellow = articular facets
and blue

1	Foramen transversarium
2	Vertebral foramen
3	Body of vertebra
4	Superior articular facet
5	Base of sacrum
6	Anterior tubercle of atlas
7	Superior articular facet of atlas
8	Transverse process
9	Posterior tubercle of atlas
10	Dens of axis
11	Superior articular surface
12	Transverse process
13	Arch of vertebra
14	Anterior tubercle of transverse process
15	Posterior tubercle of transverse process
16	Spinous process
17	Shaft of rib
18	Body of vertebra and head of rib articulating with each other (costovertebral joint)
19	Superior articular process

20	Transverse process and tubercle of rib articulating with each other (costotransverse joint)
21	Costal process
22	Auricular surface
23	Lateral part of sacrum
24	Lateral sacral crest
25	Intermediate sacral crest
26	Median sacral crest
27	Inferior articular facet
28	Superior demifacet for head of rib
29	Inferior demifacet for head of rib
30	Inferior vertebral notch
31	Superior vertebral notch
32	Apex of the sacrum
33	Sacral cornu
34	Coccyx
35	Dorsal sacral foramina
36	Mamillary process
37	Pedicle
38	Inferior articular process

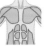

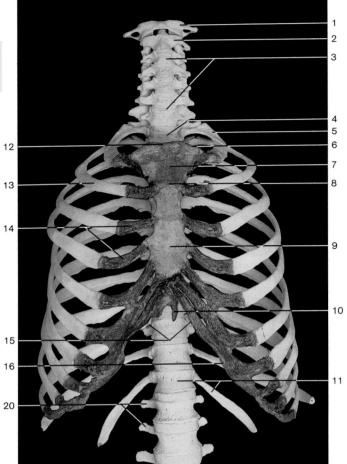

Skeleton of the thorax (anterior aspect).

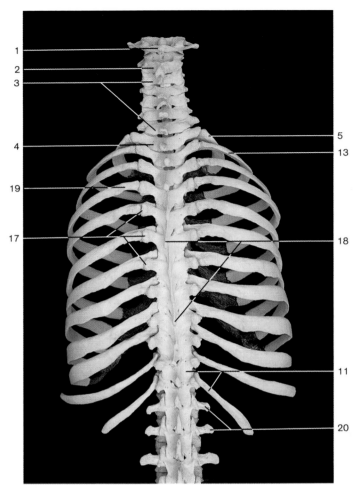

Skeleton of the thorax (posterior aspect).

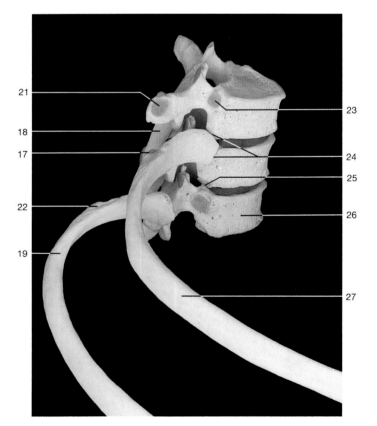

Costovertebral articulation (right lateral aspect).

1   Atlas
2   Axis
3   Cervical vertebrae
4   First thoracic vertebra
5   First rib
6   Facet for clavicle and clavicular notch
7   Manubrium sterni
8   Sternal angle
9   Body of sternum
10 Xiphoid process
11 Twelfth thoracic vertebra and rib
12 Jugular notch
13 Second rib
14 Costal cartilages
15 Infrasternal angle
16 Costal arch
17 Costotransverse joints between the transverse processes
    of thoracic vertebra and the tubercles of the ribs
18 Spinous processes
19 Costal angle
20 Costal processes of lumbar vertebrae
21 Facet for articulation with rib
22 Tubercle of rib
23 Superior facet for articulation with head of rib
24 Articulation of head of rib with two vertebrae
25 Inferior facet for articulation with head of rib
26 Body of thoracic vertebra
27 Body or shaft of rib

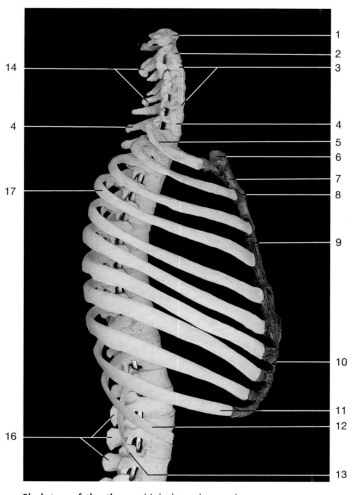

Skeleton of the thorax (right lateral aspect).

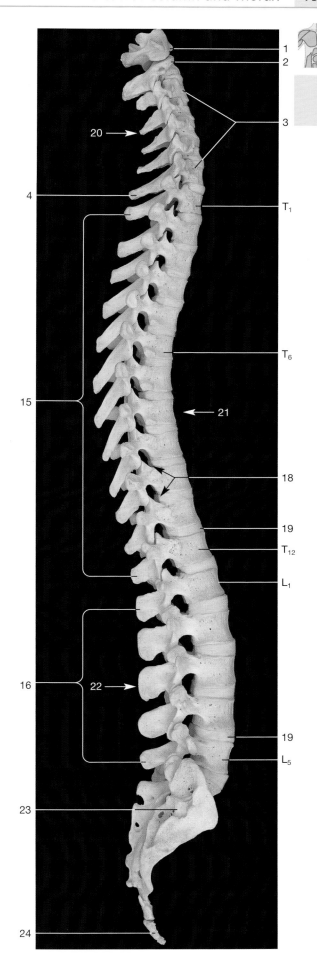

Vertebral column
(right lateral aspect).

1   Atlas
2   Axis
3   Cervical vertebrae
4   Seventh cervical vertebra (vertebra prominens)
5   First rib
6   Facet for clavicle
7   Manubrium sterni
8   Sternal angle
9   Body of sternum
10 Costal arch
11 Tenth rib
12 Eleventh rib
13 Twelfth rib
14 Spinous processes of cervical vertebrae
15 Spinous processes of thoracic vertebrae
16 Spinous processes of lumbar vertebrae
17 Costal angle
18 Intervertebral foramina
19 Intervertebral discs
20 Cervical curvature
21 Thoracic curvature
22 Lumbar curvature
23 Sacrum
24 Coccyx

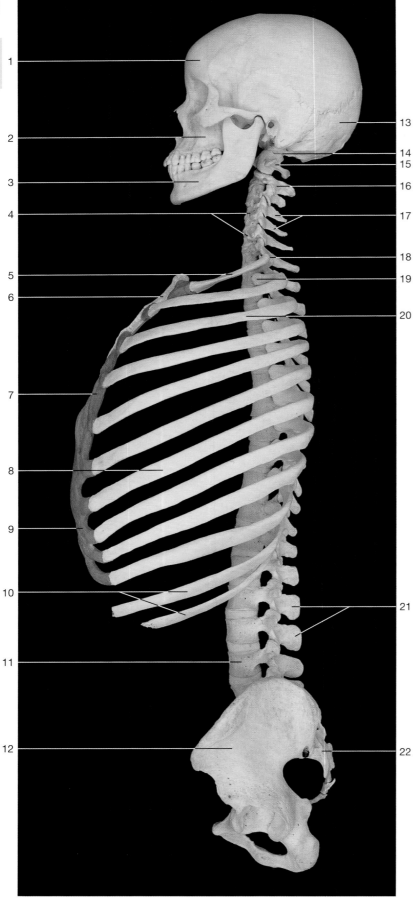

1 Frontal bone
2 Maxilla
3 Mandible
4 Bodies of cervical vertebrae
5 First rib
6 Manubrium of sternum
7 Sternum (corpus sterni)
8 Seventh rib (last of the true ribs)
9 Costal arch (arcus costalis)
10 Floating ribs (costae fluctuantes)
11 Body of fourth lumbar vertebra
12 Pelvis
13 Occipital bone
14 Atlanto-occipital joint
15 Atlas
16 Axis
17 Spinous processes of cervical vertebrae (C$_4$, C$_5$)
18 Costotransverse joint of first rib
19 Head of second rib
20 Third rib
21 Spinous processes of lumbar vertebrae (L$_2$, L$_3$)
22 Sacrum

Vertebral column and thorax in connection with head and pelvis (lateral aspect).

1   Atlas
2   Dens of axis
3   Axis
4   Body of cervical vertebra
5   Intervertebral discs
6   Sternocleidomastoid muscle
7   Scalenus muscles
8   Body of vertebra
9   Superior articular facet
10 Vertebral arch
11 Transverse process of vertebra
12 Zygapophysial joint
13 Spinous process
14 Articular facet
    of costovertebral joint
15 Transverse process
    with articular facet
    of costotransverse joint
16 Costal process of lumbar
    vertebra
17 Sacrum
18 Median sacral crest
19 Dorsal sacral foramina
20 Coccyx

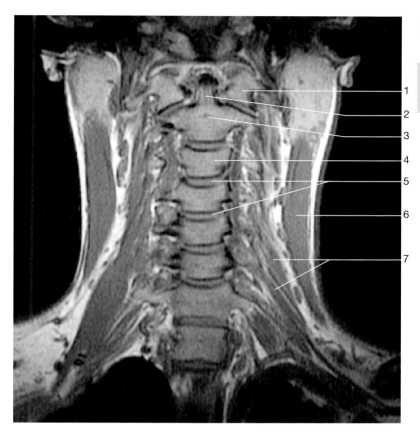

Coronal section through the neck at the level of the cervical vertebrae (MRI scan, courtesy of Prof. Heuck, Munich).

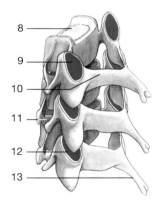

Cervical vertebrae (lateral aspect, articular facets = blue).

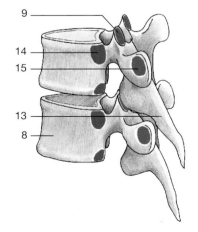

Thoracic vertebrae (lateral aspect, articular facets = blue).

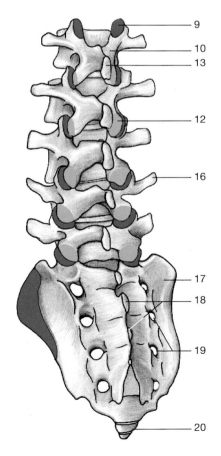

Lumbar vertebrae with sacrum and coccyx (posterior aspect, articular facets = blue).

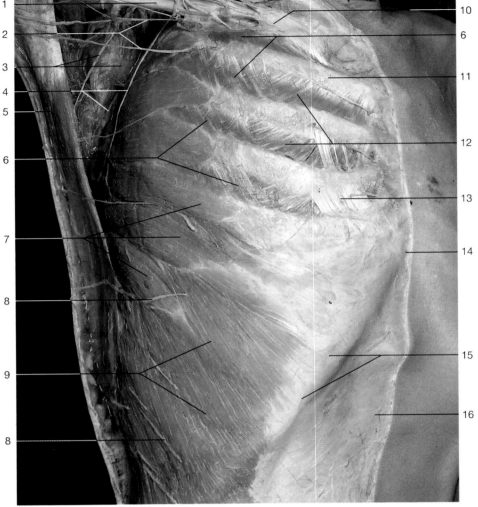

1 Axillary vein
2 Intercostobrachial nerves
3 Subscapularis muscle and
   thoracodorsal nerve
4 Long thoracic nerve, lateral
   thoracic artery and vein
5 Latissimus dorsi muscle
6 External intercostal muscles
7 Serratus anterior muscle
8 Lateral cutaneous branches of
   intercostal nerves
9 External abdominal oblique muscle
10 Clavicle (divided)
11 Second rib (costochondral
   junction)
12 Internal intercostal muscles
13 External intercostal membrane
14 Position of xiphoid process
15 Costal arch or margin
16 Anterior layer of rectus sheath

Muscles of the thorax, superficial layer (lateral aspect). Upper limb elevated.
Pectoralis major and minor muscles have been removed.

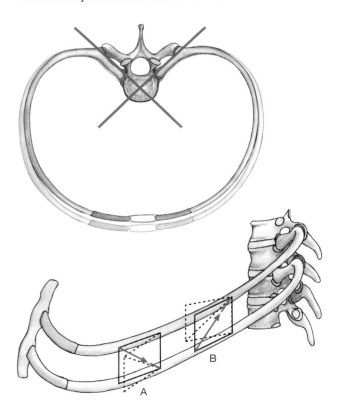

**Effect of intercostal muscles on the costovertebral and
costotransverse joints.** Axes of movement indicated by red lines;
direction of movements indicated by red arrows.
A = action of internal intercostal muscles (expiration);
B = action of external intercostal muscles (inspiration).

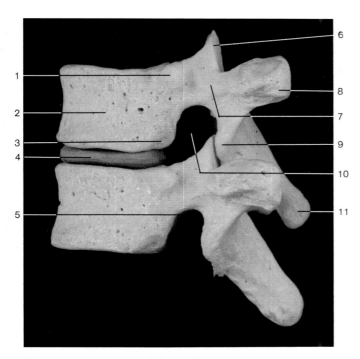

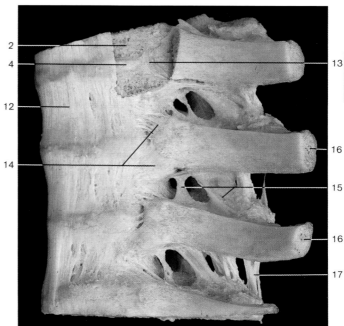

Two thoracic vertebrae (left lateral aspect).

1	Superior demifacet for head of rib	8	Transverse process and facet for tubercle of rib
2	Body of vertebra	9	Inferior articular process
3	Inferior demifacet for head of rib	10	Intervertebral foramen
4	Intervertebral disc	11	Spinous process
5	Inferior vertebral notch	12	Anterior longitudinal ligament
6	Superior articular facet and superior articular process	13	Intra-articular ligament
7	Pedicle	14	Radiate ligament

Ligaments of thoracic vertebrae and costovertebral joints (left antero-lateral aspect). In the upper joint, most of the radiate ligament and the anterior part of the head of the rib have been removed to expose the two joint cavities and the interposed intra-articular ligament.

15	Superior costotransverse ligament
16	Body of rib
17	Intertransverse ligament

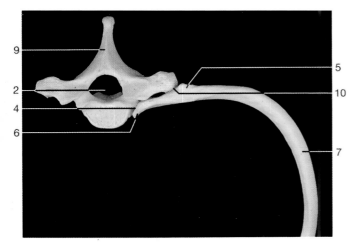

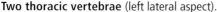

Location of costovertebral joints (superior aspect).

1	Superior articular process	7	Shaft or body of rib
2	Vertebral canal	8	Transverse process with articular facet
3	Body of thoracic vertebra	9	Spinous process
4	Costovertebral joint (articular facets)	10	Costotransverse joint (articular facets)
5	Tubercle of rib		
6	Head of rib		

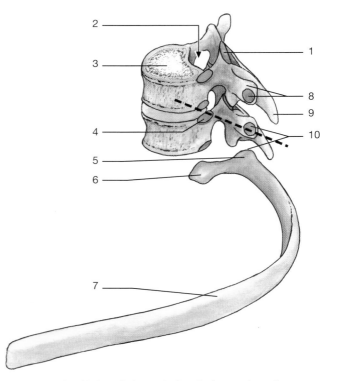

Costovertebral joints (schematic drawing). Two thoracic vertebrae with an articulating rib (separated). Axis of movement indicated by dashed line. Blue = articular facets.

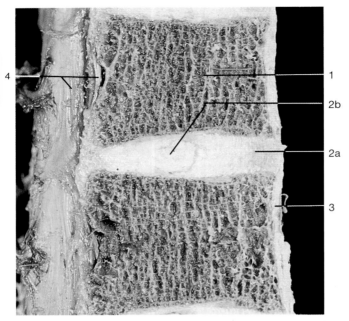

Median-sagittal section of the bodies of the vertebrae, showing the **intervertebral discs,** each of which consists of an outer laminated portion and an inner core.

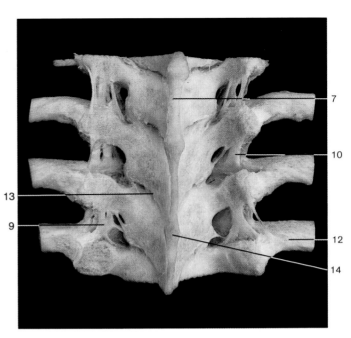

Ligaments of the vertebral column (dorsal aspect).

1 Body of vertebra
2 Intervertebral disc
  a Outer portion (anulus fibrosus)
  b Inner core (nucleus pulposus)
3 Anterior longitudinal ligament
4 Posterior longitudinal ligament and spinal dura mater
5 Costal process of lumbar vertebra
6 Sacrum
7 Supraspinous ligament

8 Interspinous ligament
9 Intertransverse ligament
10 Superior costotransverse ligament
11 Transverse process of thoracic vertebra
12 Rib
13 Ligamentum flavum
14 Spinous process
15 Intervertebral foramen

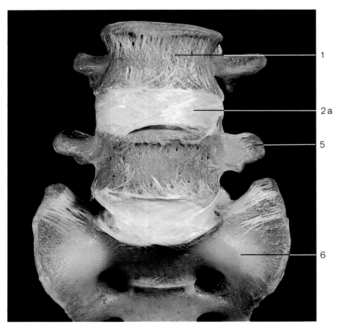

The two caudal lumbar vertebrae and the sacrum with their intervertebral discs (anterior aspect). Anterior longitudinal ligament removed.

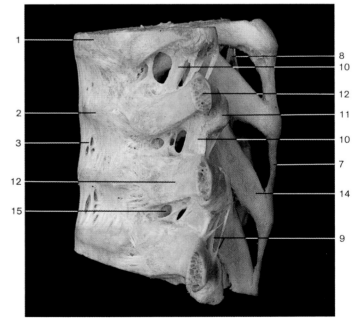

Ligaments of the vertebral column, thoracic part (left lateral aspect).

Disarticulated thorax skeleton. ▷
The twelve ribs (I–XII) are arranged
in a craniocaudal direction.

1 Anterior longitudinal ligament
2 Body of vertebra
3 Intervertebral disc
4 Intra-articular ligament
5 Radiate ligament
6 Posterior longitudinal ligament
7 Superior articular facet
8 Articular facets of
  costovertebral joints
9 Superior costotransverse ligament
10 Costovertebral joint
11 Rib
12 Interspinal ligament
13 Costotransverse joint
14 Lateral costotransverse ligament
15 Spinous process
16 Supraspinal ligament
17 Nucleus pulposus
18 Costal process
19 Vertebral arch
20 Intervertebral foramen
21 Intertransverse ligament ▽

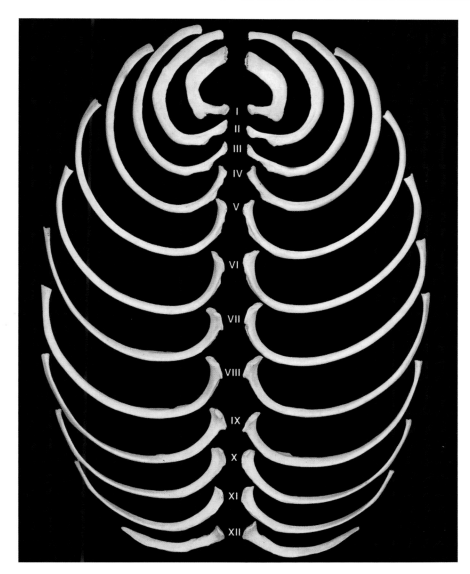

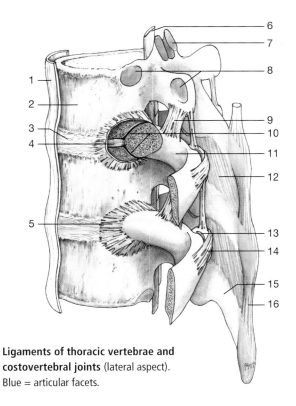

**Ligaments of thoracic vertebrae and
costovertebral joints** (lateral aspect).
Blue = articular facets.

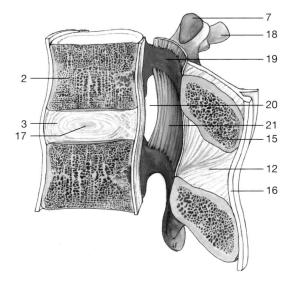

Median-sagittal section of two lumbar vertebrae showing
ligaments and vertebral discs.

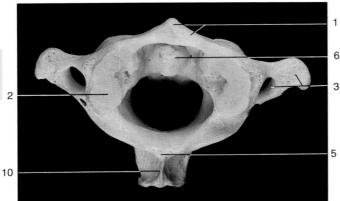

Atlas and axis (from above).

Median atlanto-axial joint and transverse ligament of atlas (from above). Dens of axis partly severed.

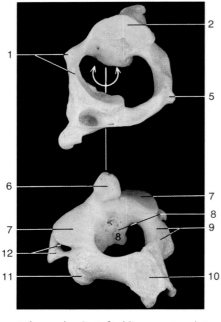

1 Anterior arch of atlas with anterior tubercle
2 Superior articular facet of atlas
3 Foramen transversarium and transverse process
4 Posterior arch of atlas and vertebral artery
5 Posterior tubercle of atlas
6 Dens of axis
7 Superior articular surface of axis
8 Body of axis
9 Pedicle and lamina of axis
10 Spinous process
11 Inferior articular process
12 Transverse process and foramen transversarium of axis
13 Median atlanto-axial joint (anterior part)

14 Articular capsule of atlanto-occipital joint
15 Transverse ligament of atlas
16 Occipital bone
17 Atlanto-occipital joint
18 Lateral atlanto-axial joint
19 Third cervical vertebra
20 Superior longitudinal band of cruciform ligament
21 Alar ligaments
22 Transverse ligament of atlas
23 Inferior longitudinal band of cruciform ligament
24 Spinous process of axis
25 Dura mater
26 Occipital bone

Atlas and axis. Left oblique postero-lateral aspect, demonstrating the articulation of the dens of axis with atlas (cf. arrows).

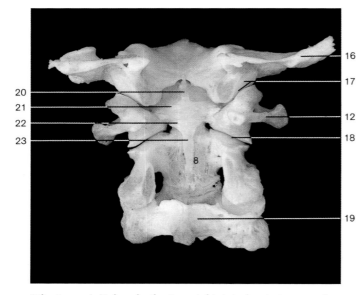

Atlanto-occipital and atlanto-axial joints (posterior aspect). Posterior part of occipital bone, posterior arch of atlas, and axis have been removed to show the cruciform ligament.

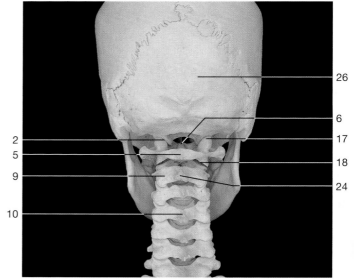

Head and cervical spine (posterior aspect). Bones of atlanto-occipital and atlanto-axial joints.

1 Cerebellum
2 Occipital condyle
3 Atlanto-occipital joint
4 Atlas
5 Lateral atlanto-axial joint
6 Intervertebral disc
7 Cistern of pons
8 Head of mandible
9 Dens of axis
10 Axis
11 Body of cervical vertebra (C$_3$)
12 External occipital protuberance
13 Foramen magnum
14 Transverse process of atlas
15 Posterior longitudinal ligament
16 Spinous process of cervical vertebra
17 Occipital bone
18 Membrana tectoria
19 Dorsum sellae
20 Clivus
21 Sella turcica
22 Superior orbital fissure
23 Internal acoustic meatus
24 Jugular foramen
25 Hypoglossal canal
26 Superior longitudinal
   band of cruciform ligament
27 Alar ligaments
28 Transverse ligament of atlas
29 Inferior longitudinal band of
   cruciform ligament

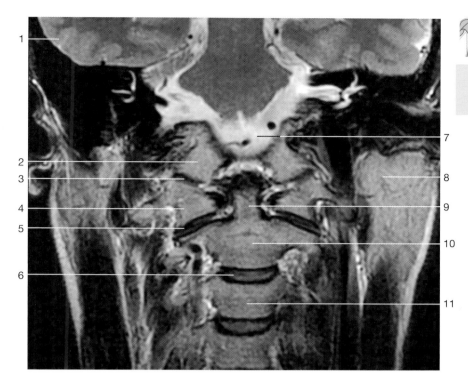

Coronal section of the neck at the level of dens of axis (MRI scan, courtesy of Prof. Heuck, Munich).

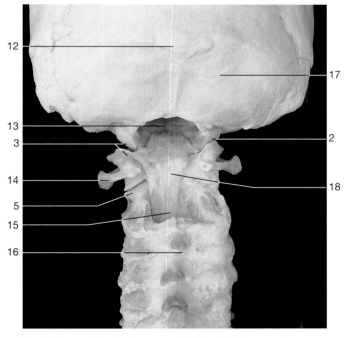

Cervical vertebral column and skull with ligaments (posterior aspect). Posterior arches of atlas and axis removed to show the membrana tectoria.

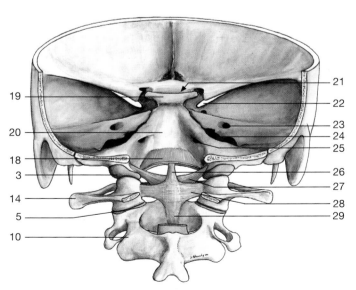

Atlanto-occipital and atlanto-axial joints with ligaments (posterior aspect). Posterior part of occipital bone and posterior arch of atlas have been removed to show the cruciform ligament.

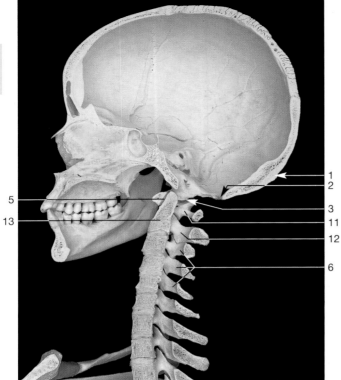

Cervical vertebral column in relation to the head (midsagittal section, medial aspect).

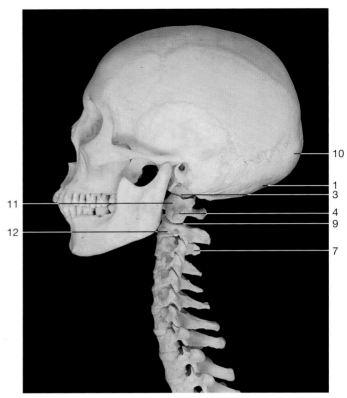

Atlas and axis in relation to the head (lateral aspect).

1	External occipital protuberance	9	Lateral atlanto-axial joint
2	Foramen magnum	10	Occipital bone
3	Atlanto-occipital joint	11	Atlas
4	Transverse process of atlas	12	Axis
5	Median atlanto-axial joint	13	Dens of axis
6	Vertebral canal	14	Hypoglossal canal
7	Spinous process of third cervical vertebra	15	Spinous process of axis
8	Occipital condyle		

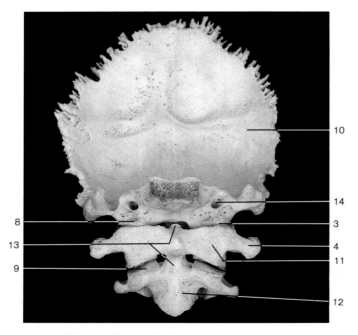

Occipital bone, atlas, and axis (anterior aspect).

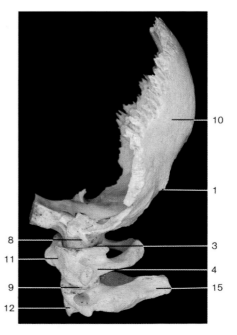

Occipital bone, atlas, and axis (left lateral aspect).

1 Pons
2 Base of skull (clivus)
3 Medulla oblongata
4 Atlas (anterior arch)
5 Dens of axis
6 Intervertebral disc
7 Body of cervical vertebra (C₄)
8 Site of larynx
9 Trachea
10 Cerebellum
11 Cerebellomedullary cistern
12 Spinal cord
13 Trapezius muscle
14 Muscles of the neck
15 Spinous process of cervical
    vertebra (C₇)
16 Internal jugular vein
17 Common carotid artery
18 Vagus nerve (n. X)
19 Larynx
20 Body of cervical vertebra
21 Vertebral artery
22 Spinal nerve with spinal ganglion
23 Transverse process of cervical vertebra
24 Spinous process of cervical vertebra

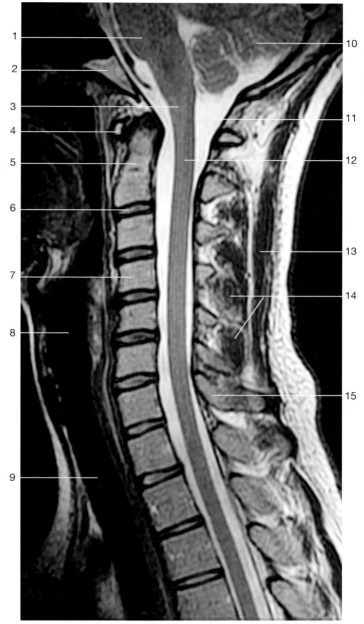

Midsagittal section of the neck showing the spinal cord in connection with medulla oblongata (MRI scan, courtesy of Prof. Heuck, Munich).

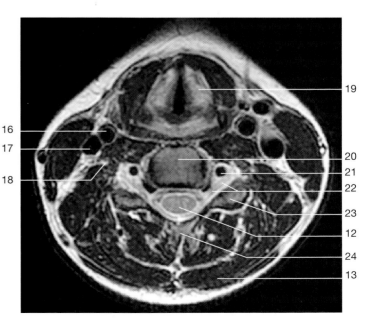

Horizontal section of the neck at the level of the larynx (MRI scan, courtesy of Prof. Heuck, Munich).

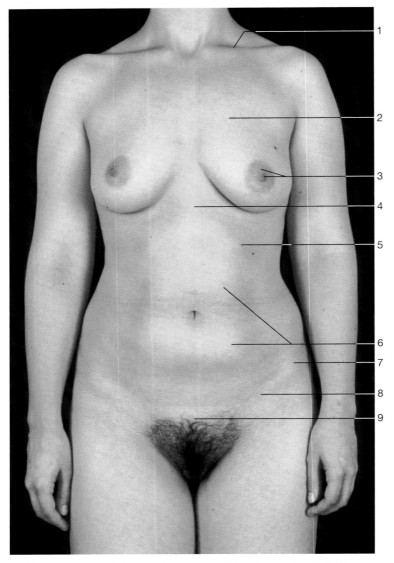

1   Clavicle
2   Pectoralis major muscle
3   Areola and nipple
4   Infrasternal angle
5   Costal arch
6   Rectus abdominis muscle
7   Anterior superior iliac spine
8   Inguinal ligament
9   Mons pubis
10 Epidermis
11 Subcutaneous layer
12 Muscles of the back
13 Kidney
14 Body of lumbar vertebra
15 External abdominal oblique muscle
16 Small intestine
17 Deltoid muscle
18 Anterior serratus muscle
19 External intercostal muscle
20 Internal abdominal oblique muscle
21 Transverse abdominal muscle
22 Rectus sheath
23 Spermatic cord
24 Pectoralis minor muscle
25 Linea alba

Surface anatomy of the anterior body wall in the female. Note the differences in thickness and structure of skin and hairs (compare with the section below).

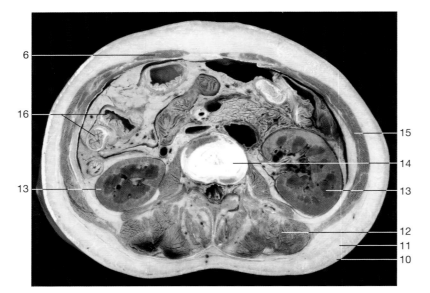

Cross section of the body at the first lumbar vertebra. Note the differences in thickness of the subcutaneous layers.

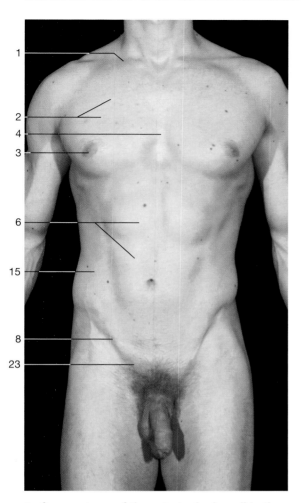

Surface anatomy of the anterior body wall in the male. Localization and structure of the muscles can be identified.

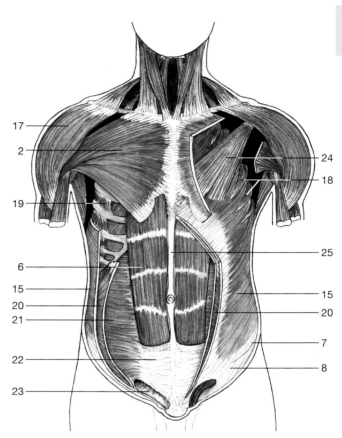

Muscles of the anterior body wall (schematic drawing).

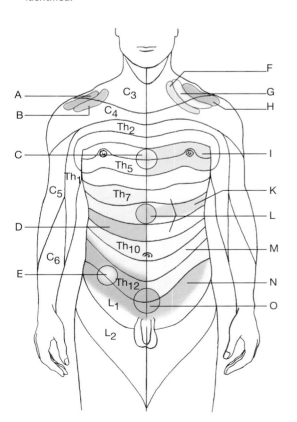

Head's areas

A = duodenum
B = gallbladder, liver (C_3–C_4)
C = esophagus (Th_4, Th_5)
D = liver, gallbladder (Th_6–Th_{11})
E = colon, vermiform appendix
      (Th_{11-12}, L_1)
F = heart
G = pancreas
H = stomach (C_3, C_4)
I = heart (Th_3, Th_4)
K = pancreas (Th_8)
L = stomach (Th_6–Th_9)
M = small intestine (Th_{10}–L_1)
N = kidney, ureter, testis (Th_{10}–L_1)
O = urinary bladder (Th_{11}–L_1)

◁ **Segments of anterior body wall.**
Head's areas are indicated.

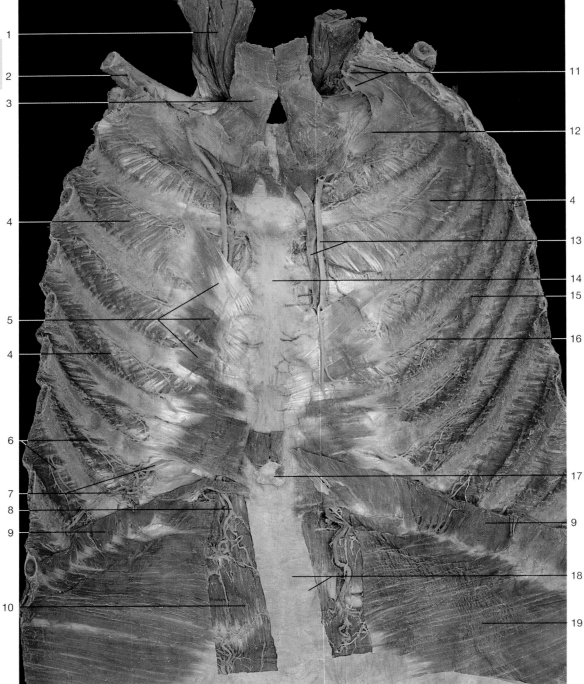

Anterior thoracic wall (posterior aspect). Diaphragm partly removed, posterior layer of rectus sheath fenestrated on both sides.

1	Sternocleidomastoid muscle (divided)	11	Subclavian artery and brachial plexus
2	Clavicle	12	First rib
3	Sternothyroid muscle	13	Internal thoracic artery and vein
4	Internal intercostal muscle	14	Sternum
5	Transversus thoracic muscle	15	Innermost intercostal muscle
6	Intercostal arteries and nerves	16	Intercostal artery and vein
7	Musculophrenic artery	17	Xiphoid process
8	Superior epigastric artery and vein	18	Linea alba and posterior layer of
9	Diaphragm (divided)		rectus sheath
10	Rectus abdominis muscle	19	Transversus abdominis muscle

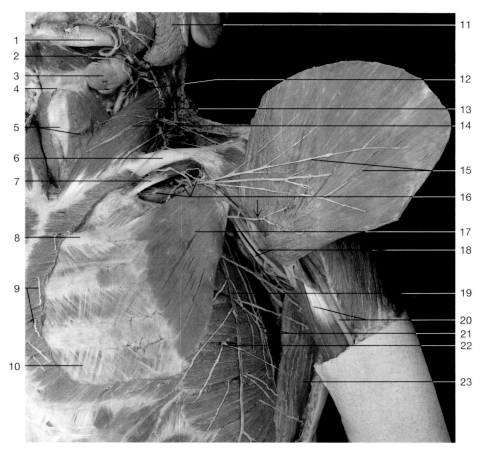

1 Mandible
2 Facial artery
3 Submandibular gland
4 Hyoid bone
5 Thyroid cartilage and sternohyoid muscle
6 Clavicle
7 Subclavius muscle
8 Second rib
9 Anterior cutaneous branches of intercostal nerves
10 External intercostal membrane
11 Parotid gland
12 External carotid artery
13 Sternocleidomastoid muscle and cutaneous branches of cervical plexus
14 Supraclavicular nerves
15 Pectoralis major muscle and lateral pectoral nerves
16 Thoraco-acromial artery and subclavian vein
17 Pectoralis minor muscle
18 Median and ulnar nerve
19 Thoraco-epigastric vein
20 Cephalic vein and long head of biceps brachii muscle
21 Lateral thoracic artery and long thoracic nerve
22 Lateral cutaneous branches of intercostal nerve
23 Latissimus dorsi muscle
24 Median nerve
25 Axillary artery
26 Intercostobrachial nerves
27 Thoracodorsal nerve
28 Long thoracic nerve
29 Latissimus dorsi muscle
30 Serratus anterior muscle
31 Thoraco-acromial artery
32 Clavicle
33 External intercostal muscle
34 Third rib
35 Internal intercostal muscle
36 Anterior intercostal artery and vein, and intercostal nerve
37 Costal arch or margin

Thoracic wall (anterior aspect). Left pectoralis major muscle has been divided and reflected. Note the connection of the cephalic vein with the subclavian vein.
Arrow: medial pectoral nerve.

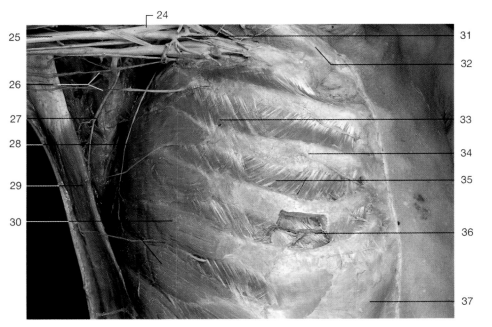

Thoracic wall (lateral aspect). Pectoralis major and minor muscles have been removed. A section of the fourth rib has been cut and removed to display the intercostal vessels and nerve.

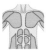

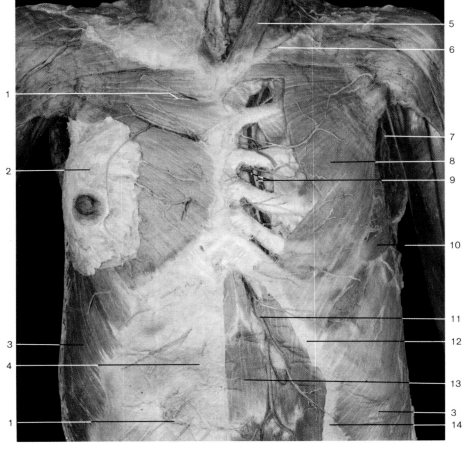

1   Anterior perforating branches of intercostal nerve
2   Mammary gland
3   External abdominal oblique muscle
4   Rectus sheath (anterior layer)
5   Sternocleidomastoid muscle
6   Clavicle
7   Lateral thoracic artery and vein
8   Pectoralis major muscle
9   Internal thoracic artery and vein
10 Serratus anterior muscle
11 Superior epigastric artery and vein
12 Costal margin
13 Rectus abdominis muscle
14 Cut edge of the anterior layer of the rectus sheath
15 Subclavian artery
16 Highest intercostal artery
17 Internal thoracic artery
18 Musculophrenic artery
19 Superficial epigastric artery
20 Deep circumflex iliac artery
21 Superior epigastric artery
22 Inferior epigastric artery
23 Superficial circumflex iliac artery

Thoracic wall (anterior aspect). Dissection of the **internal thoracic artery and vein.** Left pectoralis major muscle partly removed. Anterior lamina of the rectus sheath on the left side has been removed.

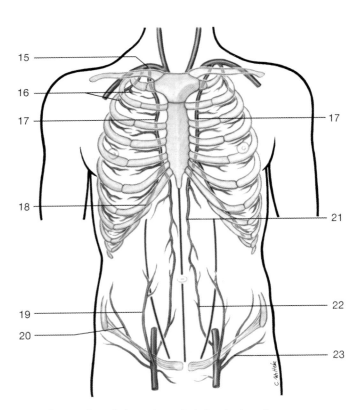

Main arteries of thoracic and abdominal walls.

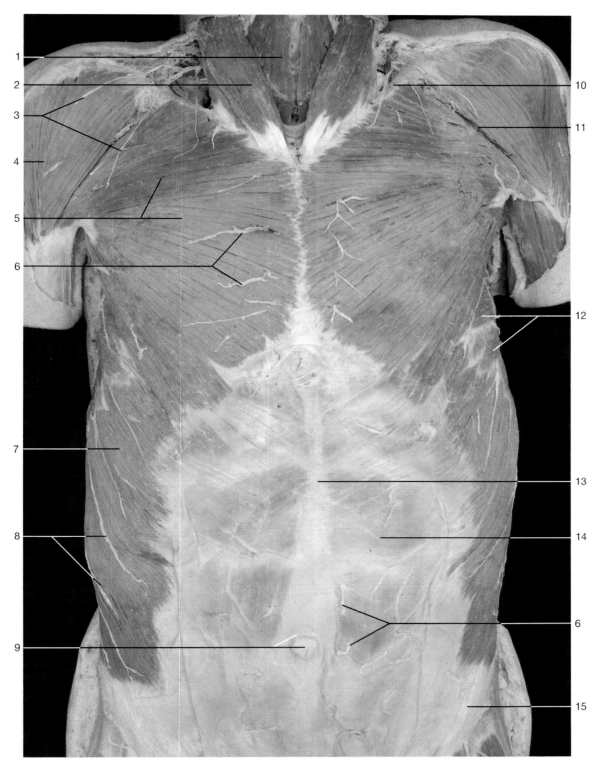

Anterior thoracic and abdominal walls with superficial muscles. The fascia of pectoralis major muscle and the abdominal wall have been removed; the anterior layer of the sheath of the rectus abdominis muscle is displayed.

1   Sternohyoid muscle
2   Sternocleidomastoid muscle
3   Supraclavicular nerves (branches of cervical plexus)
4   Deltoid muscle
5   Pectoralis major muscle
6   Anterior cutaneous branches of intercostal nerves
7   External abdominal oblique muscle
8   Lateral cutaneous branches of intercostal nerves

9   Umbilicus and umbilical ring
10 Clavicle
11 Cephalic vein
12 Serratus anterior muscle
13 Linea alba
14 Sheath of rectus abdominis muscle
     (anterior layer)
15 Inguinal ligament

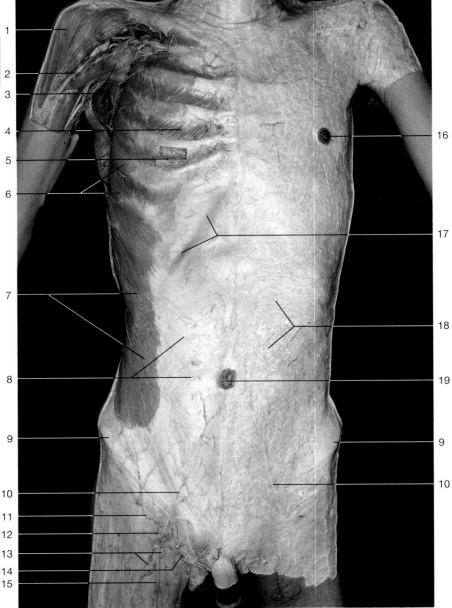

1 Deltoid muscle
2 Cephalic vein
3 Pectoralis major muscle (divided)
4 Internal intercostal muscle
5 Intercostal artery and vein (intercostal space, fenestrated)
6 Serratus anterior muscle
7 External abdominal oblique muscle
8 Anterior layer of rectus sheath
9 Iliac crest
10 Superficial epigastric vein
11 Superficial circumflex iliac vein
12 Saphenous opening
13 Superficial inguinal lymph nodes
14 Superficial external pudendal veins
15 Great saphenous vein
16 Nipple
17 Costal margin
18 Subcutaneous fatty tissue
19 Umbilicus
20 Anterior layer of rectus sheath
21 Rectus abdominis muscle
22 Posterior layer of rectus sheath
23 Internal abdominal oblique muscle
24 External abdominal oblique muscle (cut)
25 Transversus abdominis muscle
26 Transversalis fascia and peritoneum
27 Psoas major muscle
28 Body of lumbar vertebra (L$_4$)
29 Quadratus lumborum muscle
30 Medial tract of erector spinae muscle
31 Lateral tract of erector spinae muscle (longissimus and iliocostalis muscles)
32 Small intestine
33 Left ureter
34 Abdominal aorta
35 Inferior vena cava
36 Descending colon
37 Spinous process

Thoracic and abdominal walls. Right pectoralis major and minor muscles are divided. Muscles of thoracic and abdominal walls on right side are displayed.

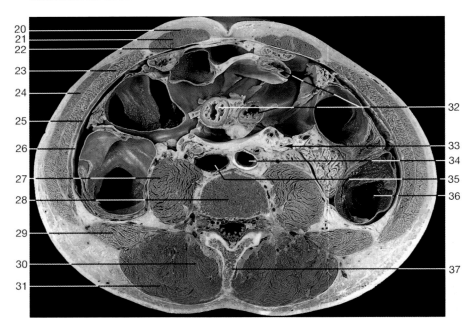

Horizontal section of the trunk at the level of the umbilicus, superior to arcuate line (inferior aspect).

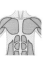

1   Deltoid muscle
2   Pectoralis major muscle (divided)
3   Internal intercostal muscle
4   Intercostal artery and vein
5   Rectus abdominis muscle
6   Tendinous intersections
7   External abdominal oblique muscle
8   Anterior superior iliac spine
9   Superficial circumflex iliac vein
10 Superficial epigastric vein
11 Great saphenous vein
12 Cephalic vein
13 Pectoralis major muscle
14 Anterior cutaneous branches of
    intercostal nerves
15 Nipple
16 Linea alba
17 Anterior layer of rectus sheath
18 Umbilicus
19 Inguinal ligament
20 Pyramidal muscle
21 Superficial inguinal ring and spermatic
    cord
22 Suspensory ligament of penis
23 Longissimus and iliocostalis muscles
24 Multifidus muscle
25 Quadratus lumborum muscle
26 Latissimus dorsi muscle
27 Psoas major muscle
28 Spinous process
29 Body of first lumbar vertebra
30 Transversus abdominis muscle
31 Internal abdominal oblique muscle

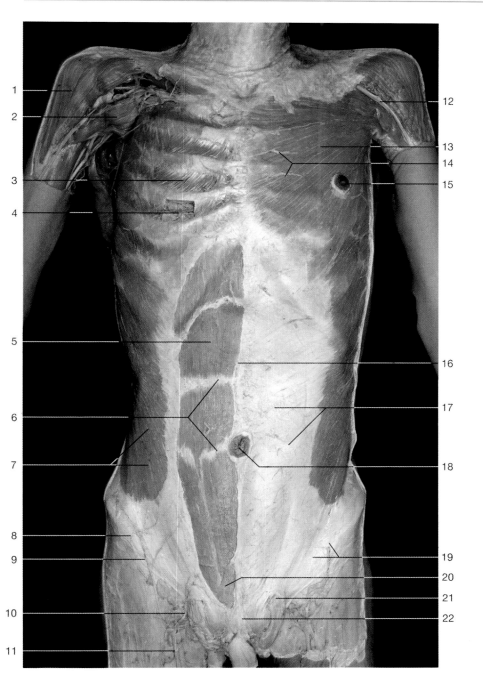

Thoracic and abdominal walls. Right pectoralis major and minor muscles and anterior layer of rectus sheath have been removed on the right side.

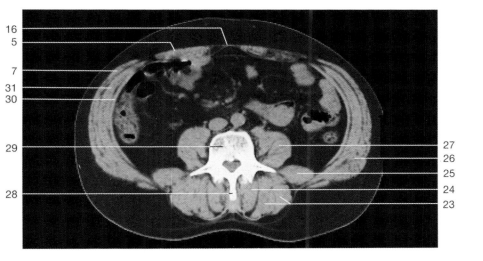

Horizontal section through the body at the level of fourth lumbar vertebra; seen from below. (CT scan.)

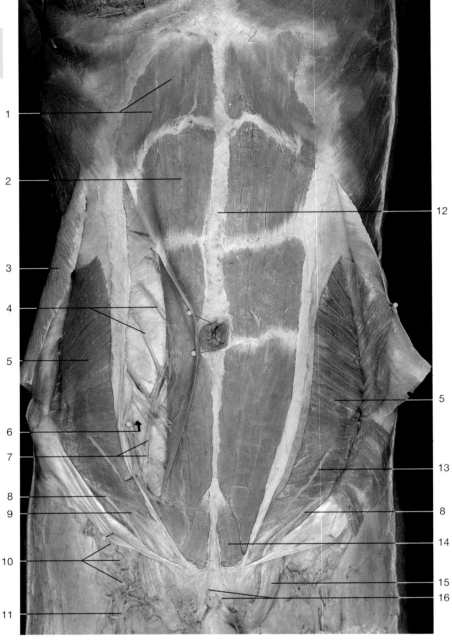

1 Costal margin
2 Rectus abdominis muscle
3 External abdominal oblique muscle (reflected)
4 Thoraco-abdominal (intercostal) nerves with accompanying vessels
5 Internal abdominal oblique muscle
6 Arcuate line (arrow)
7 Inferior epigastric artery and vein
8 Ilio-inguinal nerve
9 Position of deep inguinal ring
10 Superficial inguinal lymph nodes
11 Great saphenous vein
12 Linea alba
13 Iliohypogastric nerve
14 Pyramidal muscle
15 Spermatic cord
16 Fundiform ligament of penis

Thoracic and abdominal walls.
External abdominal oblique muscle has been divided and reflected on both sides. The right rectus muscle has been reflected medially to display the posterior layer of rectus sheath. Arrow: location of arcuate line.

1 Anterior layer of rectus sheath
2 Rectus abdominis muscle
3 Posterior layer of rectus sheath
4 Transversalis fascia
5 Transversus abdominis muscle
6 Internal oblique muscle
7 External oblique muscle
8 Thoracolumbar fascia with superficial and deep layer
9 Lateral column of erector spinae muscle
10 Medial column of intrinsic muscles of the back

Horizontal section of the trunk superior to arcuate line (schematic drawing).

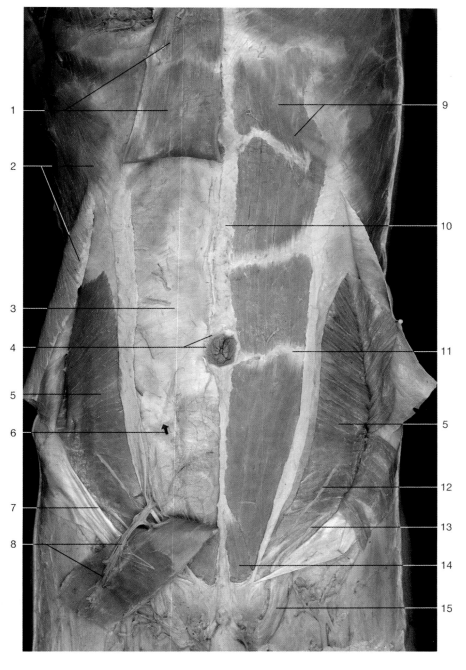

1   Rectus abdominis muscle (reflected)
2   External abdominal oblique muscle
    (divided)
3   Posterior layer of rectus sheath
4   Umbilical ring
5   Internal abdominal oblique muscle
6   Arcuate line (arrow)
7   Inguinal ligament
8   Inferior epigastric artery and vein
    and rectus abdominis muscle
    (divided and reflected)
9   Costal margin
10 Linea alba
11 Tendinous intersection
12 Iliohypogastric nerve
13 Ilio-inguinal nerve
14 Pyramidal muscle
15 Spermatic cord

Thoracic and abdominal walls.
External abdominal oblique muscle has been
divided and reflected on both sides. The right
rectus muscle has been cut and reflected
to display the posterior layer of rectus sheath.
Arrow: location of arcuate line.

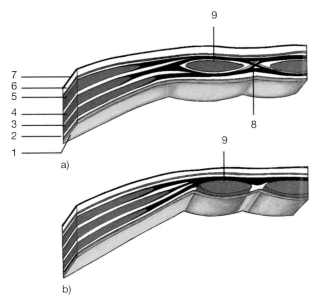

1   Peritoneum
2   Transversalis fascia (green)
3   Transversus abdominis muscle
4   Internal abdominal oblique muscle
5   External abdominal oblique muscle
6   Fascia of external abdominal oblique
    muscle (green)
7   Skin
8   Linea alba
9   Rectus abdominis muscle

**Transverse sections through the
abdominal wall** superior (a) and inferior (b)
to arcuate line.

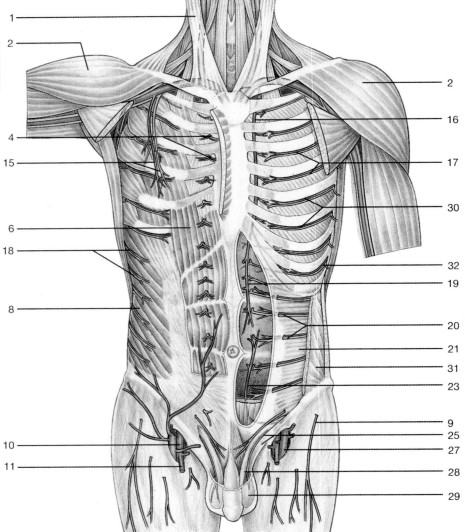

1   Sternocleidomastoid muscle
2   Deltoid muscle
3   Pectoralis major muscle
4   Anterior cutaneous branches of intercostal nerves
5   Cut edge of anterior layer of rectus sheath
6   Rectus abdominis muscle
7   Tendinous intersection
8   External abdominal oblique muscle
9   Lateral femoral cutaneous nerve
10 Femoral vein
11 Great saphenous vein
12 Medial supraclavicular nerves
13 Pectoralis minor muscle (reflected) and medial pectoral nerves
14 Axillary vein
15 Long thoracic nerve and lateral thoracic artery
16 Internal thoracic artery
17 Intercostal nerves
18 Lateral cutaneous branches of intercostal nerves
19 Superior epigastric artery
20 Thoraco-abdominal (intercostal) nerves
21 Transversus abdominis muscle
22 Posterior layer of rectus sheath
23 Inferior epigastric artery
24 Lateral femoral cutaneous nerve
25 Inguinal ligament and ilio-inguinal nerve
26 Femoral nerve
27 Femoral artery
28 Spermatic cord
29 Testis
30 Posterior intercostal arteries
31 Internal abdominal oblique muscle
32 Lateral cutaneous branch of intercostal nerve
33 Dorsal branch of spinal nerve
34 Latissimus dorsi muscle
35 Deep muscles of the back (medial and lateral tract)
36 Anterior layer of rectus sheath
37 Posterior layer of rectus sheath
38 Thoracolumbar fascia
39 Spinal cord
40 Aorta
41 Ventral root ⎫ of spinal
42 Dorsal root ⎬ nerve

Thoracic and abdominal walls (schematic drawing). Note the segmental organization of the blood vessels and nerves. Right side: superficial layers; left side: deeper layers.

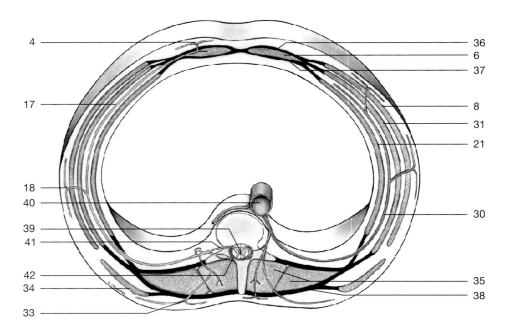

Horizontal section of the abdominal wall (from below) showing the location of the intercostal arteries (left side) and nerves (right side).

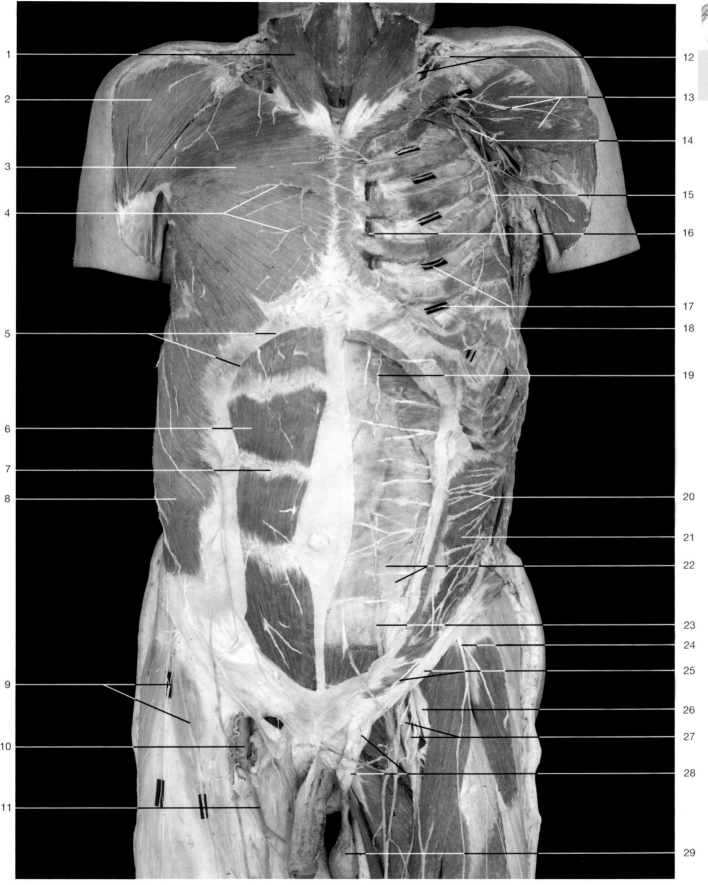

Thoracic and abdominal walls with vessels and nerves (anterior aspect). Right side: superficial layers; left side: deeper layers. Pectoralis major and minor muscles, the external and internal intercostal muscles on the left side have been removed to display the intercostal nerves. The anterior layer of rectus sheath, the left rectus abdominis muscle, and the external and internal abdominal oblique muscles have been removed to show the thoraco-abdominal nerves within the abdominal wall.

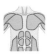

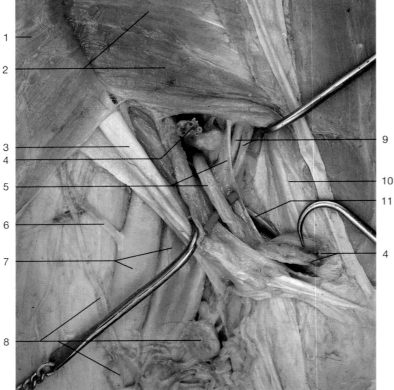

1   Internal abdominal oblique muscle (reflected)
2   Transversus abdominis muscle
3   Inguinal ligament
4   Spermatic cord with the exception of the ductus deferens (divided and reflected)
5   Ductus deferens and interfoveolar ligament
6   Superficial circumflex iliac artery
7   Femoral artery and vein
8   Superficial inguinal lymph nodes and inguinal lymph vessel
9   Inferior epigastric artery and vein
10 Falx inguinalis or conjoint tendon (cut)
11 Pubic branch of inferior epigastric artery
12 Superficial inguinal ring
13 Penis
14 External abdominal oblique muscle
15 Anterior superior iliac spine
16 Intercrural fibers
17 Fascia lata and sartorius muscle
18 Saphenous opening and great saphenous vein
19 Deep inguinal ring
20 Skin of scrotum and dartos muscle
21 Cremaster muscle
22 Internal spermatic fascia
23 Ductus deferens
24 Epididymis
25 Peritoneum (blue)
26 Remnant of processus vaginalis
27 Tunica vaginalis testis
28 Rectus abdominis muscle
29 Spermatic cord with ductus deferens covered by external spermatic fascia
30 Anterior layer of rectus sheath
31 Suspensory ligament of penis
32 Testis and epididymis
33 Ductus deferens
34 Pampiniform venous plexus and testicular artery
35 Inferior epigastric artery
36 Lateral femoral cutaneous nerve
37 Ilio-inguinal nerve
38 Femoral nerve
39 Sartorius muscle
40 Deep dorsal vein of penis

Inguinal canal in the male, right side (deep layer, anterior aspect). Spermatic cord with exception of ductus deferens (probe) has been divided and reflected.

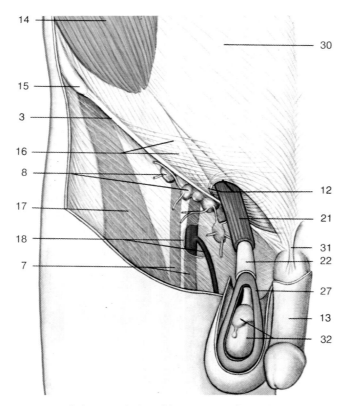

General characteristics of lower part of anterior abdominal wall and inguinal canal (schematic drawing).

Inguinal hernias may either pass through the inguinal canal lateral to the inferior epigastric artery (indirect or lateral inguinal hernias, A and C) or directly penetrate the abdominal wall through the inguinal triangle located medial to the inferior epigastric artery (direct or medial inguinal hernias, B). The lateral hernias can be congenital if the vaginal process remains open (C) or acquired (A) if the hernia develops independently of a patent processus vaginalis.

Femoral hernias generally protrude through the femoral ring below the inguinal ligament. Proper assessment of the site of herniation requires the identification of both the inguinal ligament and the epigastric artery.

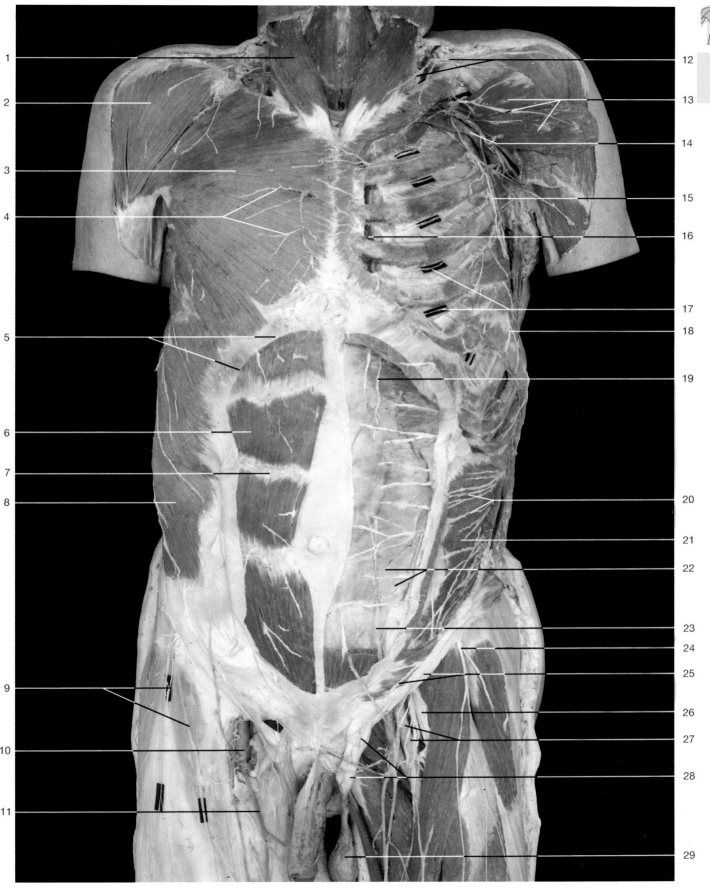

Thoracic and abdominal walls with vessels and nerves (anterior aspect). Right side: superficial layers; left side: deeper layers. Pectoralis major and minor muscles, the external and internal intercostal muscles on the left side have been removed to display the intercostal nerves. The anterior layer of rectus sheath, the left rectus abdominis muscle, and the external and internal abdominal oblique muscles have been removed to show the thoraco-abdominal nerves within the abdominal wall.

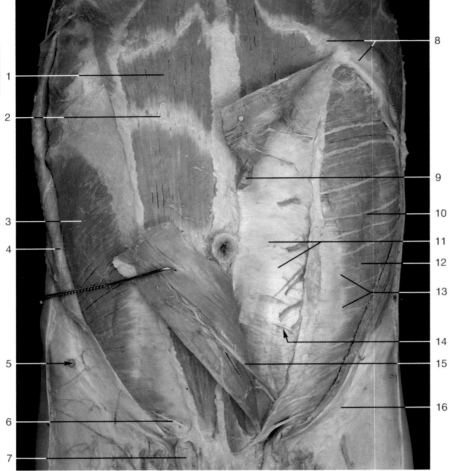

1   Rectus abdominis muscle
2   Tendinous intersection
3   Internal abdominal oblique muscle
4   External abdominal oblique muscle
     (reflected)
5   Anterior superior iliac spine
6   Ilio-inguinal nerve
7   Spermatic cord
8   Costal margin
9   Superior epigastric artery
10   Thoraco-abdominal (intercostal)
     nerves
11   Posterior layer of rectus sheath
12   Transversus abdominis muscle
13   Semilunar line
14   Arcuate line
15   Inferior epigastric artery
16   Inguinal ligament

Abdominal wall with vessels and nerves. The left rectus abdominis muscle has been divided and reflected to display the inferior epigastric vessels. The left internal abdominal oblique muscle has been removed to show the thoraco-abdominal nerves.

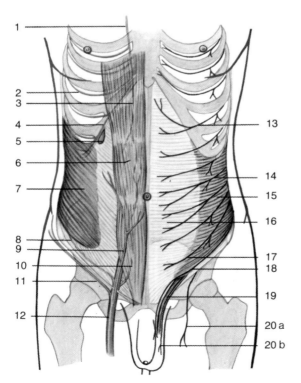

Arteries and nerves that supply the thoracic and abdominal walls.
Note their segmental arrangement (schematic drawing).

1   Internal thoracic artery
2   Intercostal artery
3   Superior epigastric artery
4   Musculophrenic artery
5   Gallbladder
6   Rectus abdominis muscle
7   External abdominal oblique muscle
8   Deep circumflex iliac artery
9   Superficial epigastric artery
10   Inferior epigastric artery
11   Superficial circumflex iliac artery
12   Femoral artery
13   Intercostal nerve
14   Thoraco-abdominal nerve (T_{10})
15   Transversus abdominis muscle
16   Posterior layer of the rectus sheath
17   Iliohypogastric nerve (L_1)
18   Ilio-inguinal nerve (L_1)
19   Spermatic cord
20   Genitofemoral nerve (L_1, L_2)
     a Femoral branch
     b Genital branch

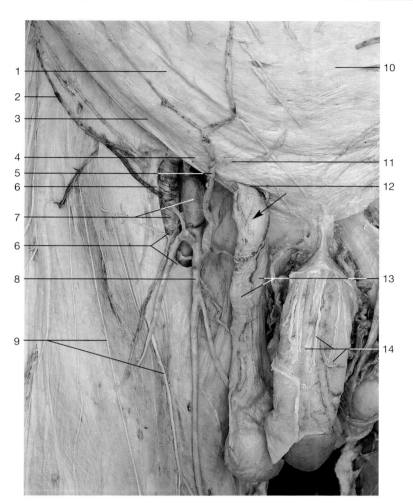

1   Aponeurosis of external abdominal oblique muscle
2   Superficial circumflex iliac vein
3   Inguinal ligament
4   Lateral crus of inguinal ring
5   Superficial epigastric vein
6   Saphenous opening
7   Femoral artery and vein
8   Great saphenous vein
9   Anterior cutaneous branches of femoral nerve
10 Anterior layer of rectus sheath
11 Intercrural fibers
12 Superficial inguinal ring
13 Spermatic cord and genital branch
    of genitofemoral nerve
14 Penis with dorsal nerves and deep dorsal vein
    of penis
15 Aponeurosis of external abdominal oblique
    muscle (divided and reflected)
16 Internal abdominal oblique muscle
17 Ilio-inguinal nerve
18 Anterior cutaneous branches of iliohypogastric
    nerve
19 Superficial external pudendal veins

Inguinal canal in the male, right side (superficial layer, anterior aspect).
There is a small inguinal hernia (arrow).

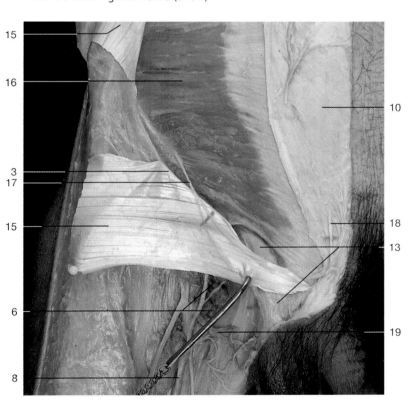

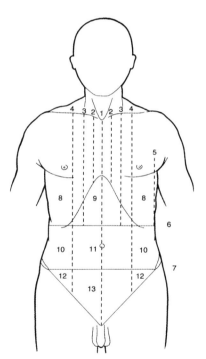

Inguinal canal in the male, right side (anterior aspect). The external
abdominal oblique muscle has been divided to display the inguinal canal.

Regions and reference lines
for delineating surface projections.
1   Median line
2   Lateral sternal line
3   Parasternal line
4   Midclavicular line
5   Axillary line
6   Transpyloric plane
7   Transtubercular plane
8   Hypochondriac region
9   Epigastric region
10 Lumbar region
11 Umbilical region
12 Iliac region
13 Hypogastric region

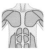

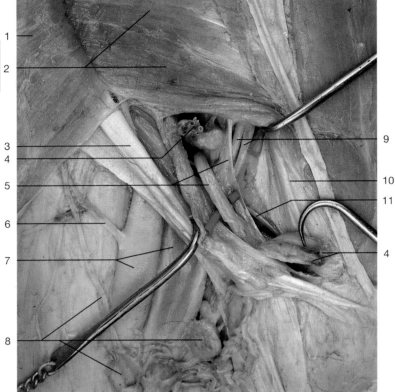

Inguinal canal in the male, right side (deep layer, anterior aspect). Spermatic cord with exception of ductus deferens (probe) has been divided and reflected.

1   Internal abdominal oblique muscle (reflected)
2   Transversus abdominis muscle
3   Inguinal ligament
4   Spermatic cord with the exception of the ductus deferens (divided and reflected)
5   Ductus deferens and interfoveolar ligament
6   Superficial circumflex iliac artery
7   Femoral artery and vein
8   Superficial inguinal lymph nodes and inguinal lymph vessel
9   Inferior epigastric artery and vein
10 Falx inguinalis or conjoint tendon (cut)
11 Pubic branch of inferior epigastric artery
12 Superficial inguinal ring
13 Penis
14 External abdominal oblique muscle
15 Anterior superior iliac spine
16 Intercrural fibers
17 Fascia lata and sartorius muscle
18 Saphenous opening and great saphenous vein
19 Deep inguinal ring
20 Skin of scrotum and dartos muscle
21 Cremaster muscle
22 Internal spermatic fascia
23 Ductus deferens
24 Epididymis
25 Peritoneum (blue)
26 Remnant of processus vaginalis
27 Tunica vaginalis testis
28 Rectus abdominis muscle
29 Spermatic cord with ductus deferens covered by external spermatic fascia
30 Anterior layer of rectus sheath
31 Suspensory ligament of penis
32 Testis and epididymis
33 Ductus deferens
34 Pampiniform venous plexus and testicular artery
35 Inferior epigastric artery
36 Lateral femoral cutaneous nerve
37 Ilio-inguinal nerve
38 Femoral nerve
39 Sartorius muscle
40 Deep dorsal vein of penis

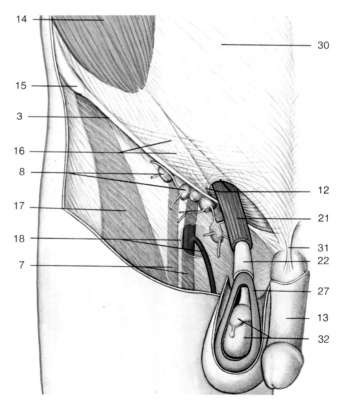

General characteristics of lower part of anterior abdominal wall and inguinal canal (schematic drawing).

Inguinal hernias may either pass through the inguinal canal lateral to the inferior epigastric artery (indirect or lateral inguinal hernias, A and C) or directly penetrate the abdominal wall through the inguinal triangle located medial to the inferior epigastric artery (direct or medial inguinal hernias, B). The lateral hernias can be congenital if the vaginal process remains open (C) or acquired (A) if the hernia develops independently of a patent processus vaginalis.
Femoral hernias generally protrude through the femoral ring below the inguinal ligament. Proper assessment of the site of herniation requires the identification of both the inguinal ligament and the epigastric artery.

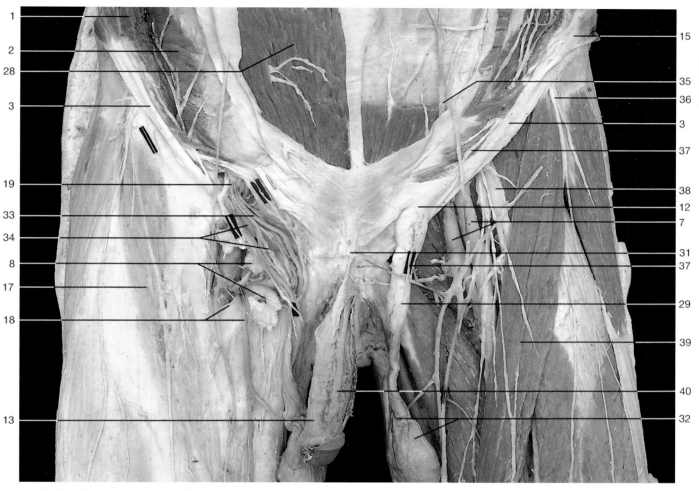

Inguinal and femoral regions in the male (anterior aspect). On the right, the spermatic cord was dissected to display the ductus deferens and the accompanying vessels and nerves. The fascia lata on the left side has been removed.

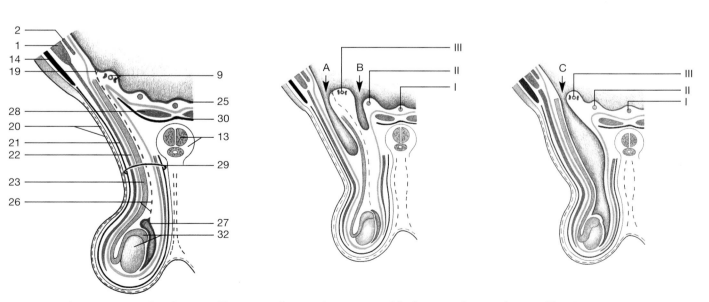

Layers of spermatic cord and types of hernias. Left: normal situation. Middle: location of acquired inguinal hernias:
A = indirect; B = direct inguinal hernia. Right: congenital indirect inguinal hernia (C); the vaginal process remained open.
I   = median umbilical fold containing urachus chord.
II = medial umbilical fold with remnants of umbilical artery.
III = lateral umbilical fold with inferior epigastric artery and vein.

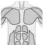

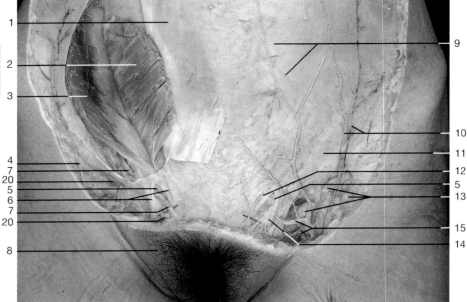

1   Aponeurosis of external abdominal oblique muscle
2   Internal abdominal oblique muscle (divided and reflected)
3   Transversus abdominis muscle
4   Superficial circumflex iliac artery and vein
5   Superficial inguinal ring with fat pad
6   Medial and lateral crural fibers
7   Round ligament (ligamentum teres uteri)
8   Labium majus pudendi
9   Anterior layer of rectus sheath
10 Superficial epigastric artery and vein
11 Inguinal ligament
12 Cutaneous branch of ilio-inguinal nerve
13 Superficial inguinal lymph nodes
14 Entrance of round ligament into the labium majus
15 External pudendal artery and vein
16 Position of deep inguinal ring
17 Ilio-inguinal nerve
18 Internal abdominal oblique muscle
19 Pubic branch of inferior epigastric artery
20 Genital branch of genitofemoral nerve
21 Fat pad of inguinal canal
22 Ilio-inguinal nerve
23 Sheath of round ligament (inguinal canal)
24 Transversalis fascia

Inguinal region in the female (anterior aspect). Left side: superficial layer; right side: external and internal abdominal oblique muscle divided and reflected.

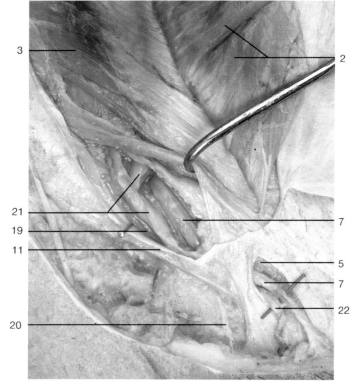

Inguinal canal of the female (anterior aspect, right side). The external abdominal oblique muscle has been divided and reflected, to display the ilio-inguinal nerve and the round ligament.

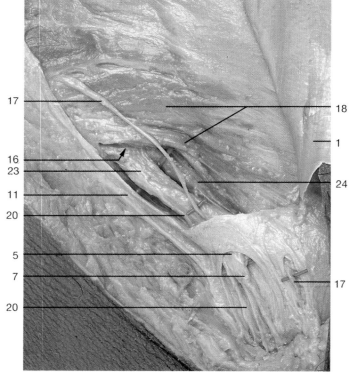

Inguinal canal of the female (anterior aspect, right side). The external and internal abdominal oblique muscle have been divided and reflected to show the content of the inguinal canal.

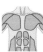

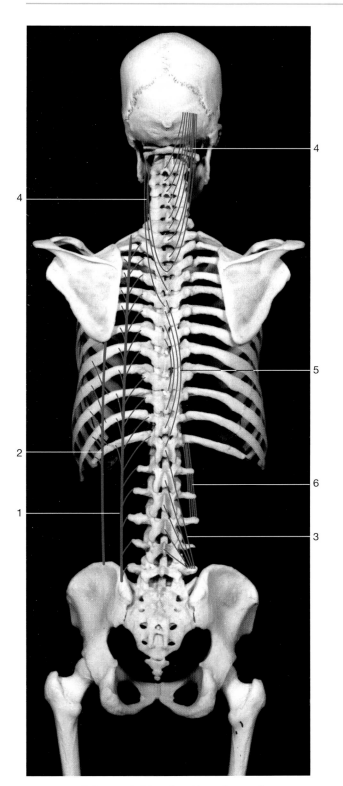

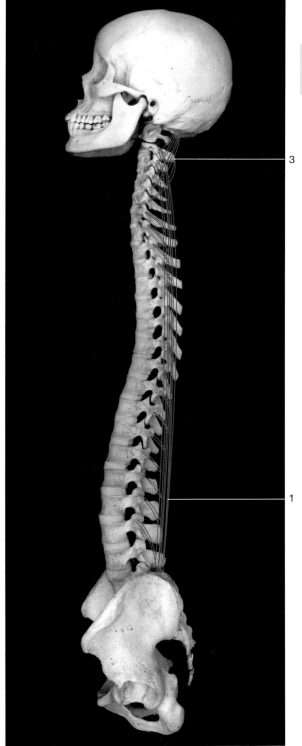

Skeleton of the trunk (dorsal and lateral aspect).
The long muscles of the back [longissimus (1) and iliocostalis (2) muscles] originate at the sacrum and pelvis and insert at the spinous or transverse processes of the vertebrae or at the ribs. There are also muscles that insert at the occipital bone.
The long muscles form the lateral tract, whereas muscles of the medial tract are situated within the groove between the spinous and transverse processes of the vertebrae [transversospinal (3) and spinotransversal (4) muscles] or between the spinous processes [spinalis muscles (5)] or between the transverse processes [intertransversarii muscles (6)] of the vertebrae.

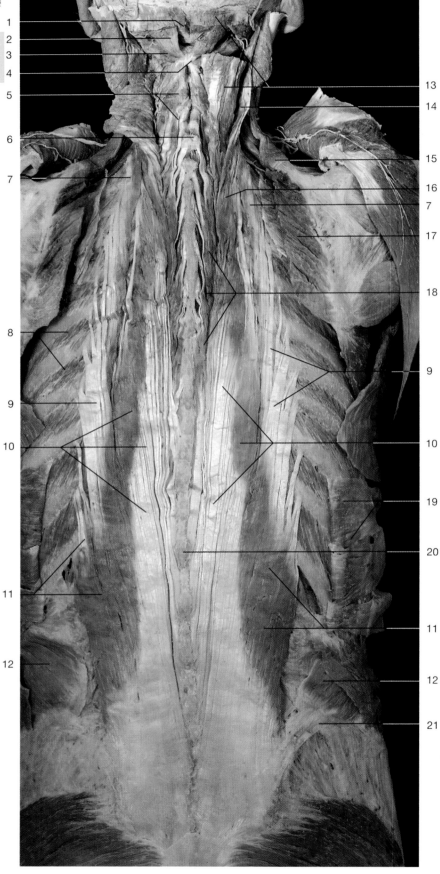

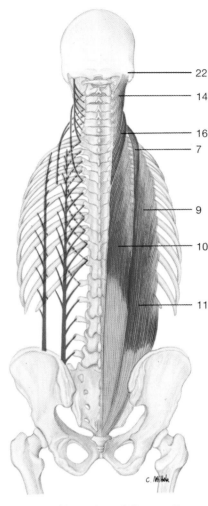

Origin and insertion of iliocostalis and longissimus muscles (schematic drawing).

1   Rectus capitis posterior minor muscle
2   Rectus capitis posterior major muscle
3   Obliquus capitis inferior muscle
4   Spinous process of axis
5   Semispinalis cervicis muscle
6   Spinous process of seventh vertebra
7   Iliocostalis cervicis muscle
8   External intercostal muscles
9   Iliocostalis thoracis muscle
10 Longissimus thoracis muscle
11 Iliocostalis lumborum muscle
12 Internal abdominal oblique muscle
13 Semispinalis capitis muscle (divided)
14 Longissimus capitis muscle
15 Levator scapulae muscle
16 Longissimus cervicis muscle
17 Rhomboid major muscle
18 Spinalis thoracis muscle
19 Serratus posterior inferior muscle (reflected)
20 Spinous process of second lumbar vertebra
21 Iliac crest
22 Mastoid process

Muscles of the back. Dissection of the erector spinae muscle (lateral column of the intrinsic back muscles).

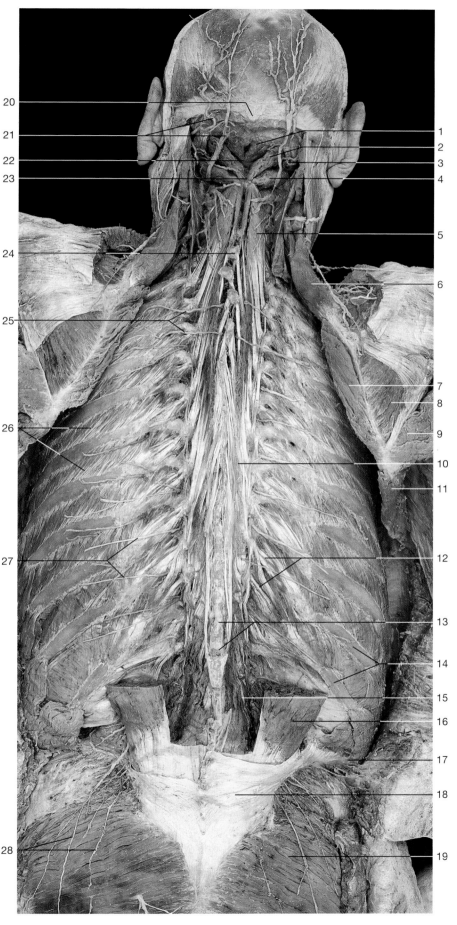

1 Rectus capitis posterior minor muscle
2 Rectus capitis posterior major muscle
3 Obliquus capitis superior muscle
4 Obliquus capitis inferior muscle
5 Semispinalis cervicis muscle
6 Levator scapulae muscle
7 Rhomboideus major muscle
8 Scapula with infraspinatus muscle
9 Teres major muscle
10 Spinalis muscle
11 Latissimus dorsi muscle
12 Levatores costarum muscles
13 Spinous processes of lumbar vertebrae
14 Ribs (Th$_{11}$, Th$_{12}$)
15 Multifidus muscle
16 Longissimus and iliocostalis
   muscles (cut)
17 Iliac crest (lumbar triangle)
18 Thoracolumbar fascia
19 Gluteus maximus muscle
20 Protuberantia occipitalis externa
21 Occipital artery and greater occipital
   nerve (C$_2$)
22 Posterior tubercle of atlas
23 Spinous process of axis
24 Spinous process of seventh cervical
   vertebra (vertebra prominens)
25 Medial branches of dorsal branches
   of spinal nerves
26 External intercostal muscles
27 Lateral branches of dorsal branches
   of spinal nerves
28 Superior cluneal nerves

Muscles of the back. Dissection of the deeper layer of the intrinsic muscles of the back (longissimus and iliocostalis muscles are cut).

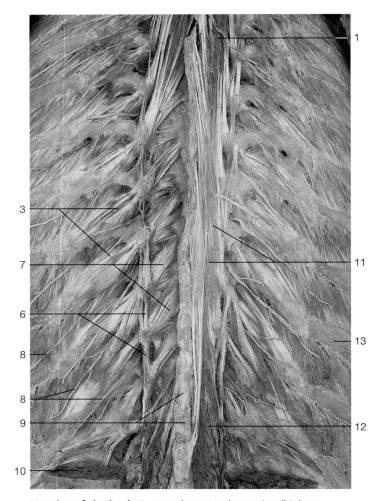

Muscles of the back. Deepest layer. Lumbar region (higher magnification).

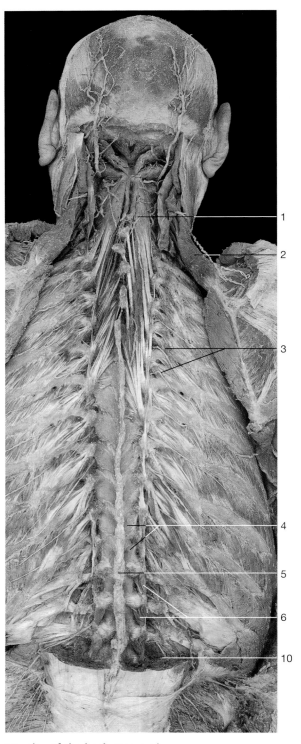

Muscles of the back. Deepest layer.

1   Semispinalis cervicis muscle
2   Levator scapulae muscle
3   Levatores costarum muscles
4   Vertebral arches of lumbar vertebrae
5   Supraspinal ligaments
6   Intertransverse lumbar muscles
7   Lumbar rotator muscles
8   Cutaneous branches of spinal nerves
9   Lumbar interspinal muscles
10   Longissimus and iliocostalis muscle (cut)
11   Spinal muscle of the back
12   Multifidus muscle
13   Tenth rib (T$_{10}$)

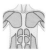

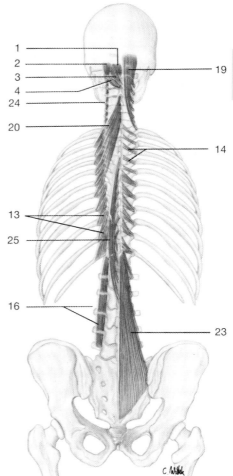

Medial column of intrinsic muscles of the back. Transversospinal and intertransversal system (schematic drawing).

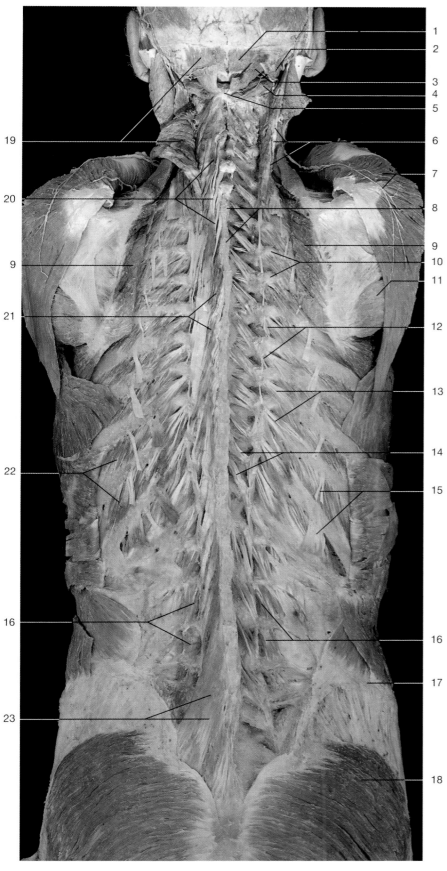

Muscles of the back. Transversospinal muscles, deepest layer on the right, where all parts of semispinalis and multifidus muscles have been removed.

1 Rectus capitis posterior minor muscle
2 Obliquus capitis superior muscle
3 Rectus capitis posterior major muscle
4 Obliquus capitis inferior muscle
5 Spinous process of axis
6 Longissimus capitis muscle
7 Trapezius muscle (reflected) and accessory nerve (n. XI)
8 Spinous processes
9 Rhomboid major muscle
10 Transverse processes of thoracic vertebrae
11 Teres major muscle
12 Intertransverse ligaments
13 Levatores costarum muscles
14 Rotatores muscles
15 Tendons of iliocostalis muscle
16 Intertransversarii lumborum muscles (lateral)
17 Iliac crest
18 Gluteus maximus muscle
19 Semispinalis capitis muscle
20 Semispinalis cervicis muscle
21 Semispinalis thoracis muscle
22 External intercostal muscles
23 Multifidus muscle
24 Posterior cervical intertransversarii muscles
25 Spinalis thoracis muscle

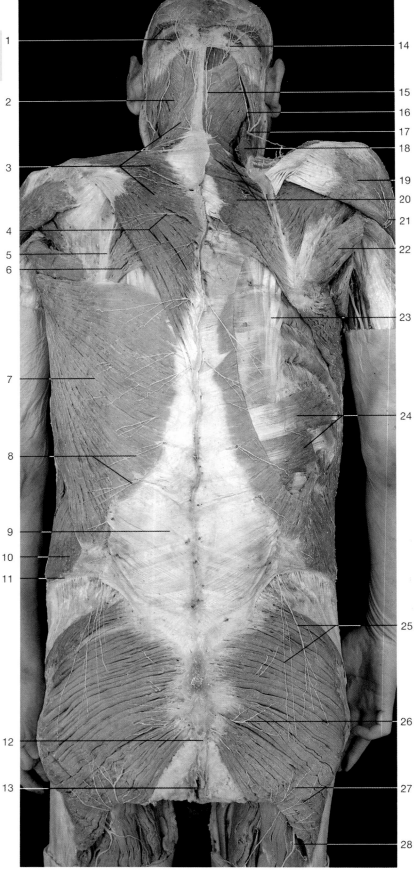

1   Occipital belly of occipitofrontalis muscle
2   Splenius capitis muscle
3   Trapezius muscle
4   Medial cutaneous branches of dorsal rami of spinal nerves
5   Medial margin of scapula
6   Rhomboid major muscle
7   Latissimus dorsi muscle
8   Lateral cutaneous branches of dorsal rami of spinal nerves
9   Thoracolumbar fascia
10 External abdominal oblique muscle
11 Iliac crest
12 Last coccygeal vertebra
13 Anus
14 Greater occipital nerve
15 Third occipital nerve
16 Lesser occipital nerve
17 Cutaneous branches of cervical plexus
18 Levator scapulae muscle
19 Deltoid muscle
20 Rhomboid major and minor muscles
21 Upper lateral cutaneous nerve of arm (branch of axillary nerve)
22 Teres major muscle
23 Iliocostalis thoracis muscle
24 Serratus posterior inferior muscle
25 Superior cluneal nerves
26 Middle cluneal nerves
27 Inferior cluneal nerves
28 Posterior femoral cutaneous nerve

Innervation of the back. Superficial (left) and deeper (right) layers. Right trapezius and latissimus dorsi muscles removed.

▷   **To page 227:**

1   Trapezius muscle
2   Infraspinatus muscle
3   Left latissimus dorsi muscle
4   Thoracolumbar fascia
5   Splenius cervicis muscle
6   Serratus posterior superior muscle
7   Medial branches of dorsal rami of thoracic spinal nerves
8   Lateral branches of dorsal rami of thoracic spinal nerves
9   Iliocostalis muscle
10 Serratus posterior inferior muscle
11 Latissimus dorsi muscle (reflected)

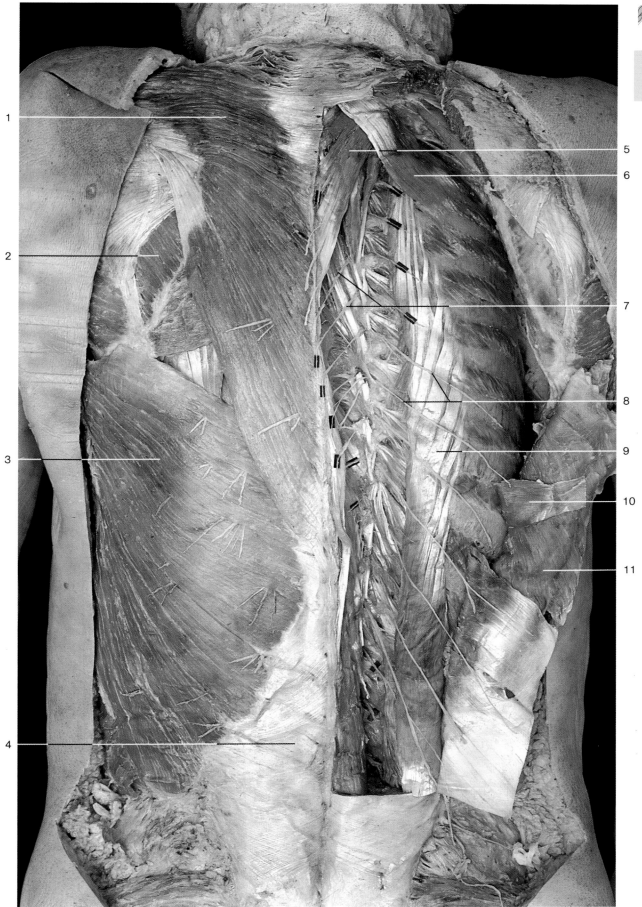

Innervation of the back. Dissection of the dorsal branches of spinal nerves. On the right, longissimus thoracis muscle has been removed and iliocostalis muscle laterally reflected.

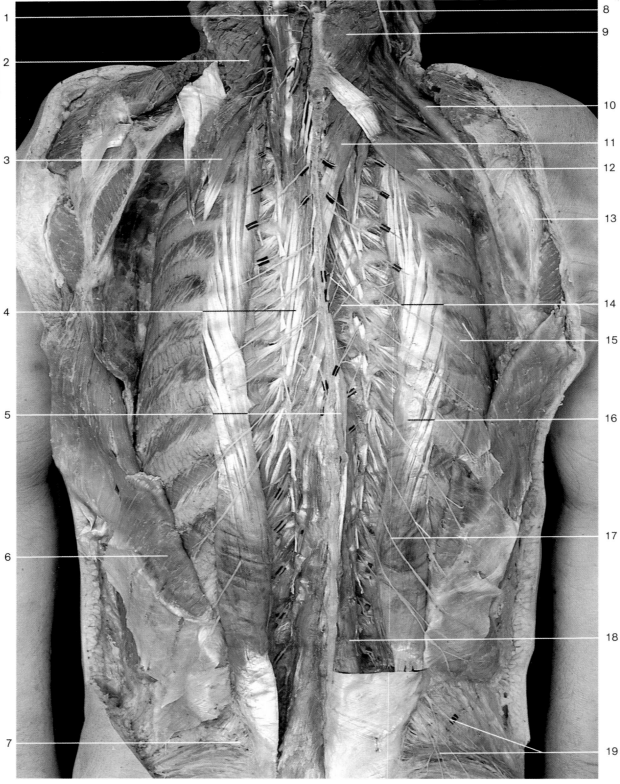

Innervation of the back. Deeper layer (dorsal aspect).

1 Semispinalis capitis muscle	7 Iliac crest	14 Medial branches of dorsal rami
2 Left splenius capitis muscle	8 Lesser occipital nerve	of spinal nerves
(cut and reflected)	9 Splenius capitis muscle	15 Rib and external intercostal muscle
3 Left splenius cervicis muscle	10 Levator scapulae muscle	16 Iliocostalis thoracis muscle
(cut and reflected)	11 Splenius cervicis muscle	17 Lateral branches of dorsal rami
4 Semispinalis thoracis muscle	12 Serratus posterior superior muscle	of spinal nerves
5 Spinalis thoracis muscle	13 Scapula	18 Multifidus muscle
6 Latissimus dorsi muscle (reflected)		19 Superior cluneal nerves

1 Greater occipital nerve (C$_2$)
2 Suboccipital nerve (C$_1$)
3 Medial branches of dorsal rami of spinal nerves
4 Lateral branches of dorsal rami of spinal nerves
5 Superior cluneal nerves (L$_1$–L$_3$)
6 Middle cluneal nerves (S$_1$–S$_3$)
7 Inferior cluneal nerves (derived from branches
   of the sacral plexus, ventral rami)
8 Lesser occipital nerve
9 Great auricular nerve
10 Trapezius muscle
11 Deltoid muscle
12 Latissimus dorsi muscle
13 Gluteus maximus muscle
14 External intercostal muscle
15 Internal intercostal muscle
16 Innermost intercostal muscle
17 Dorsal ramus of spinal nerve
18 Spinal nerve and spinal ganglion
19 Sympathetic trunk with ganglion
20 Intercostal nerve
21 Lateral cutaneous branch ⎫
22 Anterior cutaneous branch ⎬ of intercostal nerve
23 Longissimus thoracis muscle
24 Spinal cord
25 Aorta
26 Esophagus
27 Body of rib
28 Thoracic rib
29 Thoracic duct
30 Azygos vein

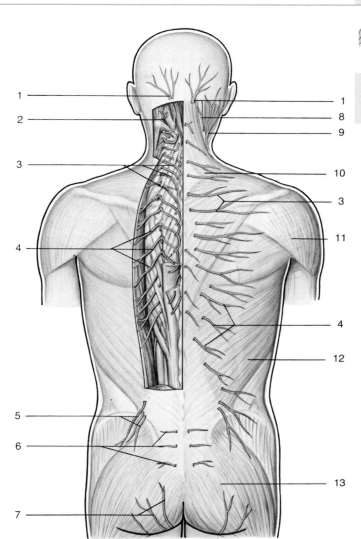

General characteristics of the innervation of the back.
Distribution of dorsal branches of spinal nerves. Note the
segmental arrangement of the innervation of the dorsal part
of the trunk (schematic drawing).

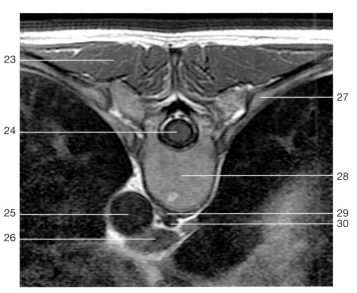

Posterior part of the thoracic wall (MRI scan, coronal section;
from Heuck et al., MRT-Atlas, 2009).

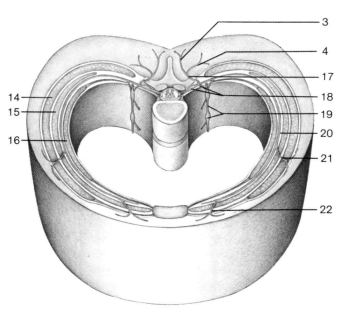

**Position and branches of spinal nerves in one segment of
thoracic wall** (schematic drawing).

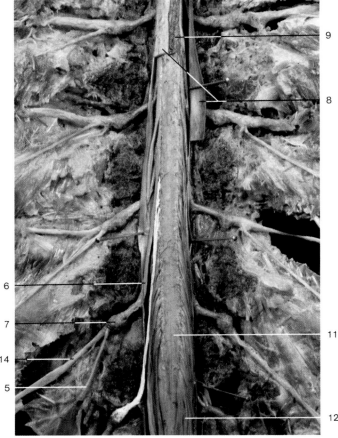

Lumbar portion of spinal cord. Note the relation between the nervous and muscular segments.

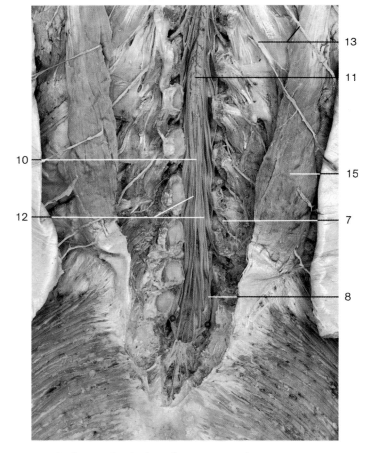

Terminal part of spinal cord. Dura removed.

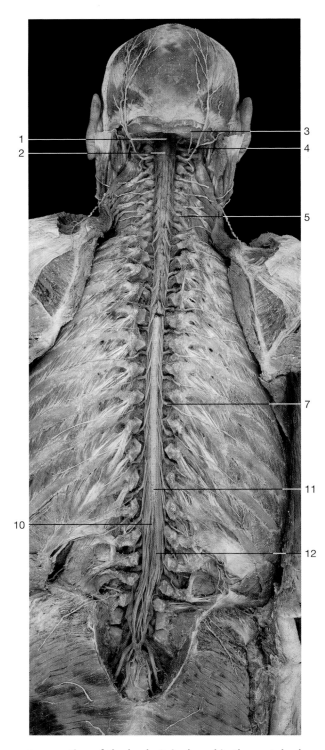

Innervation of the back. Spinal cord in the vertebral canal (opened). Longissimus dorsi and iliocostal muscles have been removed.

1	Cerebellomedullary cistern	9	Spinal arachnoid mater
2	Medulla oblongata	10	Filum terminale
3	Third cervical nerve (C_3)	11	Conus medullaris
4	Greater occipital nerve (C_2)	12	Cauda equina
5	Dorsal primary ramus	13	Lateral branches of dorsal rami of spinal nerves
6	Dorsal roots	14	Ventral ramus of spinal nerve (intercostal nerve)
7	Spinal ganglion	15	Iliocostalis muscle
8	Spinal dura mater		

1   Arch of vertebra (divided)
2   Spinal nerve with meningeal coverings
3   Dorsal roots of thoracic spinal nerves
4   Spinal cord (thoracic portion)
5   Spinal ganglia with meningeal coverings
6   Pia mater with blood vessels
7   Dura mater (opened)
8   Denticulate ligament
9   Lateral branch of dorsal ramus
10 Dorsal ramus of spinal nerve
    (dividing into a medial and lateral branch)
11 Medial branch of dorsal ramus
    of spinal nerve
12 Spinal dura mater
13 Spinal nerves of sacral segments
14 Filum terminale

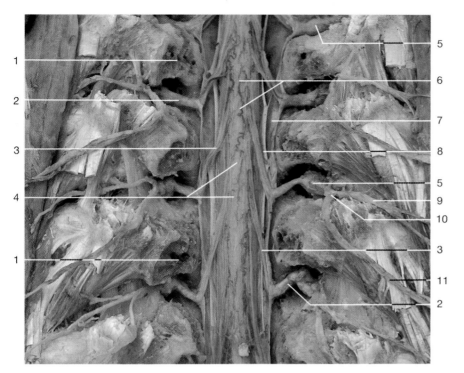

Thoracic portion of spinal cord (dorsal aspect). Vertebral canal and dura mater opened.

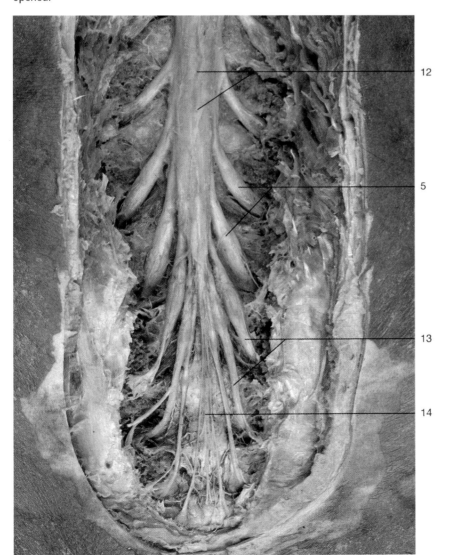

Terminal part of spinal cord with dura mater (dorsal aspect). Dorsal part of sacrum removed.

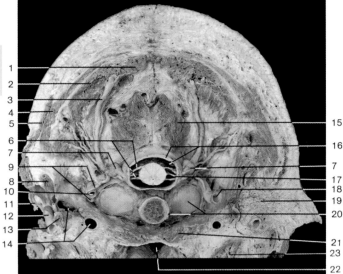

Horizontal section of the neck. Dissection of the second cervical spinal nerve. Posterior surface at top of figure.

1   Trapezius muscle
2   Semispinalis capitis muscle
3   Dorsal ramus of spinal nerve
4   Sternocleidomastoid muscle
5   Platysma muscle
6   Dorsal and ventral roots of spinal nerves
7   Spinal ganglion
8   Posterior belly of digastric muscle
9   Ventral ramus of spinal nerve
10 Vertebral artery
11 Great auricular nerve
12 Superficial temporal artery
13 Styloid process
14 Internal jugular vein and internal carotid artery
15 Rectus capitis posterior major muscle
16 Dura mater and subarachnoid space
17 Denticulate ligament
18 Vertebral artery
19 Parotid gland
20 Dens of axis (divided) and inferior articular facet of atlas
21 Longus capitis muscle
22 Pharyngeal cavity
23 Medial pterygoid muscle
24 Periosteum of vertebral canal
25 Posterior spinal arteries
26 Anterior spinal artery

Meningeal coverings
27 Dura mater
28 Subdural space
29 Extradural or epidural space with venous plexus and fatty tissue
30 Arachnoid (green)
31 Subarachnoid space
32 Pia mater (pink)
33 Nucleus pulposus
34 Crus of diaphragm
35 Intervertebral disc
36 Body of first lumbar vertebra
37 Spinal cord
38 Conus medullaris
39 Cauda equina
40 Filum terminale
41 Spinous process

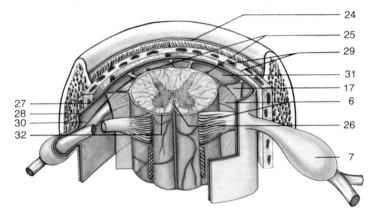

Meningeal coverings of the spinal cord (anterior aspect). (Schematic drawing.)

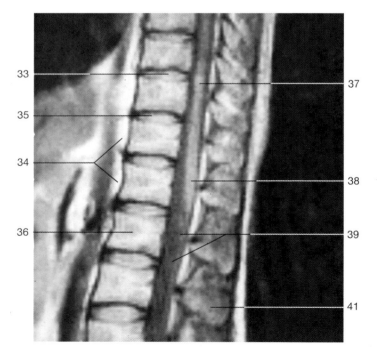

Sagittal section through the vertebral canal, T₉–L₂. (MRI scan.)

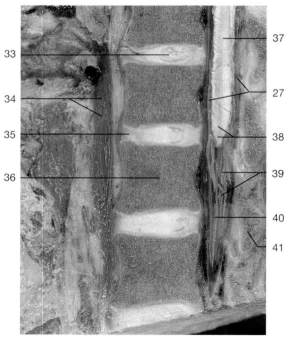

Sagittal section through the vertebral canal, T₁₂–L₂. Notice red bone marrow (unfixed).

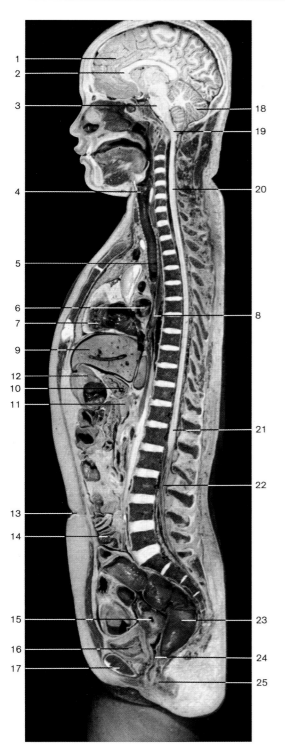

Median section of the head and trunk in the adult (female). The conus medullaris of the spinal cord is located at the level of L_1.

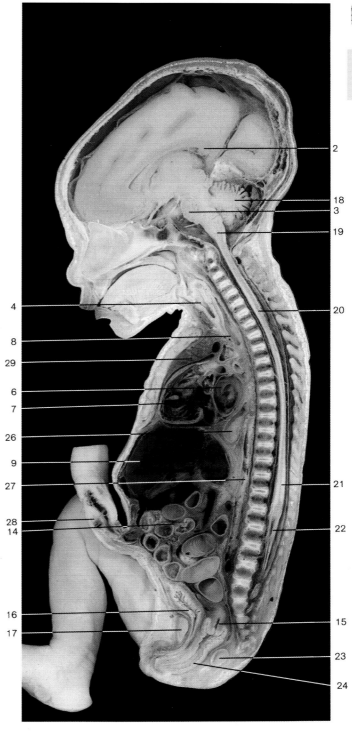

Median section of the head and trunk in the neonate.
Note that in the neonate the conus medullaris of the spinal cord extends far more caudally than in the adult.

1	Cerebrum	11	Pancreas
2	Corpus callosum	12	Transverse colon
3	Pons	13	Umbilicus
4	Larynx	14	Small intestine
5	Trachea	15	Uterus
6	Left atrium	16	Urinary bladder
7	Right ventricle	17	Pubic symphysis
8	Esophagus	18	Cerebellum
9	Liver	19	Medulla oblongata
10	Stomach	20	Spinal cord

21	Conus medullaris
22	Cauda equina
23	Rectum
24	Vagina
25	Anus
26	Inferior vena cava
27	Aorta
28	Umbilical cord
29	Thymus

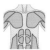

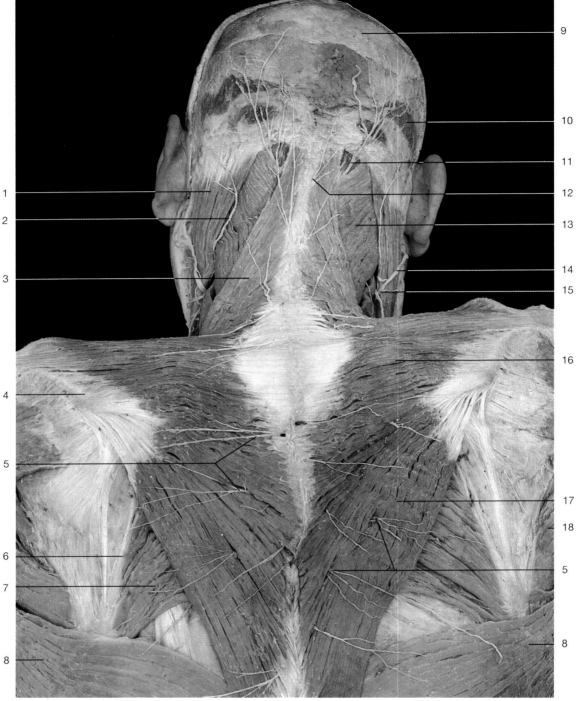

Dorsal aspect of the neck (superficial layer). Nuchal region and shoulder.

1	Sternocleidomastoid muscle	10	Occipital belly of occipitofrontalis muscle
2	Lesser occipital nerve	11	Greater occipital nerve
3	Descending fibers of trapezius muscle	12	Third occipital nerve
4	Spine of scapula	13	Splenius capitis muscle
5	Medial cutaneous branches of dorsal rami of spinal nerves	14	Great auricular nerve
6	Medial margin of scapula	15	Cutaneous nerves of cervical plexus
7	Rhomboid major muscle	16	Transverse fibers of trapezius muscle
8	Latissimus dorsi muscle	17	Ascending fibers of trapezius muscle
9	Galea aponeurotica	18	Teres major muscle

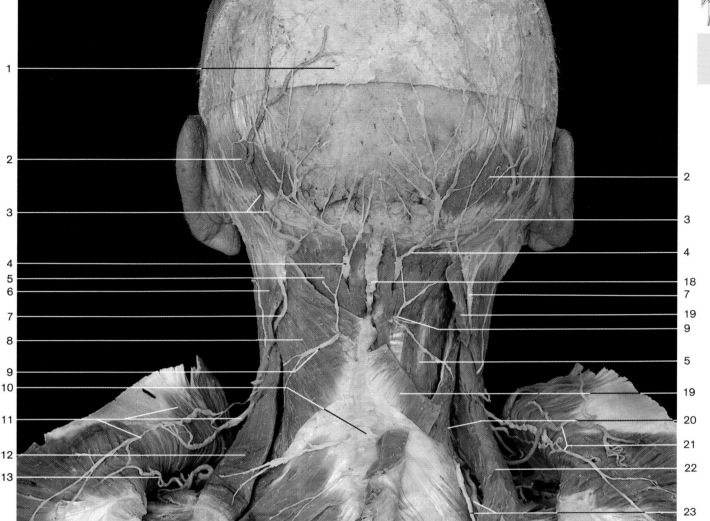

Dorsal aspect of the neck (deeper layer). The left trapezius muscle has been divided and reflected. On the right, trapezius, rhomboid, and splenius muscles have been divided. Right levator scapulae muscle has been slightly reflected.

1 Galea aponeurotica
2 Occipital belly of occipitofrontalis muscle
3 Occipital artery
4 Greater occipital nerve (C₂)
5 Semispinalis capitis muscle
6 Sternocleidomastoid muscle
7 Lesser occipital nerve
8 Left splenius capitis muscle
9 Third occipital nerve (C₃)
10 Spinous process of vertebra prominens (C₇)

11 Left trapezius muscle and accessory nerve
12 Levator scapulae muscle
13 Superficial branch of transverse cervical artery
14 Rhomboid minor muscle
15 Rhomboid major muscle
16 Medial margin of scapula
17 Medial branches of dorsal rami of spinal nerves
18 Ligamentum nuchae
19 Splenius capitis muscle (divided)

20 Splenius cervicis muscle
21 Right accessory nerve and superficial branch of transverse cervical artery
22 Right levator scapulae muscle
23 Dorsal scapular nerve and deep branch of transverse cervical artery
24 Serratus posterior superior muscle
25 Right trapezius muscle (divided and reflected)
26 Right rhomboid major muscle (divided and reflected)

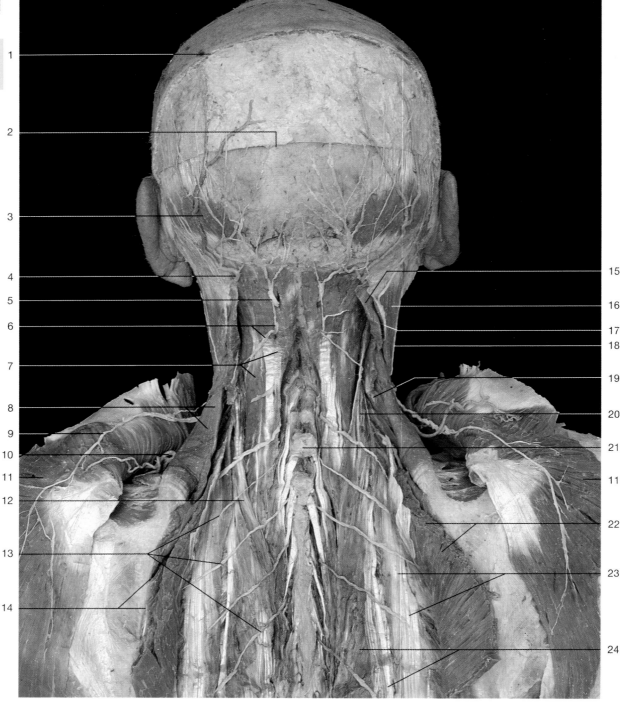

Dorsal aspect of the neck (deepest layer). Trapezius, splenius capitis, and cervicis muscles have been divided and partly removed or reflected.

1　Skin of scalp
2　Galea aponeurotica
3　Occipital belly of occipitofrontalis muscle
4　Occipital artery
5　Greater occipital nerve
6　Third occipital nerve
7　Semispinalis capitis muscle
8　Levator scapulae muscle
9　Accessory nerve (n. XI)
10　Superficial cervical artery
11　Trapezius muscle (reflected)
12　Longissimus cervicis muscle
13　Medial cutaneous branches of dorsal rami of spinal nerves
14　Medial margin of scapula
15　Splenius capitis muscle (divided)
16　Sternocleidomastoid muscle
17　Lesser occipital nerve
18　Great auricular nerve
19　Splenius cervicis muscle
20　Longissimus cervicis muscle
21　Spinous process of seventh cervical vertebra (vertebra prominens)
22　Rhomboid muscles (divided)
23　Iliocostalis thoracis muscle
24　Longissimus thoracis muscle

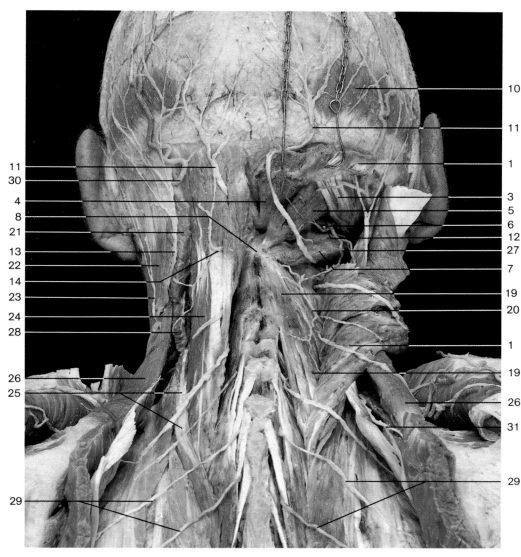

1 Semispinalis capitis muscle (divided)
2 External occipital protuberance
3 Obliquus capitis superior muscle
4 Rectus capitis posterior minor muscle
5 Rectus capitis posterior major muscle
6 Vertebral artery
7 Obliquus capitis inferior muscle
8 Spinous process of axis
9 Third cervical vertebra
10 Occipital belly of occipitofrontalis muscle
11 Greater occipital nerve
12 Suboccipital nerve (C$_1$)
13 Lesser occipital nerve
14 Third occipital nerve (C$_3$)
15 Mastoid process and splenius capitis muscle
16 Atlas
17 Axis
18 Spinous process of third cervical vertebra
19 Right semispinalis cervicis muscle
20 Deep cervical artery
21 Left splenius capitis muscle (divided)
22 Left sternocleidomastoid muscle
23 Great auricular nerve
24 Left semispinalis capitis muscle
25 Left longissimus cervicis muscle
26 Levator scapulae muscle
27 Muscular branch of vertebral artery
28 Left semispinalis cervicis muscle (divided)
29 Medial branches of dorsal rami of spinal nerves
30 Occipital artery
31 Dorsal scapular nerve

Dorsal aspect of the neck (deepest layer). **Suboccipital triangle.** Right semispinalis capitis muscle divided and reflected.

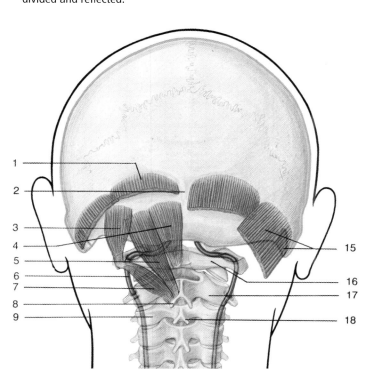

Suboccipital triangle and position of the vertebral artery (schematic drawing).

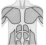

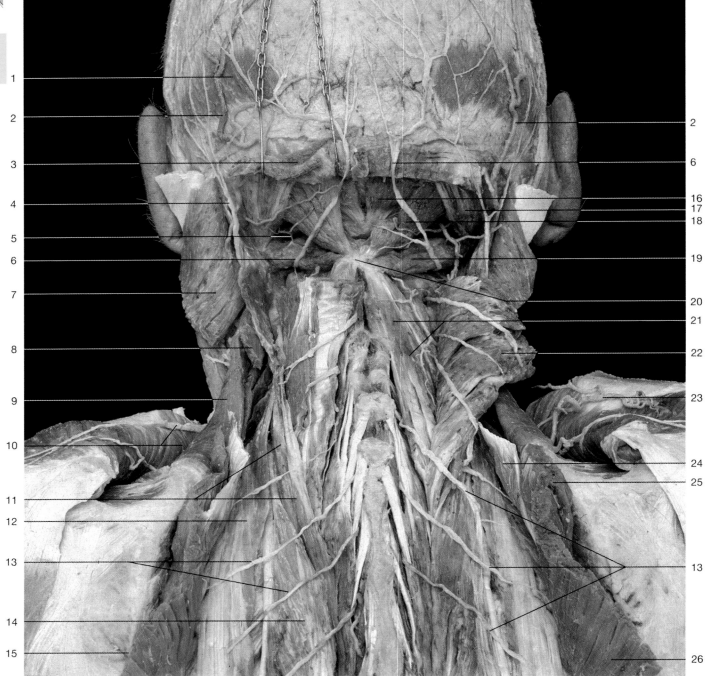

Dorsal aspect of the neck (deepest layer). Dissection of suboccipital triangle on both sides.

1 Occipital belly of occipitofrontalis muscle
2 Occipital artery
3 Insertion of semispinalis capitis muscle (divided)
4 Lesser occipital nerve (from cervical plexus)
5 Suboccipital nerve (C$_1$)
6 Greater occipital nerve (C$_2$)
7 Splenius capitis muscle (reflected)
8 Splenius cervicis muscle
9 Levator scapulae muscle
10 Accessory nerve (n. XI), trapezius muscle

11 Longissimus cervicis muscle
12 Iliocostalis cervicis muscle
13 Medial cutaneus branches of dorsal rami of spinal nerves (C$_7$, C$_8$)
14 Longissimus thoracis muscle
15 Medial margin of scapula
16 Rectus capitis posterior minor muscle
17 Obliquus capitis superior muscle
18 Rectus capitis posterior major muscle
19 Obliquus capitis inferior muscle
20 Spinous process of axis

21 Semispinalis cervicis muscle
22 Semispinalis capitis muscle (divided and reflected)
23 Transverse cervical artery (superficial branch)
24 Serratus posterior superior muscle (divided and reflected)
25 Rhomboid minor muscle (divided and reflected)
26 Rhomboid major muscle (divided and reflected)

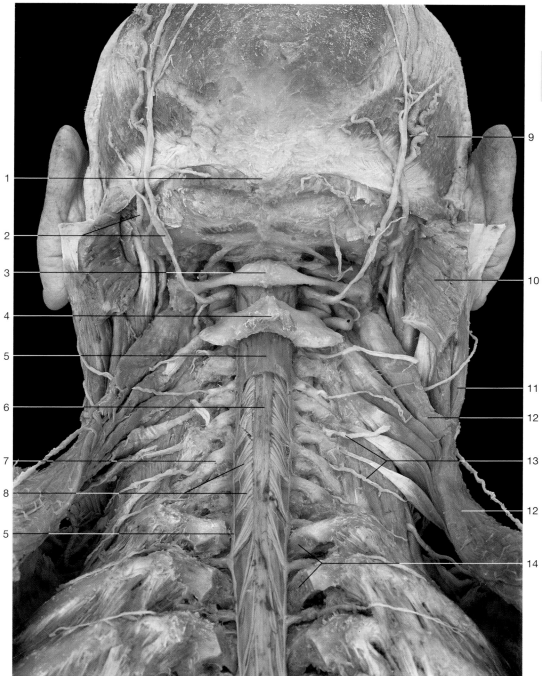

Dorsal aspect of the neck (deepest layer). The vertebral canal caudally of the atlas and axis has been opened to show the spinal cord (dura mater has been partly removed).

1 Protuberantia occipitalis externa
2 Greater occipital nerve (C₂) and occipital artery
3 Atlas (posterior arch)
4 Axis (posterior arch)
5 Dura mater
6 Spinal cord
7 Spinal ganglion

8 Posterior root filaments (fila radicularia posterior)
9 Occipital belly of occipitofrontalis muscle
10 Splenius capitis muscle (cut and reflected)
11 Sternocleidomastoid muscle
12 Levator scapulae muscle
13 Posterior branches of spinal nerves
14 Arches of cervical vertebrae (cut)

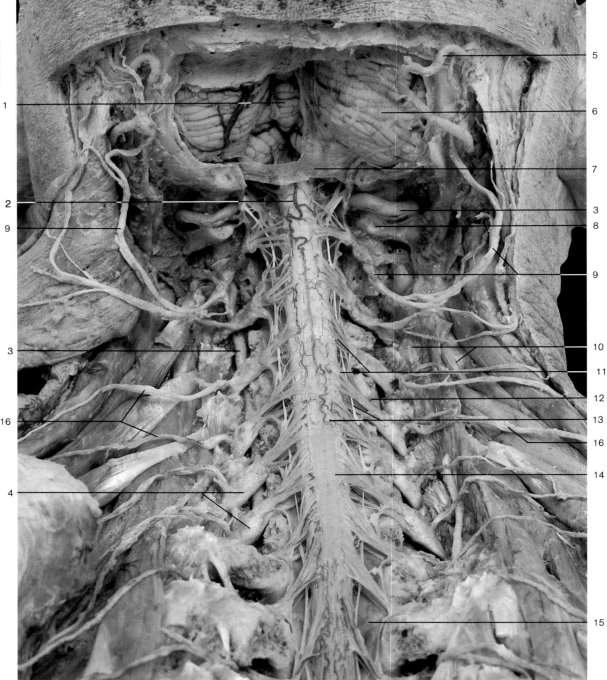

Dorsal aspect of the neck (deepest layer). Dissection of medulla oblongata and spinal cord. Cranial cavity opened.

1 Vermis of the cerebellum	9 Greater occipital nerve (C$_2$)
2 Medulla oblongata and posterior spinal artery	10 Levator scapulae muscle and intertransverse ligament
3 Vertebral artery	11 Dorsal roots of spinal nerves
4 Spinal ganglion	12 Vertebral arch
5 Occipital artery	13 Denticulate ligament and arachnoid mater
6 Cerebellum	14 Area where pia mater has been removed
7 Cerebellomedullary cistern	15 Dura mater
8 Atlas	16 Dorsal rami of spinal nerves

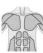

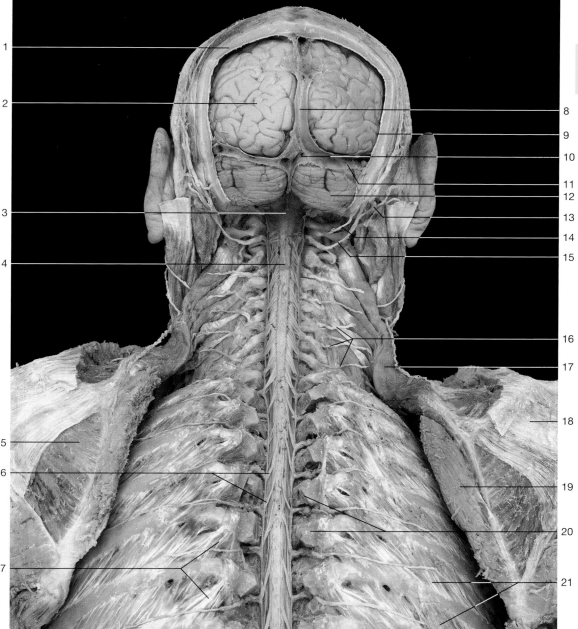

Dorsal aspect of the neck (deepest layer). Dissection of medulla oblongata and spinal cord in relation to the brain.

1	Calvaria	12	Cerebellum
2	Left hemisphere of the brain	13	Occipital artery
3	Cerebellomedullary cistern	14	Suboccipital nerve (C$_1$)
4	Spinal cord	15	Greater occipital nerve (C$_2$)
5	Scapula with infraspinous muscle	16	Posterior branches of spinal nerves
6	Root filaments (fila radicularia posterior)	17	Levator scapulae muscle
7	Levatores costarum muscles	18	Deltoid muscle
8	Falx cerebri with sinus sagittalis superior	19	Rhomboid muscles
9	Subarachnoidal space	20	Vertebral arches (cut)
10	Confluens sinuum	21	External intercostal muscle
11	Transverse sinus	22	Dura mater

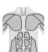

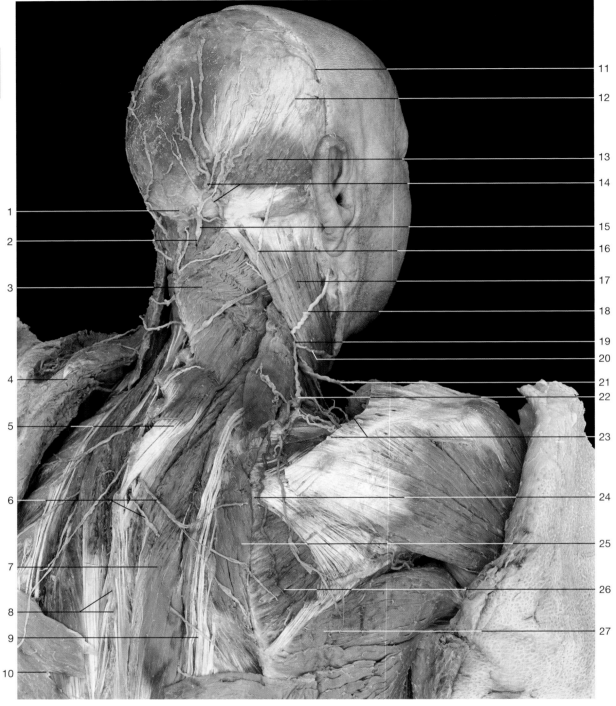

Oblique-lateral aspect of the neck and head (deeper layer). The trapezius muscle has been removed.

1 Protuberantia occipitalis externa
2 Semispinalis capitis muscle
3 Splenius capitis muscle
4 Scapula
5 Splenius cervicis muscle
6 Posterior branches of spinal nerves
7 Longissimus muscle
8 Spinous processes of thoracic vertebrae
9 Iliocostalis muscle
10 Latissimus dorsi muscle
11 Epidermis of the head (scalp)
12 Galea aponeurotica
13 Occipital belly of occipitofrontalis muscle
14 Occipital artery

15 Greater occipital nerve (C$_2$)
16 Lesser occipital nerve
17 Sternocleidomastoid muscle
18 Great auricular nerve
19 Punctum nervosum
20 Transverse cervical nerve
21 Supraclavicular nerves
22 Accessory nerve (n. XI)
23 Trapezius muscle (cut edge)
24 Medial margin of scapula
25 Rhomboid muscle
26 Infraspinous muscle
27 Teres major muscle

4 Thoracic Organs

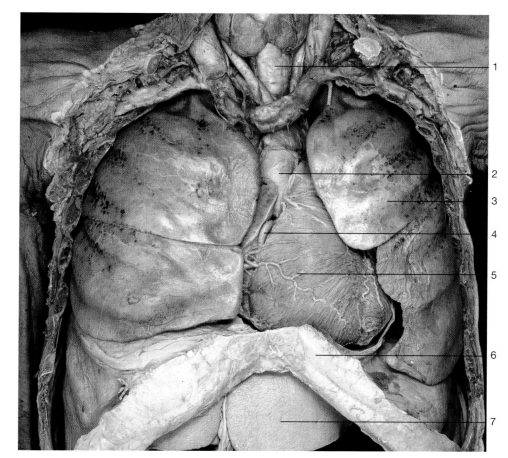

The thoracic cavity contains heart, lungs, and mediastinal organs. The thorax protects all organs but is still movable so that respiration can occur. The respiratory movements of the lung depend on the pleura covering, the thoracic wall, and the surface of the lungs.

The mediastinal organs comprise the esophagus, trachea, and the related nerves and vessels, particularly the aorta, superior vena cava, and the thoracic duct. The thoracic cavity is separated from the abdominal cavity by the diaphragm.

Thoracic organs, heart, and lungs in situ (ventral aspect). Anterior thoracic wall, parietal pleura, and pericardium have been removed.

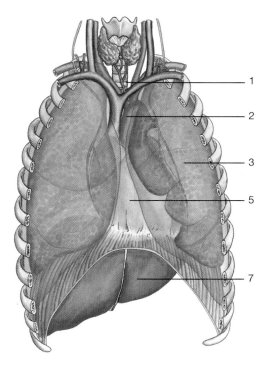

Position of lungs and heart within the thoracic cavity (schematic drawing). The anterior part of the thorax is not depicted.

1 Trachea
2 Ascending aorta
3 Left lung
4 Right coronary artery
5 Heart (right ventricle)
6 Costal arch
7 Liver

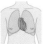

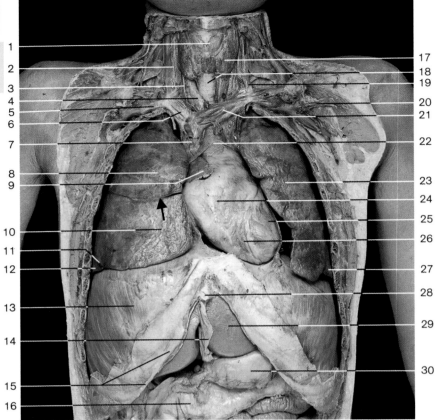

1	Cricothyroid muscle
2	Right internal jugular vein
3	Vagus nerve
4	Right common carotid artery
5	Right subclavian vein
6	Right brachiocephalic vein
7	Superior vena cava
8	Upper lobe of right lung
9	Right auricle
10	Middle lobe of right lung
11	Oblique fissure of right lung
12	Lower lobe of right lung
13	Diaphragm
14	Falciform ligament
15	Costal margin
16	Transverse colon
17	Thyroid gland
18	Trachea
19	Left internal jugular vein
20	Left cephalic vein
21	Left brachiocephalic vein
22	Pericardium (cut edge)
23	Upper lobe of left lung
24	Right ventricle
25	Left ventricle
26	Anterior interventricular sulcus
27	Lower lobe of left lung
28	Xiphoid process
29	Liver
30	Stomach
31	Pectoralis major muscle
32	Sternum
33	Left ventricle and bulb of aorta
34	Left main bronchus
35	Esophagus
36	Descending aorta
37	Spinal cord
38	Scapula
39	Right atrium
40	Right pulmonary vein
41	Right main bronchus
42	Azygos vein
43	Body of vertebra
44	Rib

Positions of thoracic organs. The anterior thoracic wall has been removed.
Arrow: horizontal fissure of right lung.

Horizontal section through the thorax at the level of the seventh thoracic vertebra (from below).

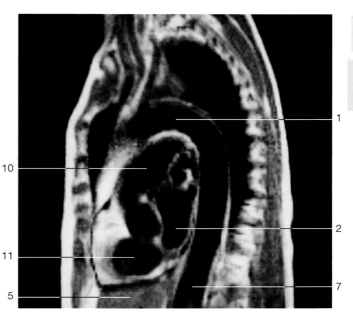

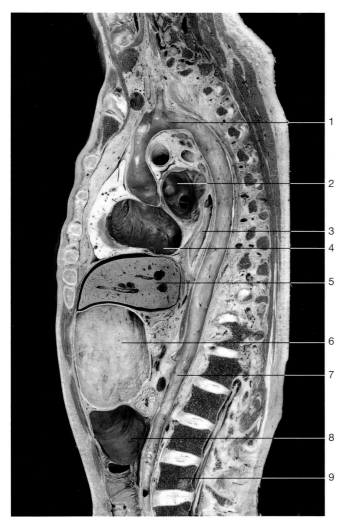

Sagittal section through the thorax, 2 cm lateral to the median plane.

Sagittal section through the thorax (MRI scan).

1   Aortic arch
2   Left atrium of the heart
3   Esophagus
4   Right atrium of the heart
5   Liver
6   Stomach
7   Abdominal aorta
8   Transverse colon (dilated)
9   Lumbar vertebral body
10   Pulmonary trunk
11   Left ventricle of the heart
12   Trachea
13   Ascending aorta
14   Right ventricle of the heart
15   Pericardium
16   Remaining parts of thymus gland

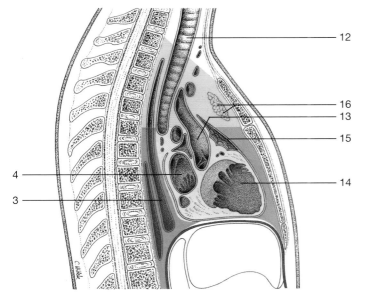

Regional anatomy of the thoracic cavity (midsagittal section). The parts of the mediastinum are indicated by colors.

Parts of mediastinum	Content
Superior mediastinum (yellow)	Trachea, brachiocephalic vein, thymus, aortic arch, esophagus, thoracic duct
Middle portion of mediastinum (light blue)	Heart, ascending aorta, pulmonary trunk, pulmonary veins, phrenic nerves
Posterior mediastinum (red)	Esophagus with vagus nerves, descending aorta, thoracic duct, sympathetic trunks
Anterior portion of mediastinum (light red)	Smaller vessels and nerves, fat and connective tissue, thymus (only in the child)

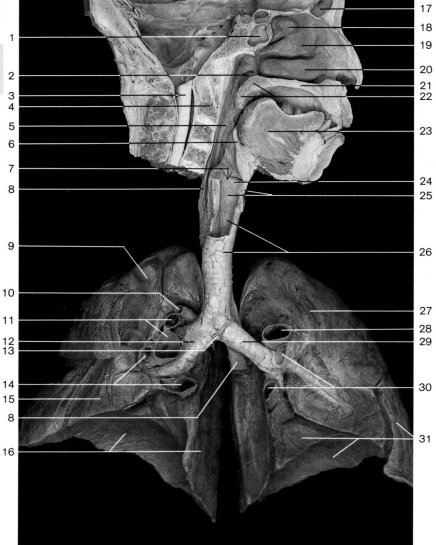

1 Sphenoid sinus
2 Pharyngeal opening of auditory tube
3 Spinal cord
4 Dens of axis
5 Oropharynx (oropharyngeal isthmus)
6 Epiglottis
7 Entrance of larynx
8 Esophagus
9 Upper lobe of right lung
10 Azygos vein
11 Branches of pulmonary artery
12 Right main bronchus
13 Bifurcation of trachea
14 Tributaries of right pulmonary veins
15 Middle lobe of right lung
16 Lower lobe of right lung
17 Frontal sinus
18 Superior nasal concha
19 Middle nasal concha
20 Inferior nasal concha
21 Hard palate
22 Soft palate with uvula
23 Tongue
24 Vocal fold
25 Larynx
26 Trachea
27 Upper lobe of left lung
28 Left pulmonary artery
29 Left main bronchus
30 Left pulmonary veins
31 Lower lobe of left lung

Respiratory system. The lungs have been fixed in expiration and turned laterally. Head bisected and turned laterally.

▷ **To page 247:**

1 Nasal cavity
2 Pharynx
3 Larynx (thyroid cartilage)
4 Trachea
5 Upper lobe of right lung
6 Bifurcation of trachea
7 Right main bronchus
8 Horizontal fissure of right lung
9 Middle lobe of right lung
10 Oblique fissures of lungs
11 Lower lobe of right lung
12 Clavicle
13 Upper lobe of left lung
14 Left main bronchus
15 Bronchi supplying bronchopulmonary segments
16 Lower lobe of left lung
17 Costal margin
18 Hyoid bone
19 Right superior lobe bronchus
20 Right middle lobe bronchus
21 Right inferior lobe bronchus
22 Left superior lobe bronchus
23 Left inferior lobe bronchus
24 Segmental bronchi
25 Branches of pulmonary arteries
26 Branches of pulmonary veins

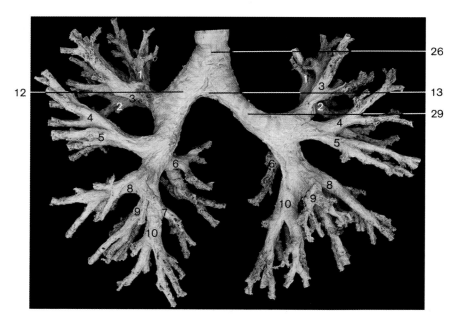

Bronchial tree (ventral aspect). The lung tissue has been removed. The bronchopulmonary segments are numbered 1–10.

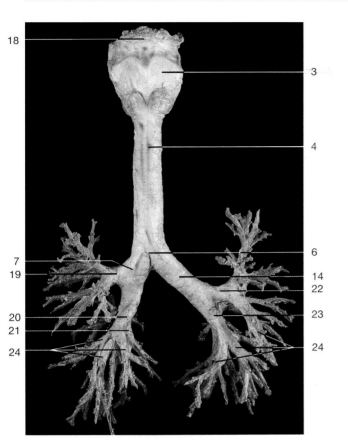

Larynx, trachea, and bronchial tree (anterior aspect).

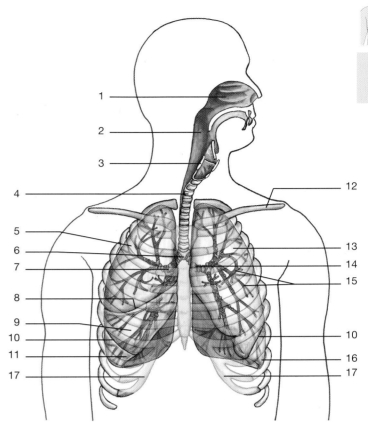

Organization and positions of respiratory organs (schematic drawing).

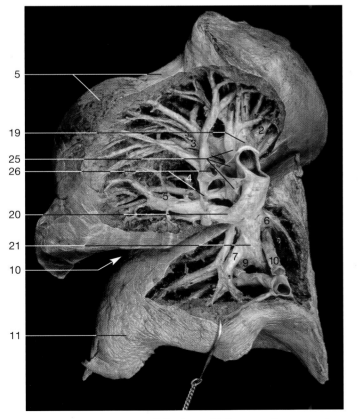

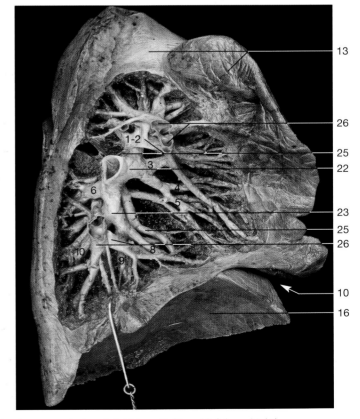

Mediastinal dissection of the bronchial tree, pulmonary veins, and pulmonary arteries of right lung (left) and left lung (right) (medial aspect). The bronchopulmonary segments are numbered 1–10.

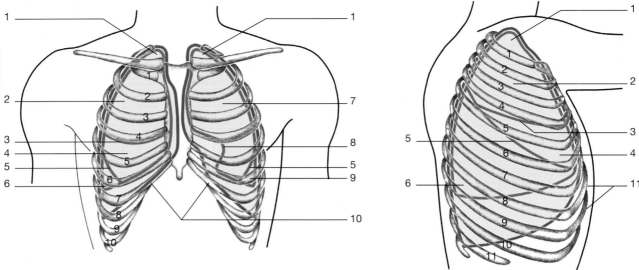

Surface projections of lungs and pleura on the thoracic wall. Left: anterior aspect; right: right-lateral aspect.
Red = margins of the lung; blue = margins of pleura. The numbers indicate ribs.

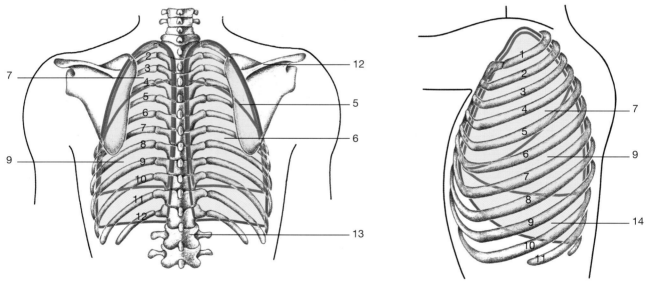

Surface projections of lungs and pleura on the thoracic wall. Left: posterior aspect; right: left-lateral aspect.
Red = margins of lung; blue = margins of pleura. The numbers indicate ribs.

1 Apex of lung	6 Lower lobe of right lung	11 Costal margin
2 Upper lobe of right lung	7 Upper lobe of left lung	12 Spine of scapula
3 Horizontal fissure of right lung	8 Cardiac notch of left lung	13 First lumbar vertebra
4 Middle lobe of right lung	9 Lower lobe of left lung	14 Space between border of lung and pleura
5 Oblique fissures of lungs	10 Infrasternal angle	(costodiaphragmatic recess)

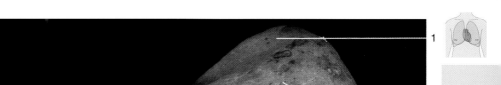

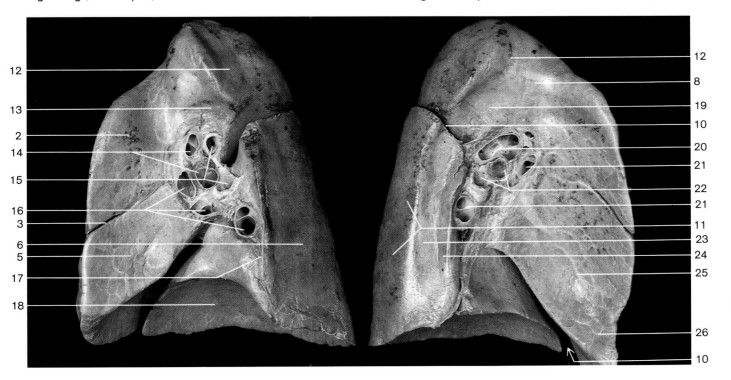

Right lung (lateral aspect).

Left lung (lateral aspect).

Right lung (medial aspect).

Left lung (medial aspect).

1	Apex of lung	8	Upper lobe of left lung	15	Bronchi	22	Left secondary bronchi
2	Upper lobe of right lung	9	Impressions of ribs	16	Right pulmonary veins	23	Groove of thoracic aorta
3	Horizontal fissure of right lung	10	Oblique fissure of left lung	17	Pulmonary ligament	24	Groove of esophagus
4	Oblique fissure of right lung	11	Lower lobe of left lung	18	Diaphragmatic surface	25	Cardiac impression
5	Middle lobe of right lung	12	Groove of subclavian artery	19	Groove of aortic arch	26	Lingula
6	Lower lobe of right lung	13	Groove of azygos arch	20	Left pulmonary artery		
7	Inferior border	14	Branches of right pulmonary artery	21	Branches of left pulmonary veins		

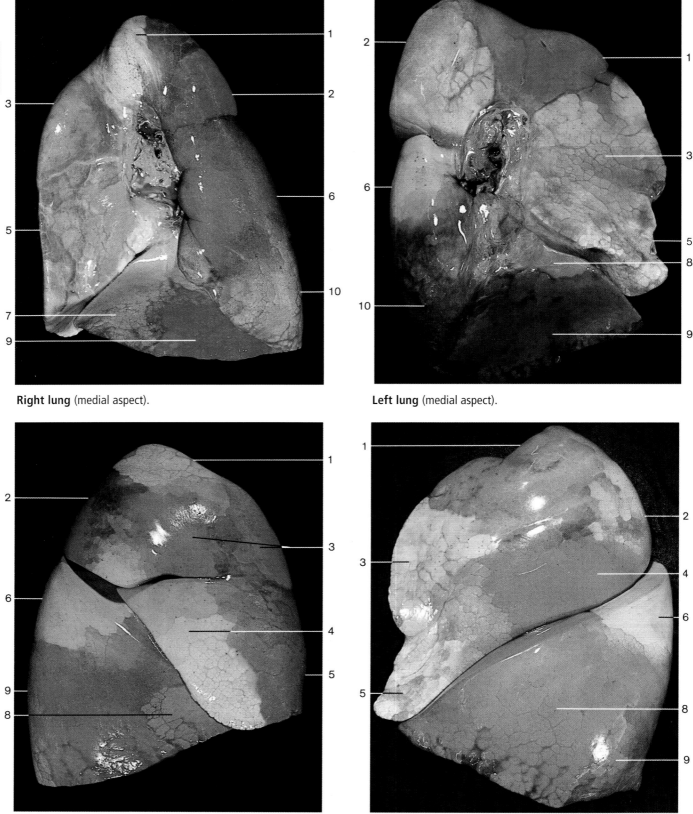

Right lung (medial aspect).

Left lung (medial aspect).

Right lung (lateral aspect).

Left lung (lateral aspect).

The bronchopulmonary segments of the lungs are differentiated by the various colors. Notice that there is no segment in the left lung that corresponds to the seventh segment of the right lung. Compare with the schematic drawing on the facing page.

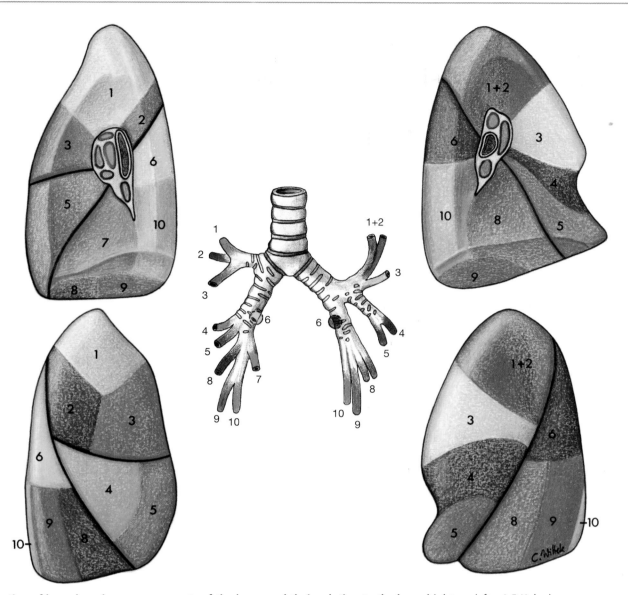

Distribution of bronchopulmonary segments of the lungs and their relation to the bronchial tree (after J. F. Huber).

The bronchopulmonary segments are morphologically and functionally separate, independent respiratory units of the lung tissue. Each segment is surrounded by connective tissue that is continuous with the visceral pleura. The segmental bronchi are centrally located in each segment and are closely accompanied by branches of the pulmonary arteries, whereas the tributaries of the pulmonary veins run **between** the segments. Thus, the veins serve two adjacent segments that drain for the most part into more than one vein. A bronchopulmonary segment is therefore not a complete vascular unit, but segmentation is the result of a specific architecture of the lung vasculature.

Right lung			Left lung			
1 Apical segment	Upper lobe bronchus		1+2 Apicoposterior segment	Superior division		Upper lobe bronchus
2 Posterior segment						
3 Anterior segment			3 Anterior segment			
4 Lateral segment	Middle lobe bronchus		4 Superior lingular segment	Inferior division		
5 Medial segment			5 Inferior lingular segment			
6 Superior (apical) segment	Lower lobe bronchus		6 Superior (apical) segment	Lower lobe bronchus		
7 Medial basal segment			7 Absent			
8 Anterior basal segment			8 Anteromedial basal segment			
9 Lateral basal segment			9 Lateral basal segment			
10 Posterior basal segment			10 Posterior basal segment			

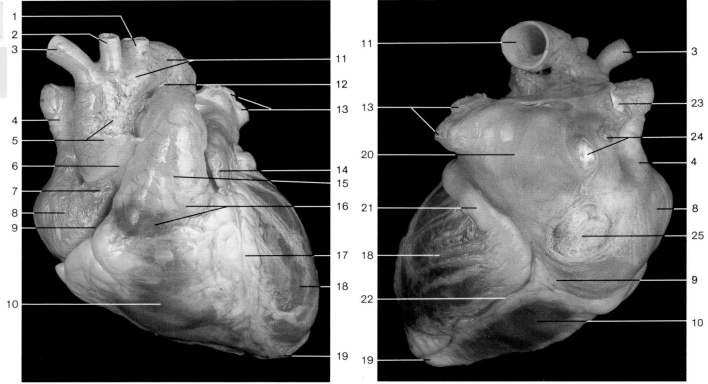

Heart of 30-year-old woman (anterior aspect).

Heart of 30-year-old woman (oblique-posterior view).

1	Left subclavian artery	9	Coronary sulcus	18	Left ventricle
2	Left common carotid artery	10	Right ventricle	19	Apex of the heart
3	Brachiocephalic trunk	11	Aortic arch	20	Left atrium
4	Superior vena cava	12	Ligamentum arteriosum	21	Epicardial fat overlying coronary sinus
5	Ascending aorta	13	Left pulmonary veins	22	Posterior interventricular sulcus
6	Bulb of the aorta	14	Left auricle	23	Right pulmonary artery
7	Right auricle	15	Pulmonary trunk	24	Right pulmonary veins
8	Right atrium	16	Sinus of pulmonary trunk	25	Inferior vena cava
		17	Anterior interventricular sulcus		

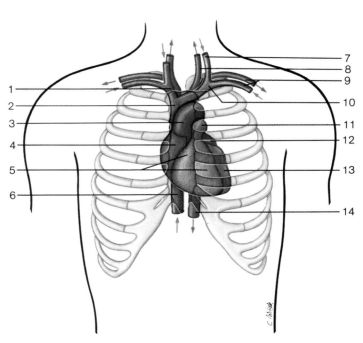

Position of heart and its vessels within the thorax (schematic drawing).

1	Right brachiocephalic vein
2	Superior vena cava
3	Ascending aorta
4	Right atrium
5	Right ventricle
6	Inferior vena cava
7	Left internal jugular vein
8	Left common carotid artery
9	Left axillary artery and vein
10	Left brachiocephalic vein
11	Pulmonary trunk
12	Left auricle
13	Left ventricle
14	Descending aorta

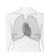

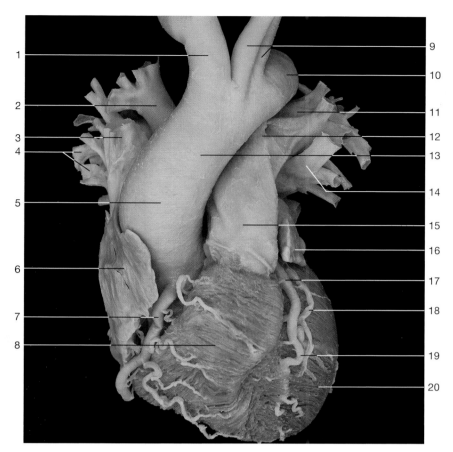

1   Brachiocephalic trunk
2   Right pulmonary artery
3   Superior vena cava
4   Right pulmonary veins
5   Ascending aorta
6   Right atrium
7   Right coronary artery
8   Right ventricle
9   Left common carotid artery and left
    subclavian artery
10 Descending aorta (thoracic part)
11 Ligamentum arteriosum (remnant of
    ductus arteriosus Botalli)
12 Left pulmonary artery
13 Aortic arch
14 Left pulmonary veins
15 Pulmonary trunk
16 Left atrium
17 Left coronary artery
18 Diagonal branch of left coronary artery
19 Interventricular branch of left coronary
    artery
20 Left ventricle
21 Right brachiocephalic vein
22 Thoracic wall
23 Liver
24 Aortic valve
25 Chordae tendineae
26 Papillary muscles
27 Stomach

Heart with related vessels. Dissection of coronary arteries (anterior aspect, systolic phase of heart action).

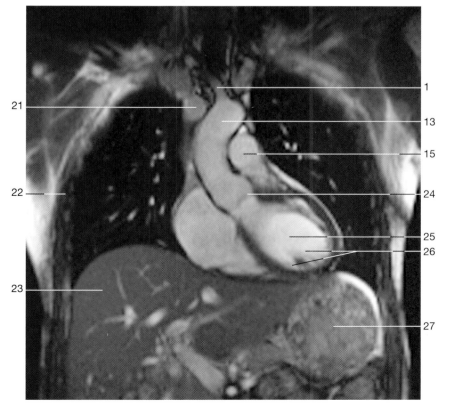

Coronal section through the thorax at the level of the ascending aorta (MRI scan, courtesy of Prof. W. Bautz and R. Janka, M. D., University of Erlangen, Germany).

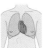

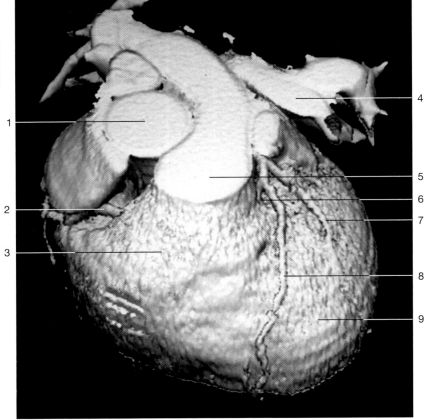

1   Ascending aorta
2   Right coronary artery
3   Right ventricle
4   Left atrium
5   Pulmonary trunk
6   Septal branch of left coronary artery
7   Diagonal branch
8   Anterior interventricular branch of left
    coronary artery
9   Left ventricle
10 Aortic root
11 Superior vena cava
12 Circumflex branch of left coronary artery
13 Sternum

Human heart (3-D reconstruction of electron beam CT scans as "Shaded Surface Display" [1]).

Electron beam tomographic image of the human heart (axial section after injection of contrast medium[1]).

[1] Courtesy of Drs. W. Moshage, S. Achenbach, and D. Ropers, Dept. of Internal Medicine II, University of Erlangen-Nürnberg, Germany.

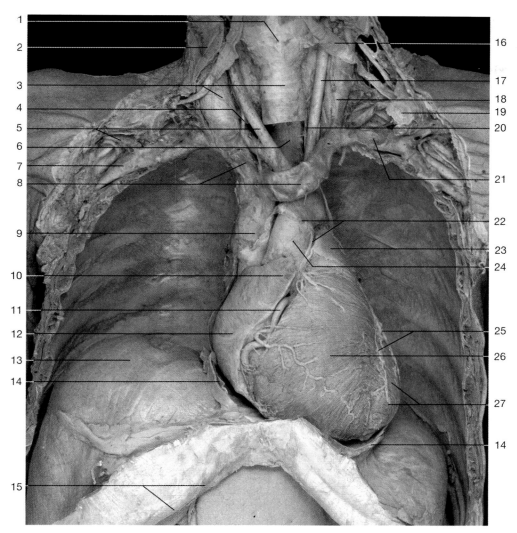

1	Larynx (thyroid cartilage)
2	Sternocleidomastoid muscle (divided)
3	Trachea (divided) and right internal jugular vein
4	Vagus nerve
5	Right common carotid artery and cephalic vein
6	Esophagus
7	Right axillary vein
8	Right and left brachiocephalic veins
9	Superior vena cava
10	Right auricle
11	Right coronary artery
12	Right atrium
13	Diaphragm
14	Pericardium (cut edges)
15	Costal margin
16	Omohyoid muscle
17	Left common carotid artery
18	Left internal jugular vein
19	Clavicle (divided)
20	Left recurrent laryngeal nerve
21	Subclavian vein
22	Pericardial reflection
23	Pulmonary trunk
24	Ascending aorta
25	Anterior interventricular sulcus and anterior interventricular branch of left coronary artery
26	Right ventricle
27	Left ventricle
28	Aortic valve
29	Tricuspid or right atrioventricular valve
30	Inferior vena cava
31	Pulmonary veins
32	Pulmonary valve
33	Left atrioventricular (bicuspid or mitral) valve

Heart and related vessels in situ (anterior aspect). Anterior thoracic wall, pericardium, and epicardium have been removed; trachea divided.

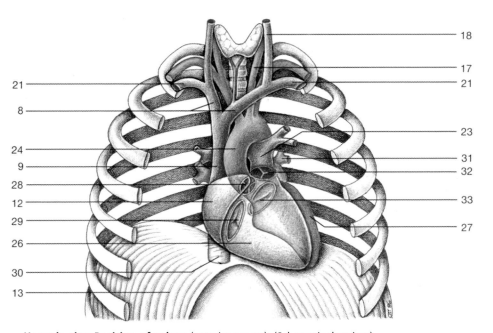

Heart in situ. Position of valves (anterior aspect). (Schematic drawing.)

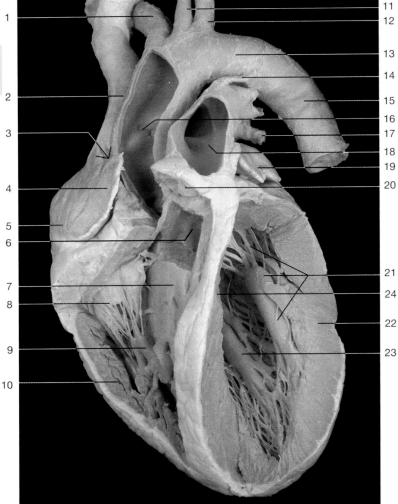

1 Brachiocephalic trunk
2 Superior vena cava
3 Sulcus terminalis
4 Right auricle
5 Right atrium
6 Aortic valve
7 Conus arteriosus (interventricular septum)
8 Right atrioventricular (tricuspid) valve
9 Anterior papillary muscle
10 Myocardium of right ventricle
11 Left common carotid artery
12 Left subclavian artery
13 Aortic arch
14 Ligamentum arteriosum (remnant of ductus arteriosus)
15 Thoracic aorta (descending aorta)
16 Ascending aorta
17 Left pulmonary vein
18 Pulmonary trunk
19 Left auricle
20 Pulmonic valve
21 Anterior papillary muscle with chordae tendineae
22 Myocardium of left ventricle
23 Posterior papillary muscle
24 Interventricular septum
25 Right and left brachiocephalic veins
26 Chordae tendineae
27 Papillary muscles of right ventricle
28 Left atrium
29 Infundibulum
30 Anterior papillary muscle of left ventricle
31 Left atrioventricular (bicuspid or mitral) valve and chordae tendineae
32 Apex of heart
33 Inferior vena cava
34 Liver
35 Aorta (pars abdominalis)

Anterior aspect of the heart. Dissection of the four valves.

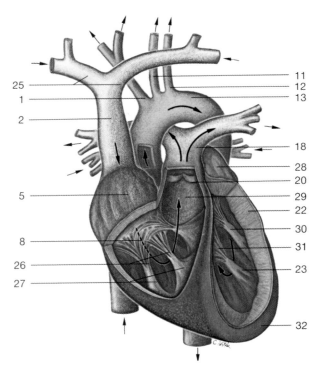

Circulation within the heart (anterior aspect).
Arrows = direction of blood flow.

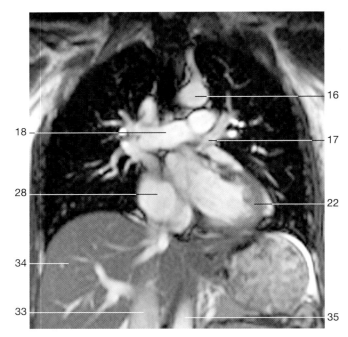

MRI scan of the heart (coronal section at the level of the left atrium; courtesy of Prof. W. Bautz and R. Janka, M. D., University of Erlangen, Germany).

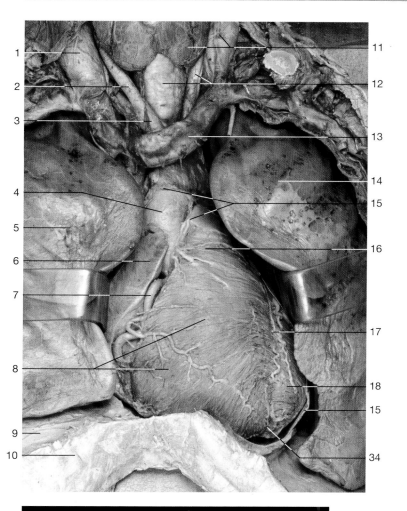

Heart in situ. Myocardium and coronary arteries (anterior aspect).

1   Internal jugular vein
2   Common carotid artery
3   Brachiocephalic trunk
4   Ascending aorta
5   Right lung
6   Right auricle
7   Right coronary artery
8   Myocardium of right ventricle
9   Diaphragm
10 Costal margin
11 Thyroid gland and internal jugular vein
12 Trachea and left common carotid artery
13 Left brachiocephalic vein
14 Left lung
15 Pericardium (cut edge)
16 Pulmonary trunk
17 Anterior interventricular artery
18 Myocardium of left ventricle
19 Muscular vortex (right ventricle)
20 Posterior interventricular sulcus
21 Anterior interventricular sulcus
22 Muscular vortex (left ventricle)
23 Aortic arch
24 Left atrium
25 Coronary sinus
26 Superior vena cava
27 Right pulmonary vein
28 Right atrium
29 Inferior vena cava
30 Coronary sulcus
31 Myocardium of left ventricle
32 Left pulmonary artery
33 Left pulmonary vein
34 Apex of heart

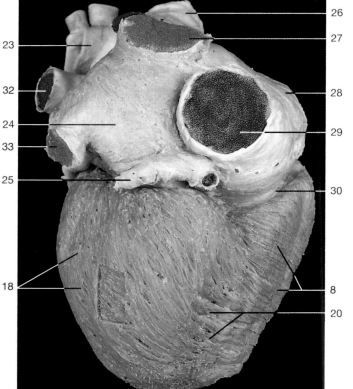

Heart (posterior aspect). The myocardium of the left ventricle has been fenestrated to show the muscle fiber bundles of the deeper layer with their more circular course.

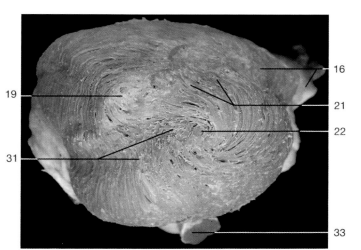

Vortex of cardiac muscle fibers (from below).

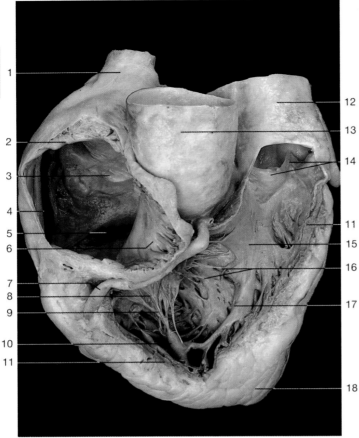

1 Superior vena cava
2 Crista terminalis
3 Fossa ovalis
4 Opening of inferior vena cava
5 Opening of coronary sinus
6 Right auricle
7 Right coronary artery and coronary sulcus
8 Anterior cusp of tricuspid valve
9 Chordae tendineae
10 Anterior papillary muscle
11 Myocardium
12 Pulmonary trunk
13 Ascending aorta
14 Pulmonic valve
15 Conus arteriosus (interventricular septum)
16 Septal papillary muscles
17 Septomarginal trabecula or moderator band
18 Apex of heart
19 Left auricle
20 Aortic valve
21 Left ventricle
22 Pulmonary veins
23 Position of fossa ovalis
24 Left atrium
25 Left atrioventricular (bicuspid or mitral) valve
26 Right atrium
27 Pericardium
28 Posterior papillary muscle
29 Right ventricle
30 Interventricular septum

Right heart (anterior aspect). Anterior wall of right atrium and ventricle removed.

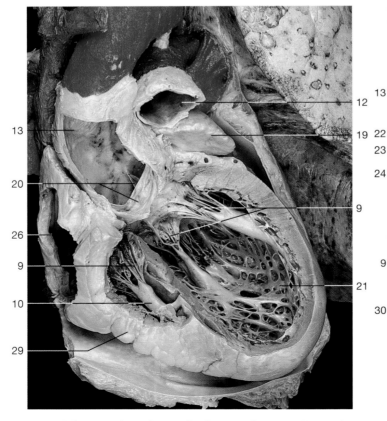

Heart, left ventricle with mitral valve, papillary muscles, and aortic valve (anterior portion of the heart removed).

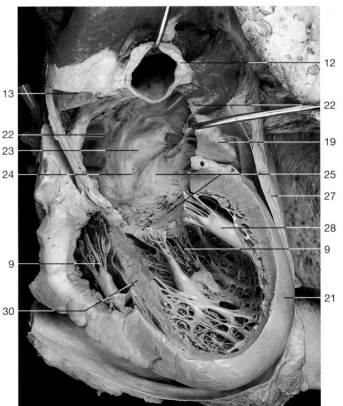

Heart, left ventricle, and atrium (opened) showing the posterior part of the mitral valve with papillary muscles.

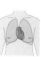

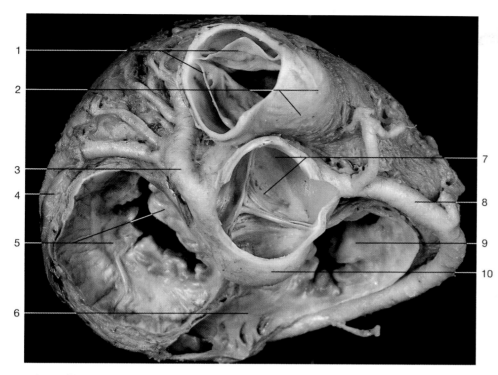

1	Pulmonic valve
2	Sinus of pulmonary trunk
3	Left coronary artery
4	Great cardiac vein
5	Left atrioventricular (mitral) valve
6	Coronary sinus
7	Aortic valve
8	Right coronary artery
9	Right atrioventricular (tricuspid) valve
10	Bulb of aorta
11	Anterior semilunar cusp of pulmonic valve
12	Left semilunar cusp of pulmonic valve
13	Right semilunar cusp of pulmonic valve
14	Left semilunar cusp of aortic valve
15	Right semilunar cusp of aortic valve
16	Posterior semilunar cusp of aortic valve
17	Right atrium
18	Anterior cusp of tricuspid valve
19	Chordae tendineae
20	Trabeculae carneae
21	Interventricular septum
22	Septal cusp of tricuspid valve
23	Anterior papillary muscle
24	Myocardium of right ventricle

Valves of heart (superior aspect). Left and right atria removed. Dissection of coronary arteries. Above: anterior wall of the heart.

Pulmonic and aortic valves (from above). Anterior wall of the heart at the top. Both valves are closed.

Right atrioventricular (tricuspid) valve (anterior aspect after removal of the anterior wall of the right ventricle).

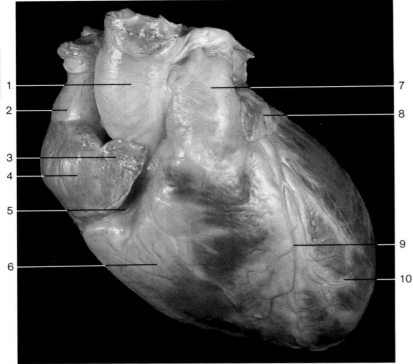

1 Ascending aorta
2 Superior vena cava
3 Right auricle
4 Right atrium
5 Coronary sulcus
6 Right ventricle
7 Pulmonary trunk
8 Left auricle
9 Anterior interventricular sulcus
10 Left ventricle
11 Right pulmonary artery
12 Sulcus terminalis with sinu-atrial node
13 Line indicating plane of position of valves
14 Myocardium of right atrium
15 Inferior vena cava
16 Valve of pulmonary trunk
17 Tricuspid valve
18 Myocardium of right ventricle

Heart, fixed in **diastole** (anterior aspect). The ventricles are relaxed, atria contracted.

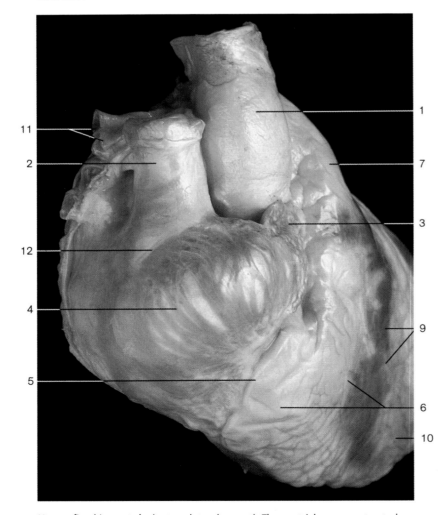

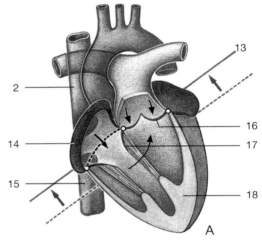

Heart, fixed in **systole** (antero-lateral aspect). The ventricles are contracted, atria dilated.

Morphological changes during heart movements.
Note the changes in position of the valves (red arrows). Contracted portions of heart are indicated in black.
A. **Diastole:** muscles of the ventricles relaxed, atrioventricular valves open, semilunar valves closed.
B. **Systole:** muscles of ventricles contracted, atrioventricular valves closed, semilunar valves open.

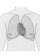

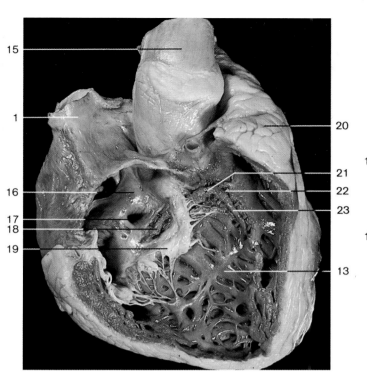

Right ventricle, dissection of **atrioventricular node, atrioventricular bundle (bundle of His),** and **right limb or bundle branch** (probes).

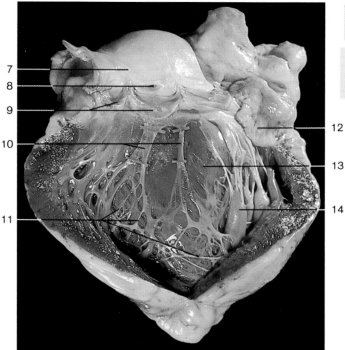

Left ventricle, dissection of left **limb or bundle branch of conducting system** (probes).

1 Superior vena cava	5 Muscle fiber bundles of right atrium
2 Sulcus terminalis	6 Coronary sulcus (with right coronary artery)
3 Bulb of aorta	7 Aortic sinus
4 Sinu-atrial node (arrows)	8 Entrance to left coronary artery

9 Aortic valve
10 Branches of left bundle branch
11 Purkinje fibers
12 Left auricle
13 Interventricular septum
14 Papillary muscles
15 Ascending aorta
16 Right atrium
17 Opening of coronary sinus
18 Atrioventricular node
19 Septal cusp of tricuspid valve
20 Pulmonary trunk
21 Atrioventricular bundle (bundle of His)
22 Bifurcation of atrioventricular bundle
23 Right bundle branch
24 Inferior vena cava
25 Left atrium
26 Left bundle branch
27 Papillary muscles with Purkinje fibers

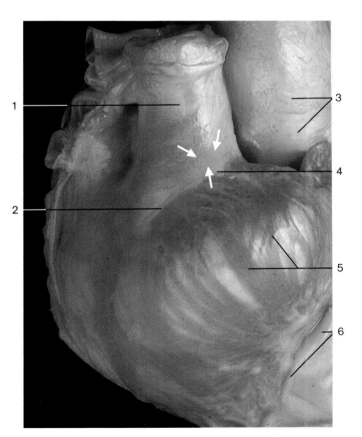

Right atrium, anterior wall, showing the location of the **sinu-atrial node** (arrows).

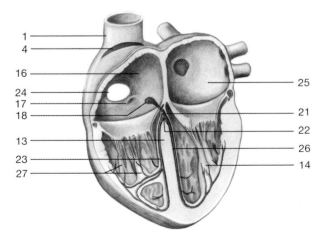

Conducting system of the heart (schematic drawing).

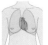

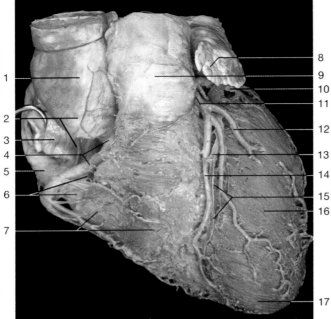

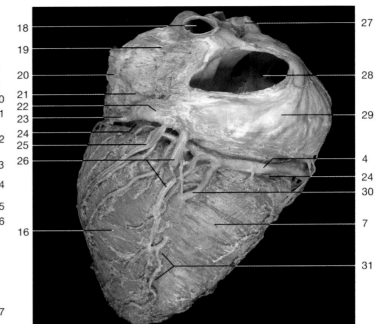

Coronary arteries (anterior aspect). The epicardium and subepicardial fatty tissue have been removed. The arteries have been injected with red resin from the aorta.

Right coronary artery and veins of the heart (dorsal aspect). The epicardium and subepicardial fatty tissue have been removed.

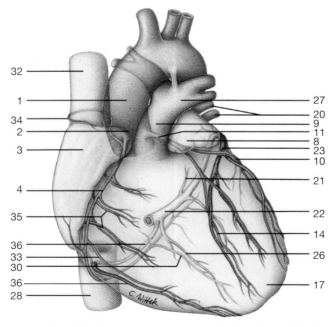

Vessels of the heart. Coronary arteries (red) and veins (blue) of the heart (anterior aspect).

1   Ascending aorta
2   Aortic bulb and (in the above specimen) sinu-atrial branch of right coronary artery
3   Right auricle
4   Right coronary artery
5   Right atrium
6   Coronary sulcus
7   Right ventricle
8   Left auricle
9   Pulmonary trunk
10 Circumflex branch of left coronary artery
11 Left coronary artery
12 Diagonal branch of left artery
13 Great cardiac vein
14 Anterior interventricular artery
15 Anterior interventricular sulcus
16 Left ventricle
17 Apex of heart
18 Right pulmonary vein
19 Left atrium
20 Left pulmonary veins
21 Oblique vein of left atrium (Marshall's vein)
22 Coronary sinus
23 Great cardiac vein
24 Coronary sulcus (posterior portion)
25 Posterior vein of left ventricle
26 Middle cardiac vein
27 Left pulmonary artery
28 Inferior vena cava
29 Right atrium
30 Posterior interventricular branch of right coronary artery
31 Posterior interventricular sulcus
32 Superior vena cava
33 Right marginal branch
34 Branch of sinu-atrial node
35 Minimal cardiac veins
36 Small cardiac vein

1 Brachiocephalic trunk
2 Superior vena cava
3 Right atrium
4 Right coronary artery
5 Right ventricle
6 Connection of one of the bypass vessels with the anterior interventricular artery
7 Left subclavian artery
8 Left common carotid artery
9 Ductus arteriosus (Botalli) (still open)
10 Ascending aorta with three bypass vessels implanted
11 Pulmonary trunk
12 Left atrium
13 Circumflex branch of left coronary artery
14 Anterior interventricular branch of left coronary artery
15 Left ventricle
16 Apex of heart
17 Sternum
18 Right ventricle
19 Liver
20 Spinal cord
21 Trachea
22 Aorta
23 Body of thoracic vertebrae
24 Pulmonary artery
25 Inferior vena cava
26 Hepatic vein

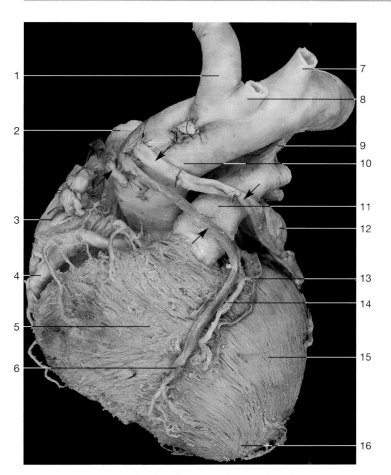

Heart, coronary vessels after implantation of three bypass vessels (anterior aspect). The ductus arteriosus (9) is still open.

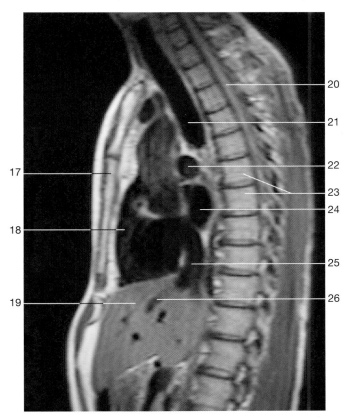

Sagittal section through the thoracic cavity (MRI scan, courtesy of Prof. W. Bautz and R. Janka, M. D., University of Erlangen, Germany).

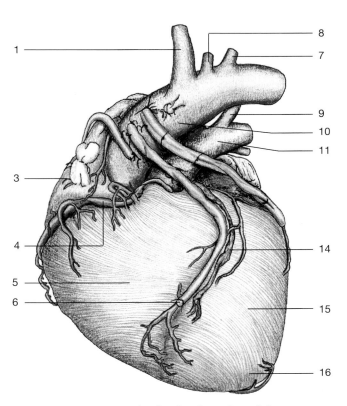

Heart, coronary vessels after implantation of three bypass vessels (yellow) (schematic drawing of the specimen above).

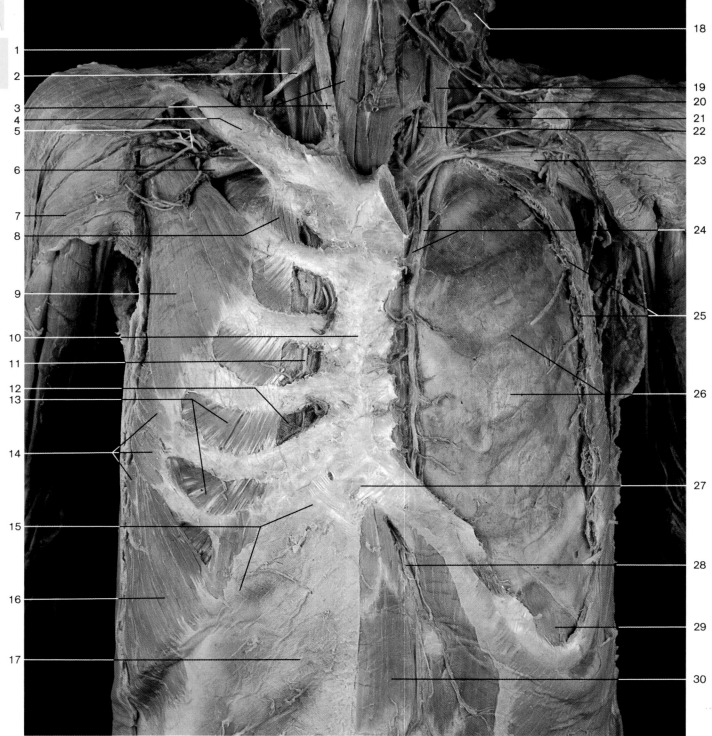

Thoracic organs (ventral aspect). The left clavicle and ribs have been partially removed, and the right intercostal spaces have been opened to show the internal thoracic vein and artery.

1	Right internal jugular vein	11	Right internal thoracic artery and vein	21	Brachial plexus
2	Omohyoid muscle	12	Fascicles of transversus thoracis muscle	22	Vagus nerve
3	Sternohyoid muscle and external jugular vein	13	Internal intercostal muscles	23	Left axillary vein
4	Clavicle	14	Serratus anterior muscle	24	Left internal thoracic artery and vein
5	Thoraco-acromial artery	15	Costal margin	25	Ribs and thoracic wall (cut)
6	Right subclavian vein	16	External abdominal oblique muscle	26	Costal pleura
7	Pectoralis major muscle	17	Anterior sheath of rectus abdominis muscle	27	Xiphoid process
8	External intercostal muscle	18	Sternocleidomastoid muscle	28	Superior epigastric artery
9	Pectoralis minor muscle	19	Left internal jugular vein	29	Diaphragm
10	Body of sternum	20	Transverse cervical artery	30	Rectus abdominis muscle

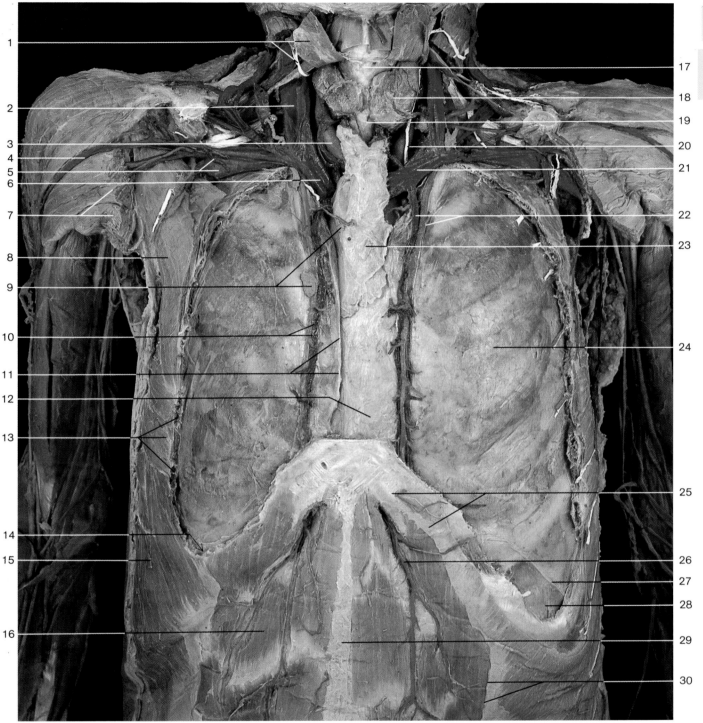

Thoracic organs, anterior mediastinum, and pleura (ventral aspect). Ribs, clavicle, and sternum have been partly removed.
Red = arteries; blue = veins; green = lymph vessels and nodes.

1 Sternothyroid muscle and its nerve (a branch of the ansa cervicalis)	11 Anterior margin of costal pleura	21 Left brachiocephalic vein
2 Right internal jugular vein	12 Pericardium	22 Left internal thoracic artery and vein
3 Right common carotid artery	13 Fifth and sixth ribs (divided) and serratus anterior muscle	23 Thymus
4 Cephalic vein	14 Costodiaphragmatic recess	24 Costal pleura
5 Right subclavian vein	15 External abdominal oblique muscle	25 Costal margin
6 Right brachiocephalic vein	16 Rectus abdominis muscle	26 Superior epigastric artery
7 Pectoralis major muscle (divided)	17 Larynx (thyroid cartilage)	27 Margin of costal pleura
8 Pectoralis minor muscle (divided)	18 Thyroid gland	28 Diaphragm
9 Parasternal lymph nodes	19 Trachea	29 Linea alba
10 Internal thoracic artery and vein	20 Left vagus nerve	30 Cut edge of anterior sheath of rectus abdominis muscle

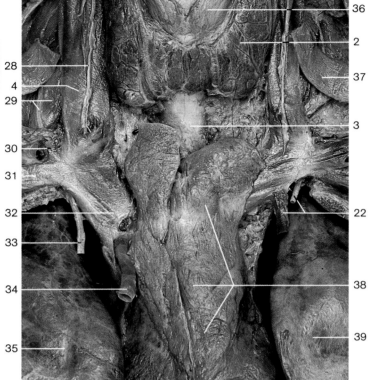

1   Larynx (thyroid cartilage)
2   Thyroid gland
3   Trachea
4   Internal jugular vein
5   Brachial plexus
6   Right brachiocephalic vein and common carotid artery
7   Right phrenic nerve
8   Ascending aorta
9   Pectoralis minor muscle (divided)
10 Pulmonary trunk (covered by pericardium)
11 Costal pleura
12 Pericardium and heart
13 Serratus anterior muscle
14 Xiphoid process
15 Costal margin
16 External abdominal oblique muscle
17 Sternothyroid muscle (divided and reflected)
18 Vagus nerve
19 Left common carotid artery
20 Left sympathetic trunk
21 Left recurrent laryngeal nerve
22 Left internal thoracic artery and vein (divided)
23 Margin of costal pleura
24 Intercostal nerves and vessels
25 Superior epigastric artery
26 Rectus abdominis muscle
27 Diaphragm
28 Ansa cervicalis
29 Phrenic nerve and scalenus anterior muscle
30 External jugular vein (divided)
31 Right subclavian vein
32 Right brachiocephalic vein
33 Internal thoracic artery (divided)
34 Internal thoracic vein (divided)
35 Right lung
36 Cricothyroid muscle
37 Omohyoid muscle
38 Thymus
39 Left lung

The **thymus** above the heart, showing its position and size.

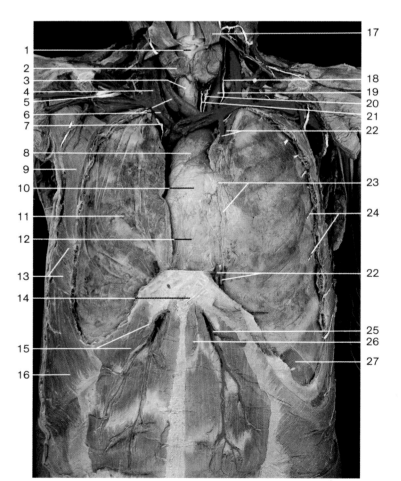

Thoracic organs (ventral aspect). The internal thoracic vessels have been removed, and the anterior margins of the pleura and lungs have been slightly reflected to display the anterior and middle mediastinum, including the heart and great vessels.

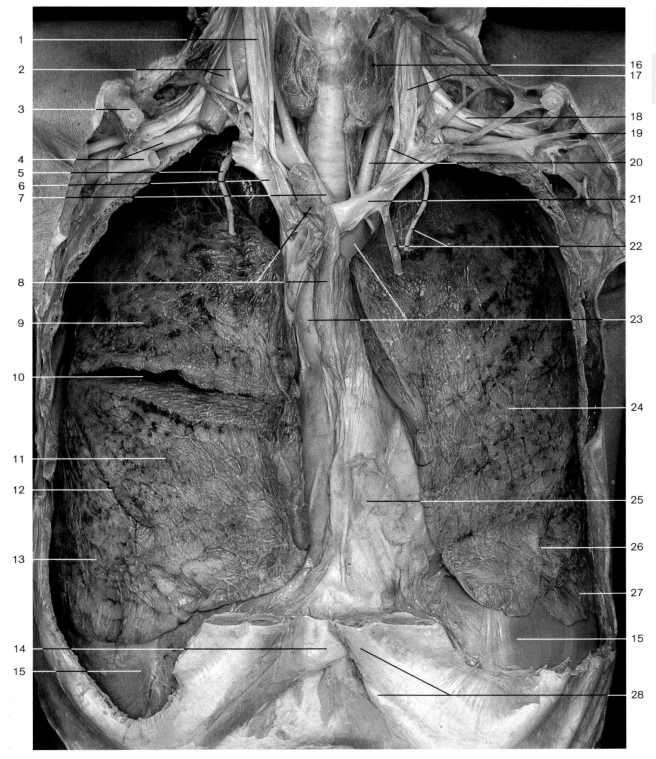

Thoracic organs (ventral aspect). The pleura has been opened and the lungs exposed. Remnants of the thymus and pericardium are seen.

1 Right internal jugular vein	11 Middle lobe of right lung	20 Left common carotid artery and
2 Phrenic nerve and scalenus anterior muscle	12 Oblique fissure of right lung	vagus nerve
3 Clavicle (divided)	13 Lower lobe of right lung	21 Left brachiocephalic vein
4 Right subclavian artery and vein	14 Xiphoid process	22 Internal thoracic artery and vein (divided)
5 Internal thoracic artery	15 Diaphragm	23 Ascending aorta and aortic arch
6 Right brachiocephalic vein	16 Thyroid gland	24 Upper lobe of left lung
7 Brachiocephalic trunk	17 Left internal jugular vein	25 Pericardium
8 Thymus (atrophic)	18 Brachial plexus	26 Oblique fissure of left lung
9 Upper lobe of right lung	19 Left cephalic vein	27 Lower lobe of left lung
10 Horizontal fissure of right lung (incomplete)		28 Costal margin

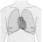

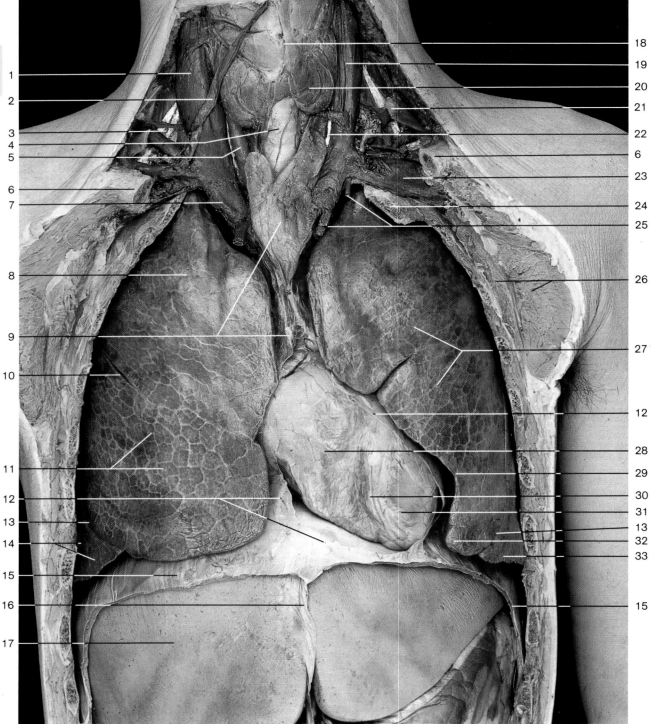

Thoracic organs (ventral aspect). The thoracic wall, costal pleura, pericardium, and diaphragm have been partly removed.

1	Internal jugular vein	13	Oblique fissure of lung	25	Internal thoracic artery and vein
2	External jugular vein (displaced medially)	14	Lower lobe of right lung	26	Pectoralis major and pectoralis minor muscles (cut edges)
3	Brachial plexus	15	Diaphragm	27	Upper lobe of left lung
4	Trachea	16	Falciform ligament	28	Right ventricle
5	Right common carotid artery	17	Liver	29	Cardiac notch of left lung
6	Clavicle (divided)	18	Location of larynx	30	Interventricular sulcus of heart
7	Right brachiocephalic vein	19	Left internal jugular vein	31	Left ventricle
8	Upper lobe of right lung	20	Thyroid gland	32	Lingula
9	Thymus (atrophic)	21	Omohyoid muscle (divided)	33	Lower lobe of left lung
10	Horizontal fissure of right lung	22	Vagus nerve		
11	Middle lobe of right lung	23	Left subclavian vein		
12	Pericardium (cut edges)	24	First rib (divided)		

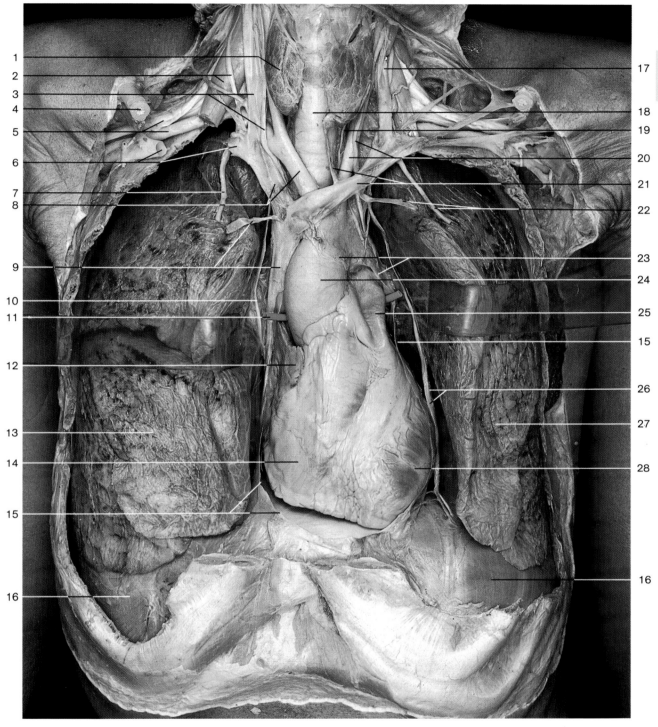

Thoracic organs (ventral aspect). Position of the heart and middle mediastinum. The anterior wall of the thorax, the costal pleura, and the pericardium have been removed and the lungs slightly reflected.

1 Thyroid gland	11 Transverse pericardial sinus (probe)	21 Left brachiocephalic vein and inferior thyroid vein
2 Phrenic nerve and scalenus anterior muscle	12 Right auricle	22 Left internal thoracic artery and vein (divided)
3 Vagus nerve and internal jugular vein	13 Middle lobe of right lung	23 Upper margin of pericardial sac
4 Clavicle (divided)	14 Right ventricle	24 Ascending aorta
5 Brachial plexus and subclavian artery	15 Cut edge of pericardium	25 Pulmonary trunk
6 Subclavian vein	16 Diaphragm	26 Left phrenic nerve and left peri-cardiacophrenic artery and vein
7 Internal thoracic artery	17 Internal jugular vein	27 Upper lobe of left lung
8 Brachiocephalic trunk and right brachiocephalic vein	18 Trachea	28 Left ventricle
9 Superior vena cava and thymic vein	19 Left recurrent laryngeal nerve	
10 Right phrenic nerve	20 Left common carotid artery and vagus nerve	

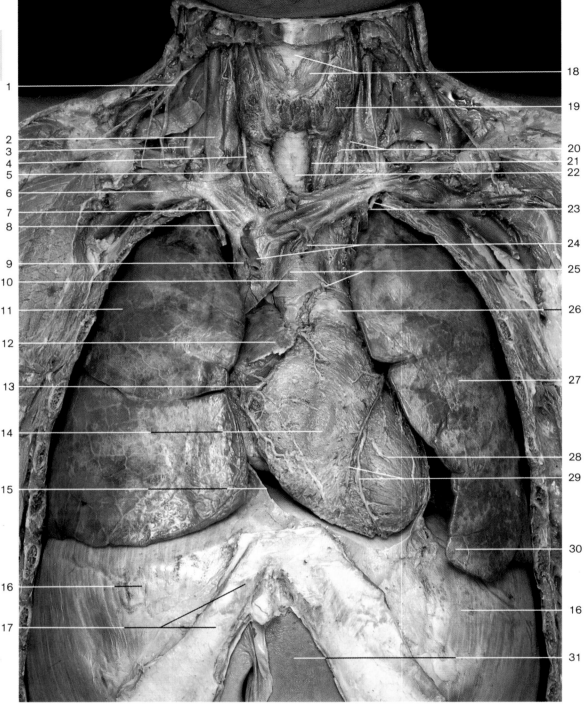

Thoracic organs (ventral aspect). Position of heart, dissection of coronary vessels in situ. The anterior wall of thorax, costal pleura, and pericardium have been removed.

1	Intermediate supraclavicular nerve	13	Right coronary artery and small cardiac vein	21	Left recurrent laryngeal nerve
2	Internal jugular vein	14	Right ventricle	22	Trachea
3	Right phrenic nerve	15	Cut edge of pericardium	23	Left internal thoracic artery and vein (divided)
4	Right vagus nerve	16	Diaphragm	24	Thymic veins
5	Right common carotid artery	17	Costal margin	25	Margin of pericardial sac
6	Right subclavian vein	18	Larynx (cricothyroid muscle and thyroid cartilage)	26	Pulmonary trunk
7	Right brachiocephalic vein	19	Thyroid gland	27	Left lung
8	Right internal thoracic artery	20	Left common carotid artery and left vagus nerve	28	Left ventricle
9	Superior vena cava			29	Anterior interventricular artery and vein
10	Ascending aorta			30	Lingula
11	Right lung			31	Liver
12	Right atrium				

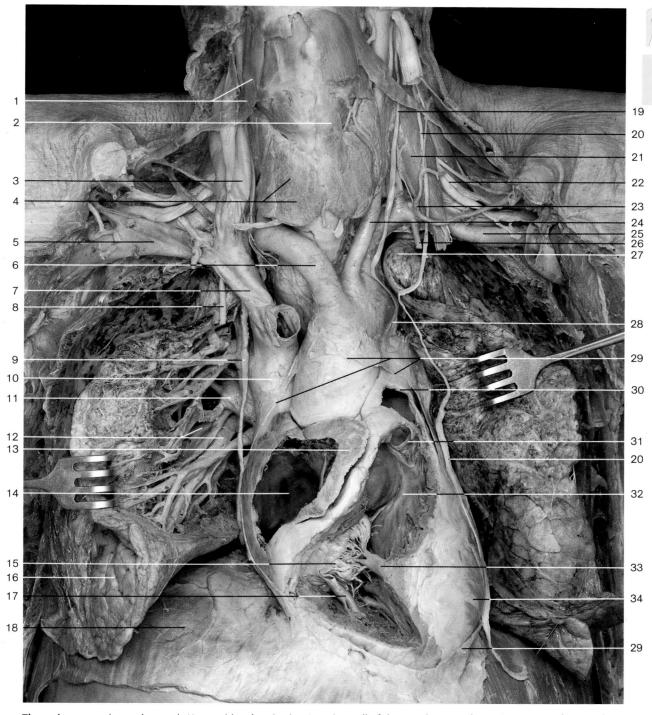

Thoracic organs (ventral aspect). Heart with valves in situ. Anterior wall of thorax, pleura, and anterior portion of pericardium have been removed. The right atrium and ventricle have been opened to show the right atrioventricular and pulmonary valves.

1 Omohyoid muscle	13 Right auricle	24 Left common carotid artery
2 Pyramidal lobe of thyroid gland	14 Right atrium	25 Left subclavian artery
3 Internal jugular vein	15 Right atrioventricular (tricuspid) valve	26 Left internal thoracic artery
4 Thyroid gland	16 Right lung	27 Apex of left lung
5 Right subclavian vein	17 Posterior papillary muscle	28 Left recurrent laryngeal nerve
6 Brachiocephalic trunk	18 Diaphragm	29 Cut edge of pericardium
7 Right brachiocephalic vein	19 Left vagus nerve	30 Pulmonary trunk (fenestrated)
8 Right internal thoracic artery	20 Left phrenic nerve	31 Pulmonic valve
9 Right phrenic nerve	21 Scalenus anterior muscle	32 Supraventricular crest
10 Superior vena cava	22 Brachial plexus	33 Anterior papillary muscle
11 Pulmonary vein	23 Thyrocervical trunk	34 Left ventricle
12 Branches of pulmonary artery		

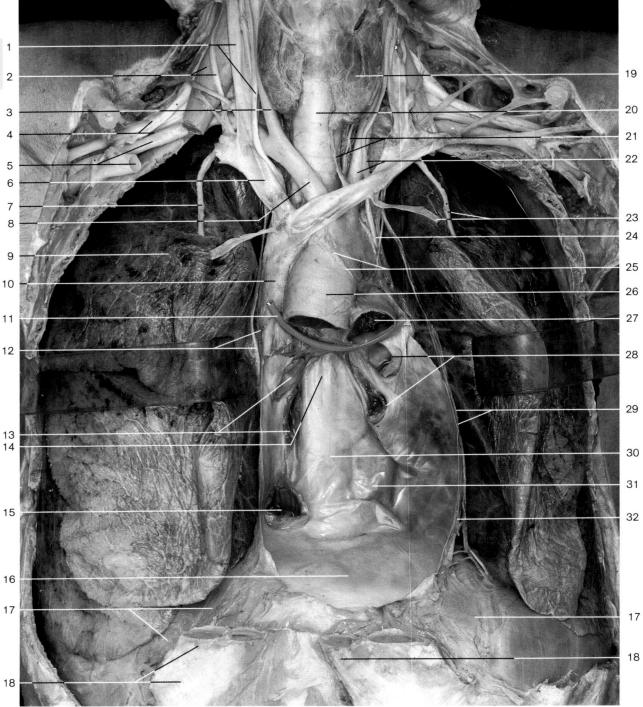

Thoracic organs (ventral aspect). Pericardium and mediastinum. Anterior wall of thorax and heart have been removed and the lungs slightly reflected. Note probe within transverse pericardial sinus.

1 Right internal jugular vein and right vagus nerve
2 Right phrenic nerve and scalenus anterior muscle
3 Right common carotid artery
4 Brachial plexus
5 Right subclavian artery and vein
6 Right brachiocephalic vein
7 Right internal thoracic artery (divided)
8 Brachiocephalic trunk
9 Upper lobe of right lung
10 Superior vena cava
11 Transverse pericardial sinus (probe)

12 Right phrenic nerve and right pericardiacophrenic artery and vein
13 Right pulmonary veins
14 Oblique sinus of pericardium
15 Inferior vena cava
16 Diaphragmatic part of pericardium
17 Diaphragm
18 Costal margin
19 Thyroid gland
20 Trachea
21 Left recurrent laryngeal nerve and inferior thyroid vein

22 Left common carotid artery and left vagus nerve
23 Left internal thoracic artery and vein (divided)
24 Vagus nerve at aortic arch
25 Cut edge of pericardium
26 Ascending aorta
27 Pulmonary trunk (divided)
28 Left pulmonary veins
29 Left phrenic nerve and left pericardiacophrenic artery and vein
30 Contour of esophagus beneath pericardium
31 Contour of aorta beneath pericardium
32 Pericardium (cut edge)

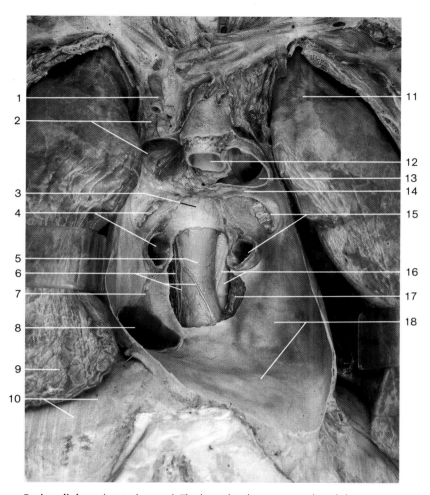

1   Internal thoracic vein
2   Superior vena cava
3   Oblique sinus of pericardium
4   Right pulmonary veins
5   Esophagus
6   Branches of right vagus nerve
7   Mesocardium
8   Inferior vena cava
9   Middle lobe of right lung
10 Diaphragm
11 Upper lobe of left lung
12 Ascending aorta
13 Pulmonary trunk
14 Transverse pericardial sinus
15 Left pulmonary veins
16 Descending aorta and left vagus nerve
17 Left lung (adjacent to pericardium)
18 Pericardium
19 Left subclavian artery
20 Vagus nerve
21 Left recurrent laryngeal nerve
22 Descending aorta
23 Pulmonary artery
24 Left atrium
25 Left ventricle
26 Coronary sinus
27 Left common carotid artery
28 Brachiocephalic trunk
29 Azygos arch
30 Right atrium
31 Right ventricle
32 Aortic arch

Pericardial sac (ventral aspect). The heart has been removed, and the posterior wall of the pericardium has been opened to show the adjacent esophagus and aorta.

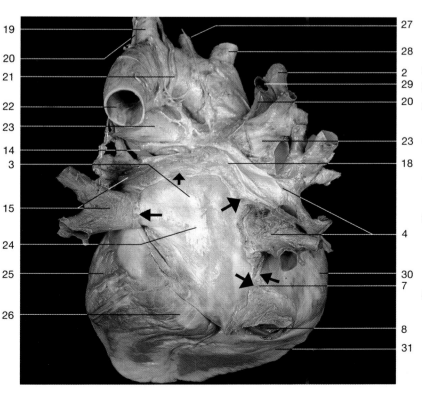

Heart with epicardium (posterior aspect). Arrows: oblique sinus.

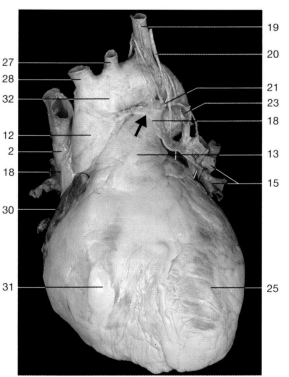

Heart with epicardium (anterior aspect). Arrow: pericardial reflection.

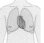

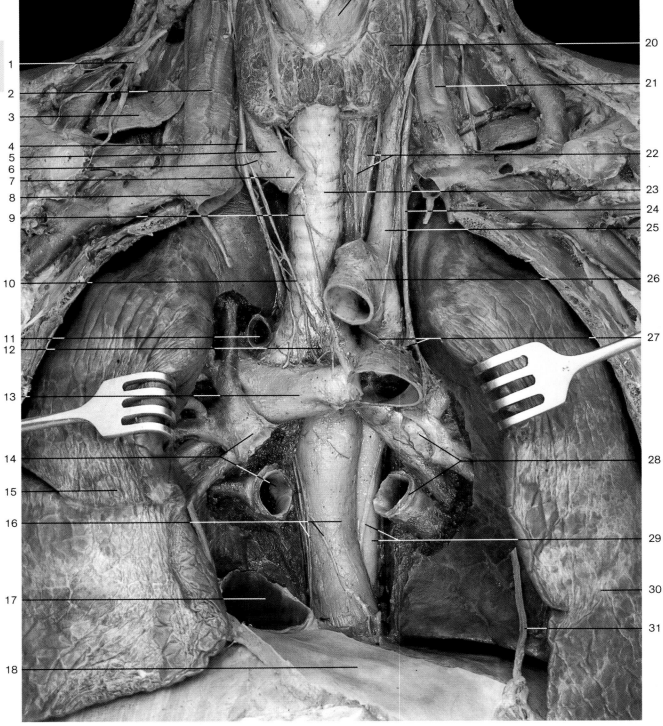

Mediastinal organs after removal of heart and pericardium (ventral aspect). Both lungs have been slightly reflected.

1 Supraclavicular nerves	11 Azygos arch (divided)	22 Esophagus and left recurrent laryngeal nerve
2 Internal jugular vein	12 Bifurcation of trachea	23 Trachea
3 Omohyoid muscle	13 Right pulmonary artery	24 Left vagus nerve
4 Right vagus nerve	14 Right pulmonary veins	25 Left common carotid artery
5 Right common carotid artery	15 Right lung	26 Aortic arch
6 Right subclavian artery	16 Esophagus and branches of right vagus nerve	27 Left recurrent laryngeal nerve branching off from vagus nerve
7 Brachiocephalic trunk	17 Inferior vena cava	28 Left pulmonary veins
8 Right brachiocephalic vein	18 Pericardium	29 Thoracic aorta and left vagus nerve
9 Superior cervical cardiac branch of vagus nerve	19 Larynx (thyroid cartilage, cricothyroid muscle)	30 Left lung
10 Inferior cervical cardiac branches of vagus nerve	20 Thyroid gland	31 Left phrenic nerve (divided)
	21 Internal jugular vein	

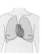

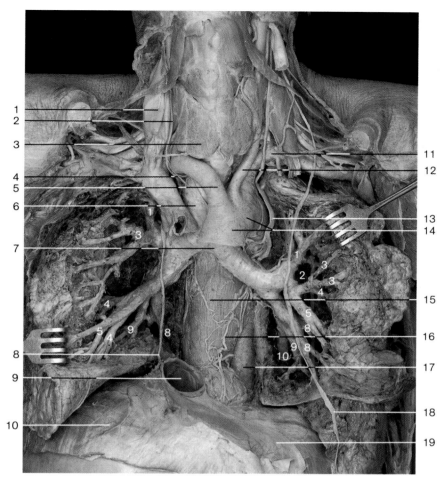

1   Internal jugular vein
2   Right vagus nerve
3   Thyroid gland
4   Right recurrent laryngeal nerve
5   Brachiocephalic trunk
6   Trachea
7   Bifurcation of trachea
8   Right phrenic nerve
9   Inferior vena cava
10   Diaphragm
11   Left subclavian artery
12   Left common carotid artery
13   Left vagus nerve
14   Aortic arch
15   Esophagus
16   Esophageal plexus
17   Thoracic aorta
18   Left phrenic nerve
19   Pericardium at the central tendon of diaphragm
20   Right pulmonary artery
21   Left pulmonary artery
22   Tracheal lymph nodes
23   Superior tracheobronchial lymph nodes
24   Bronchopulmonary lymph nodes

Bronchial tree in situ (ventral aspect). Heart and pericardium have been removed; the bronchi of the bronchopulmonary segments are dissected.
1–10 = numbers of segments (cf. p. 246 and 251).

Relation of aorta, pulmonary trunk, and esophagus to trachea and bronchial tree (schematic drawing).
1–10 = numbers of segments (cf. p. 246 and 251).

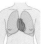

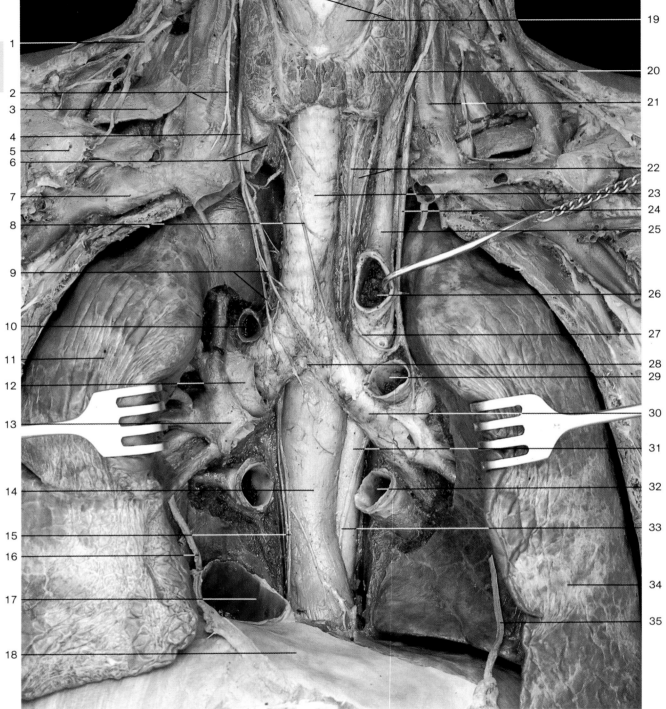

Mediastinal organs (ventral aspect). The heart with the pericardium has been removed, and the lungs and aortic arch have been slightly reflected to show the vagus nerves and their branches.

1 Supraclavicular nerves	12 Right pulmonary artery	24 Left vagus nerve
2 Right internal jugular vein with ansa cervicalis	13 Right pulmonary veins	25 Left common carotid artery
3 Omohyoid muscle	14 Esophagus	26 Aortic arch
4 Right vagus nerve	15 Esophageal plexus	27 Left recurrent laryngeal nerve
5 Clavicle	16 Right phrenic nerve (divided)	28 Bifurcation of trachea
6 Right subclavian artery and recurrent laryngeal nerve	17 Inferior vena cava	29 Left pulmonary artery
7 Right subclavian vein	18 Pericardium covering the diaphragm	30 Left primary bronchus
8 Superior cervical cardiac branch of vagus nerve	19 Larynx (thyroid cartilage and cricothyroid muscle)	31 Descending aorta
9 Inferior cervical cardiac branch of vagus nerve	20 Thyroid gland	32 Left pulmonary veins
10 Azygos arch (divided)	21 Left internal jugular vein	33 Branch of left vagus nerve
11 Right lung	22 Esophagus and left recurrent laryngeal nerve	34 Left lung
	23 Trachea	35 Left phrenic nerve (divided)

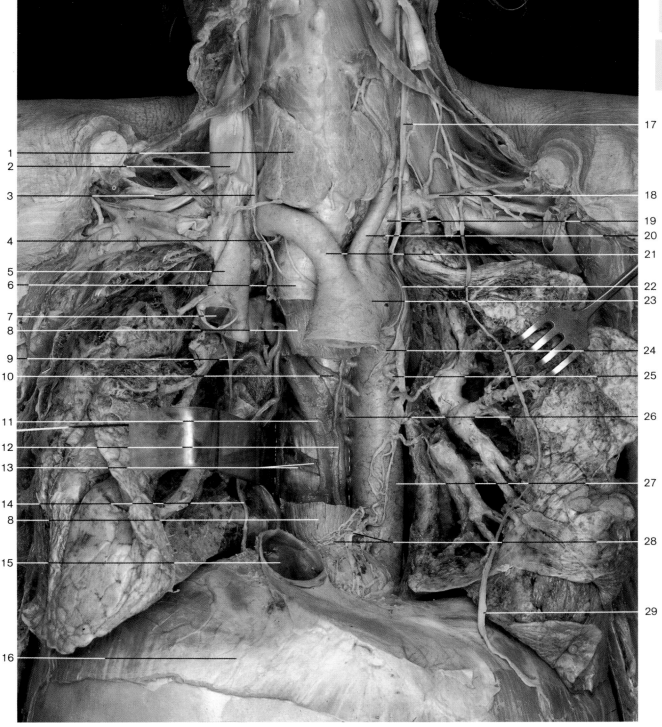

Mediastinal organs (ventral aspect). Heart and distal part of esophagus have been removed to display the vessels and nerves of the posterior mediastinum.

1 Thyroid gland	11 Azygos vein	21 Brachiocephalic trunk
2 Right internal jugular vein	12 Thoracic duct	22 Left vagus nerve
3 Right vagus nerve	13 Posterior intercostal artery and vein	23 Aortic arch
4 Point where right recurrent laryngeal nerve	(in front of the vertebral column)	24 Left recurrent laryngeal nerve
is branching off the vagus nerve	14 Right phrenic nerve	25 Left bronchial artery
5 Right brachiocephalic vein	15 Inferior vena cava	26 Lymph node
6 Trachea	16 Diaphragm	27 Thoracic aorta
7 Left brachiocephalic vein (reflected)	17 Left vagus nerve	28 Esophageal plexus
8 Esophagus	18 Thyrocervical trunk	29 Left phrenic nerve
9 Right bronchial artery	19 Left subclavian artery	
10 Posterior intercostal artery	20 Left common carotid artery	

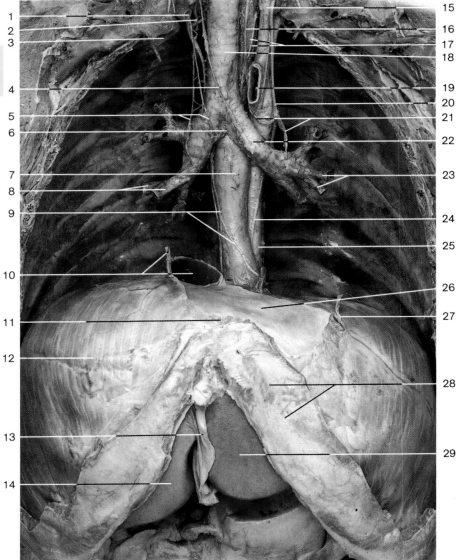

Diaphragm and organs of mediastinum (anterior aspect). Heart and lungs have been removed; the costal margin remains in place. Note the different courses of left and right vagus.

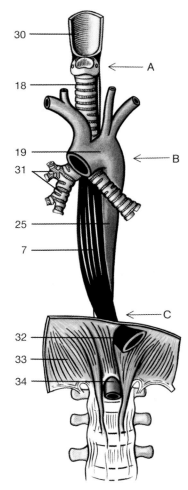

Organs of posterior mediastinum (ventral aspect, schematic drawing). Three regions in which the esophagus is narrowed are shown:

A = termed upper sphincter (at the level of the cricoid cartilage);

B = termed middle sphincter (at the level of the aortic arch);

C = termed lower sphincter (at the level of the diaphragm).

1 Right subclavian artery	11 Sternal part of diaphragm	23 Superior and inferior lingular bronchi
2 Right recurrent laryngeal nerve	12 Costal part of diaphragm	24 Esophageal plexus of left vagus nerve
3 Right brachiocephalic vein	13 Falciform ligament of liver	25 Descending aorta
4 Superior cervical cardiac nerve	14 Liver (quadrate lobe)	26 Central tendon of diaphragm
5 Inferior cervical cardiac nerves and pulmonary branches	15 Left common carotid artery	covered with pericardium
6 Bifurcation of trachea	16 Left recurrent laryngeal nerve	27 Left phrenic nerve (divided)
7 Esophagus (thoracic part)	17 Esophageal branches of left vagus nerve and esophagus	28 Costal margin
8 Bronchi of lateral and medial segments of middle lobe	18 Trachea	29 Liver, left lobe
9 Esophageal plexus and branches of right vagus nerve	19 Aortic arch	30 Pharynx
10 Inferior vena cava and right phrenic nerve (cut)	20 Left vagus nerve	31 Secondary bronchi
	21 Left recurrent laryngeal nerve with inferior cardiac nerve	32 Esophagus (abdominal part)
	22 Left primary bronchus	33 Diaphragm
		34 Abdominal aorta

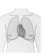

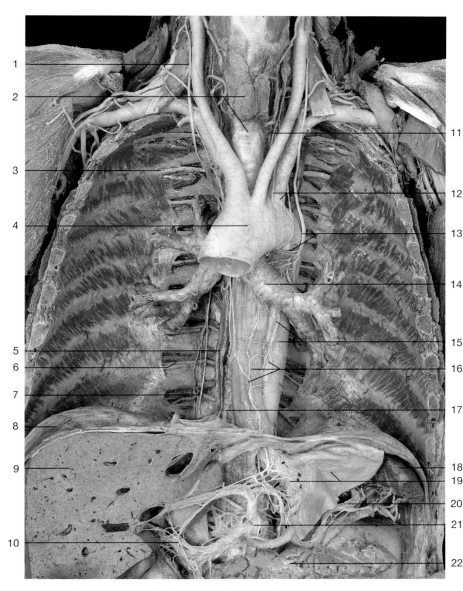

Organs of posterior mediastinum (anterior aspect).

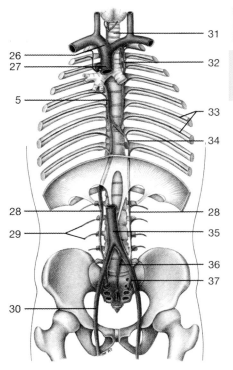

Veins of the posterior wall of thoracic and abdominal cavity (schematic drawing).

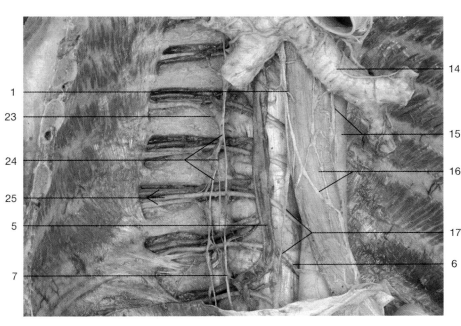

Inferior segment of posterior mediastinum (anterior aspect).

1   Right vagus nerve
2   Thyroid gland and trachea
3   Intercostal nerve
4   Aortic arch
5   Azygos vein
6   Posterior intercostal artery
7   Greater splanchnic nerve
8   Diaphragm
9   Liver
10 Proper hepatic artery and hepatic plexus
11 Left recurrent laryngeal nerve
12 Inferior cervical cardiac nerves
13 Left vagus nerve and left recurrent laryngeal nerve
14 Left primary bronchus
15 Thoracic aorta and left vagus nerve
16 Esophagus and esophageal plexus
17 Thoracic duct
18 Spleen
19 Anterior gastric plexus and stomach (divided)
20 Splenic artery and splenic plexus
21 Celiac trunk and celiac plexus
22 Pancreas
23 Ramus communicans
24 Sympathetic trunk and sympathetic ganglion
25 Posterior intercostal vein and artery and intercostal nerve
26 Right brachiocephalic vein
27 Superior vena cava
28 Ascending lumbar vein
29 Lumbar veins
30 Right external iliac vein
31 Trachea
32 Accessory hemiazygos vein
33 Posterior intercostal veins
34 Hemiazygos vein
35 Inferior vena cava
36 Median sacral vein
37 Internal iliac vein

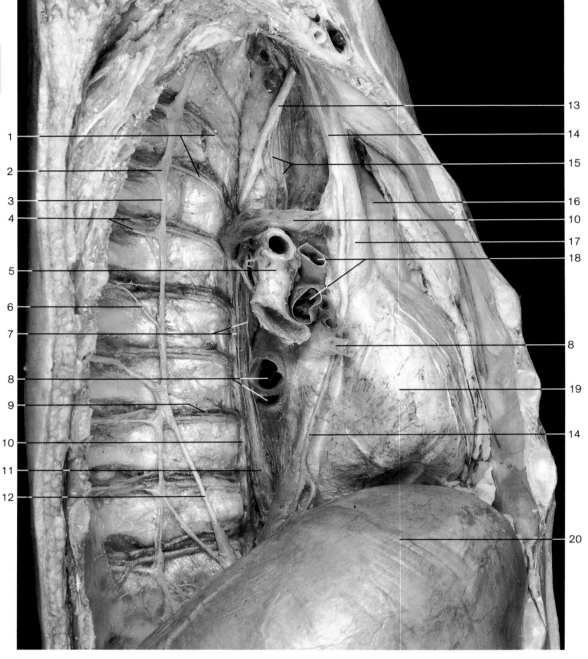

Mediastinal organs (right lateral aspect). Right lung and pleura of right half of the thorax have been removed.

1 Posterior intercostal arteries
2 Ganglion of sympathetic trunk
3 Sympathetic trunk
4 Vessels and nerves of the intercostal space (from above: posterior intercostal vein and artery and intercostal nerve)
5 Right primary bronchus
6 Ramus communicans of sympathetic trunk
7 Esophageal plexus (branches of right vagus nerve)
8 Pulmonary veins
9 Posterior intercostal vein
10 Azygos vein
11 Esophagus
12 Greater splanchnic nerve
13 Right vagus nerve
14 Right phrenic nerve
15 Inferior cervical cardiac branches of vagus nerve
16 Aortic arch
17 Superior vena cava
18 Right pulmonary artery
19 Heart with pericardium
20 Diaphragm

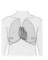

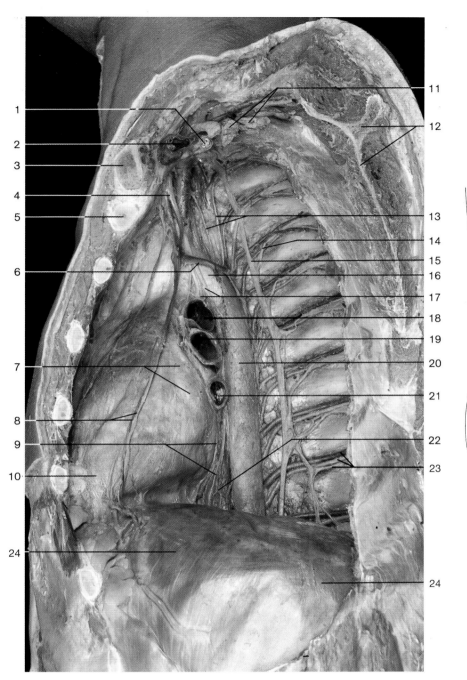

Organs of posterior and superior mediastinum (left lateral aspect).

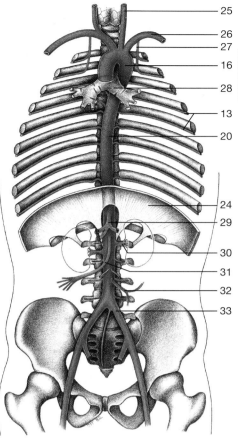

Main branches of descending aorta (schematic drawing).

1	Subclavian artery	12	Scapula (divided)
2	Subclavian vein	13	Posterior intercostal arteries
3	Clavicle (divided)	14	White ramus communicans of sympathetic trunk
4	Left vagus nerve	15	Sympathetic trunk
5	First rib (divided)	16	Aortic arch
6	Left superior intercostal vein	17	Left vagus nerve and left recurrent laryngeal nerve
7	Left atrium with pericardium	18	Left pulmonary artery
8	Left phrenic nerve and pericardiacophrenic artery and vein	19	Left primary bronchus
9	Esophageal plexus (branches derived from left vagus nerve)	20	Thoracic aorta
10	Apex of heart with pericardium	21	Pulmonary vein
11	Brachial plexus	22	Esophagus (thoracic part)

23	Posterior intercostal artery and vein and intercostal nerve
24	Diaphragm
25	Common carotid artery
26	Subclavian artery
27	Highest intercostal artery
28	Bifurcation of trachea
29	Celiac trunk
30	Renal artery
31	Superior mesenteric artery
32	Inferior mesenteric artery
33	Common iliac artery

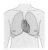

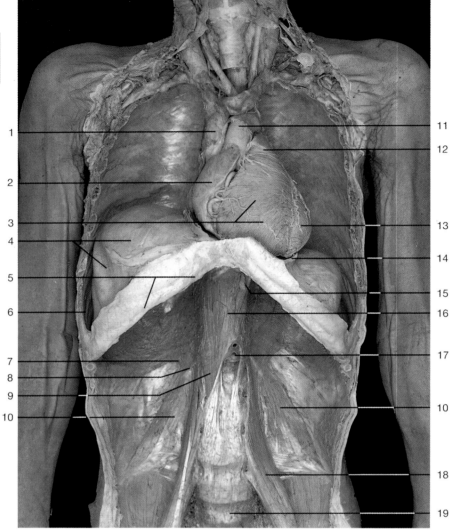

1   Superior vena cava
2   Right atrium
3   Right ventricle
4   Costal part of diaphragm
5   Costal margin
6   Position of costodiaphragmatic recess
7   Lateral arcuate ligament
8   Medial arcuate ligament
9   Right crus of lumbar part of diaphragm
10 Quadratus lumborum muscle
11 Ascending aorta
12 Pulmonary trunk
13 Left ventricle
14 Pericardium, diaphragm
15 Esophageal hiatus and abdominal
    part of esophagus (cut)
16 Lumbar part of diaphragm
17 Aortic hiatus
18 Psoas major muscle
19 Lumbar vertebra

Diaphragm in situ (anterior aspect). Anterior walls of thoracic and abdominal cavities have been removed. Natural position of the heart above the central tendon on the diaphragm is shown.

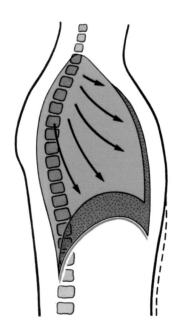

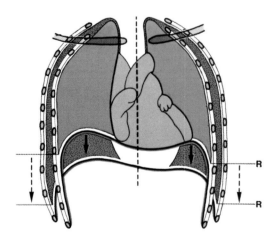

Changes in the position of the diaphragm and thoracic cage during respiration. Left: lateral aspect; right: anterior aspect. During inspiration the diaphragm moves downwards and the lower part of the thoracic cage expands forward and laterally, causing the costodiaphragmatic recess (R) to enlarge (cf. dotted arrows).

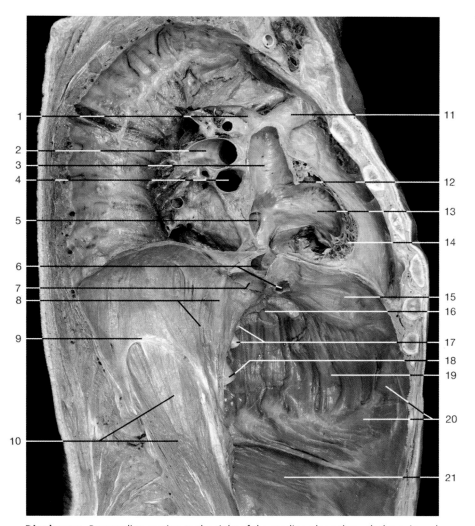

1 Azygos venous arch
2 Right pulmonary artery
3 Superior vena cava
4 Right pulmonary vein
5 Fossa ovalis
6 Hepatic veins
7 Inferior vena cava
8 Right crus of lumbar part of diaphragm
9 Medial arcuate ligament
10 Psoas major muscle
11 Left brachiocephalic vein
12 Terminal crista
13 Right atrium
14 Right auricle
15 Central tendon of diaphragm
16 Esophagus
17 Celiac trunk and superior mesenteric artery
18 Aorta
19 Costal part of diaphragm
20 Costal margin
21 Transversus abdominis muscle

Diaphragm. Paramedian section to the right of the median plane through thoracic and upper abdominal cavities. The plane passes through the superior and inferior vena cava just to the right of the vertebral bodies. Most of the heart remains in situ to the left of this plane (viewed from the right side).

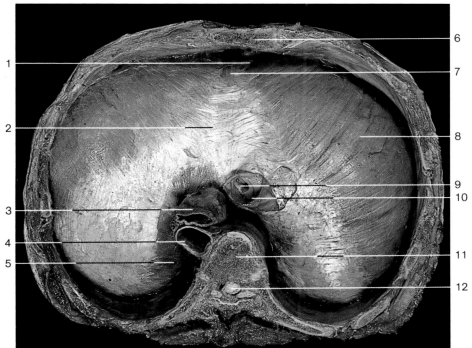

Diaphragm (superior aspect). The pleura and pericardium have been removed.

1 Sternocostal triangle
2 Central tendon (from above)
3 Esophagus
4 Aorta
5 Lumbar part of diaphragm
6 Sternum
7 Sternal part of diaphragm
8 Costal part of diaphragm
9 Entrance of hepatic veins
10 Inferior vena cava
11 Body of 9th thoracic vertebra
12 Spinal cord

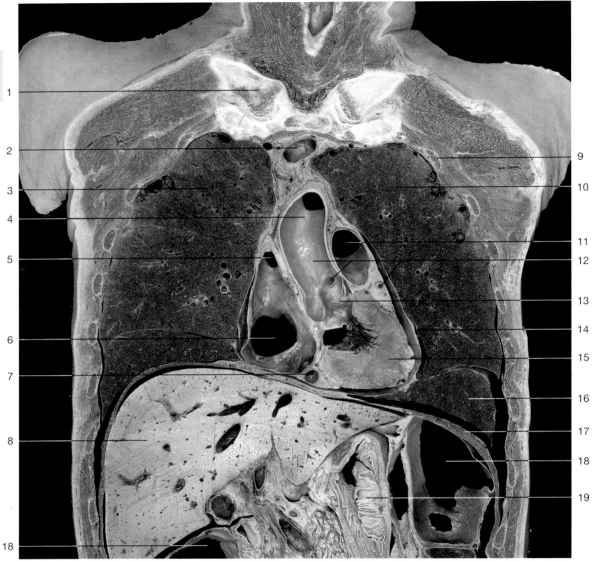

Coronal section through the thorax at the level of ascending aorta (anterior aspect).

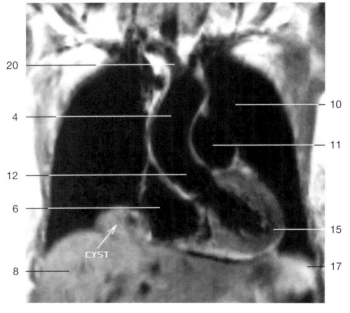

Coronal section through the thorax at the level of ascending aorta (MRI scan).

1 Clavicle
2 Left brachiocephalic vein
3 Upper lobe of right lung
4 Aortic arch
5 Superior vena cava
6 Right atrium (entrance of inferior vena cava)
7 Coronary sinus
8 Liver
9 Second rib
10 Upper lobe of left lung
11 Pulmonary trunk
12 Ascending aorta and left coronary artery
13 Aortic valve
14 Pericardium
15 Myocardium of left ventricle
16 Lower lobe of left lung
17 Diaphragm
18 Colic flexures
19 Stomach
20 Brachiocephalic trunk

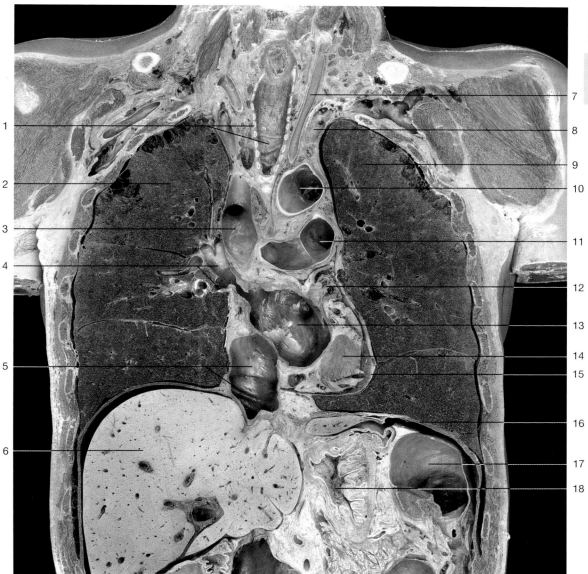

Coronal section through the thorax at the level of superior and inferior vena cava (anterior aspect).

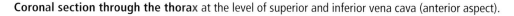

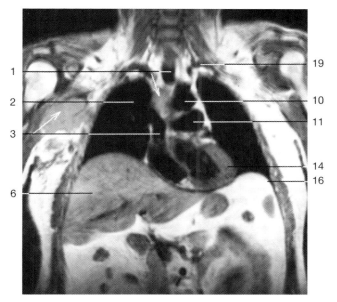

Coronal section through the thorax at the level of superior vena cava (MRI scan). Arrows = metastases of tumor.

1   Trachea
2   Upper lobe of right lung
3   Superior vena cava
4   Right pulmonary veins
5   Inferior vena cava and right atrium
6   Liver
7   Left common carotid artery
8   Left subclavian vein
9   Upper lobe of left lung
10 Aortic arch
11 Left pulmonary artery
12 Left auricle
13 Left atrium with orifices
    of pulmonary veins
14 Left ventricle (myocardium)
15 Pericardium
16 Diaphragm
17 Left colic flexure
18 Stomach
19 Left subclavian artery

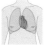

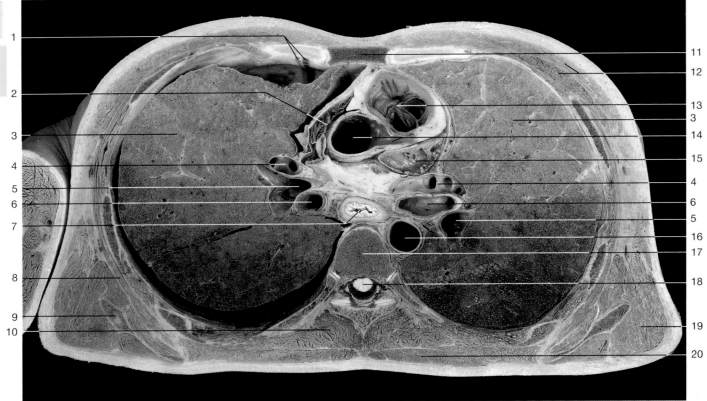

Horizontal section through the thorax at level 1 (from below).

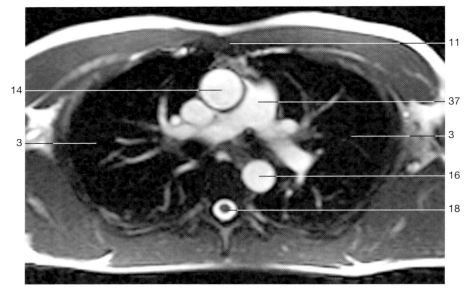

Horizontal section through the thorax at level 1 (from below). (MRI scan, courtesy of Prof. W. Bautz and R. Janka, M. D., University of Erlangen, Germany.)

1	Internal thoracic artery and vein	12	Pectoralis major and minor muscles
2	Right atrium	13	Conus arteriosus (right ventricle),
3	Lung		pulmonic valve
4	Pulmonary artery	14	Ascending aorta and left coronary artery
5	Pulmonary vein		(only in upper figure)
6	Primary bronchus	15	Left atrium
7	Esophagus	16	Descending aorta
8	Serratus anterior muscle	17	Thoracic vertebra
9	Scapula	18	Spinal cord
10	Longissimus thoracis muscle	19	Latissimus dorsi muscle
11	Sternum	20	Trapezius muscle

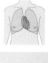

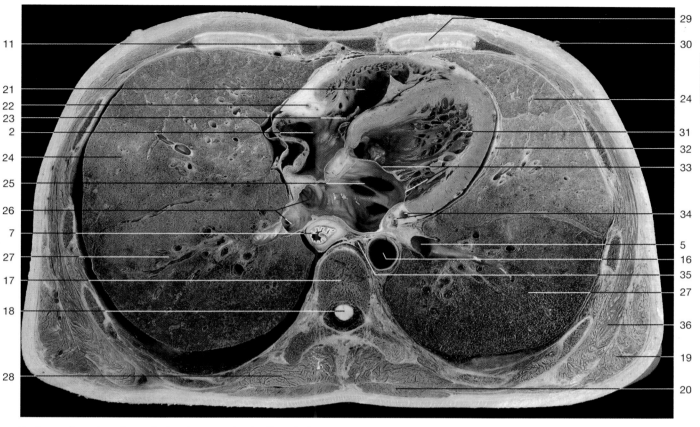

Horizontal section through the thorax at level 2 (from below).

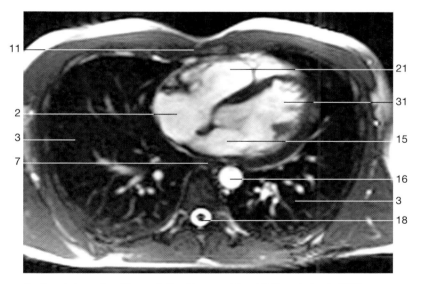

Horizontal section through the thorax at level 2 (from below). (MRI scan, courtesy of Prof. W. Bautz and R. Janka, M. D., University of Erlangen, Germany.)

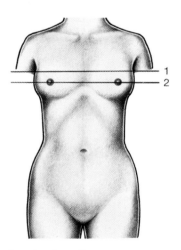

Levels of sections.

21 Right ventricle	30 Nipple
22 Right coronary artery	31 Left ventricle
23 Right atrioventricular valve	32 Pericardium
24 Lung (upper lobe)	33 Left atrioventricular valve
25 Left atrium	34 Left coronary artery and coronary sinus
26 Pulmonary veins	35 Accessory hemiazygos vein
27 Lung (lower lobe)	36 Serratus anterior muscle
28 Erector muscle of spine	37 Pulmonary trunk
29 Third costal cartilage	

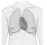

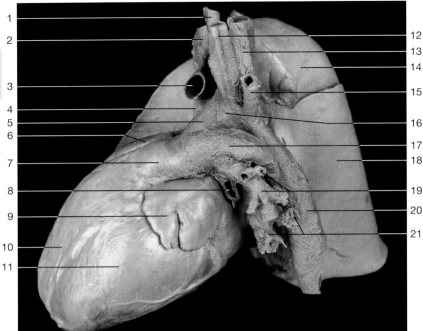

Heart and right lung of the fetus (viewed from left side). The left lung has been removed. Note the ductus arteriosus (Botalli).

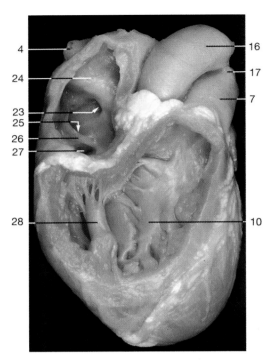

Heart of the fetus (anterior aspect). Right atrium and ventricle opened.

Shunts in the fetal circulation system		
1. Ductus venosus (of Arantius)	between umbilical vein and inferior vena cava	bypass of liver circulation
2. Foramen ovale	between right and left atrium	bypass of pulmonary circulation
3. Ductus arteriosus (Botalli)	between pulmonary trunk and aorta	

1   Right common carotid artery
2   Right brachiocephalic vein
3   Left brachiocephalic vein
4   Superior vena cava
5   Ascending aorta
6   Right auricle
7   Pulmonary trunk
8   Left primary bronchus
9   Left auricle
10 Right ventricle
11 Left ventricle
12 Left common carotid artery
13 Trachea
14 Superior lobe of right lung
15 Left subclavian artery
16 Aortic arch
17 Ductus arteriosus (Botalli)
18 Inferior lobe of right lung
19 Left pulmonary artery with branches to the left lung
20 Descending aorta
21 Left pulmonary veins
22 Inferior vena cava
23 Foramen ovale
24 Right atrium
25 Opening of inferior vena cava
26 Valve of inferior vena cava (Eustachian valve)
27 Opening of coronary sinus
28 Anterior papillary muscle of right ventricle

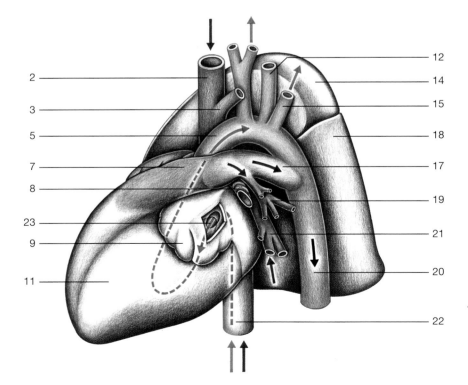

◁ **Heart of the fetus** (schematic drawing). Direction of blood flow indicated by arrows. Note the change in oxygenation of blood after ductus arteriosus entry into aorta.

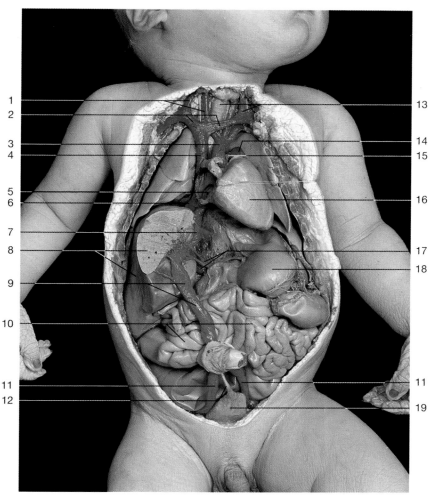

1   Internal jugular vein and right common carotid artery
2   Right and left brachiocephalic vein
3   Aortic arch
4   Superior vena cava
5   Foramen ovale
6   Inferior vena cava
7   Ductus venosus
8   Liver
9   Umbilical vein
10 Small intestine
11 Umbilical artery
12 Urachus
13 Trachea and left internal jugular vein
14 Left pulmonary artery
15 Ductus arteriosus (Botalli)
16 Right ventricle
17 Hepatic arteries (red) and portal vein (blue)
18 Stomach
19 Urinary bladder
20 Portal vein
21 Pulmonary veins
22 Descending aorta
23 Placenta

Thoracic and abdominal organs in the newborn (anterior aspect). The right atrium has been opened to show the foramen ovale. The left lobe of the liver has been removed.

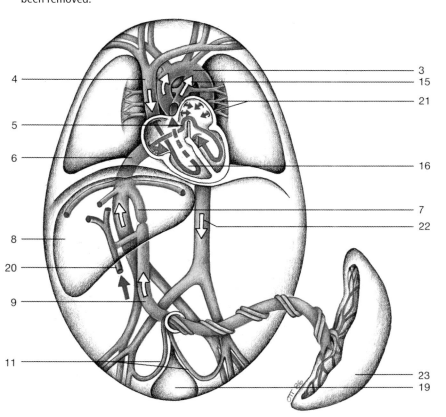

◁ **Fetal circulatory system** (schematic drawing). The oxygen gradient is indicated by color.

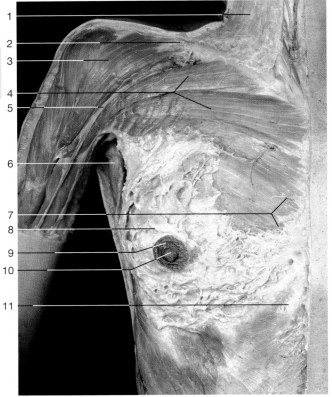

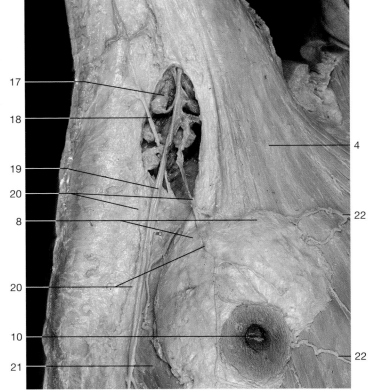

Dissection of mammary gland (anterior aspect).

Dissection of mammary gland and axillary lymph nodes.

1	Platysma muscle	8	Breast tissue	16	Apical lymph nodes
2	Clavicle	9	Areola	17	Axillary lymph nodes
3	Deltoid muscle	10	Nipple (papilla)	18	Intercostobrachial nerve
4	Pectoralis major muscle	11	Costal margin	19	Lateral thoracic vein
5	Deltopectoral groove	12	Pectoral fascia	20	Lymph vessels
	and cephalic vein	13	Mammary gland	21	Serratus anterior muscle
6	Latissimus dorsi muscle	14	Serratus anterior muscle	22	Medial branches of intercostal
7	Medial mammarian branches		(insertion)		arteries
	of intercostal nerves	15	Lactiferous sinus	23	Pectoralis minor muscle

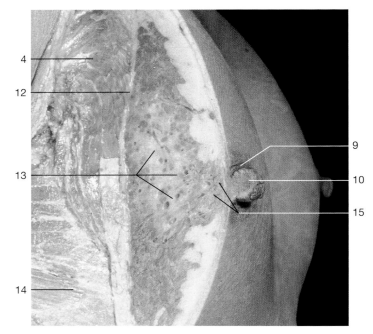

Mammary gland (sagittal section) of a pregnant female.

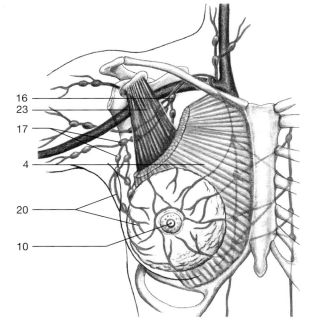

Lymphatics of the breast and axilla. Most lymph vessels drain into the axillary lymph nodes.

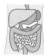

5 Abdominal Organs

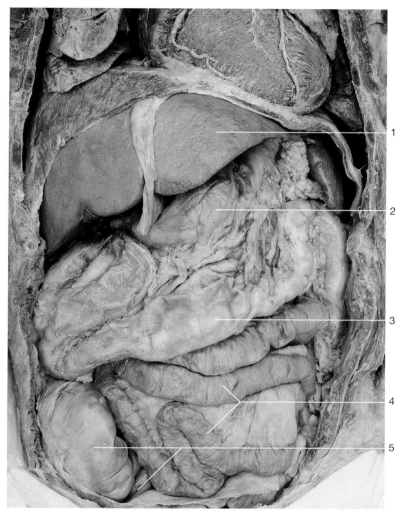

The abdominal cavity located underneath the diaphragm contains the main organs of the digestive system (liver, spleen, stomach, intestine). The greater omentum partly fixed to the transverse colon covers the small intestine.

The liver, stomach, and superior part of the duodenum are connected to the lesser omentum covering the omental bursa, the entrance of which is the epiploic foramen.

The hepatoduodenal ligament contains the portal vein, the common bile duct, and the hepatic arteries. The spleen is located dorsally underneath the diaphragm.

Abdominal organs in situ (anterior aspect). The greater omentum and part of the diaphragm have been removed. The heart is in contact with the diaphragm (from Lütjen-Drecoll, Rohen, Innenansichten des menschlichen Körpers, 2010).

1 Liver
2 Stomach
3 Transverse colon
4 Small intestine
5 Hindgut (cecum) with vermiform appendix
6 Esophagus
7 Duodenum
8 Rectum

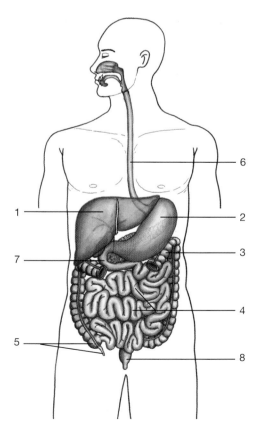

Organization of the digestive system (anterior aspect). Position of the abdominal organs.

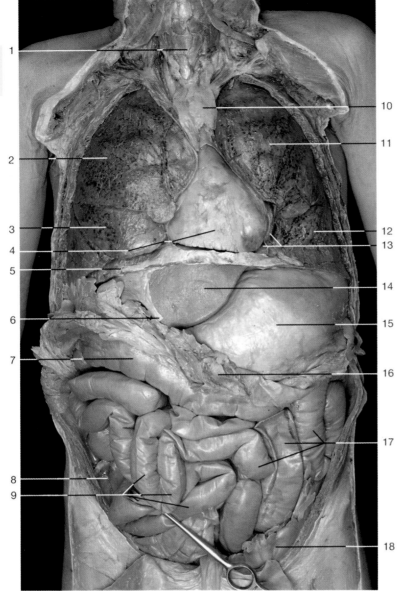

1   Thyroid gland
2   Upper lobe of right lung
3   Middle lobe of right lung
4   Heart
5   Diaphragm
6   Round ligament of liver (ligamentum teres)
7   Transverse colon
8   Cecum
9   Small intestine (ileum)
10 Thymus
11 Upper lobe of left lung
12 Lower lobe of left lung
13 Pericardium (cut edge)
14 Liver (left lobe)
15 Stomach
16 Greater omentum
17 Small intestine (jejunum)
18 Sigmoid colon
19 Rectus abdominis muscle
20 Small intestine (section)
21 Rib
22 Common bile duct, duodenum, and pancreas
23 Inferior vena cava
24 Liver
25 Body of second lumbar vertebra
26 Right kidney
27 Cauda equina and dura mater
28 Linea alba
29 Stomach and pylorus
30 Superior mesenteric artery and vein
31 Abdominal aorta
32 Left renal artery and vein
33 Left kidney
34 Psoas major muscle
35 Deep muscles of the back
36 Pancreas adjacent to lesser sac
     (omental bursa)
37 Falciform ligament with ligamentum teres

Abdominal organs in situ. The greater omentum has been partly removed or reflected.

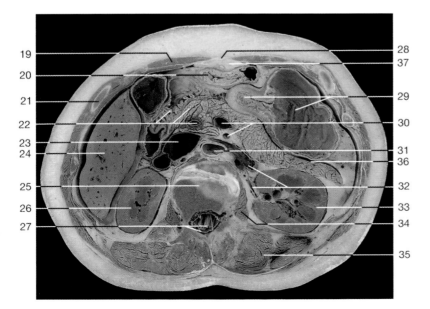

Transverse section through the abdominal cavity at the level of the second lumbar vertebra (from below).

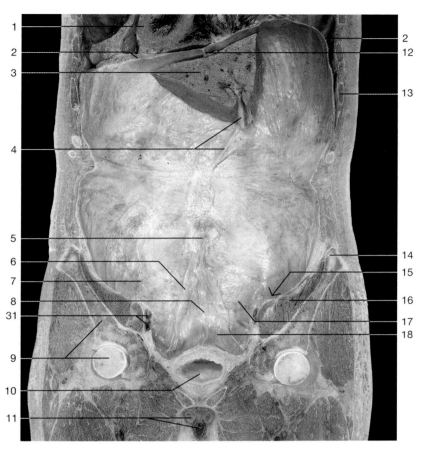

Anterior abdominal wall with pelvic cavity and thigh (frontal section, male) (internal aspect).

1 Left ventricle with pericardium
2 Diaphragm
3 Remnant of liver
4 Ligamentum teres
   (free margin of falciform ligament)
5 Site of umbilicus
6 Medial umbilical fold
   (containing the obliterated umbilical artery)
7 Lateral umbilical fold (containing inferior
   epigastric artery and vein)
8 Median umbilical fold
   (containing remnant of urachus)
9 Head of femur and pelvic bone
10 Urinary bladder
11 Root of penis
12 Falciform ligament of liver
13 Rib (divided)
14 Iliac crest (divided)
15 Site of deep inguinal ring and
   lateral inguinal fossa
16 Iliopsoas muscle (divided)
17 Medial inguinal fossa
18 Supravesical fossa
19 Posterior layer of rectus sheath
20 Transversus abdominis muscle
21 Umbilicus and arcuate line
22 Inferior epigastric artery
23 Femoral nerve
24 Iliopsoas muscle
25 Remnant of umbilical artery
26 Femoral artery and vein
27 Tendinous intersection of rectus abdominis
   muscle
28 Rectus abdominis muscle
29 Interfoveolar ligament
30 Pubic symphysis (divided)
31 External iliac artery and vein

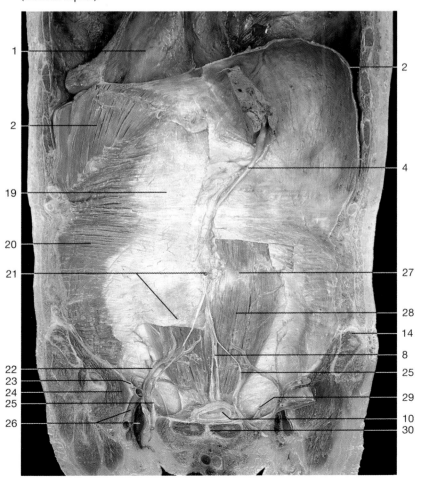

Anterior abdominal wall (male) (internal aspect). The peritoneum and parts of the posterior layer of rectus sheath have been removed. Dissection of inferior epigastric arteries and veins.

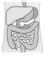

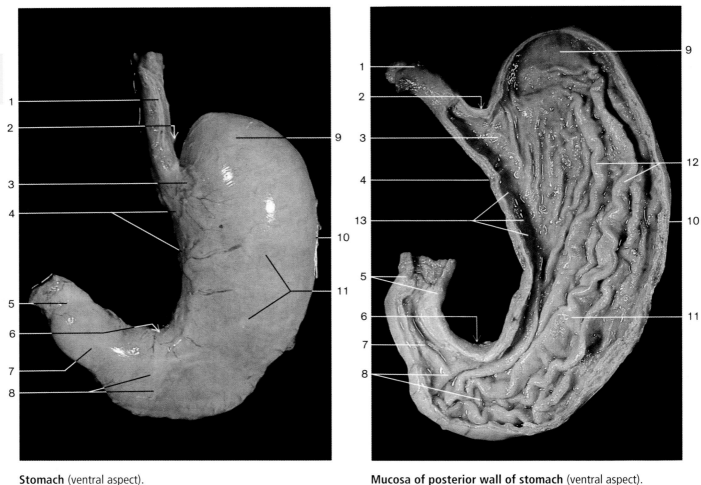

Stomach (ventral aspect).

Mucosa of posterior wall of stomach (ventral aspect).

Position of the stomach. Parasagittal section through upper part of left abdominal cavity 3.5 cm lateral to median plane.

1   Esophagus
2   Cardial notch
3   Cardial part of stomach
4   Lesser curvature of stomach
5   Pyloric sphincter
6   Angular notch (incisura angularis)
7   Pyloric canal
8   Pyloric antrum
9   Fundus of stomach
10 Greater curvature of stomach
11 Body of stomach
12 Folds of mucous membrane (gastric rugae)
13 Gastric canal
14 Right ventricle of heart
15 Diaphragm (cut edge)
16 Abdominal portion of esophagus
17 Liver
18 Cardial part of stomach (cut edge)
19 Position of pyloric canal
20 Body of stomach
21 Transverse colon
22 Small intestine
23 Lung (cut edge)
24 Fundus of stomach (section)
25 Lumbar portion of diaphragm (cut edge)
26 Suprarenal gland
27 Splenic vein
28 Pancreas
29 Superior mesenteric artery and vein
30 Intervertebral disc

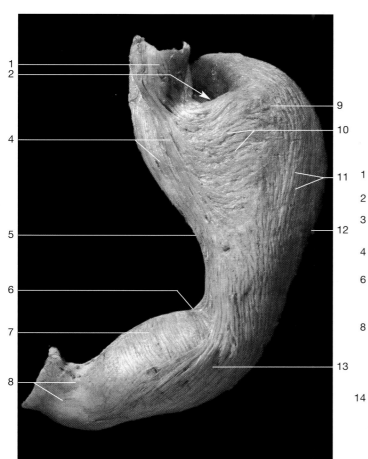

Muscular coat of stomach, outer layer (ventral aspect).

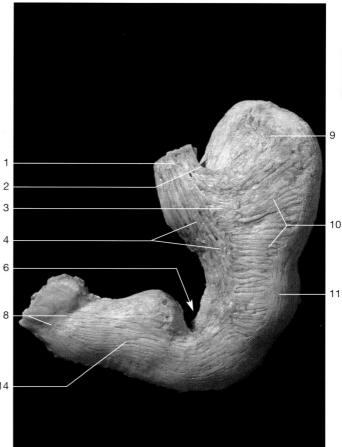

Muscular coat of stomach, middle layer (ventral aspect).

1 Esophagus (abdominal part)
2 Cardial notch
3 Cardial part of stomach
4 Longitudinal muscle layer at lesser curvature of stomach
5 Lesser curvature
6 Incisura angularis
7 Circular muscle layer of pyloric part of stomach
8 Pyloric sphincter muscle
9 Fundus of stomach
10 Circular muscle layer of fundus of stomach
11 Longitudinal muscle layer of greater curvature of stomach
12 Greater curvature of stomach
13 Longitudinal muscle layer (transition from body to pyloric part of stomach)
14 Pyloric part of stomach
15 Oblique muscle fibers

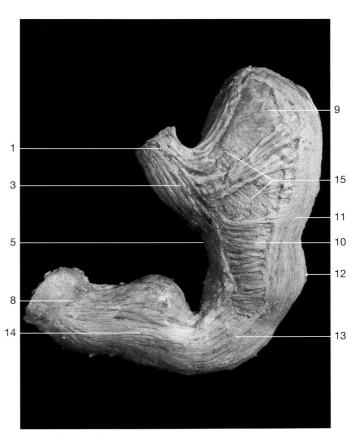

Muscular coat of stomach, inner layer (ventral aspect).

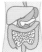

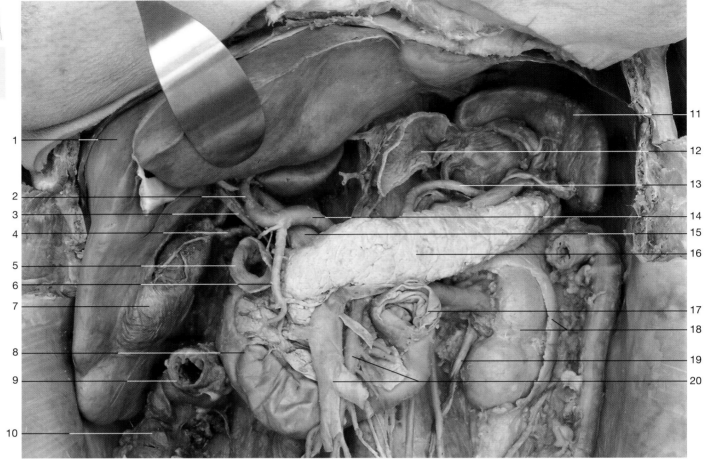

Upper abdominal organs. Pancreas, duodenum, and left kidney are shown. Stomach and transverse colon have been removed, liver elevated; superior mesenteric vein is slightly enlarged.

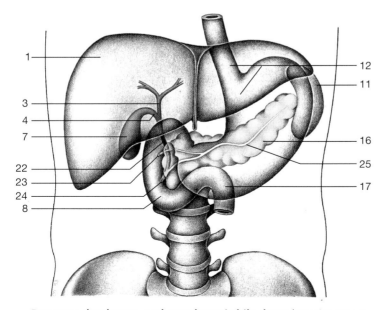

Pancreas, duodenum, and extrahepatic bile ducts (anterior aspect, schematic drawing).

1 Liver
2 Hepatic artery proper
3 Hepatic duct
4 Cystic duct
5 Pylorus
6 Gastroduodenal artery
7 Gallbladder
8 Duodenum
9 Transverse colon (cut)
10 Ascending colon
11 Spleen
12 Cardia
13 Splenic artery
14 Common hepatic artery
15 Portal vein
16 Pancreas (body)
17 Duodenojejunal flexure
18 Kidney (with capsula adiposa)
19 Ureter
20 Superior mesenteric artery and vein
21 Aorta (abdominal part)
22 Common bile duct
23 Lesser duodenal papilla
24 Greater duodenal papilla
25 Pancreatic duct

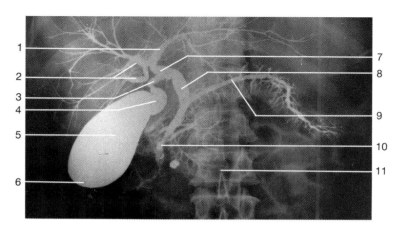

1   Left hepatic duct
2   Right hepatic duct
3   Cystic duct
4   Neck of gallbladder
5   Body of gallbladder
6   Fundus of gallbladder
7   Common hepatic duct
8   Common bile duct
9   Pancreatic duct
10   Greater duodenal papilla
11   Second lumbar vertebra
12   Folds of mucous membrane of gallbladder
13   Muscular coat of gallbladder
14   Neck of gallbladder (opened)
15   Cystic duct with spiral fold
16   Lesser duodenal papilla
17   Accessory pancreatic duct
18   Uncinate process
19   Plica circularis of duodenum (Kerckring's fold)
20   Head of pancreas
21   Body of pancreas
22   Tail of pancreas
23   Descending part of duodenum
24   Incisure of pancreas

Radiograph of biliary ducts, gallbladder, and pancreatic duct (antero-posterior view).

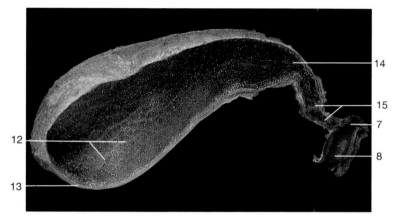

Isolated gallbladder and cystic duct (anterior aspect).
The gallbladder has been opened to display the mucous membrane.

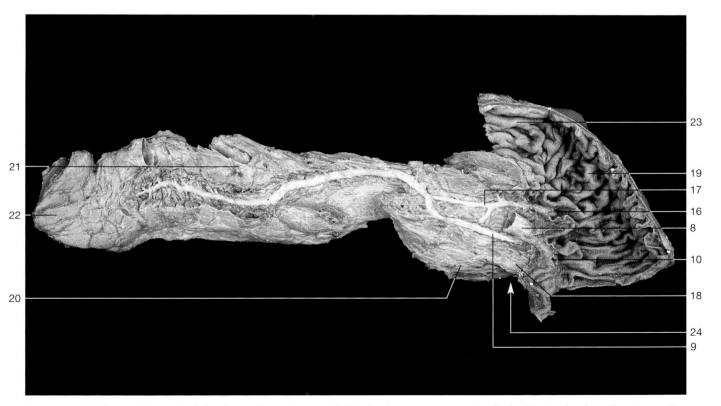

Pancreas with descending part of duodenum (posterior aspect). The duodenum was opened to display the duodenal papillae. Pancreatic duct has been dissected, the common bile duct has been divided. The sphincter of Oddi is shown.

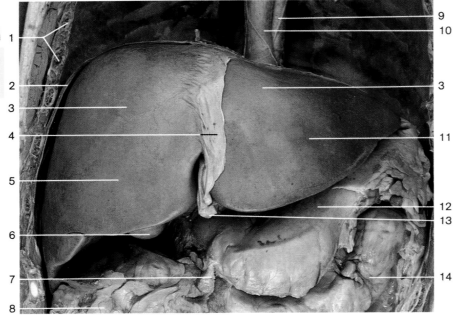

Liver in situ (ventral aspect). Part of the diaphragm has been removed.

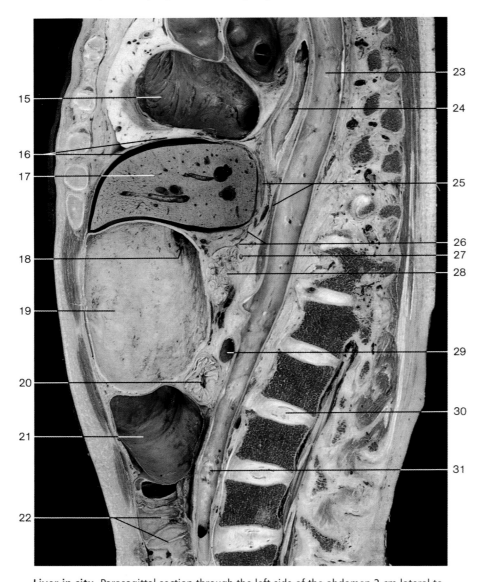

Liver in situ. Parasagittal section through the left side of the abdomen 2 cm lateral to median plane.

1 Ribs (cut edges)
2 Diaphragm
3 Diaphragmatic surface of liver
4 Falciform ligament of liver
5 Right lobe of liver
6 Fundus of gallbladder
7 Gastrocolic ligament
8 Greater omentum
9 Aorta
10 Esophagus
11 Left lobe of liver
12 Stomach
13 Ligamentum teres
14 Transverse colon
15 Right atrium of heart
16 Central tendon and sternal portion of diaphragm
17 Liver (cut edge)
18 Entrance to duodenum (pylorus)
19 Stomach
20 Duodenum
21 Transverse colon (divided, dilated)
22 Small intestine
23 Thoracic aorta (longitudinally divided)
24 Esophagus (longitudinally divided)
25 Esophageal hiatus of diaphragm
26 Omental bursa (lesser sac)
27 Splenic artery
28 Pancreas
29 Left renal vein
30 Intervertebral disc
31 Abdominal aorta (longitudinally divided)

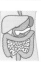

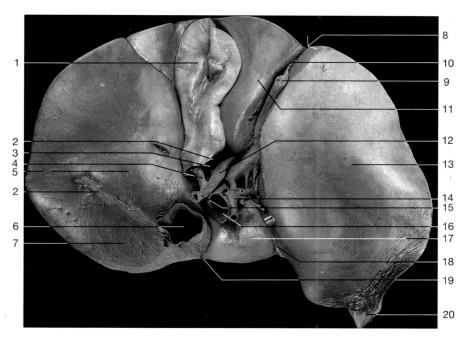

1 Fundus of gallbladder
2 Peritoneum (cut edges)
3 Cystic artery
4 Cystic duct
5 Right lobe of liver
6 Inferior vena cava
7 Bare area of liver
8 Notch for ligamentum teres and falciform ligament
9 Ligamentum teres
10 Falciform ligament of liver
11 Quadrate lobe of liver
12 Common hepatic duct
13 Left lobe of liver
14 Hepatic artery proper ⎫
15 Common bile duct   ⎬ Portal triad
16 Portal vein   ⎭
17 Caudate lobe of liver
18 Ligamentum venosum
19 Ligament of inferior vena cava
20 Appendix fibrosa (left triangular ligament)
21 Coronary ligament of liver
22 Hepatic veins
23 Porta hepatis

Liver (inferior aspect). Dissection of porta hepatis. Gallbladder partly collapsed. Ventral margin of liver above.

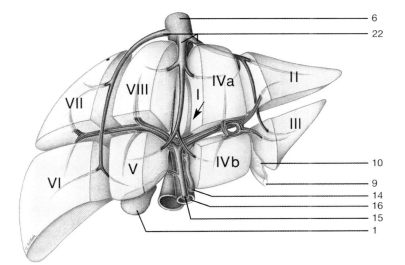

Segmentation of the liver (anterior aspect). Liver segments indicated by Roman numerals.

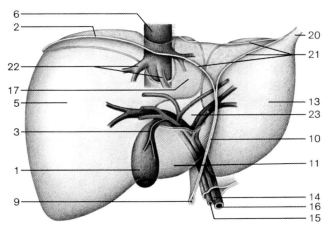

Liver (ventral aspect) (transparent drawing illustrating margins of peritoneal folds).

It should be noted that the anatomical left and right lobes of the liver do not reflect the internal distribution of the hepatic artery, portal vein, and biliary ducts. With these structures, used as criteria, the left lobe includes both the caudate and quadrate lobes, and thus the line dividing the liver into left and right functional lobes passes through the gallbladder and inferior vena cava. The three main hepatic veins drain segments of the liver that have no visible external markings.

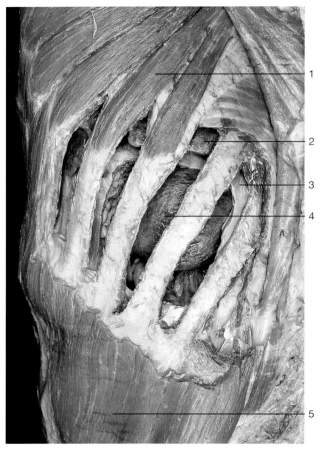

1 Serratus anterior muscle
2 Left lung
3 Diaphragm
4 Spleen
5 External abdominal oblique muscle
6 Gastrosplenic ligament
7 Splenic artery
8 Pancreas tail
9 Superior margin of spleen
10 Anterior border of spleen
11 Liver
12 Hepatic artery proper
13 Cystic duct
14 Gallbladder
15 Lesser duodenal papilla (probe)
16 Greater duodenal papilla (probe)
17 Duodenum (fenestrated)
18 Cardia
19 Pancreas and pancreatic duct
20 Kidney (with capsula adiposa, capsular fat, adipose tissue)
21 Common bile duct
22 Superior mesenteric artery and vein
23 Ureter
24 Aorta with celiac trunk
25 Suprarenal gland
26 Inferior mesenteric vein

Location of the spleen in situ (left-lateral aspect).
Intercostal spaces and diaphragm have been fenestrated.

Spleen (visceral surface), hilum of spleen with vessels, nerves, and ligaments.

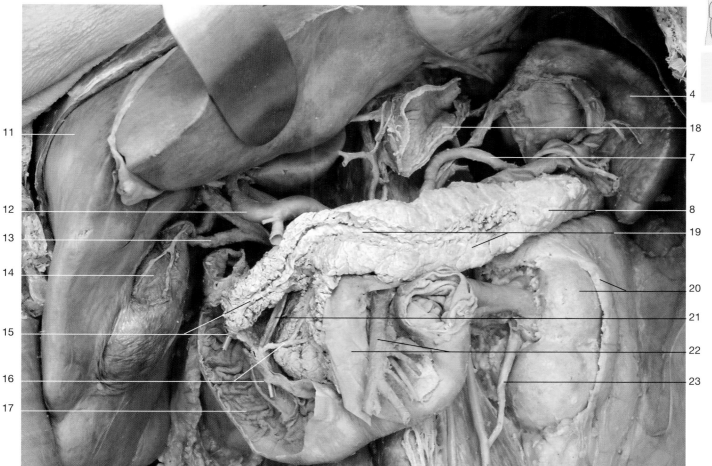

Upper abdominal organs (anterior aspect). Stomach and transverse colon have been removed, the duodenum fenestrated. The liver has been elevated to show the extrahepatic bile ducts. In this case the accessory pancreatic duct represents the main excretory duct of the pancreas.

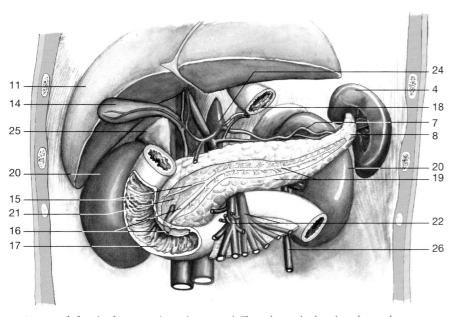

Upper abdominal organs (anterior aspect). The schematic drawing shows the most common situation of the pancreatic ducts.

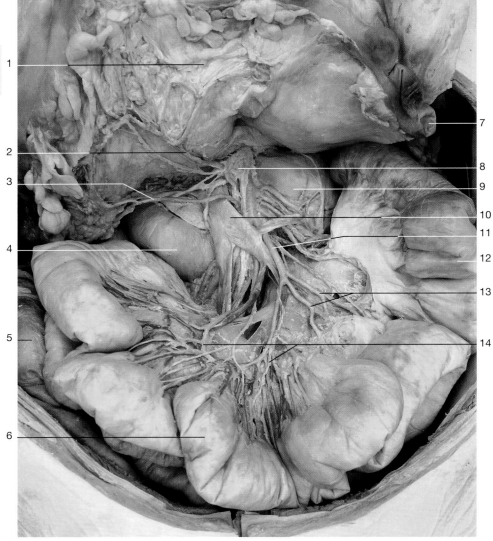

1 Greater omentum
2 Middle colic artery
3 Right colic artery
4 Duodenum
5 Ascending colon
6 Ileum
7 Transverse colon
8 Celiac ganglion
9 Duodenojejunal flexure
10 Superior mesenteric vein
11 Superior mesenteric artery
12 Jejunum
13 Jejunal arteries
14 Ileal arteries
15 Liver
16 Celiac trunk and abdominal aorta
17 Gallbladder
18 Pancreas
19 Ileocolic artery
20 Stomach
21 Spleen
22 Left colic flexure
23 Appendicular artery
24 Vermiform appendix

Vessels of abdominal organs, dissection of superior mesenteric artery and vein.
Greater omentum and transverse colon are reflected.

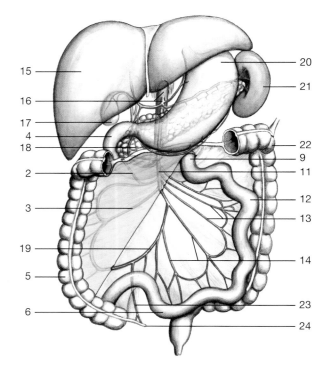

Main branches of superior mesenteric artery
(schematic drawing).

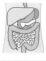

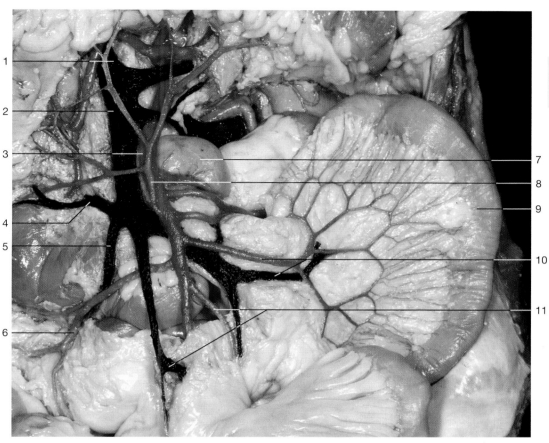

Tributaries of portal vein (blue) **and branches of superior mesenteric artery** (red) (anterior aspect).

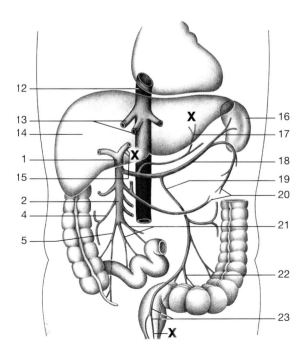

Main tributaries of portal vein (blue).
Inferior vena cava = violet; X = sites of portocaval anastomoses.

1   Portal vein
2   Superior mesenteric vein
3   Superior mesenteric artery
4   Right colic vein
5   Ileocolic vein
6   Ileocolic artery
7   Duodenojejunal flexure
8   Middle colic artery
9   Jejunum
10 Jejunal arteries and veins
11 Ileal arteries and veins
12 Inferior vena cava
13 Hepatic veins
14 Liver
15 Para-umbilical veins
    (located within the
    ligamentum teres)
16 Spleen
17 Left gastric vein with
    esophageal branches
18 Splenic vein
19 Inferior mesenteric vein
20 Gastro-omental veins
21 Ileal veins
22 Sigmoid veins
23 Superior rectal vein

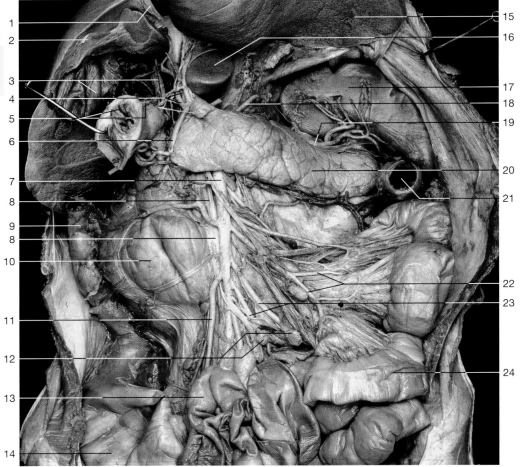

1	Ligamentum teres
2	Liver
3	Gallbladder and common bile duct
4	Hepatic artery proper and portal vein
5	Right gastric artery and pylorus
6	Gastroduodenal artery
7	Superior mesenteric artery
8	Superior mesenteric vein
9	Ascending colon
10	Duodenum
11	Ileocolic artery
12	Lymph nodes
13	Ileum
14	Cecum
15	Left lobe of liver
16	Caudate lobe of liver
17	Spleen
18	Left gastric artery
19	Splenic artery
20	Pancreas
21	Left colic flexure (cut)
22	Jejunal arteries
23	Ileal arteries
24	Jejunum
25	Middle colic artery
26	Right colic artery
27	Appendicular artery
28	Transverse mesocolon
29	Duodenojejunal flexure
30	Inferior mesenteric artery
31	Left colic artery
32	Sigmoid arteries
33	Superior rectal artery
34	Inferior vena cava
35	Abdominal aorta
36	Descending colon
37	Ileum
38	Sigmoid colon
39	Vermiform appendix
40	Cecum

Superior mesenteric artery in relation to pancreas and duodenum. Stomach and transverse colon have been removed and the liver elevated. Note the location of the spleen. A yellow probe is inserted through the omental foramen.

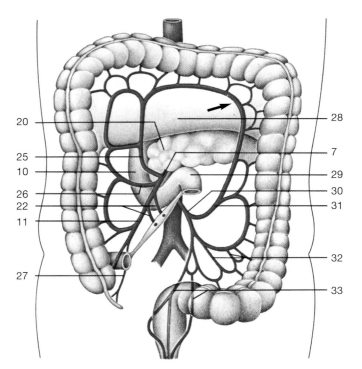

Main branches of superior and inferior mesenteric arteries (schematic drawing). Arrow = Riolan's anastomosis.

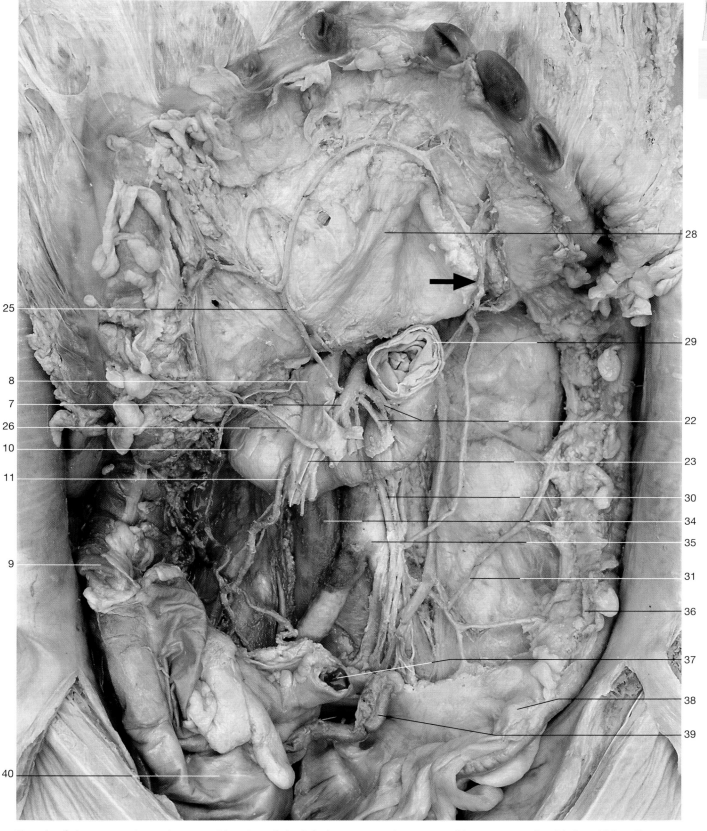

Vessels of the retroperitoneal organs. Direction of the inferior mesenteric artery and its anastomosis with the middle colic artery (arrow = Riolan's anastomosis). Greater omentum and transverse colon have been reflected, the intestine partly removed. The normally retrocecally located vermiform appendix has been replaced anteriorly. The right common iliac artery is partly obstructed by a blood thrombus.

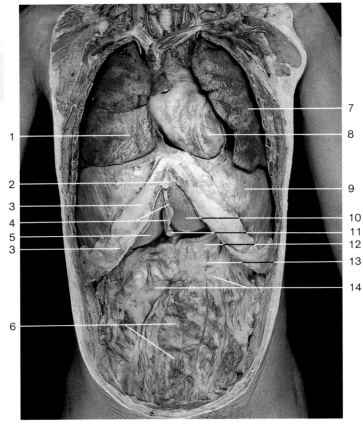

1 Middle lobe of right lung
2 Xiphoid process
3 Costal margin
4 Falciform ligament of liver
5 Quadrate lobe of liver
6 Greater omentum
7 Upper lobe of left lung
8 Heart
9 Diaphragm
10 Left lobe of liver
11 Ligamentum teres
12 Stomach
13 Gastrocolic ligament
14 Transverse colon
15 Taenia coli
16 Appendices epiploicae
17 Cecum
18 Taenia coli
19 Ileum
20 Transverse mesocolon
21 Jejunum
22 Sigmoid colon
23 Position of root of mesentery
24 Vermiform appendix
25 Duodenojejunal flexure
26 Mesentery

Abdominal organs. The anterior thoracic and abdominal walls have been removed.

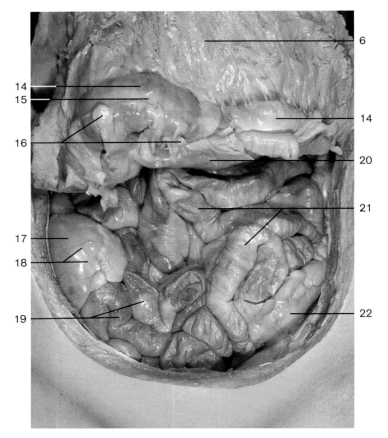

Abdominal organs (anterior aspect). The greater omentum, which is fixed to the transverse colon, has been raised.

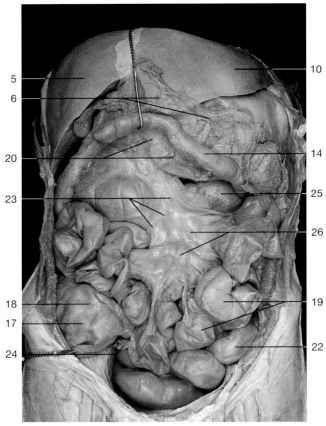

Abdominal organs (anterior aspect). The transverse colon has been reflected.

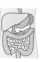

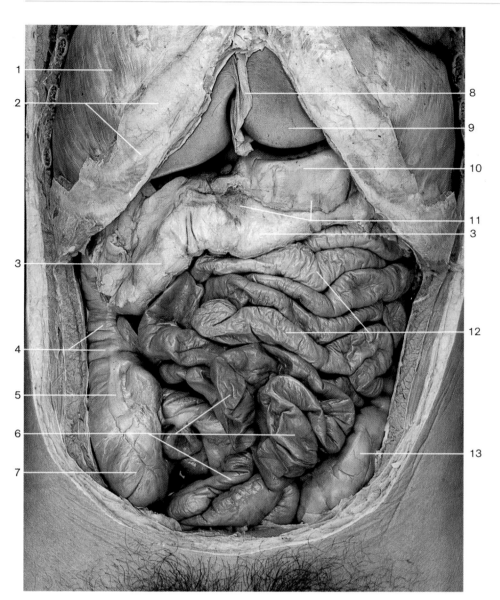

1 Diaphragm
2 Costal margin
3 Transverse colon
4 Ascending colon with haustra
5 Free taenia of cecum
6 Ileum
7 Cecum
8 Falciform ligament of liver
9 Liver
10 Stomach
11 Gastrocolic ligament
12 Jejunum
13 Sigmoid colon
14 Vermiform appendix
15 Terminal ileum
16 Meso-appendix
17 Mesentery

Abdominal organs in situ. The greater omentum has been removed.

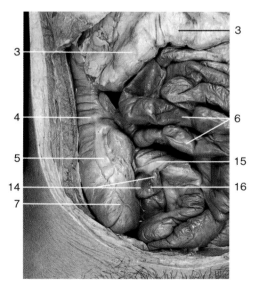

Ascending colon, cecum, and vermiform appendix (detail of the preceding figure).

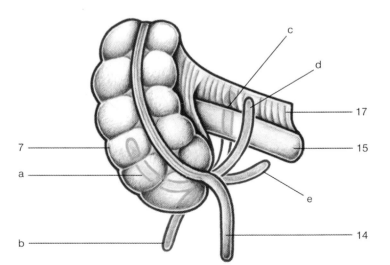

Variations in the position of the vermiform appendix.
a = retrocecal; b = paracolic; c = retro-ileal; d = pre-ileal;
e = subcecal.

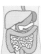

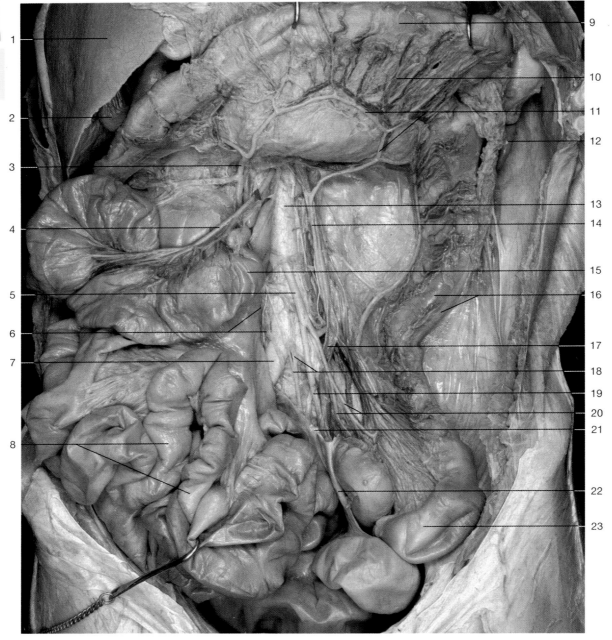

Abdominal organs. Dissection of inferior mesenteric artery and autonomic plexus. The transverse colon with mesocolon has been raised and the small intestine reflected.

1	Liver	12	Spleen
2	Gallbladder	13	Abdominal aorta
3	Middle colic artery	14	Left colic artery
4	Jejunal artery	15	Duodenojejunal flexure
5	Inferior mesenteric artery	16	Descending colon (free taenia of colon)
6	Sympathetic nerves and ganglia	17	Inferior mesenteric vein
7	Right common iliac artery	18	Superior hypogastric plexus
8	Small intestine (ileum)	19	Superior rectal artery
9	Transverse colon (reflected)	20	Sigmoid arteries
10	Transverse mesocolon	21	Peritoneum (cut edge)
11	Anastomosis between middle and left colic artery	22	Sigmoid mesocolon
		23	Sigmoid colon

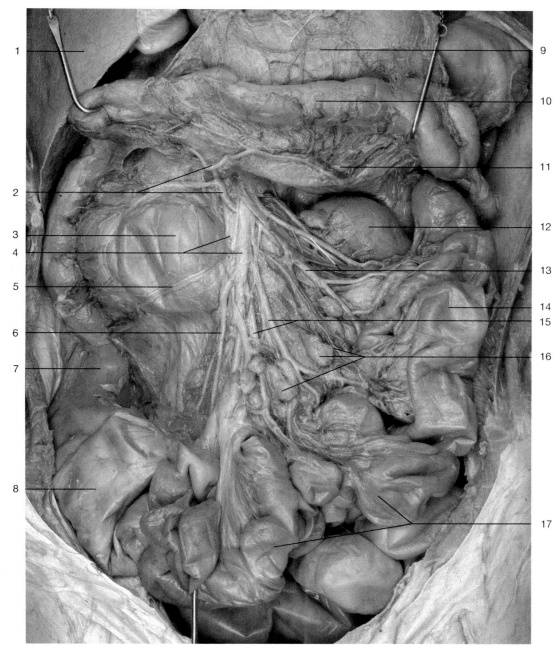

1 Liver
2 Middle colic artery
3 Horizontal part of
   duodenum (extended)
4 Superior mesenteric
   artery and vein
5 Right colic artery
6 Ileocolic artery
7 Ascending colon
8 Cecum
9 Greater omentum
   (reflected)
10 Transverse colon
11 Transverse
   mesocolon
12 Duodenojejunal
   flexure
13 Jejunal arteries
14 Jejunum
15 Ileal arteries
16 Mesenteric lymph
   nodes and lymph
   vessels
17 Ileum
18 Abdominal aorta
19 Inferior vena cava
20 Stomach
21 Spleen
22 Splenic artery
23 Head of pancreas
24 Superior mesenteric
   artery

Abdominal organs. Superior mesenteric artery. Mesenteric lymph nodes. Transverse colon reflected.

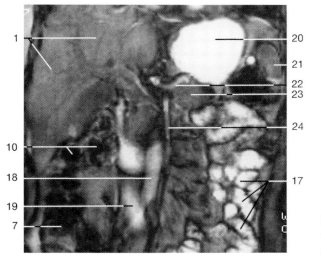

Frontal section through the abdominal cavity (MRI scan; the intestinal tract and vessels are filled with a paramagnetic substance [Gadolinium]; courtesy of Dr. W. Rödl, Erlangen, Germany).

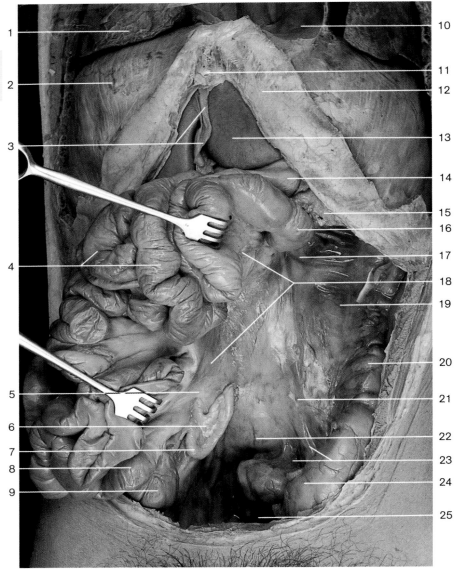

1	Lung
2	Diaphragm
3	Falciform ligament of liver
4	Jejunum
5	Ileocecal fold
6	Meso-appendix
7	Vermiform appendix
8	Ileocecal junction
9	Cecum
10	Pericardial sac
11	Xiphoid process
12	Costal margin
13	Liver
14	Stomach
15	Transverse colon
16	Duodenojejunal flexure
17	Inferior duodenal fold
18	Mesentery
19	Position of left kidney
20	Descending colon
21	Position of left common iliac artery
22	Sacral promontory
23	Sigmoid mesocolon
24	Sigmoid colon
25	Rectum
26	Beginning of jejunum
27	Peritoneum of posterior abdominal wall
28	Transverse mesocolon
29	Superior duodenal fold
30	Superior duodenal recess
31	Retroduodenal recess
32	Free taenia of ascending colon
33	Ileocecal valve
34	Frenulum of ileocecal valve
35	Orifice of vermiform appendix (probe)
36	Ileocolic artery
37	Vermiform appendix with appendicular artery
38	Ascending colon

Abdominal cavity. Mesenteries. The small intestine has been reflected laterally to demonstrate the mesentery.

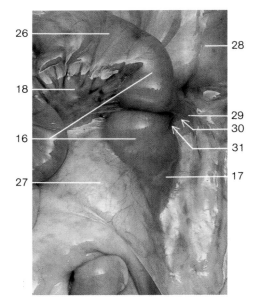

Duodenojejunal flexure
(enlargement of preceding figure).

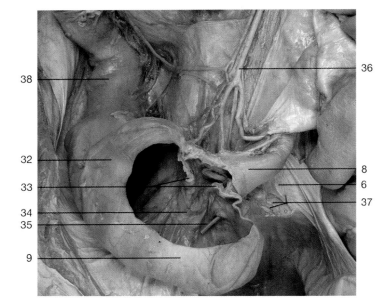

Ileocecal valve (ventral aspect). The cecum and terminal part of the ileum have been opened.

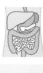

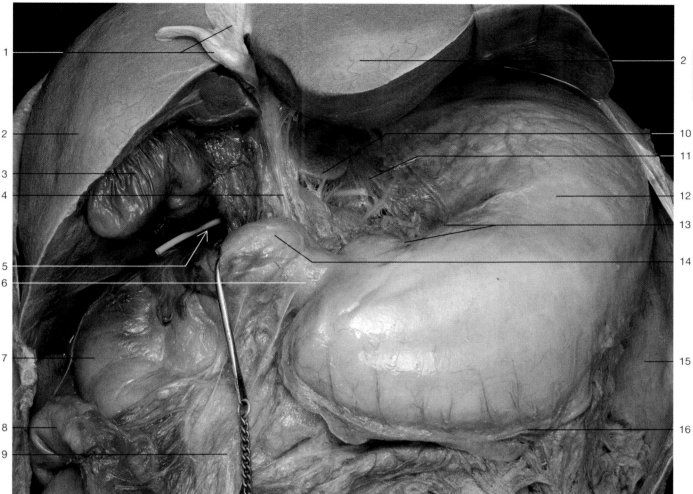

Upper abdominal organs (anterior aspect). Thorax and anterior part of diaphragm have been removed and the liver raised to display the lesser omentum. A probe has been inserted into the epiploic foramen and lesser sac.

1   Falciform ligament and ligamentum teres
2   Liver
3   Gallbladder (fundus)
4   Hepatoduodenal ligament
5   Epiploic foramen (probe)
6   Pylorus
7   Descending part of duodenum
8   Right colic flexure
9   Gastrocolic ligament
10 Caudate lobe of liver (behind lesser omentum)
11 Lesser omentum
12 Stomach
13 Lesser curvature of stomach
14 Superior part of duodenum
15 Diaphragm
16 Greater curvature of stomach with gastro-omental vessels
17 Twelfth thoracic vertebra
18 Right kidney
19 Right suprarenal gland
20 Inferior vena cava
21 Falciform ligament of liver
22 Abdominal aorta
23 Spleen
24 Lienorenal ligament
25 Gastrosplenic ligament
26 Pancreas
27 Lesser sac (omental bursa)

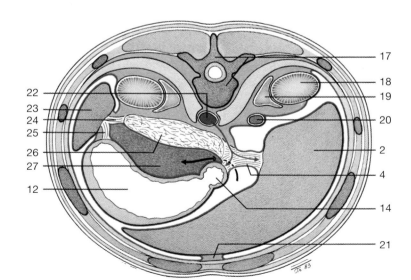

Horizontal section through the lesser sac above the level of epiploic foramen (black arrow). Viewed from above. Red arrows: routes of the arterial branches of celiac trunk to liver, stomach, duodenum, and pancreas (posterior aspect).

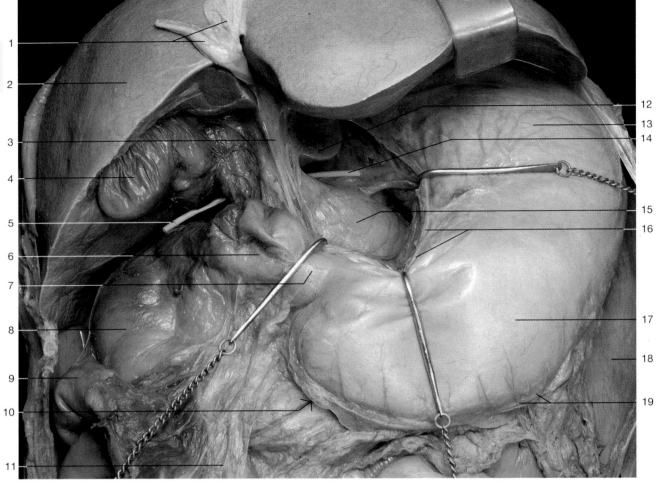

Upper abdominal organs (anterior aspect). **Lesser sac.** Lesser omentum partly removed, liver and stomach slightly reflected.

1 Falciform ligament and ligamentum teres	18 Diaphragm
2 Liver	19 Greater curvature with gastro-omental vessels
3 Hepatoduodenal ligament	20 Head of pancreas and gastropancreatic fold
4 Gallbladder	21 Spleen
5 Probe within the epiploic foramen	22 Tail of pancreas
6 Superior part of duodenum	23 Left colic flexure
7 Pylorus	24 Root of transverse mesocolon
8 Descending part of duodenum	25 Transverse mesocolon
9 Right colic flexure	26 Gastrocolic ligament (cut edge)
10 Gastrocolic ligament	27 Transverse colon
11 Greater omentum	28 Umbilicus
12 Caudate lobe of liver	29 Small intestine
13 Fundus of stomach	30 Lesser omentum
14 Probe at the level of the vestibule of lesser sac (through epiploic foramen)	31 Lesser sac (omental bursa)
15 Head of pancreas	32 Duodenum
16 Lesser curvature of stomach	33 Mesentery
17 Body of stomach	34 Sigmoid colon

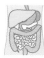

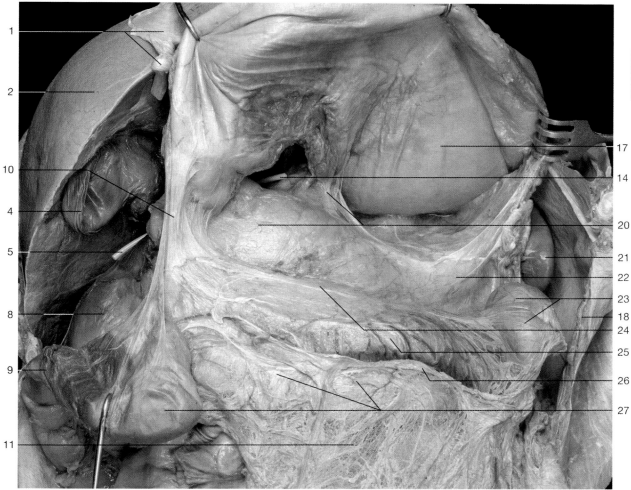

Upper abdominal organs (anterior aspect). **Lesser sac.** The gastrocolic ligament has been divided and the whole stomach raised to display the posterior wall of the lesser sac.

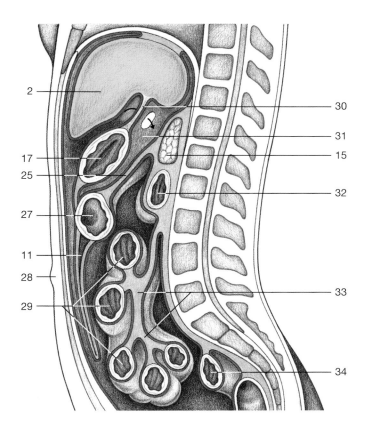

Midsagittal section through abdominal cavity, demonstrating the site of lesser sac (blue). (Schematic drawing.) The epiploic foramen, entrance to the lesser sac, is indicated by an arrow. Red = peritoneum.

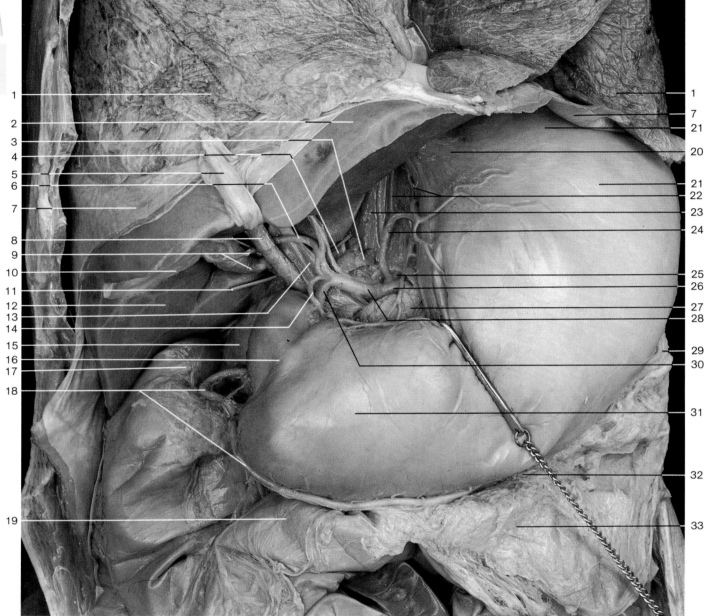

Arteries of upper abdominal organs (anterior aspect). **Dissection of celiac trunk.** The lesser omentum has been removed and the lesser curvature of the stomach reflected to display the branches of the celiac trunk. The probe is situated within the epiploic foramen.

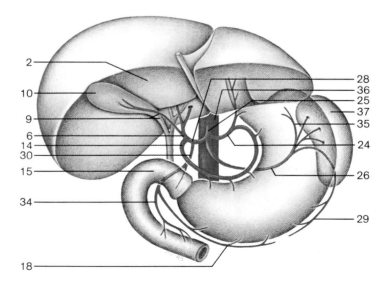

Branches of celiac trunk (schematic drawing).

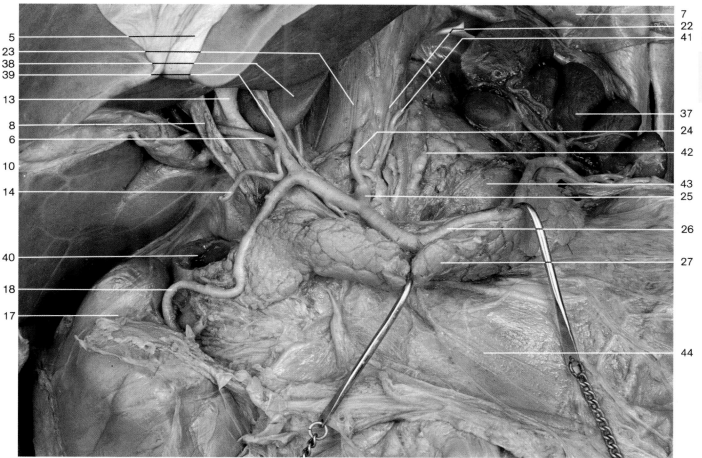

Arteries of upper abdominal organs (anterior aspect). **Branches of celiac trunk; blood supply of liver, pancreas, and spleen.**
The stomach, superior part of duodenum, and celiac ganglion have been removed to reveal the anterior aspect of the posterior wall of the lesser sac (omental bursa) and the vessels and ducts of the hepatoduodenal ligament. The pancreas has been slightly reflected anteriorly.

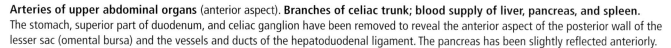

1	Lung	23	Lumbar part of diaphragm
2	Liver (visceral surface)	24	Left gastric artery
3	Lymph node	25	Celiac trunk
4	Inferior vena cava	26	Splenic artery
5	Ligamentum teres (reflected)	27	Pancreas
6	Right branch of hepatic artery proper	28	Common hepatic artery
7	Diaphragm	29	Left gastro-omental (gastro-epiploic) artery
8	Common hepatic duct (dilated)	30	Gastroduodenal artery
9	Cystic duct and artery	31	Pyloric part of stomach
10	Gallbladder	32	Greater curvature of stomach
11	Probe in epiploic foramen	33	Gastrocolic ligament
12	Right lobe of liver	34	Superior pancreaticoduodenal artery
13	Portal vein	35	Short gastric arteries
14	Right gastric artery	36	Aorta
15	Duodenum	37	Spleen
16	Pylorus	38	Caudate lobe of liver
17	Right colic flexure	39	Left branch of hepatic artery proper
18	Right gastro-omental (gastro-epiploic) artery	40	Descending part of duodenum (cut)
19	Transverse colon	41	Left inferior phrenic artery
20	Abdominal part of esophagus (cardiac part of stomach)	42	Suprarenal gland
21	Fundus of stomach	43	Kidney
22	Esophageal branches of left gastric artery	44	Transverse mesocolon

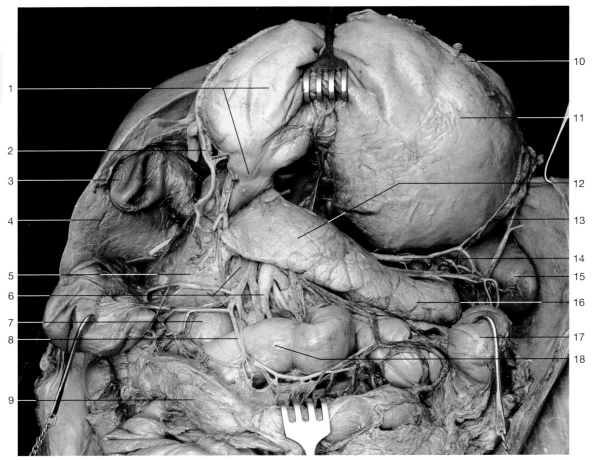

Posterior abdominal wall with pancreas and extrahepatic bile ducts in situ (anterior aspect). The gastrocolic ligament has been divided, the transverse colon and the stomach replaced to display the pancreas and superior mesenteric vessels.

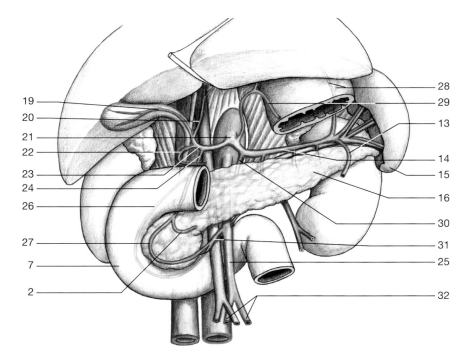

Blood supply of upper abdominal organs (branches of the celiac trunk and superior mesenteric artery). (Schematic drawing.)

1   Stomach (pyloric part) and pylorus
2   Right gastro-omental (gastro-epiploic) artery
3   Fundus of gallbladder
4   Liver (right lobe)
5   Head of pancreas
6   Superior mesenteric artery and vein
7   Duodenum
8   Middle colic artery
9   Transverse colon
10 Greater curvature of stomach
    (remnants of gastrocolic ligament)
11 Body of stomach
12 Body of pancreas
13 Left gastro-omental (gastro-epiploic) artery
14 Splenic artery
15 Spleen
16 Tail of pancreas
17 Left colic flexure
18 Jejunum
19 Cystic artery
20 Hepatic artery proper
21 Celiac trunk
22 Right gastric artery
23 Common hepatic artery
24 Gastroduodenal artery
25 Superior mesenteric artery
26 Superior posterior pancreaticoduodenal artery
27 Superior anterior pancreaticoduodenal artery
28 Short gastric arteries
29 Left gastric artery
30 Posterior pancreatic branch of splenic artery
31 Inferior pancreaticoduodenal artery
32 Jejunal arteries

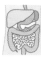

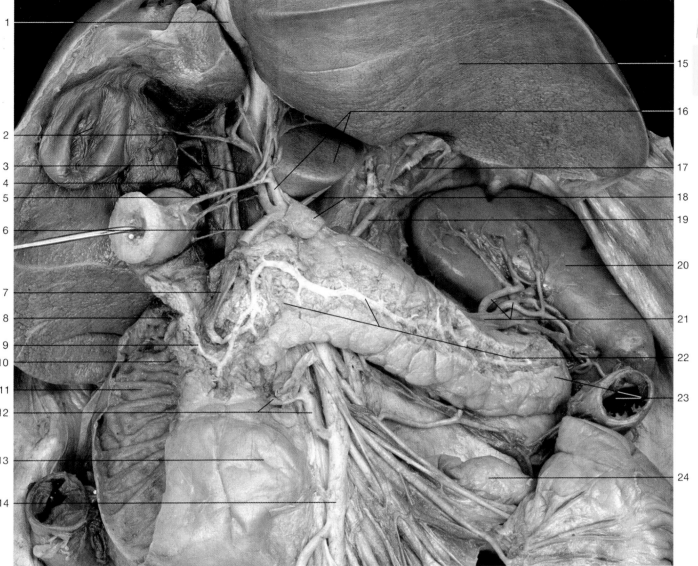

Posterior abdominal wall with duodenum, pancreas, and spleen (anterior aspect). Dissection of pancreatic and common bile duct. The stomach has been removed, the liver raised, and the duodenum anteriorly opened.

1 Ligamentum teres	13 Horizontal part of duodenum (distended)
2 Gallbladder and cystic artery	14 Superior mesenteric artery
3 Common hepatic duct and portal vein	15 Liver (left lobe)
4 Cystic duct	16 Caudate lobe of liver and hepatic artery proper
5 Right gastric artery (pylorus with superior part of duodenum, cut and reflected)	17 Abdominal part of esophagus (cut)
6 Gastroduodenal artery	18 Probe in epiploic foramen and lymph node
7 Common bile duct	19 Left gastric artery
8 Probe within the minor duodenal papilla	20 Spleen
9 Accessory pancreatic duct	21 Splenic vein and branches of splenic artery
10 Probe within the major duodenal papilla	22 Main pancreatic duct and head of pancreas
11 Descending part of duodenum (opened)	23 Left colic flexure and tail of pancreas
12 Middle colic artery and inferior pancreaticoduodenal artery	24 Duodenojejunal flexure

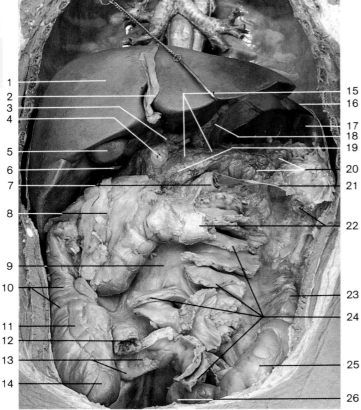

1 Liver
2 Falciform ligament
3 Hepatoduodenal ligament
4 Pylorus (divided)
5 Gallbladder
6 Probe within the epiploic foramen
7 Duodenojejunal flexure (divided)
8 Greater omentum
9 Root of mesentery
10 Ascending colon
11 Free colic taenia
12 End of ileum (divided)
13 Vermiform appendix with meso-appendix
14 Cecum
15 Pancreas and site of lesser sac
16 Diaphragm
17 Spleen
18 Cardia (part of stomach, divided)
19 Head of pancreas
20 Body and tail of pancreas
21 Transverse mesocolon
22 Transverse colon (divided)
23 Descending colon
24 Cut edge of mesentery
25 Sigmoid colon
26 Rectum
27 Attachment of bare area of liver
28 Inferior vena cava
29 Kidney
30 Attachment of right colic flexure
31 Root of transverse mesocolon
32 Junction between descending and horizontal parts of duodenum
33 Bare surface for ascending colon
34 Ileocecal recess
35 Retrocecal recess
36 Root of meso-appendix
37 Superior recess ⎫
38 Isthmus (opening) ⎬ of lesser sac (omental bursa)
39 Splenic recess ⎭
40 Superior duodenal recess
41 Inferior duodenal recess
42 Bare surface for descending colon
43 Paracolic recesses
44 Root of mesentery
45 Root of mesosigmoid
46 Intersigmoid recess
47 Hepatic veins
48 Duodenojejunal flexure
49 Attachment of left colic flexure
50 Esophagus
51 Entrance to lesser sac through the epiploic foramen

Abdominal cavity after removal of stomach, jejunum, ileum, and part of the transverse colon. Liver has been slightly raised.

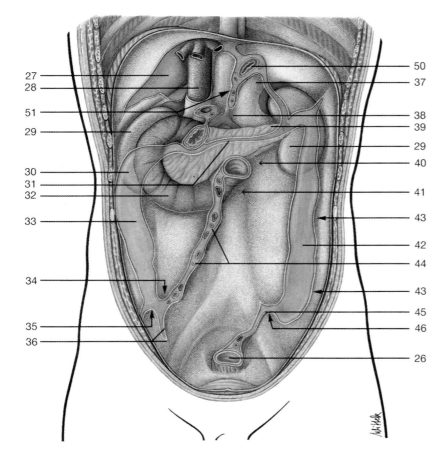

Peritoneal reflections from organs and the position of root of mesentery and peritoneal recesses on the posterior abdominal wall (schematic drawing).

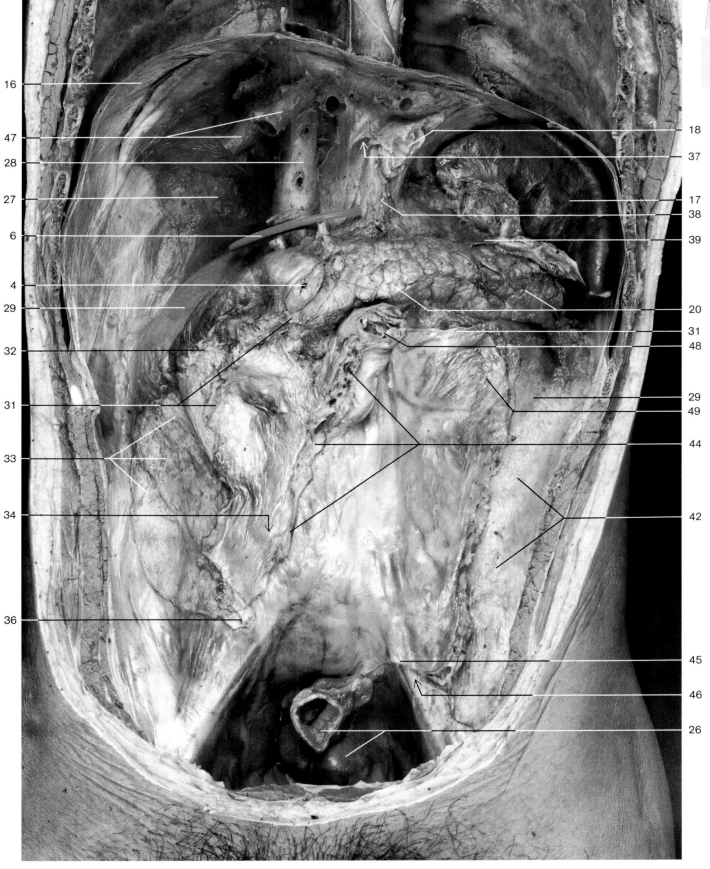

Peritoneal recesses on the posterior abdominal wall. The liver, stomach, jejunum, ileum, and colon have been removed. The duodenum, pancreas, and spleen have been left in place.

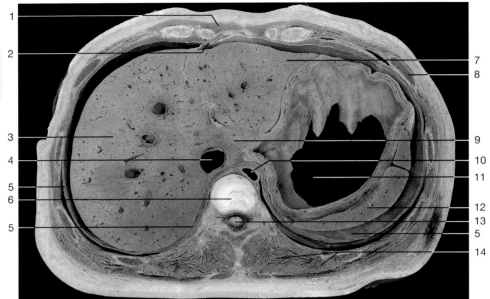

Horizontal section through the abdominal cavity at level 1 (from below).

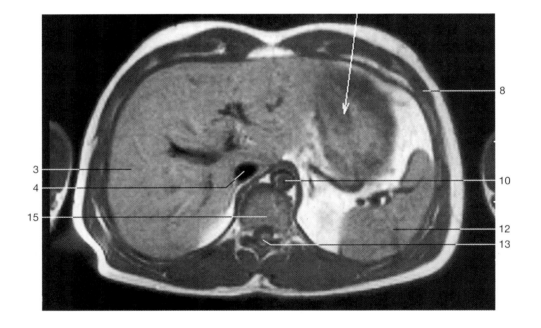

Horizontal section through the abdominal cavity (MRI scan, corresponding to level 1). Arrow: stomach.

1	Rectus abdominis muscle	20	Greater duodenal papilla
2	Falciform ligament	21	Duodenum
3	Liver (right lobe)	22	Suprarenal gland and ureter
4	Inferior vena cava	23	Kidney
5	Diaphragm	24	Round ligament of liver
6	Intervertebral disc	25	Superior mesenteric artery and vein
7	Liver (left lobe)	26	Psoas major muscle
8	Rib	27	Descending colon
9	Liver (caudate lobe)	28	Quadratus lumborum muscle
10	Abdominal (descending) aorta	29	Cauda equina
11	Stomach	30	Right renal vein
12	Spleen	31	Small intestine
13	Spinal cord	32	Iliacus muscle
14	Longissimus and iliocostalis muscles	33	Ilium
15	Body of vertebra	34	Ileocecal valve
16	Rectus abdominis muscle	35	Cecum
17	External abdominal oblique muscle	36	Common iliac artery and vein
18	Transverse colon	37	Gluteus medius muscle
19	Head of pancreas	38	Vertebral canal and dura mater

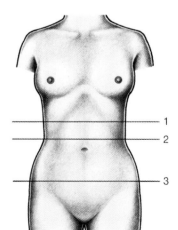

Levels of sections.

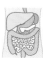

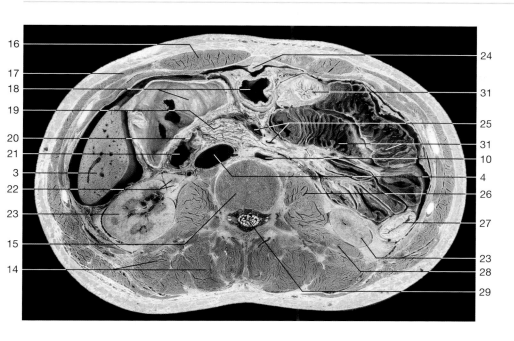

16
17
18
19
20
21
3
22
23
15
14

24
31
25
31
10
4
26
27
23
28
29

Horizontal section through the abdominal cavity at the level of greater duodenal papilla (from below).

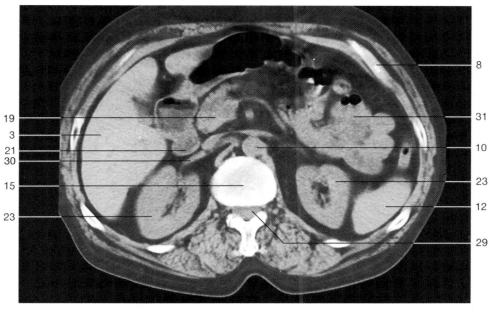

19
3
21
30
15
23

8
31
10
23
12
29

Horizontal section through the abdominal cavity (CT scan, corresponding to level 2).

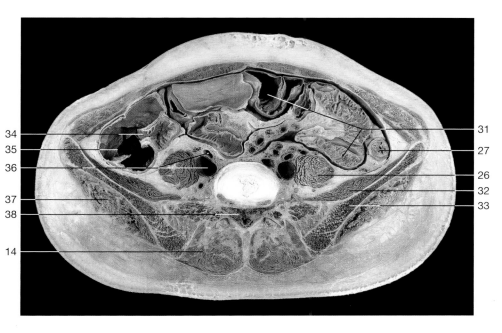

34
35
36
37
38
14

31
27
26
32
33

Horizontal section through the abdominal cavity at level 3 (from below).

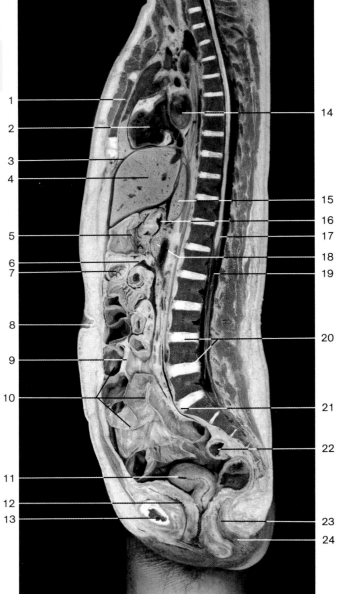

Midsagittal section through the trunk (female).

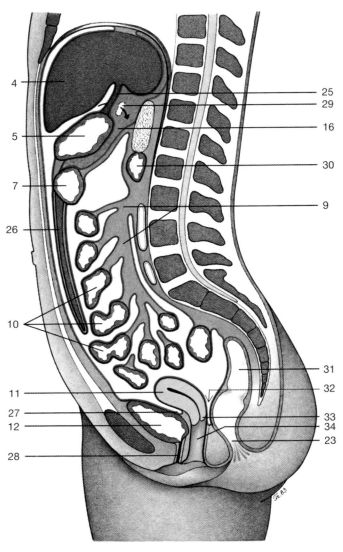

Midsagittal section through the trunk (female).
(Schematic drawing.) Blue = omental bursa; red = peritoneum.

1	Sternum	13	Pubic symphysis	24	Anus
2	Right ventricle of heart	14	Left atrium of heart	25	Lesser omentum
3	Diaphragm	15	Caudate lobe of liver	26	Greater omentum
4	Liver	16	Omental bursa or lesser sac	27	Vesico-uterine pouch
5	Stomach	17	Conus medullaris	28	Urethra
6	Transverse mesocolon	18	Pancreas	29	Epiploic (omental) foramen
7	Transverse colon	19	Cauda equina	30	Duodenum
8	Umbilicus	20	Intervertebral discs (lumbar vertebral column)	31	Rectum
9	Mesentery	21	Sacral promontory	32	Recto-uterine pouch
10	Small intestine	22	Sigmoid colon	33	Vaginal part of cervix of uterus
11	Uterus	23	Anal canal	34	Vagina
12	Urinary bladder				

6 Retroperitoneal Organs

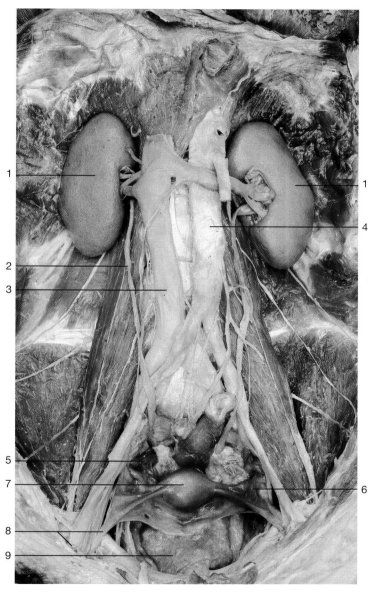

Retroperitoneal organs of the female (anterior aspect). View of the female pelvis showing uterus with uterine ligaments, ovary, and urinary bladder (from Lütjen-Drecoll, Rohen, Innenansichten des menschlichen Körpers, 2010).

1 Kidney
2 Ureter
3 Inferior vena cava
4 Abdominal aorta
5 Ovary
6 Uterine tube
7 Uterus
8 Round ligament and inguinal canal
9 Urinary bladder
10 Vagina

The organs of the urinary system (kidney, ureter, and, in the female, genital organs) are located together with vessels and nerves (aorta, inferior vena cava, plexus solaris, etc.) within the retroperitoneal space.

The upper part of the kidneys reaches the level of the margin of the lung. During respiration, the kidneys move slightly within their fasciae of Gerota. Parallel with the vertebral column, the ureter runs towards the urinary bladder. The great center of the autonomic nervous system, the solar plexus (celiac ganglion, etc.), is located in front of the abdominal aorta.

The genital organs of the female (uterus, uterine tube, ovary) are located within the pelvic cavity. In the male, the testis has moved out of the abdominal cavity and penetrated the inguinal canal to be finally located within the extragenital organs.

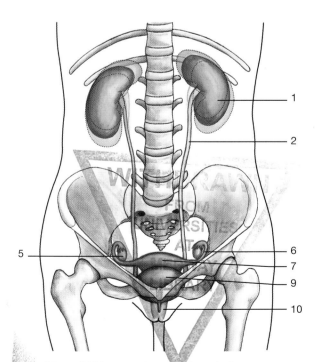

Position of kidneys, urinary and genital organs in the female (anterior aspect, schematic drawing). The excursions of the kidneys with the respiratory movements of the diaphragm are indicated.

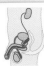

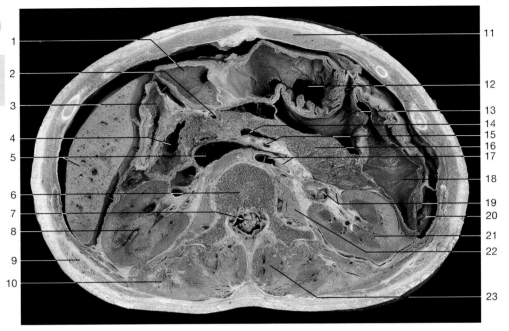

1 Pyloric antrum
2 Gastroduodenal artery
3 Descending part of duodenum
4 Vestibule of lesser sac
5 Inferior vena cava and liver
6 Body of first lumbar vertebra
7 Cauda equina
8 Right kidney
9 Latissimus dorsi muscle
10 Iliocostalis muscle
11 Rectus abdominis muscle
12 Stomach
13 Lesser sac
14 Splenic vein
15 Superior mesenteric artery
16 Pancreas
17 Aorta and left renal artery
18 Transverse colon
19 Renal artery and vein
20 Spleen
21 Left kidney
22 Psoas major muscle
23 Multifidus muscle
24 Margin of lung
25 Margin of pleura
26 Renal pelvis
27 Left ureter
28 Descending colon
29 Rectum
30 Right suprarenal gland
31 Twelfth rib
32 Ascending colon
33 Right ureter
34 Cecum
35 Vermiform appendix
36 Urinary bladder
37 Liver
38 Anterior layer of renal fascia
39 Duodenum
40 Perirenal fatty tissue
41 Posterior layer of renal fascia
42 Abdominal cavity

Horizontal section through the abdominal cavity at the level of the first lumbar vertebra (from below).

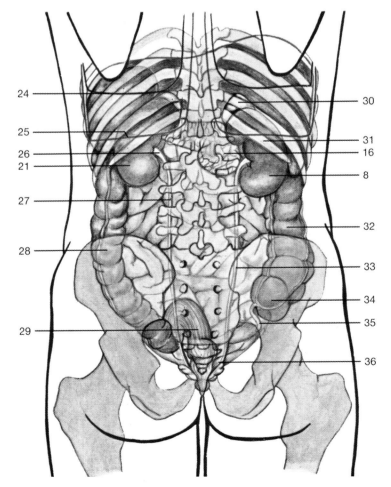

Positions of urinary organs (posterior aspect, schematic drawing). Notice that the upper part of the kidney reaches the level of the margin of pleura and lung.

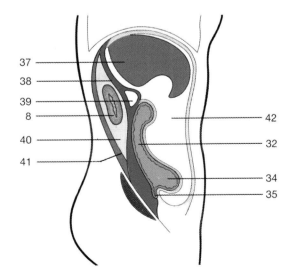

Retroperitoneal tissue, position of the right kidney (schematic drawing).
Yellow = adipose capsule of kidney.

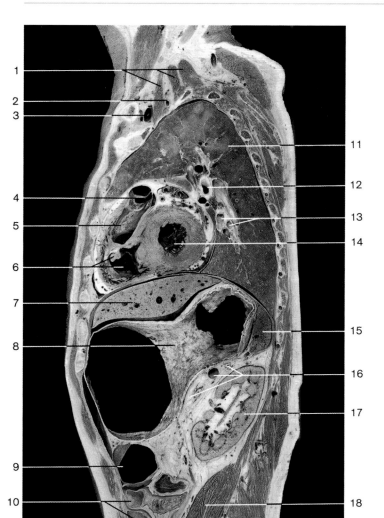

1   Scalenus anterior, medius, and posterior muscles
2   Left subclavian artery
3   Left subclavian vein
4   Pulmonic valve
5   Arterial cone
6   Right ventricle of heart
7   Liver
8   Stomach
9   Transverse colon
10 Small intestine
11 Left lung
12 Left main bronchus
13 Branches of pulmonary vein
14 Left ventricle of heart
15 Spleen
16 Splenic artery and vein and pancreas
17 Left kidney
18 Psoas major muscle
19 Inferior vena cava
20 Renal vein
21 Body of twelfth thoracic vertebra and vertebral canal
22 Right kidney
23 Superior mesenteric artery
24 Superior mesenteric vein
25 Pancreas
26 Abdominal aorta
27 Left psoas major and quadratus lumborum muscles
28 Anterior layer of renal fascia ⎫
29 Posterior layer of renal fascia ⎬ of Gerota
30 Perirenal fatty tissue
31 Abdominal cavity
32 Descending and sigmoid colon

Parasagittal section through the thoracic and abdominal cavities at the level of the left kidney (5.5 cm left of median plane).

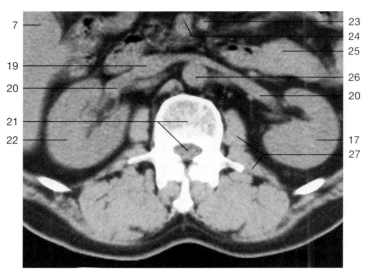

Horizontal section through the retroperitoneal region at the level of 12th thoracic vertebra (CT scan, from below).

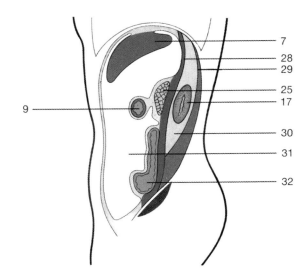

Retroperitoneal tissue, position of the left kidney (schematic drawing).

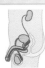

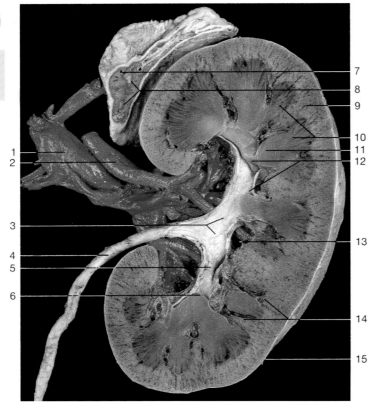

1 Renal vein
2 Renal artery
3 Renal pelvis
4 Abdominal part of ureter
5 Major renal calyx
6 Cribriform area of renal papilla
7 Cortex of suprarenal gland
8 Medulla of suprarenal gland
9 Cortex of kidney
10 Medulla of kidney
11 Renal papilla
12 Minor renal calyx
13 Renal sinus
14 Renal columns
15 Fibrous capsule of kidney

Coronal section through right kidney and suprarenal gland
(posterior aspect). The renal pelvis has been opened and the fatty
tissue removed to display the renal vessels.

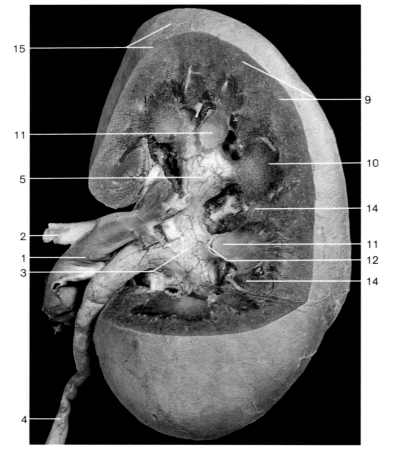

Each kidney can be divided into five segments
supplied by individual interlobar arteries
known as end arteries. Thus, obstruction leads
to infarcts marking the trace of segment
borders. The anterior kidney surface reveals
four segments; the posterior, only three (Nos.
1, 4, and 5).

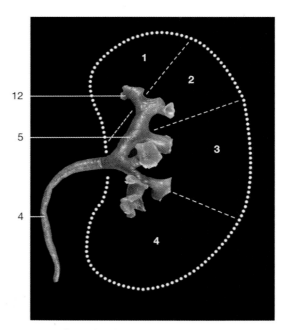

Right kidney (posterior aspect). Partial coronal section to expose
internal aspect of the kidney.

Cast of renal pelvis and calices.
1–4 = Renal segments on anterior surface.

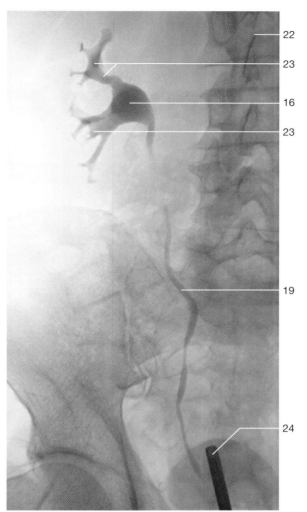

Renal pelvis with calices and ureter (X-ray, retrograde injection; by courtesy of Prof. Herrlinger, Fürth, Germany).

1   Hepatic vein
2   Anterior and posterior vagal trunk
3   Inferior vena cava
4   Lumbar part of diaphragm
5   Right greater and lesser splanchnic nerves
6   Celiac trunk
7   Celiac ganglion and plexus
8   Superior mesenteric artery
9   Left renal vein
10 Right sympathetic trunk and ganglion
11 Abdominal aorta
12 Left sympathetic trunk
13 Esophagus (cut),
    left greater splanchnic nerve
14 Left suprarenal gland
15 Left renal artery
16 Renal pelvis
17 Renal papilla with minor calyx
18 Left testicular vein
19 Ureter
20 Psoas major muscle
21 Quadratus lumborum muscle
22 Lumbar vertebra (L$_2$)
23 Renal calyx
24 Catheter

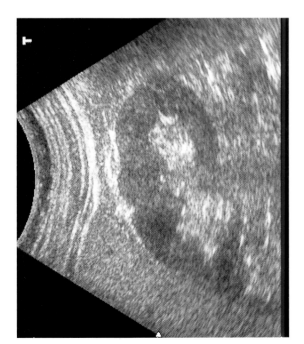

Right kidney (ultrasound image; by courtesy of Prof. Herrlinger, Fürth, Germany).

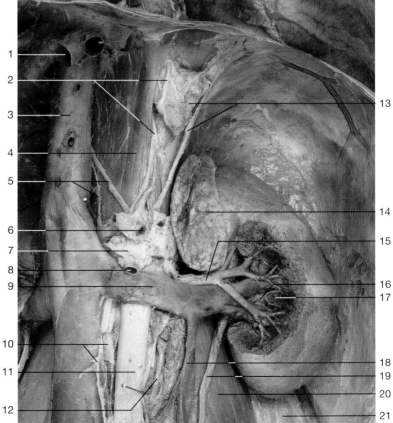

Left kidney and suprarenal gland in situ. The anterior cortical layer of the kidney has been removed to display the renal pelvis and papillae.

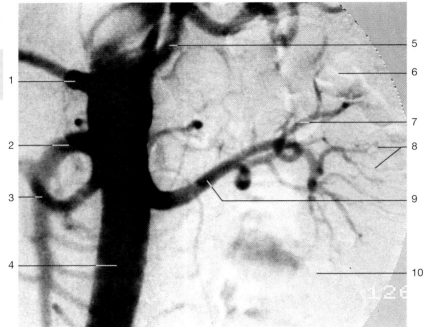

1 Celiac trunk
2 Superior mesenteric artery
3 Middle colic artery
4 Abdominal aorta (with catheter)
5 Splenic artery
6 Upper pole of kidney
7 Anterior branch of renal artery
8 Interlobular arteries
9 Left renal artery
10 Lower pole of kidney
11 Body of first lumbar vertebra
12 Posterior branch of renal artery
13 Anterior inferior segmental artery
14 Superior suprarenal artery
15 Upper capsular artery
16 Perforating artery
17 Lower capsular artery
18 Ureter
19 Right inferior phrenic artery
20 Left inferior phrenic artery
21 Middle suprarenal artery
22 Inferior suprarenal artery
23 Renal artery
24 Left testicular (or ovarian) artery
25 Inferior mesenteric artery

Abdominal aorta (subtraction angiography).

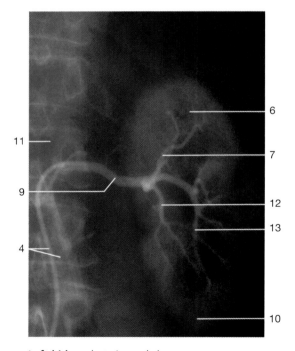

Left kidney (arteriography).

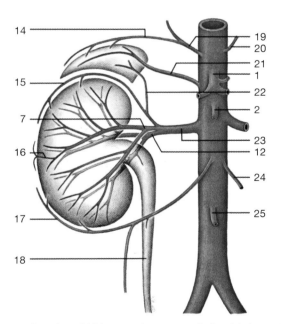

Arteries of kidney and suprarenal gland (schematic drawing).

The kidneys are perfused by app. 1.500–1.800 l of blood per day via the renal arteries. Out of more than 1.2 million renal corpuscles (glomeruli), 1% of this volume (id 150–180 l) is filtered as a cell free fluid. In the tubular system, 99% of this fluid, together with useful substances like glucose and ions, are reabsorbed. Only 1–1.5 l of urine containing waste material is excreted.

Diseases of the renal vascular system may impair the filtering process and thereby the composition of the blood.

1 Diaphragm
2 Hepatic veins
3 Inferior vena cava
4 Common hepatic artery
5 Suprarenal gland
6 Celiac trunk
7 Right renal vein
8 Kidney
9 Abdominal aorta
10 Subcostal nerve
11 Iliohypogastric nerve
12 Central tendon of diaphragm
13 Inferior phrenic artery
14 Cardic part of stomach
15 Spleen
16 Splenic artery
17 Superior renal artery
18 Superior mesenteric artery
19 Psoas major muscle
20 Inferior mesenteric artery
21 Ureter
22 Glomerulus
23 Afferent arteriole of glomerulus
24 Glomeruli
25 Radiating cortical artery
26 Subcortical or arcuate artery
27 Subcortical or arcuate vein
28 Interlobular vein
29 Interlobular artery
30 Interlobar artery and vein
31 Vessels of renal capsule
32 Efferent arteriole of glomerulus
33 Vasa recta of renal medulla
34 Spiral arteries of renal pelvis

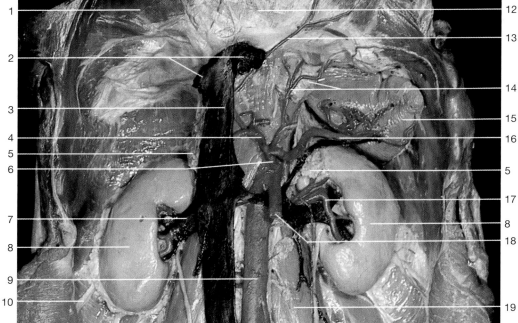
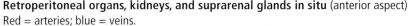

Retroperitoneal organs, kidneys, and suprarenal glands in situ (anterior aspect).
Red = arteries; blue = veins.

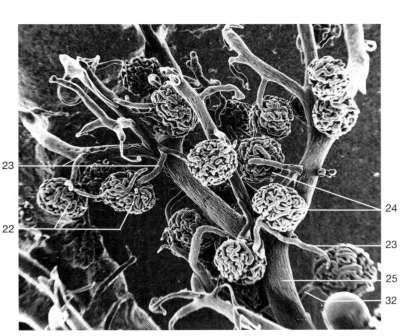

Glomeruli (210 ×). Scanning electron micrograph showing glomeruli and associated arteries.

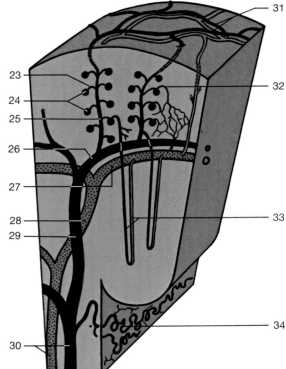

Architecture of vascular system of kidney (schematic drawing).

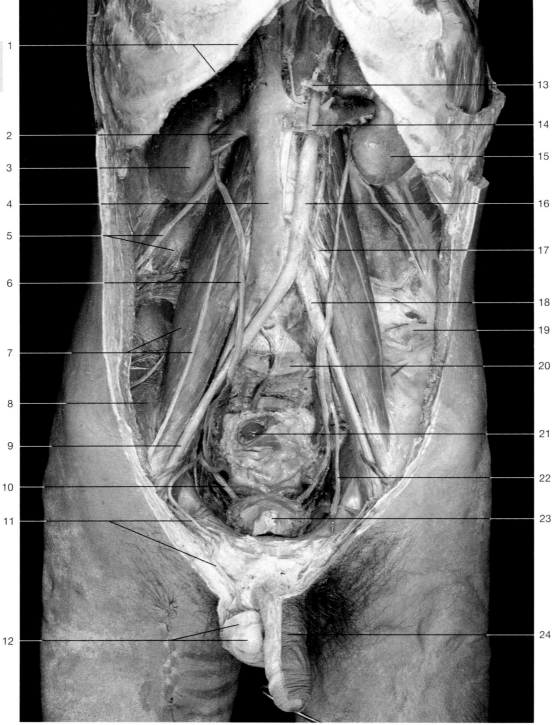

Retroperitoneal organs, urinary system in the male (anterior aspect). The peritoneum has been removed.

1	Costal arch	8	Iliacus muscle	17	Inferior mesenteric artery
2	Right renal vein	9	External iliac artery	18	Common iliac artery
3	Right kidney	10	Ureter (pelvic part)	19	Iliac crest
4	Inferior vena cava	11	Ductus deferens	20	Sacral promontory
5	Iliohypogastric nerve and quadratus lumborum muscle	12	Testis and epididymis	21	Rectum (cut)
6	Ureter (abdominal part)	13	Celiac trunk	22	Medial umbilical ligament
7	Psoas major muscle and genitofemoral nerve	14	Superior mesenteric artery	23	Urinary bladder
		15	Left kidney	24	Penis
		16	Abdominal aorta		

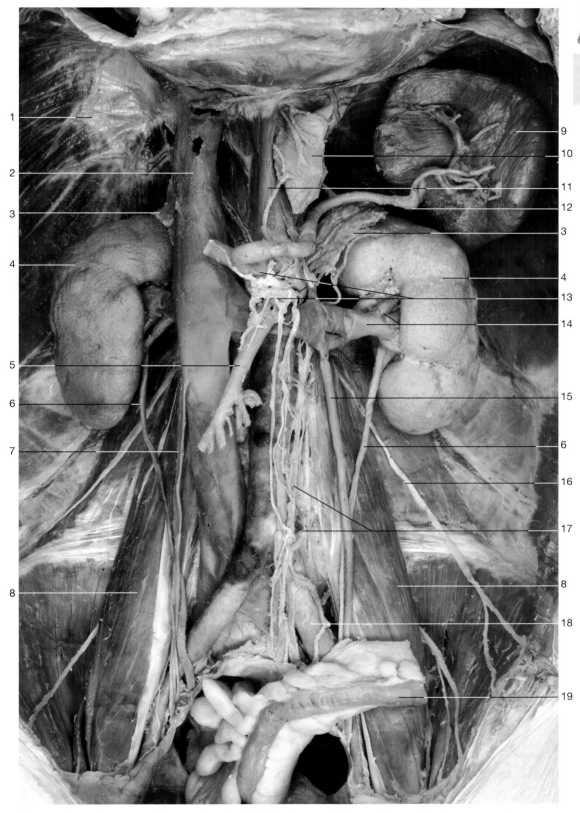

Retroperitoneal organs, urinary system in situ (anterior aspect). The peritoneum has been removed. Note the autonomic plexus and ganglia at the abdominal aorta.

1 Diaphragm	7 Right spermatic vein	11 Abdominal aorta	16 Ilio-inguinal nerve
2 Inferior vena cava	8 Psoas major	12 Splenic artery	17 Superior hypogastric
3 Suprarenal gland	muscle	13 Celiac trunk and	plexus and ganglion
4 Kidney	9 Spleen	celiac ganglion	18 Left common iliac
5 Superior mesenteric artery	10 Cardiac part of	14 Renal artery and vein	artery
6 Ureter	stomach	15 Left spermatic vein	19 Sigmoid colon

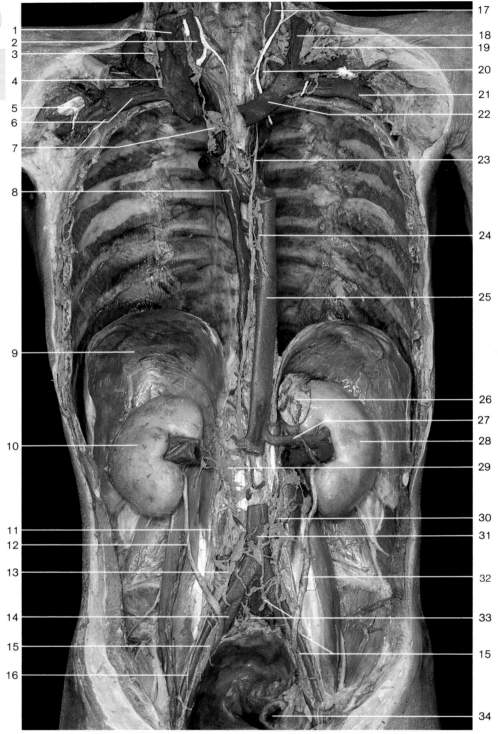

Lymph vessels and lymph nodes of the posterior wall of thoracic and abdominal cavities (anterior aspect). Green = lymph vessels and nodes; blue = veins; red = arteries; white = nerves.

1	Internal jugular vein	9	Diaphragm	18	Internal jugular vein	27	Left renal artery
2	Right common carotid artery and right vagus nerve	10	Right kidney	19	Deep cervical lymph nodes	28	Left kidney
		11	Right lumbar trunk	20	Thoracic duct entering left jugular angle	29	Cisterna chyli
3	Jugulo-omohyoid lymph node	12	Right ureter			30	Lumbar lymph nodes
		13	Common iliac lymph nodes	21	Left subclavian vein	31	Abdominal aorta
4	Right lymphatic duct	14	Right internal iliac artery	22	Left brachiocephalic vein	32	Left ureter
5	Subclavian trunk	15	External iliac lymph nodes	23	Thoracic duct	33	Sacral lymph nodes
6	Right subclavian vein	16	Right external iliac artery	24	Mediastinal lymph nodes	34	Rectum (cut edge)
7	Bronchomediastinal trunk	17	Left common carotid artery and left vagus nerve	25	Thoracic aorta		
8	Azygos vein			26	Left suprarenal gland		

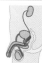

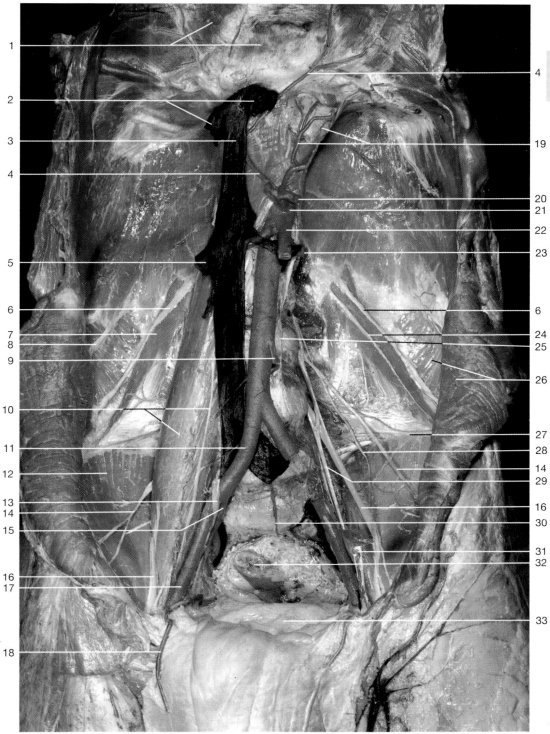

Vessels and nerves of posterior abdominal wall (anterior aspect). Part of the left psoas major muscle has been removed to display the lumbar plexus. Red = arteries; blue = veins.

1	Diaphragm	11	Common iliac artery	20	Splenic artery	31	Psoas major muscle
2	Hepatic veins	12	Iliacus muscle	21	Celiac trunk		(divided) with supplying
3	Inferior vena cava	13	Right ureter (divided)	22	Superior mesenteric artery		artery
4	Inferior phrenic artery	14	Lateral femoral cutaneous nerve	23	Left renal artery	32	Rectum (cut)
5	Right renal vein	15	Internal iliac artery	24	Ilio-inguinal nerve	33	Urinary bladder
6	Iliohypogastric nerve	16	Femoral nerve	25	Sympathetic trunk		
7	Quadratus lumborum muscle	17	External iliac artery	26	Transversus abdominis muscle		
8	Subcostal nerve	18	Inferior epigastric artery	27	Iliac crest		
9	Inferior mesenteric artery	19	Cardiac part of stomach and	28	Left genitofemoral nerve		
10	Right genitofemoral nerve		esophageal branches of left	29	Left obturator nerve		
	and psoas major muscle		gastric artery	30	Median sacral artery		

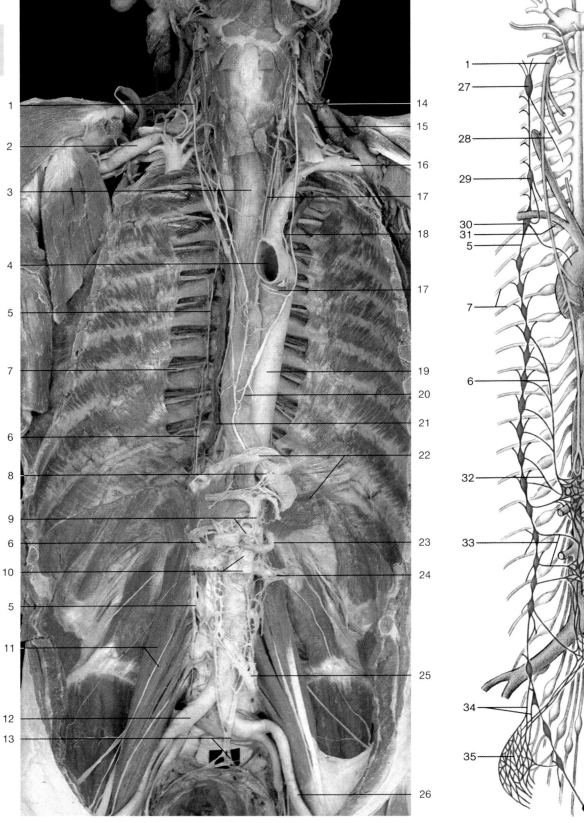

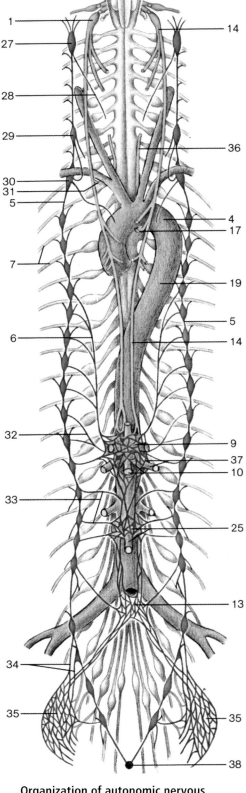

Posterior wall of thoracic and abdominal cavities with sympathetic trunk, vagus nerve, and autonomic ganglia (anterior aspect). Thoracic and abdominal organs removed, except for the esophagus and aorta.

Organization of autonomic nervous system (after Mattuschka). (Schematic drawing.) Yellow = parasympathetic nerves; green = sympathetic nerves.

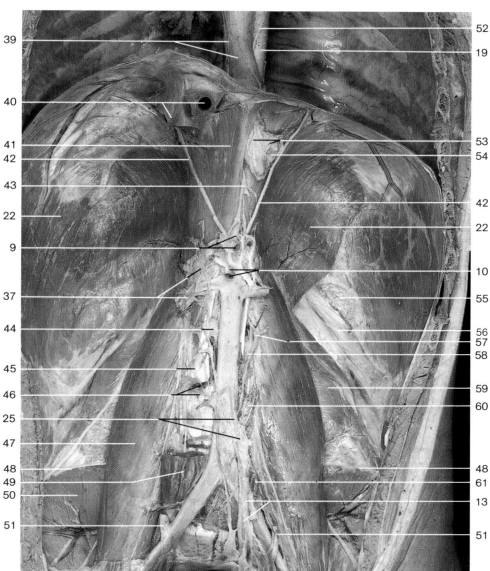

Ganglia and plexus of the autonomic nervous system within the retroperitoneal space (anterior aspect). The kidneys and the inferior vena cava with its tributaries have been removed.

1	Right vagus nerve	16	Left subclavian artery
2	Right subclavian artery	17	Left recurrent laryngeal nerve
3	Esophagus	18	Inferior cervical cardiac nerve
4	Aortic arch	19	Thoracic aorta
5	Sympathetic trunk	20	Esophageal plexus
6	Greater splanchnic nerve	21	Azygos vein
7	Intercostal nerve	22	Diaphragm
8	Abdominal part of esophagus and vagal trunk	23	Splenic artery
		24	Left renal artery and plexus
9	Celiac trunk with celiac ganglion	25	Inferior mesenteric ganglion and artery
10	Superior mesenteric artery and ganglion	26	Left external iliac artery
		27	Superior cervical ganglion of sympathetic trunk
11	Psoas major muscle and genitofemoral nerve	28	Superior cardiac branch of sympathetic trunk
12	Common iliac artery	29	Middle cervical ganglion of sympathetic trunk
13	Superior hypogastric plexus and ganglion	30	Inferior cervical ganglion of sympathetic trunk
14	Left vagus nerve		
15	Brachial plexus		

31	Right recurrent laryngeal nerve	46	Lumbar artery and vein
32	Lesser splanchnic nerve	47	Psoas major muscle
33	Lumbar splanchnic nerves	48	Iliac crest
34	Sacral splanchnic nerves	49	Inferior vena cava
35	Inferior hypogastric ganglion and plexus	50	Iliacus muscle
		51	Ureter
36	Left recurrent laryngeal nerve	52	Left vagus nerve forming the esophageal plexus
37	Aorticorenal plexus and renal artery	53	Left vagus nerve forming the gastric plexus
38	Ganglion impar	54	Esophagus continuing into the cardiac part of stomach
39	Esophagus with branches of vagus nerve	55	Lumbocostal triangle
40	Hepatic veins	56	Position of twelfth rib
41	Right crus of diaphragm	57	Left lumbar lymph trunk
42	Inferior phrenic artery	58	Ganglion of sympathetic trunk
43	Right vagus nerve entering the celiac ganglion	59	Quadratus lumborum muscle
44	Right lumbar lymph trunk	60	Lumbar part of left sympathetic trunk
45	Lumbar part of right sympathetic trunk	61	Iliac lymph vessels

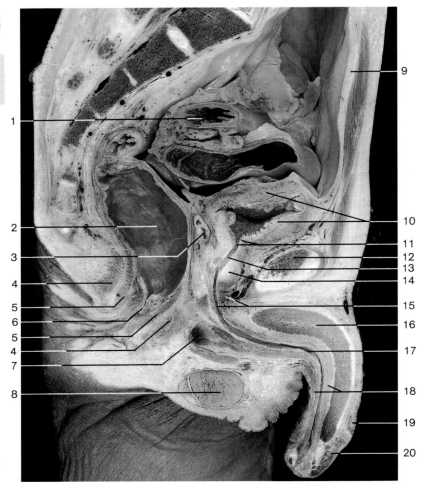

1	Sigmoid colon
2	Ampulla of rectum
3	Ampulla of ductus deferens
4	External anal sphincter muscle
5	Internal anal sphincter muscle
6	Anal canal
7	Bulb of penis
8	Testis (cut surface)
9	Median umbilical ligament
10	Urinary bladder
11	Internal urethral orifice and sphincter
12	Pubic symphysis
13	Prostatic part of urethra
14	Prostate gland
15	Membranous part of urethra and external urethral sphincter
16	Corpus cavernosum of penis
17	Spongy urethra
18	Corpus spongiosum of penis
19	Foreskin or prepuce
20	Glans penis
21	Kidney
22	Renal pelvis
23	Abdominal part of ureter
24	Pelvic part of ureter
25	Seminal vesicle
26	Ejaculatory duct
27	Bulbo-urethral or Cowper's gland
28	Ductus deferens
29	Epididymis
30	Umbilicus
31	Trigone of bladder and ureteric orifice
32	Navicular fossa of urethra
33	External urethral orifice
34	Testis

Male urogenital system, midsagittal section through the pelvis.

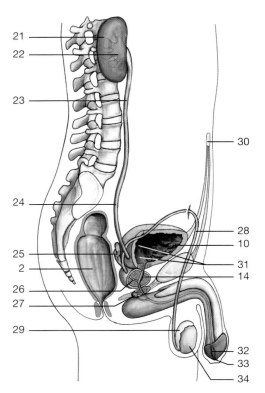

Male urogenital system (schematic drawing).

The **prostate** is located between the bladder and urogenital diaphragm. The penis includes the **urethra** and thus serves for both ejaculation and micturition. The internal (involuntary) and external (voluntary) urethral sphincters are widely separated. The **ureter,** having crossed the ductus deferens, enters the urinary bladder at its base. The peritoneum is reflected off of the posterior surface of the bladder and onto the rectum, thus forming the rectovesical pouch.

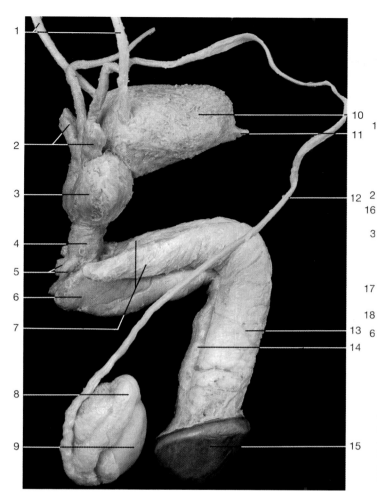

Male genital organs, isolated (right lateral aspect).

Male genital organs in situ (right lateral aspect).

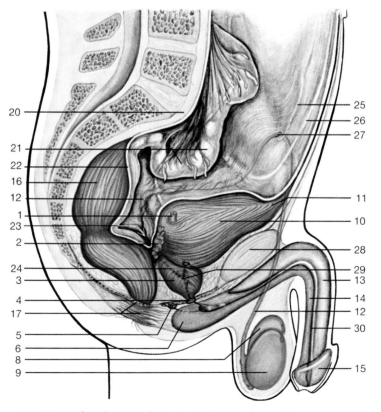

Positions of male genital organs (right lateral aspect).
(Schematic drawing.)

1 Ureter
2 Seminal vesicle
3 Prostate gland
4 Urogenital diaphragm and membranous part of urethra
5 Bulbo-urethral or Cowper's gland
6 Bulb of penis
7 Left and right crus penis
8 Epididymis
9 Testis
10 Urinary bladder
11 Apex of urinary bladder
12 Ductus deferens
13 Corpus cavernosum of penis
14 Corpus spongiosum of penis
15 Glans penis
16 Ampulla of rectum
17 Levator ani muscle
18 Anal canal and external anal sphincter muscle
19 Spermatic cord (cut)
20 Sacral promontory
21 Sigmoid colon
22 Peritoneum (cut edge)
23 Rectovesical pouch
24 Ejaculatory duct
25 Lateral umbilical fold
26 Medial umbilical fold
27 Deep inguinal ring and ductus deferens
28 Pubic symphysis
29 Prostatic part of urethra
30 Spongy urethra

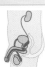

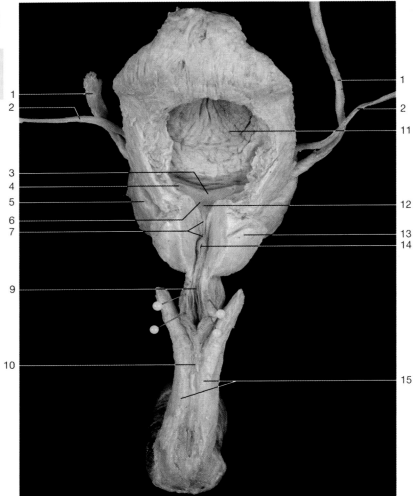

1 Ureter
2 Ductus deferens
3 Interureteric fold
4 Ureteric orifice
5 Seminal vesicle
6 Trigone of bladder
7 Prostatic urethra with seminal colliculus
   and urethral crest
8 Deep transverse perineal muscle
9 Membranous urethra
10 Spongy urethra
11 Mucous membrane of urinary bladder
12 Internal urethral orifice and uvula of bladder
13 Prostate
14 Prostatic utricle
15 Right and left corpus cavernosum of penis
16 Ejaculatory duct
17 Sphincter urethrae muscle
18 Median umbilical fold with remnant of urachus
19 Medial umbilical fold with remnant of
   umbilical artery
20 Urinary bladder
21 Rectovesical pouch
22 Rectum
23 Sacrum
24 Deep iliac circumflex artery
25 Deep inguinal ring and ductus deferens
26 External iliac artery and vein
27 Femoral nerve
28 Obturator nerve and internal iliac artery
29 Ilium and sacrum
30 Inferior epigastric artery
31 Iliopsoas muscle

Male urogenital organs, isolated (anterior aspect). Urinary bladder, prostate, and urethra have been opened. The urinary bladder is contracted.

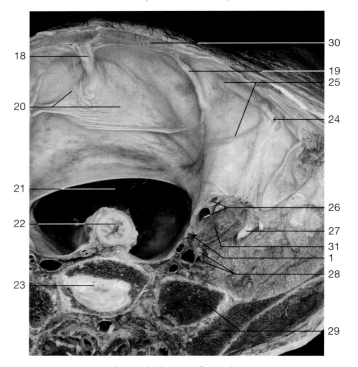

Pelvic cavity in the male (viewed from above).

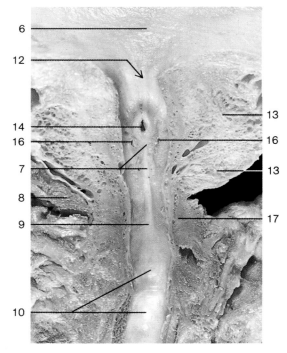

Posterior half of male urethra and prostate in continuity with neck of bladder (anterior aspect).

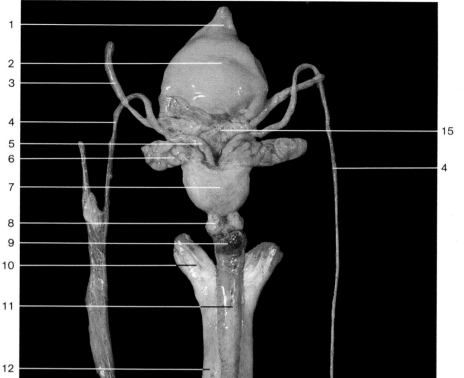

1   Apex of urinary bladder with urachus
2   Urinary bladder
3   Ureter
4   Ductus deferens
5   Ampulla of ductus deferens
6   Seminal vesicle
7   Prostate
8   Bulbo-urethral or Cowper's gland
9   Bulb of penis
10 Crus penis
11 Corpus spongiosum of penis
12 Corpus cavernosum of penis
13 Testis and epididymis with coverings
14 Glans penis
15 Fundus of bladder
16 Head of epididymis
17 Testis
18 Mucous membrane of bladder
19 Trigone of bladder
20 Ureteric orifice
21 Internal urethral orifice
22 Seminal colliculus
23 Prostate
24 Prostatic urethra
25 Membranous urethra
26 Spongy (penile) urethra
27 Skin of penis
28 Deep dorsal vein of penis (unpaired)
29 Dorsal artery of penis (paired)
30 Tunica albuginea of corpora cavernosa
31 Septum of penis
32 Deep artery of penis
33 Tunica albuginea of corpus spongiosum
34 Deep fascia of penis

Male genital organs, isolated (posterior aspect).

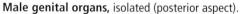

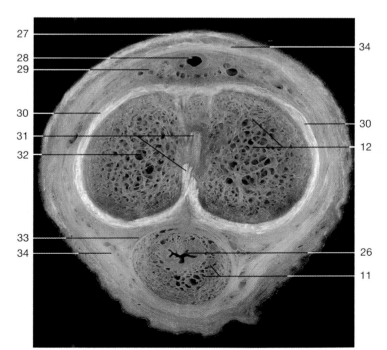

Urinary bladder, urethra, and penis (anterior aspect, opened longitudinally).

Cross section of penis (inferior aspect).

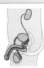

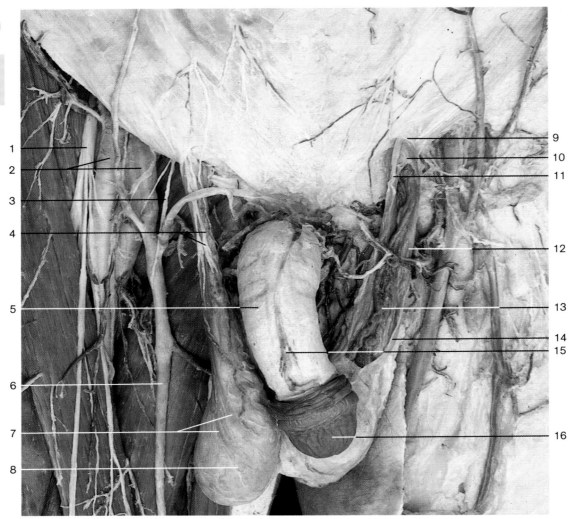

Male external genital organs with penis, testis, and spermatic cord, superficial layers (anterior aspect).

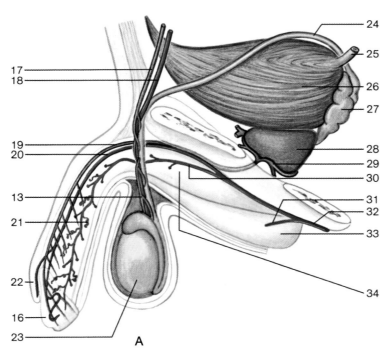

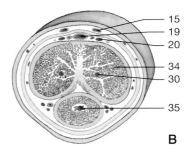

B

A

Vessels of male genital organs (schematic drawing).
A = lateral aspect; B = cross section of penis.

1 Femoral nerve
2 Femoral artery and vein
3 Femoral branch of genitofemoral nerve
4 Spermatic cord with genital branch of genitofemoral nerve
5 Penis with deep fascia
6 Great saphenous vein
7 Cremaster muscle
8 Testis with cremaster muscle
9 Superficial inguinal ring
10 Internal spermatic fascia (cut edge)
11 Ilio-inguinal nerve
12 Left spermatic cord
13 Pampiniform venous plexus
14 External spermatic fascia
15 Superficial dorsal vein of penis

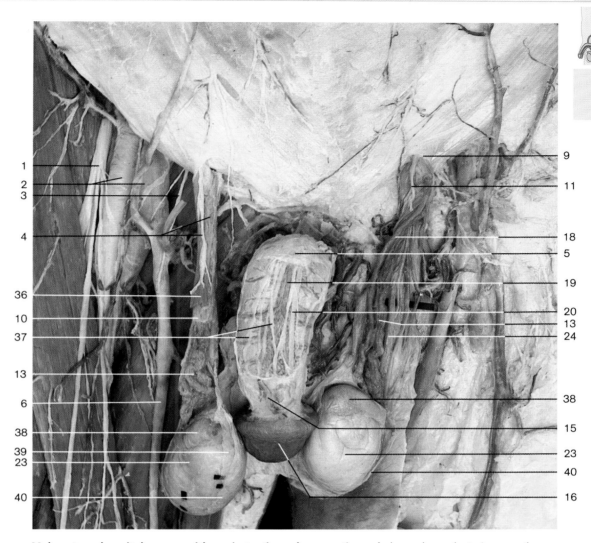

Male external genital organs with penis, testis, and spermatic cord, deeper layers (anterior aspect).
The deep fascia of the penis has been opened to display the dorsal nerves and vessels.

16 Glans penis
17 Testicular vein
18 Testicular artery
19 Deep dorsal vein of penis
20 Dorsal artery of penis
21 Helicine arteries
22 Prepuce
23 Testis with tunica albuginea
24 Ductus deferens
25 Ureter
26 Urinary bladder
27 Seminal vesicle
28 Prostate
29 Vesicoprostatic venous plexus
30 Deep artery of penis
31 Artery of bulb of penis
32 Internal pudendal artery
33 Corpus spongiosum of penis
34 Corpus cavernosum of penis
35 Urethra
36 Cremasteric fascia with cremaster muscle
37 Dorsal nerve of penis
38 Epididymis
39 Tunica vaginalis (visceral layer)
40 Tunica vaginalis (parietal layer)
41 Testis with vascular loops

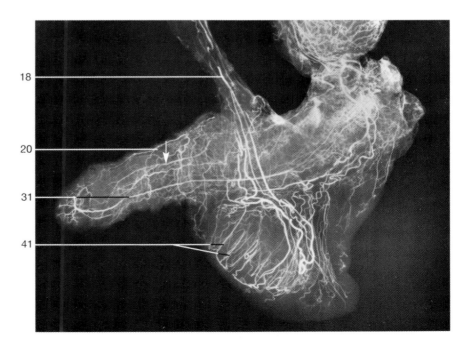

Male genital organs (arteriography, lateral aspect). Arrow = helicine artery.

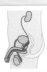

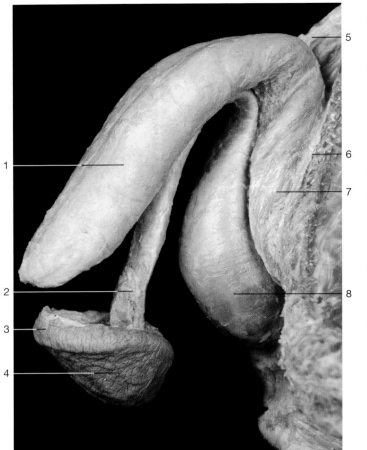

Male external genital organs (lateral aspect). The corpus spongiosum of the penis with the glans penis has been isolated and reflected.

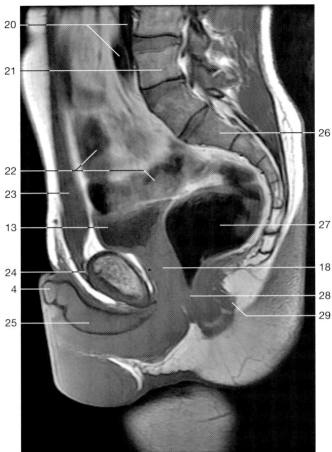

Sagittal section of the pelvic cavity with the male genital organs (MRI scan; from Heuck et al., MRT-Atlas, 2009).

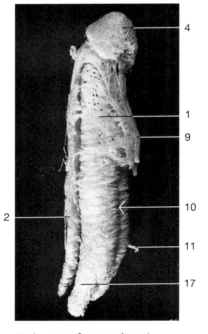

Resin cast of erected penis.

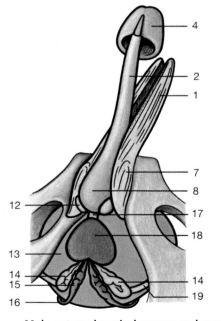

Male external genital organs and accessory glands (schematic drawing).

1   Corpus cavernosum of penis
2   Corpus spongiosum of penis
3   Corona of glans penis
4   Glans penis
5   Suspensory ligament of penis
6   Inferior pubic ramus
7   Crus penis
8   Bulb of penis
9   Deep dorsal vein of penis
10 Septum pectiniforme
11 Dorsal artery of penis
12 Bulbo-urethral or Cowper's gland
13 Urinary bladder
14 Seminal vesicle
15 Ampulla of ductus deferens
16 Ductus deferens
17 Membranous urethra
18 Prostate
19 Ureter
20 Common iliac artery and vein
21 Fifth lumbar vertebral body
22 Intestinal loops
23 Rectus abdominis muscle
24 Pubic symphysis
25 Root of penis
26 Sacral bone
27 Ampulla of rectum
28 Anal canal
29 External anal sphincter muscle

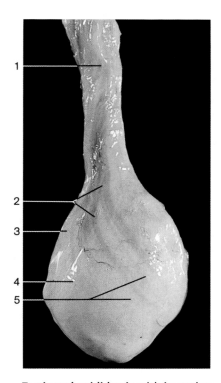

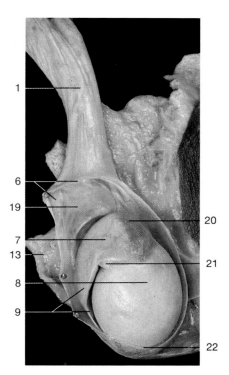

Testis and epididymis with investing layers (lateral aspect).

Testis and epididymis (lateral aspect). The tunica vaginalis has been opened.

Testis, epididymis, and spermatic cord (left side, posterolateral aspect). Dissection of spermatic cord and ductus deferens.

1 Spermatic cord covered with cremasteric fascia
2 Cremaster muscle
3 Position of epididymis
4 Internal spermatic fascia
5 Position of testis
6 Internal spermatic fascia with adjacent investing layers of testis (cut surface)
7 Head of epididymis

8 Testis with tunica vaginalis (visceral layer)
9 Body of epididymis
10 Pampiniform venous plexus (anterior veins)
11 Testicular artery
12 Tunica vaginalis (parietal layer, cut edge)
13 Skin and dartos muscle (reflected)
14 Ductus deferens

15 Artery of ductus deferens
16 Posterior veins of pampiniform plexus
17 Tail of epididymis
18 Transition of epididymal duct to ductus deferens and venous plexus
19 Parietal layer of tunica vaginalis
20 Appendix of epididymis
21 Appendix of testis
22 Gubernaculum testis

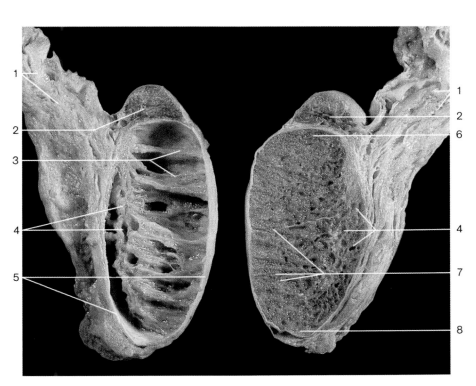

Longitudinal section through testis and epididymis. The left figure shows the testicular septa after removal of the seminiferous tubules.

1 Spermatic cord (cut surface)
2 Head of epididymis (cut surface)
3 Septa of testis
4 Mediastinum testis
5 Tunica albuginea
6 Superior pole of testis
7 Convoluted seminiferous tubules
8 Inferior pole of testis

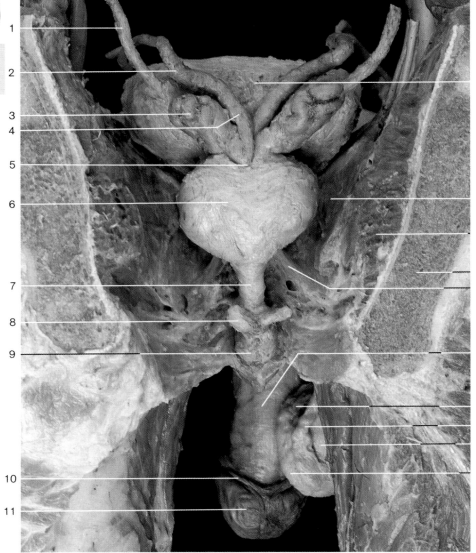

1	Ureter
2	Ductus deferens
3	Seminal vesicle
4	Ampulla of ductus deferens
5	Ejaculatory duct (proximal portion)
6	Prostate
7	Membranous urethra
8	Bulbo-urethral or Cowper's gland
9	Bulb of penis
10	Penis
11	Glans penis
12	Urinary bladder
13	Levator ani muscle
14	Obturator internus muscle
15	Pelvic bone (cut edge)
16	Puboprostatic ligament
17	Corpus spongiosum of penis
18	Head of epididymis
19	Beginning of ductus deferens
20	Testis
21	Tail of epididymis
22	Corpus cavernosum of penis
23	Spermatic cord
24	Pectineus and adductor muscles
25	Pubic bone
26	Prostatic part of urethra (seminal colliculus)
27	Rectum
28	Sciatic nerve
29	Great saphenous vein
30	Sartorius muscle
31	Femoral artery and vein
32	Rectus femoris muscle
33	Tensor fasciae latae muscle
34	Pectineus muscle
35	Iliopsoas muscle
36	Vastus lateralis muscle
37	Obturator externus muscle
38	Femur
39	Ischial tuberosity
40	Gluteus maximus muscle

Accessory glands of male genital organs in situ. Coronal section through the pelvic cavity. Posterior aspect of urinary bladder, prostate, and seminal vesicles.

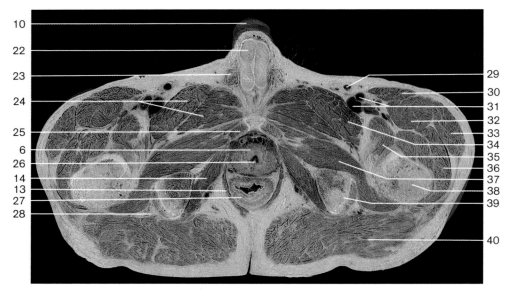

Horizontal section through pelvic cavity at the level of prostate.

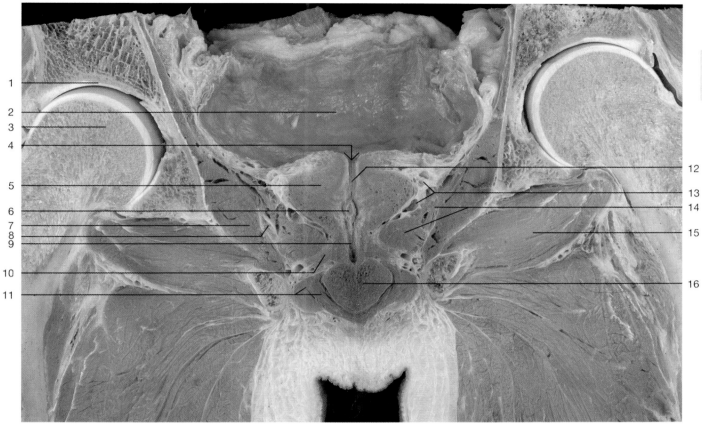

Coronal section through pelvic cavity at the level of prostate and hip joint (anterior aspect).

1	Acetabulum of hip joint	10	Deep transverse perineus muscle	19	Seminal vesicle
2	Urinary bladder	11	Crus penis and ischiocavernosus muscle	20	Internal anal sphincter muscle
3	Head of femur	12	Prostatic part of urethra	21	External anal sphincter muscle
4	Internal urethral orifice	13	Prostatic plexus	22	Anus
5	Prostate	14	Levator ani muscle	23	Psoas major muscle
6	Seminal colliculus	15	Obturator externus muscle	24	Intervertebral disc
7	Obturator internus muscle	16	Bulb of penis	25	Ilium
8	Ischiorectal fossa	17	Ampulla of rectum	26	Ligament of the head of the femur
9	Membranous urethra	18	Anal canal	27	Sacral promontory

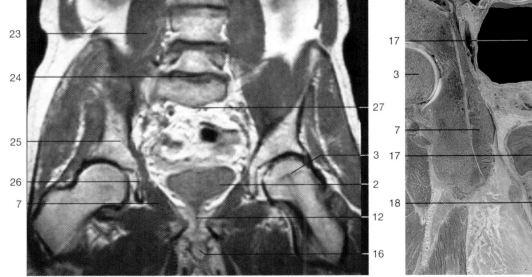

Coronal section through pelvic cavity (MRI scan).

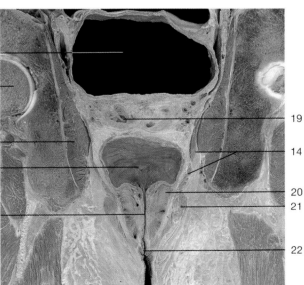

Coronal section through anal canal.

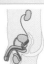

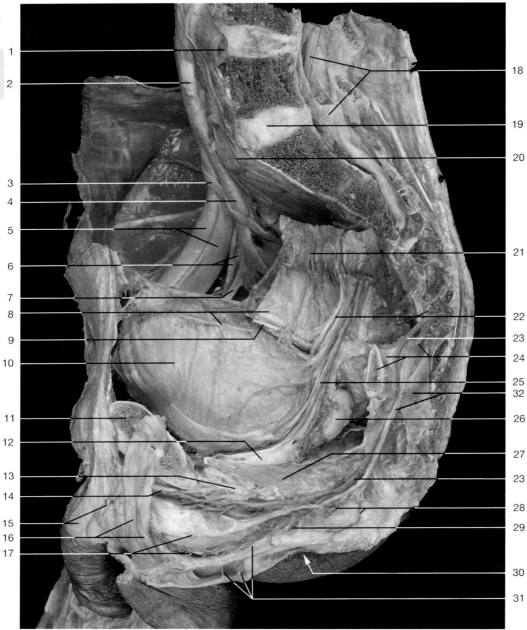

Pelvic cavity in the male (right half of parasagittal section). The arteries have been injected with red resin. The parietal layer of peritoneum has been removed. The urinary bladder is filled to a great extent.

1 Left common iliac artery
2 Right common iliac artery
3 Right ureter
4 Right internal iliac artery
5 Right external iliac artery and vein
6 Right obturator artery and nerve
7 Umbilical artery
8 Sigmoid and superior vesical artery
9 Left ductus deferens
10 Urinary bladder
11 Pubic bone (cut)
12 Prostate
13 Vesicoprostatic venous plexus
14 Deep dorsal vein of penis and
   dorsal artery of penis
15 Penis and superficial dorsal vein
16 Spermatic cord and testicular artery
17 Bulb of penis and deep artery of penis

18 Cauda equina and dura mater (divided)
19 Intervertebral disc between fifth
   lumbar vertebra and sacrum
20 Sacral promontory
21 Mesosigmoid
22 Left ureter
23 Left internal pudendal artery
24 Ischial spine (cut), sacrospinal ligament,
   inferior gluteal artery
25 Left inferior vesical artery
26 Seminal vesicle
27 Levator ani muscle
28 Branches of inferior rectal artery
29 Perineal artery
30 Anus
31 Posterior scrotal branches
32 Pudendal nerve and sacrotuberal ligament

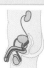

1   Internal iliac artery
2   External iliac artery
3   Ureter
4   Obturator nerve
5   Umbilical artery
6   Anulus inguinalis profundus
    (deep inguinal ring)
7   Urinary bladder (vesica urinaria)
8   Symphysis
9   Prostatic part of urethra
10 Sphincter muscle of urethra
11 Urethra (spongy part)
12 Cavernous body of penis
13 Glans penis
14 Sacrum
15 Promontory
16 Lateral sacral artery
17 Plexus sacralis
18 Inferior gluteal artery
19 Internal pudendal artery
20 Obturator artery
21 Inferior hypogastric plexus
22 Ductus deferens
23 Seminal vesicle (vesicula seminalis)
24 Rectum
25 Prostatic venous plexus
26 Prostate
27 Anal canal
28 Spongy part of penis
29 Pampiniform plexus
30 Testis and epididymis
31 Common iliac artery
32 Umbilical artery
33 Medial umbilical ligament
34 Branches of superior vesical artery
35 Urogenital diaphragm
36 Deep artery of penis
37 Dorsal artery of penis
38 Penis
39 Iliolumbar artery
40 Superior gluteal artery
41 Middle rectal artery
42 Levator ani muscle
43 Inferior rectal artery
44 Inferior vesical artery

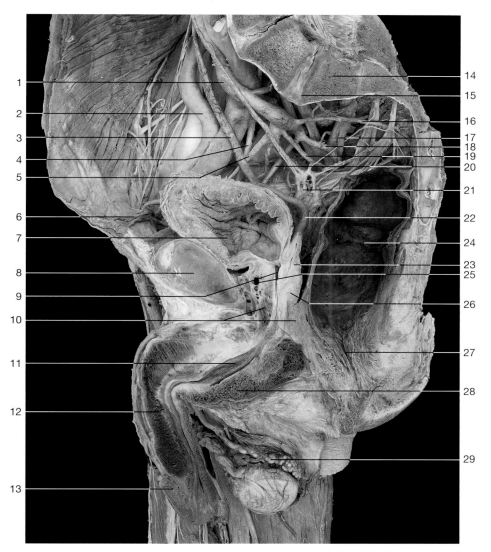

Vessels of the pelvic cavity in the male (medial aspect, midsagittal section). The gluteus maximus muscle has been removed.

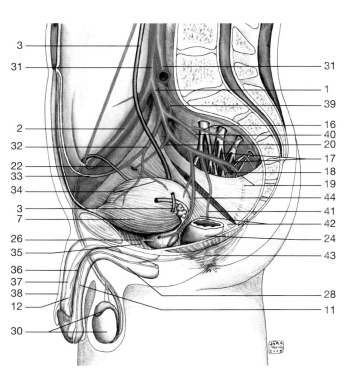

Main branches of internal iliac artery in the male (schematic drawing).

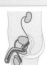

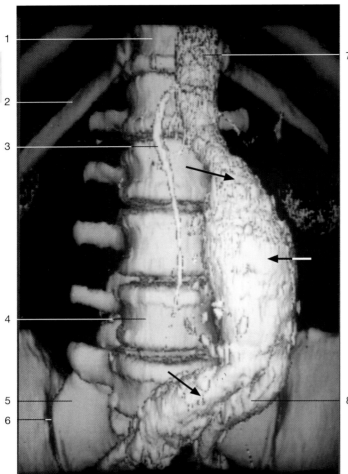

1   Twelfth thoracic vertebra (T_{12})
2   Twelfth rib (rib XII)
3   Inferior mesenteric artery
4   Fourth lumbar vertebra (L_4)
5   Sacrum
6   Sacro-iliac articulation
7   Aorta (abdominal part)
8   Left common iliac artery (included into the aneurysm)
9   Aorta with aneurysm
10   Body of lumbar vertebra
11   Intrinsic muscles of the back
12   Thrombotic part of the aneurysm (green)
13   Inferior vena cava (compressed, blue)
14   Iliopsoas muscle
15   Vertebral canal
16   Aneurysm of the aorta (red)

Abdominal part of the aorta showing an infrarenal aneurysm with involvement of both iliac arteries (arrows) (3-D reconstruction, courtesy of Prof. H. Rupprecht and Dr. M. Rexer, Klinikum Fürth, Germany).

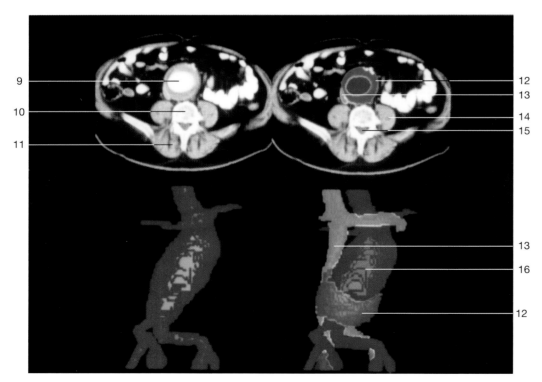

Abdominal part of the aorta with an aneurysm, after injection of contrast medium. Above = horizontal sections through the abdominal cavity, showing different contrast medium concentrations within the aorta and the aneurysm; below = 3-D reconstruction of the aneurysm; red = aorta; green = thrombotic areas; blue = vein (vena cava inferior, partly compressed).

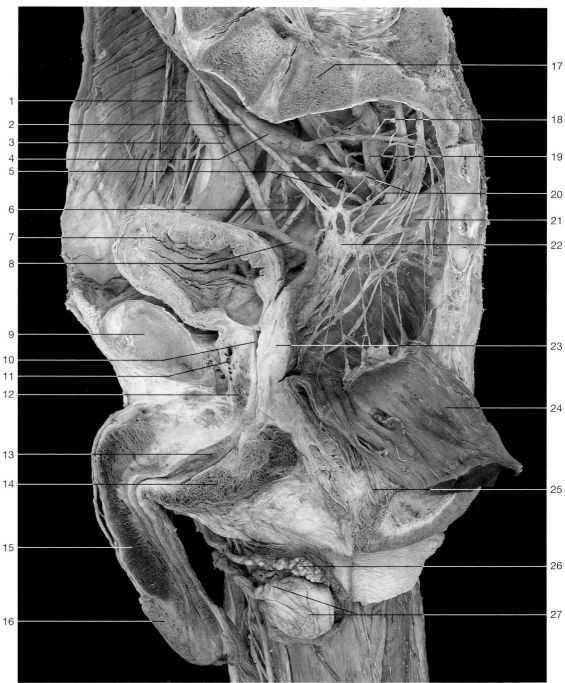

Vessels and nerves of the pelvic cavity in the male (medial aspect, midsagittal section). Rectum reflected to display the inferior hypogastric plexus.

1 External iliac artery	10 Prostatic part of urethra	20 Pelvic splanchnic nerves (nervi erigentes)
2 Right hypogastric nerve	11 Prostatic venous plexus	21 Levator ani muscle
3 Ureter	12 Sphincter urethrae muscle	22 Inferior hypogastric plexus
4 Internal iliac artery	13 Spongy part of urethra	(pelvic plexus)
5 Inferior gluteal artery and internal	14 Corpus spongiosum penis	23 Prostate
pudendal artery	15 Corpus cavernosum penis	24 Rectum (reflected)
6 Obturator artery	16 Glans penis	25 Anal canal and external anal sphincter
7 Urinary bladder	17 Sacrum	26 Pampiniform plexus continuous with
8 Ductus deferens	18 Lateral sacral artery	testicular vein
9 Symphysis pubica	19 Sacral plexus	27 Testis and epididymis

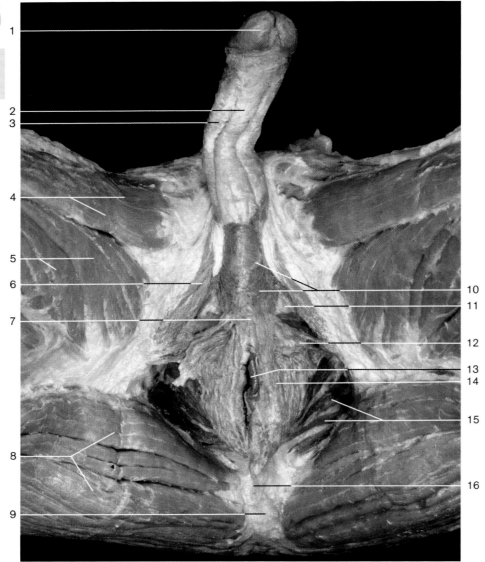

1 Glans penis
2 Corpus spongiosum of penis
3 Corpus cavernosum of penis
4 Gracilis muscle
5 Adductor muscles
6 Ischiocavernosus muscle overlying crus of penis
7 Perineal body
8 Gluteus maximus muscle
9 Coccyx
10 Bulbospongiosus muscle
11 Deep transverse perineus muscle covered by inferior fascia of urogenital diaphragm
12 Superficial transverse perineus muscle
13 Anus
14 External anal sphincter muscle
15 Levator ani muscle
16 Anococcygeal ligament
17 Obturator internus muscle
18 Urethra
19 Deep transverse perineus muscle

Muscles of urogenital and pelvic diaphragms in the male (from below).

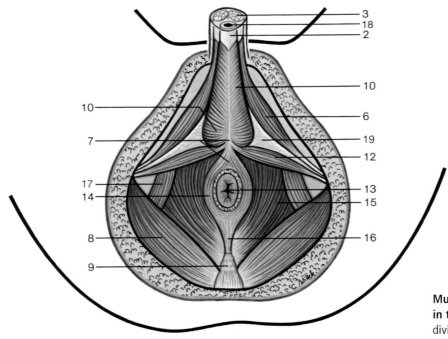

Muscles of urogenital and pelvic diaphragms in the male (from below). The penis has been divided (schematic drawing).

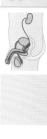

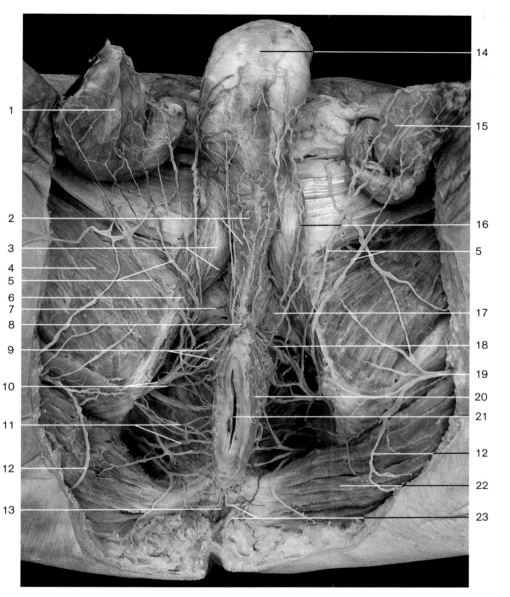

1   Right testis (reflected laterally and upward)
2   Bulbospongiosus muscle
3   Ischiocavernosus muscle
4   Adductor magnus muscle
5   Posterior scrotal nerves and superficial perineal arteries
6   Posterior scrotal artery and vein
7   Right artery of bulb of penis
8   Perineal body
9   Perineal branches of pudendal nerve
10 Pudendal nerve and internal pudendal artery
11 Inferior rectal arteries and nerves
12 Inferior cluneal nerve
13 Coccyx (location)
14 Penis
15 Left testis (reflected laterally)
16 Left posterior scrotal artery
17 Deep transverse perineal muscle
18 Left artery of bulb of penis
19 Posterior femoral cutaneous nerve
20 External anal sphincter muscle
21 Anus
22 Gluteus maximus muscle
23 Anococcygeal nerves
24 Acetabulum (femur removed)
25 Ligament of femoral head
26 Body of ischium (cut)
27 Sciatic nerve
28 Coccygeus muscle
29 Levator ani muscle
    a iliococcygeus muscle
    b pubococcygeus muscle
    c puborectalis muscle
30 Prostatic venous plexus
31 Body of pubis
32 Testis

Urogenital diaphragm and external genital organs in the male with vessels and nerves (from below). The testes have been reflected laterally.

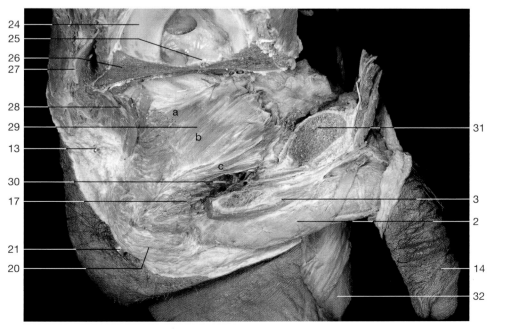

Pelvic diaphragm and external genital organs in the male. The right half of the pelvis including the obturator internus muscle and femur have been removed to display the right half of the levator ani muscle.

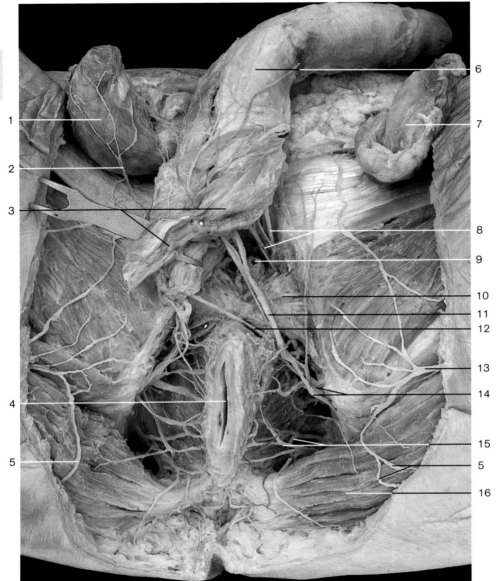

1 Right testis (reflected)
2 Posterior scrotal nerves
3 Left crus penis with
   ischiocavernosus muscle
4 Anus
5 Inferior cluneal nerves
6 Penis
7 Left testis (reflected)
8 Dorsal artery and nerve of
   penis
9 Urethra
10 Deep transverse perineus
   muscle
11 Perineal branch of pudendal
   nerve
12 Artery of bulb of penis
   (reflected)
13 Branch of posterior femoral
   cutaneous nerve
14 Internal pudendal artery and
   pudendal nerve
15 Inferior rectal arteries and
   nerves
16 Gluteus maximus muscle
17 Dorsal nerve of penis
18 Posterior femoral cutaneous
   nerve
19 Perineal branches of pudendal
   nerve
20 Inferior rectal nerves
21 Bulbospongiosus muscle
   (inside: dorsal artery of penis)
22 Perineal artery
23 External anal sphincter muscle
24 Inferior rectal artery and veins

Urogenital diaphragm and external genital organs in the male (from below). The left crus penis has been isolated and reflected laterally together with the bulb of the penis. The urethra has been cut.

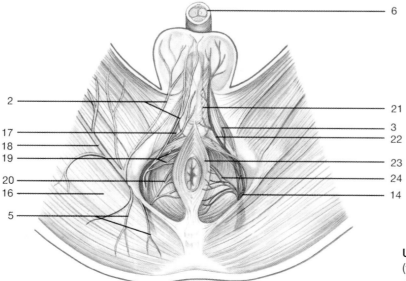

Urogenital and anal region in the male (from below). Right side: nerves; left side: arteries and veins.

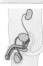

1 Right testis (reflected)
2 Corpus spongiosum of penis
3 Corpus cavernosum of penis
4 Perineal branch of posterior femoral cutaneous nerve
5 Posterior scrotal arteries and nerves
6 Deep artery of penis
7 Deep transverse perineal muscle
8 Right perineal nerves
9 Inferior rectal nerves
10 Inferior cluneal nerve
11 Anococcygeal nerves
12 Left spermatic cord
13 Left testis (cut surface)
14 Dorsal artery and nerve of penis
15 Deep dorsal vein of penis
16 Urethra (cut)
17 Artery of bulb of penis
18 Superficial transverse perineus muscle
19 Left artery of bulb of penis
20 Perineal branch of pudendal nerve
21 Anus
22 External anal sphincter muscle
23 Gluteus maximus muscle
24 Internal pudendal artery and pudendal nerve
25 Sacrotuberous ligament
26 Coccyx
27 Urogenital diaphragm (deep transverse perineus muscle)
28 Tendinous center of perineum (perineal body)
29 Levator ani muscle
30 Anococcygeal ligament
31 Obturator internus muscle
32 Dorsal artery of penis

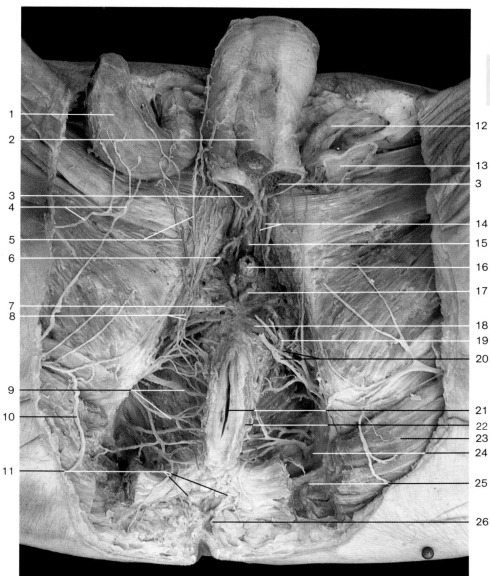

Urogenital diaphragm and external genital organs in the male (from below). The root of the penis has been cut. Dissection of the urogenital diaphragm.

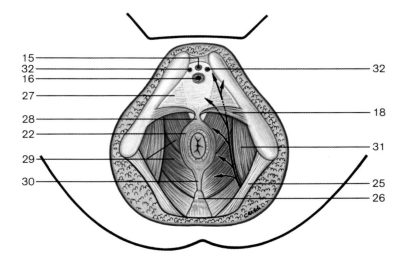

Urogenital and pelvic diaphragms in the male (from below). The penis has been removed. The arrows indicate the course of vessels and nerves (schematic drawing).

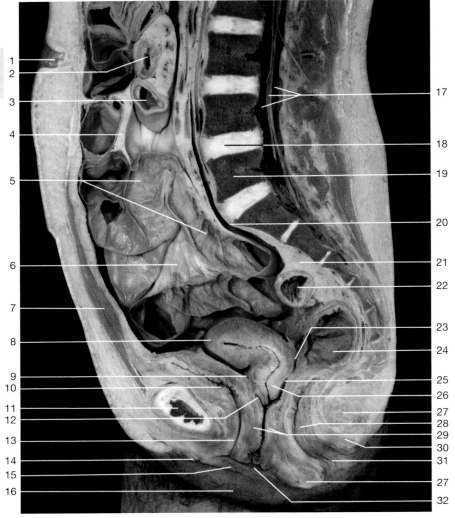

1   Umbilicus
2   Duodenum
3   Ascending part of duodenum
4   Root of mesentery
5   Small intestine
6   Mesentery
7   Rectus abdominis muscle
8   Uterus
9   Vesico-uterine pouch
10 Urinary bladder (collapsed)
11 Pubic symphysis
12 Anterior fornix of vagina
13 Urethra
14 Clitoris
15 Labium minus
16 Labium majus
17 Vertebral canal with cauda equina
18 Intervertebral disc
19 Body of fifth lumbar vertebra
20 Sacral promontory
21 Mesosigmoid
22 Sigmoid colon
23 Recto-uterine pouch
    (of Douglas)
24 Ampulla of rectum
25 Posterior fornix of vagina
26 Cervix of uterus
27 External anal sphincter muscle
28 Anal canal
29 Vagina
30 Internal anal sphincter muscle
31 Anus
32 Hymen
33 Left ureter
34 Peritoneum (cut edge)
35 Right ureter (divided)
36 Median umbilical fold
    with urachus
37 Infundibulum of uterine tube
38 Fimbriae of uterine tube
39 Ovary
40 Uterine tube (isthmus)
41 Round ligament of uterus

Female urogenital system, midsagittal section through the trunk. The urinary bladder is empty, position and shape of the uterus are normal.

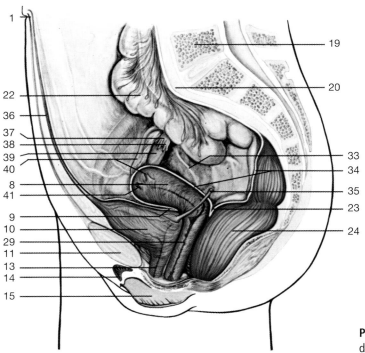

Positions of female genital organs (medial aspect, schematic drawing).

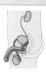

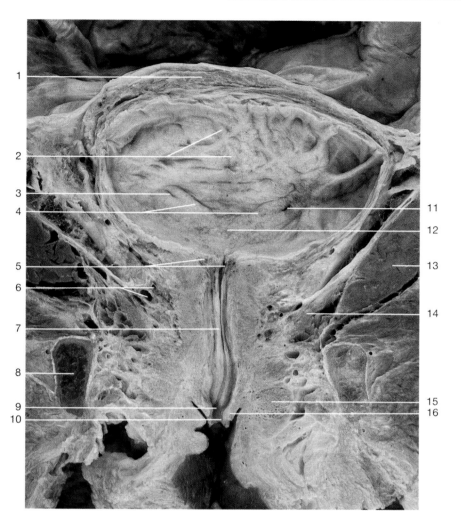

1   Muscular coat of urinary bladder
2   Folds of mucous membrane of urinary
    bladder
3   Right ureteric orifice
4   Interureteric fold
5   Internal urethral orifice
6   Vesico-uterine venous plexus
7   Urethra
8   Pubic bone (cut edge)
9   External urethral orifice
10 Vestibule of vagina
11 Left ureteric orifice
12 Trigone of bladder
13 Obturator internus muscle
14 Levator ani muscle
15 Bulb of the vestibule
16 Left labium minus
17 Psoas major muscle
18 Ampulla of rectum
19 Uterus
20 Urinary bladder
21 Promontory
22 Sigmoid colon
23 Uterine tube
24 Head of femur
25 Vagina

Coronal section through the female urinary bladder and urethra (anterior aspect).

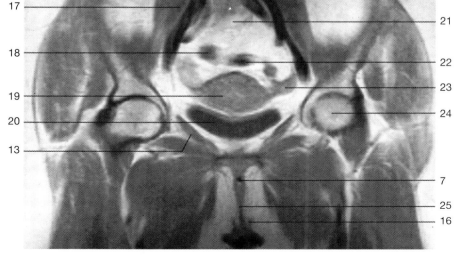

Coronal section through the pelvic cavity of the female (MRI scan).

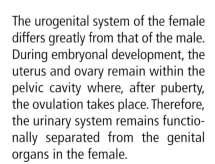

The urogenital system of the female differs greatly from that of the male. During embryonal development, the uterus and ovary remain within the pelvic cavity where, after puberty, the ovulation takes place. Therefore, the urinary system remains functionally separated from the genital organs in the female.

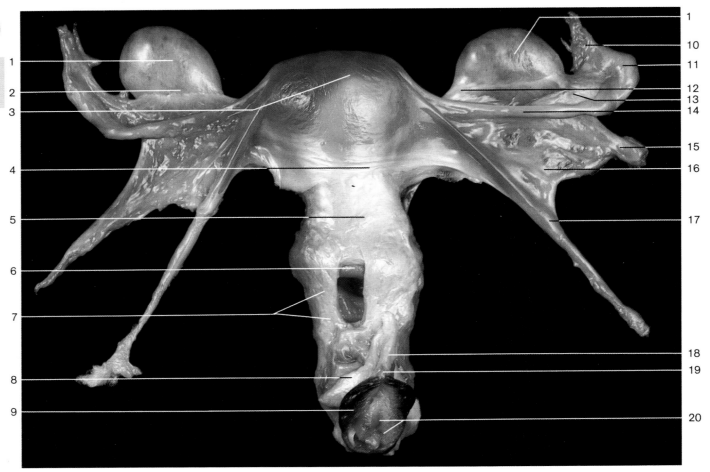

Female genital organs, isolated (anterior aspect). The anterior wall of the vagina has been opened to display the vaginal portion of the cervix.

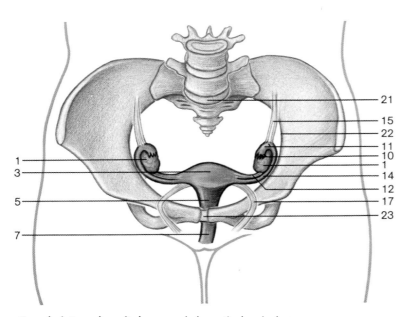

Female internal genital organs (schematic drawing).

1	Ovary
2	Mesovarium
3	Fundus of uterus
4	Vesico-uterine pouch
5	Cervix of uterus
6	Vaginal portion of cervix
7	Vagina
8	Crus of clitoris
9	Labium minus
10	Fimbriae of uterine tube
11	Infundibulum of uterine tube
12	Ligament of the ovary
13	Mesosalpinx
14	Uterine tube
15	Suspensory ligament of ovary (caudally displaced)
16	Broad ligament of uterus
17	Round ligament of uterus
18	Corpus cavernosum of clitoris
19	Glans of clitoris
20	Hymen, vaginal orifice
21	Promontory
22	Linea terminalis of pelvis
23	Pubic symphysis

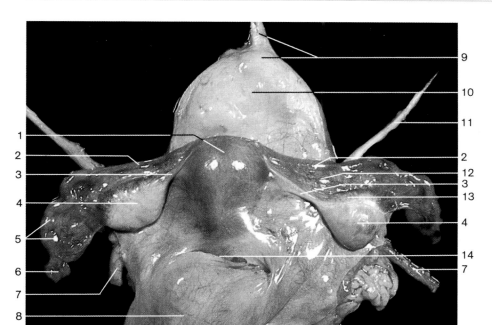

1 Fundus of uterus
2 Uterine tube
3 Ligament of the ovary
4 Ovary
5 Infundibulum of uterine tube
6 Fimbriae of uterine tube
7 Ureter
8 Rectum
9 Apex of urinary bladder and
  median umbilical ligament
10 Urinary bladder
11 Round ligament of uterus
12 Mesosalpinx
13 Mesovarium
14 Recto-uterine pouch (of Douglas)
15 Suspensory ligament of ovary
16 Scarring of ovary (following
  ovulation)
17 Abdominal opening of uterine
  tube
18 Body of uterus
19 Cervical canal
20 Vaginal portion of cervix of uterus
  (congestion)
21 Vagina
22 Mucous membrane of uterus
23 Anterior fornix of vagina

Female genital organs, isolated (supero-posterior aspect).

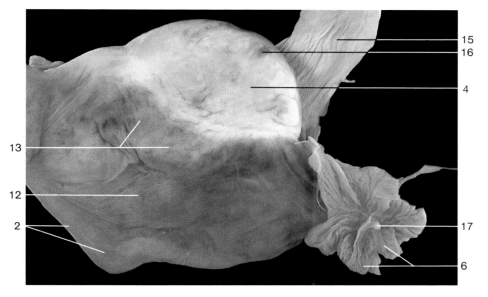

Right ovary and uterine tube, isolated (supero-posterior aspect). The fimbriae of the
uterine tube have been reflected to show the abdominal ostium.

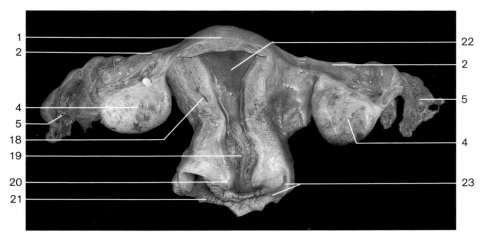

Uterus and related organs (posterior aspect). The posterior wall of the uterus has been
opened.

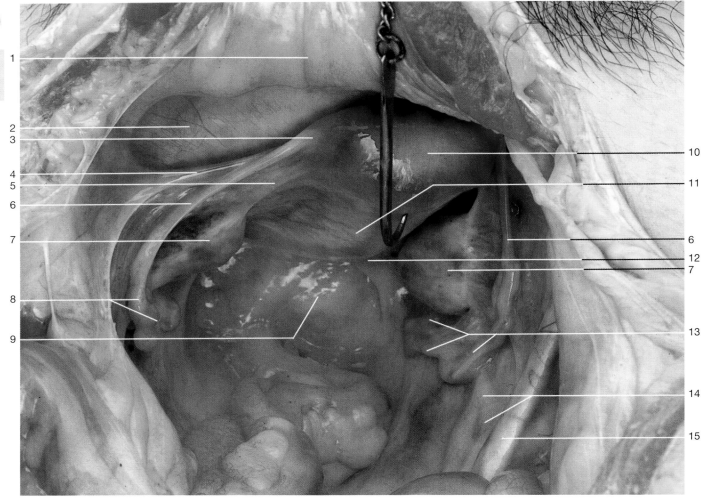

1
2
3
4
5
6
7
8
9
10
11
6
12
7
13
14
15

Female internal genital organs. Pelvic cavity (seen from above). The uterus has been reflected to the right.

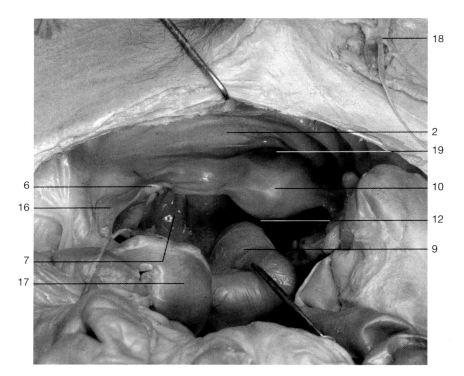

18
2
19
6
10
16
12
7
9
17

1 Median umbilical fold with urachus
2 Urinary bladder
3 Insertion of uterine tube
   at fundus of uterus
4 Round ligament of uterus
5 Ligament of ovary
6 Uterine tube (isthmus)
7 Ovary
8 Ampulla of uterine tube
9 Rectum
10 Uterus
11 Vagina
12 Recto-uterine pouch
   (of Douglas)
13 Fimbriae of uterine tube
14 Suspensory ligament of ovary
15 Right common iliac artery
   (covered by peritoneum)
16 Mesosalpinx
17 Sigmoid colon
18 Saphenous opening
19 Vesico-uterine pouch

Female internal genital organs. Pelvic cavity (seen from above).

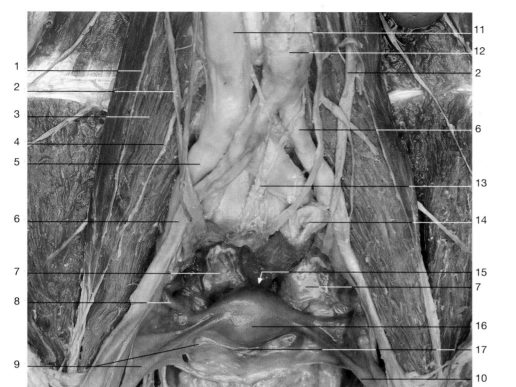

1 Ilio-inguinal nerve
2 Ureter
3 Psoas major muscle
4 Genitofemoral nerve
5 Common iliac vein
6 Common iliac artery
7 Ovary
8 Uterine tube
9 Peritoneum
10 Round ligament of uterus
11 Inferior vena cava
12 Abdominal aorta
13 Superior hypogastric plexus
14 Rectum
15 Recto-uterine pouch
    (of Douglas)
16 Uterus
17 Vesico-uterine pouch
18 Urinary bladder
19 Iliac crest
20 Pubic symphysis
21 Placenta
22 Amnion and chorion
23 Adnexa of uterus
    (uterine tube and ovaries)
24 Myometrium
25 Internal orifice of uterus
26 Cervix of uterus
27 Umbilical cord

**View of the female pelvis
showing uterus and related
organs** (superior aspect).

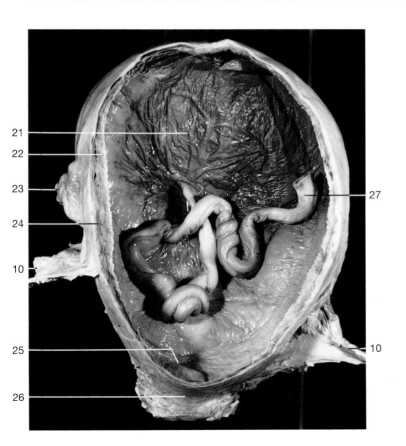

Fullterm uterus with placenta (anterior aspect).
The anterior wall of the uterus has been removed to
show the location of the placenta.

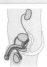

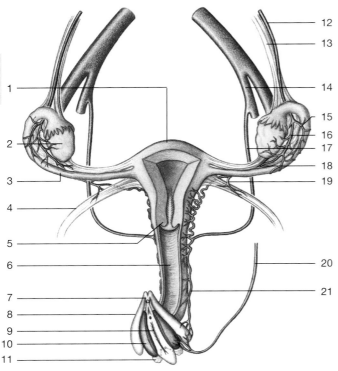

Arteries of female genital organs (schematic drawing).

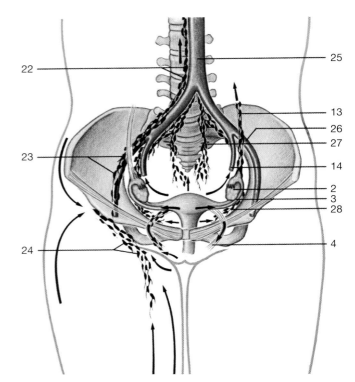

Main drainage routes of lymph vessels of uterus and its adnexa (indicated by arrows). (Schematic drawing.) Red = arteries; black = lymph vessels and nodes.

1 Uterus	10 Bulb of vestibule	19 Artery of round ligament	28 Internal iliac lymph nodes
2 Ovary	11 Greater vestibular gland	20 Internal pudendal artery	29 Superior gluteal artery
3 Uterine tube	12 Ovarian artery	21 Vaginal artery	30 Obturator artery
4 Round ligament of uterus	13 Suspensory ligament of ovary	22 Lumbar lymph nodes	31 Inferior gluteal artery
5 Vaginal portion of cervix of uterus	14 Internal iliac artery	23 External iliac lymph nodes	32 Middle sacral artery
6 Vagina	15 Tubal branch of ovarian artery	24 Inguinal lymph nodes	33 Femoral artery
7 Clitoris	16 Ovarian branch of ovarian artery	25 Abdominal aorta	34 Vessels of labium majus
8 Corpus cavernosum of clitoris	17 Uterine artery	26 External iliac artery	35 Femur
9 Vaginal orifice	18 Ovarian branch of uterine artery	27 Sacral lymph nodes	

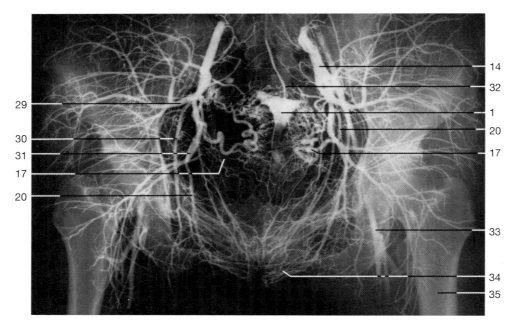

Pelvic vessels in the female (arteriography, antero-posterior view).

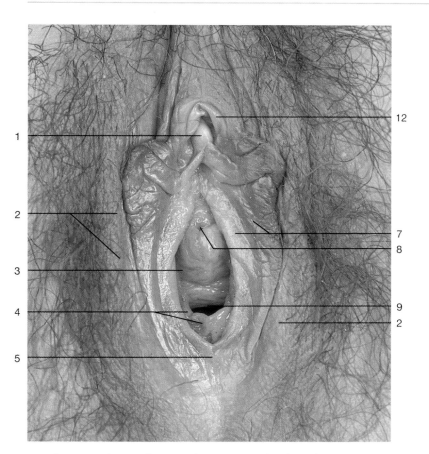

1 Glans of clitoris
2 Labium majus
3 Vestibule of vagina
4 Hymen
5 Posterior labial commissure
6 Body of clitoris
7 Labium minus
8 External orifice of urethra
9 Vaginal orifice
10 Ureter
11 Adnexa of uterus
12 Prepuce of clitoris
13 Crus of clitoris
14 Greater vestibular glands
15 Anus and internal anal sphincter muscle
16 Median umbilical ligament containing urachus
17 Urinary bladder
18 Infundibulum of uterine tube
19 Ovary
20 Ampulla of uterine tube
21 Suspensory ligament of the ovary
22 Bulbospongiosus muscle and bulb of vestibule
23 Central tendon of perineum (perineal body)
24 External anal sphincter muscle

Female external genital organs (anterior aspect). Labia reflected.

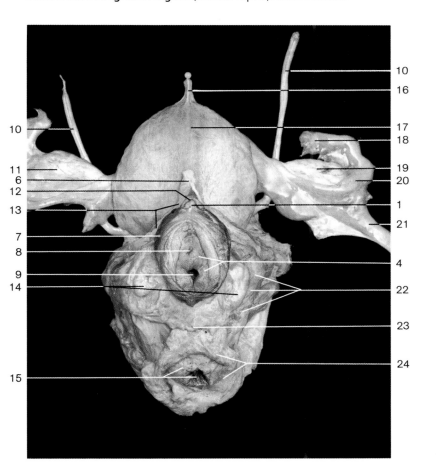

Female external genital organs in relation to internal genital organs and urinary system, isolated (anterior aspect).

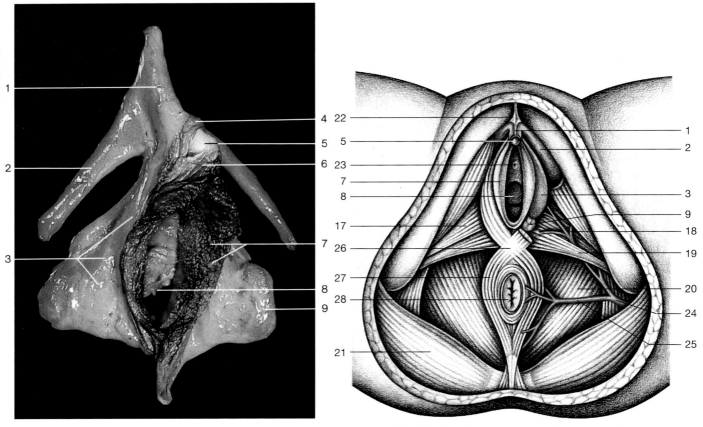

Cavernous tissue of female external genital organs, isolated (anterior aspect).

Urogenital and pelvic diaphragms (anterior aspect, schematic drawing). Blue = cavernous tissue of clitoris and bulb of vestibule.

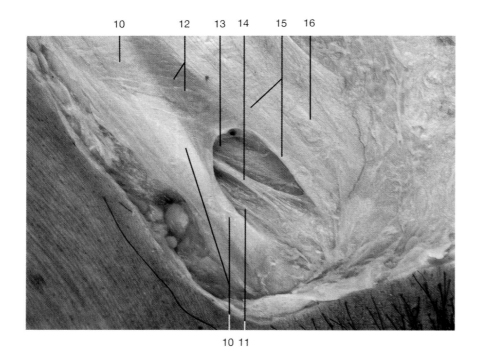

Inguinal canal and round ligament of uterus in situ (right side, ventral aspect).

1   Body of clitoris
2   Crus of clitoris
3   Bulb of vestibule
4   Prepuce of clitoris
5   Glans of clitoris
6   Frenulum of clitoris
7   Labium minus
8   Vaginal orifice
9   Greater vestibular gland
10 Lateral crus of superficial inguinal ring
11 Ilio-inguinal nerve
12 Intercrural fibers
13 Superficial inguinal ring
14 Round ligament of uterus
15 Medial crus of superficial inguinal ring
16 Aponeurosis of external abdominal
    oblique muscle
17 Deep transverse perineal muscle with
    fascia
18 Deep artery of clitoris
19 Superficial transverse perineus muscle
20 Levator ani muscle
21 Gluteus maximus muscle
22 Suspensory ligament of clitoris
23 External orifice of urethra
24 Internal pudendal artery
25 Inferior rectal artery
26 Perineal body
27 External anal sphincter muscle
28 Anus

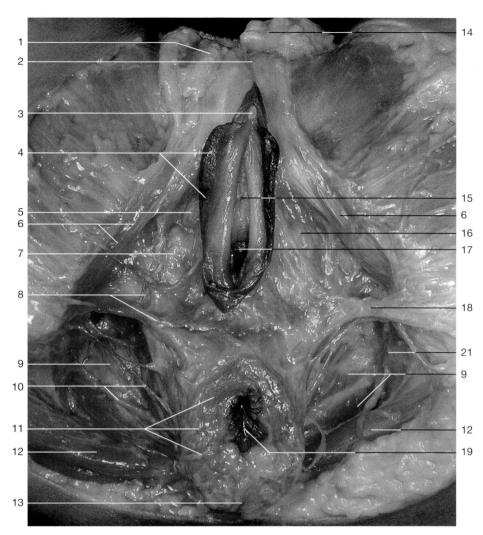

Urogenital diaphragm and external genital organs in the female, superficial layer (from below).

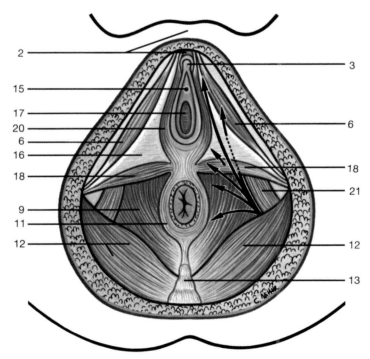

Muscles of pelvic and urogenital diaphragms in the female (from below, schematic drawing).

1   Fatty tissue encasing round ligament
2   Position of pubic symphysis
3   Clitoris
4   Labium minus
5   Bulb of vestibule
6   Ischiocavernosus muscle
7   Greater vestibular gland
8   Perineal branches of pudendal nerve
9   Levator ani muscle
10   Inferior rectal nerves
11   External anal sphincter muscle
12   Gluteus maximus muscle
13   Coccyx
14   Fatty tissue of mons pubis
15   External orifice of urethra
16   Urogenital diaphragm with fascia of deep transverse perineus muscle
17   Vaginal orifice
18   Superficial transverse perineal muscle
19   Anus
20   Bulbospongiosus muscle
21   Obturator internus muscle

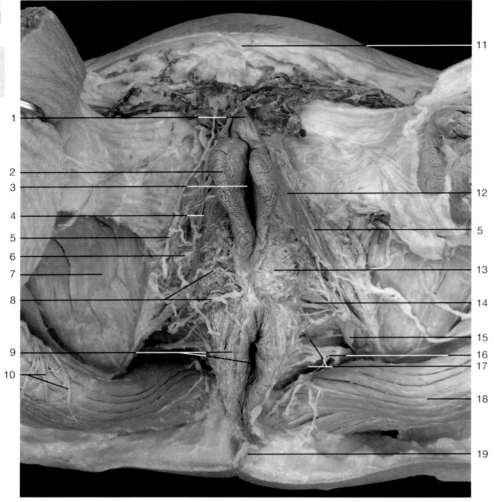

Urogenital diaphragm and external genital organs in the female, superficial layer (from below). On the right side the bulb of vestibule has been removed.

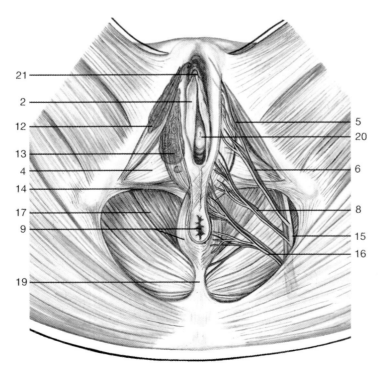

External female genital organs. Position of arteries and nerves; bulb of vestibule in blue (schematic drawing).

1 Prepuce of clitoris
2 Labium minus
3 Vaginal orifice
4 Deep transverse perineus muscle
5 Dorsal nerve of clitoris
6 Posterior labial nerves
7 Great adductor muscle
8 Perineal branches of pudendal nerve
9 Anus and external anal sphincter muscle
10 Inferior cluneal nerves
11 Mons pubis
12 Crus of clitoris with ischiocavernosus muscle
13 Bulb of vestibule
14 Superficial transverse perineus muscle
15 Pudendal nerve and internal pudendal artery
16 Inferior rectal nerves
17 Levator ani muscle
18 Gluteus maximus muscle
19 Anococcygeal ligament
20 External urethral orifice
21 Glans of clitoris

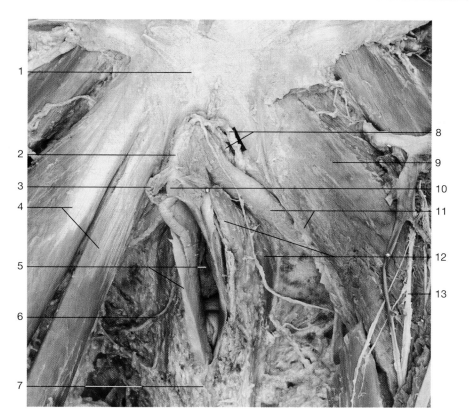

1 Position of pubic symphysis
2 Body of clitoris
3 Prepuce of clitoris
4 Adductor longus and gracilis muscles
5 External orifice of vagina and labium minus
6 Posterior labial nerve
7 Perineal body
8 Deep artery of clitoris and dorsal nerve of clitoris
9 Adductor brevis muscle
10 Glans of clitoris
11 Crus of clitoris and ischiocavernosus muscle
12 Bulb of vestibule and bulbospongiosus muscle
13 Anterior branch of obturator nerve
14 Labium minus
15 Vaginal orifice
16 Posterior labial nerves
17 Branches of pudendal nerve
18 External sphincter of anus
19 Anus
20 Bulb of vestibule (divided)
21 Dorsal artery of clitoris
22 Superficial transverse perineus muscle
23 Perineal branch of posterior femoral cutaneous nerve
24 Levator ani muscle
25 Pudendal nerve and internal pudendal artery
26 Inferior rectal nerves
27 Gluteus maximus muscle
28 Anococcygeal ligament

External genital organs in the female (inferior aspect). The clitoris has been dissected and slightly reflected to the right. The prepuce of clitoris has been divided to display the glans.

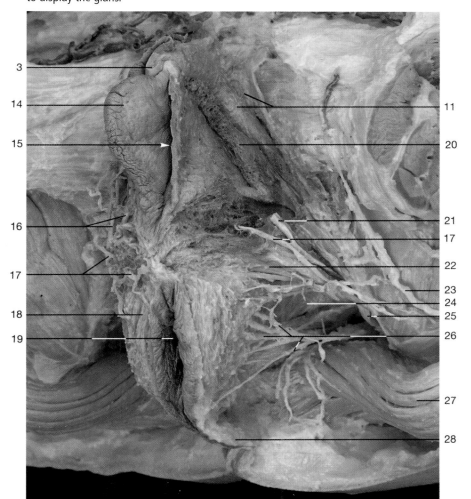

Urogenital diaphragm and external genital organs in the female (latero-inferior aspect). The bulb of vestibule has partly been removed; the left labium minus was cut away.

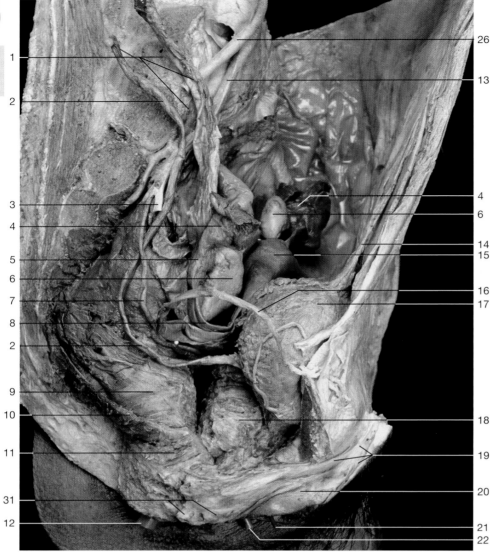

1   Body of fifth lumbar vertebra,
    suspensory ligament of ovary,
    and sacral promontory
2   Ureter
3   Medial umbilical ligament
    (remnant of umbilical artery)
    (cut)
4   Infundibulum of uterine tube
5   Ampulla of uterine tube
6   Ovary
7   Uterine artery
8   Uterine tube
9   Rectum
10 Levator ani muscle
    (pelvic diaphragm – cut edge)
11 External anal sphincter muscle
12 Anus (probe)
13 Internal iliac artery
14 Remnant of urachus
    (median umbilical ligament)
15 Uterus
16 Round ligament of uterus
17 Urinary bladder
18 Vagina
19 Clitoris
20 Labium minus
21 External orifice of urethra
    (red probe)
22 Vaginal orifice (green probe)
23 Lateral umbilical ligament
24 Inferior epigastric artery
25 Obturator artery, vein, and nerve
26 External iliac artery
27 Recto-uterine pouch (of Douglas)
28 Recto-uterine fold
29 Vesico-uterine pouch
30 Suspensory ligament of ovary
31 Greater vestibular gland and bulb
    of the vestibule

Pelvic cavity in the female, internal genital organs in situ (lateral aspect). Right half of the pelvis and sacrum have been removed.

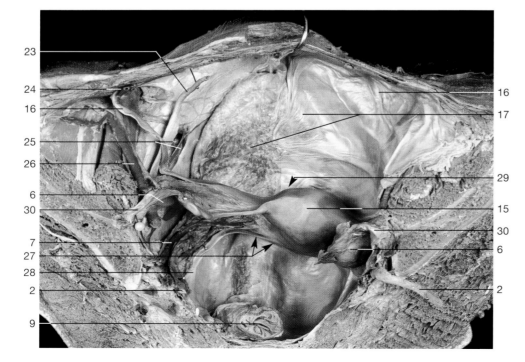

Pelvic cavity in the female, internal genital organs in situ (seen from above). The peritoneum at the left half of pelvic cavity has been removed to display uterine tube, vessels, and nerves.

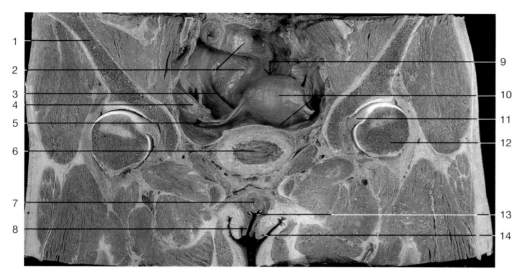

Coronal section through the pelvic cavity of the female (cf. MRI scan on p. 355).

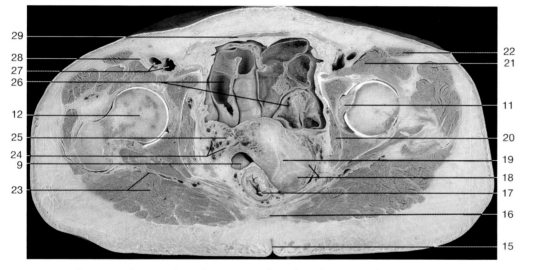

Horizontal section through the pelvic cavity of the female at level of uterus (from below). The uterus is retroverted to the left.

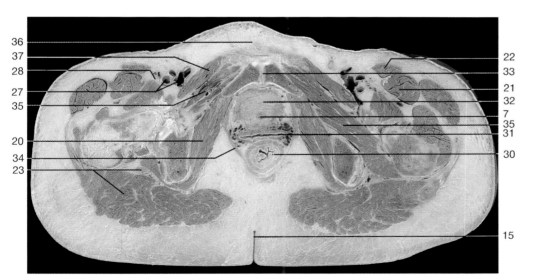

Horizontal section through the pelvic cavity of the female at level of the urethral sphincter and vagina (from below).

1　Ilium
2　Rectum
3　Recto-uterine fold
4　Ovary
5　Uterine tube
6　Urinary bladder
7　Urethra
8　Labium minus
9　Recto-uterine pouch of Douglas
10　Uterus (uterovesical pouch)
11　Ligament of the head of the femur
12　Head of femur
13　Vestibule of vagina
14　Labium majus
15　Anal cleft
16　Coccyx
17　Rectum
18　Myometrium of uterus
19　Uterine cavity
20　Obturator internus muscle
21　Iliopsoas muscle
22　Sartorius muscle
23　Sciatic nerve and gluteus maximus muscle
24　Uterine venous plexus
25　Broad ligament
26　Small intestine
27　Femoral artery and vein
28　Femoral nerve
29　Pyramidalis muscle
30　Rectum (anal canal)
31　Vagina
32　Urethral sphincter muscle (base of urinary bladder)
33　Pubic symphysis
34　Levator ani muscle
35　Obturator externus muscle
36　Mons pubis
37　Pectineus muscle

7 Upper Limb

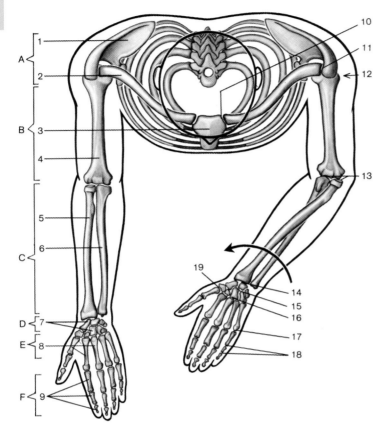

A = Shoulder girdle
B = Arm
C = Forearm
D = Wrist
E = Palm of hand
F = Finger

Bones
1 Scapula
2 Clavicle
3 Sternum
4 Humerus
5 Radius
6 Ulna
7 Carpal bones
8 Metacarpal bones
9 Phalanges

Joints
10 Sternoclavicular joint
11 Acromioclavicular joint
12 Shoulder joint
13 Elbow joint
14 Wrist joint
15 Midcarpal joint
16 Carpometacarpal joint
17 Metacarpophalangeal joint
18 Interphalangeal joints of the hand
19 Carpometacarpal joint of thumb

Organization of shoulder girdle and upper limb (superior aspect). The two positions of the forearm essential to manual skills in the human, supination (right arm) and pronation (left arm), are shown.

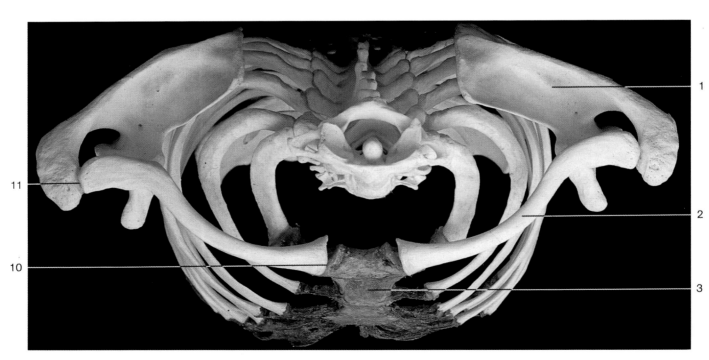

Bones of shoulder girdle articulated with the thorax (superior aspect).

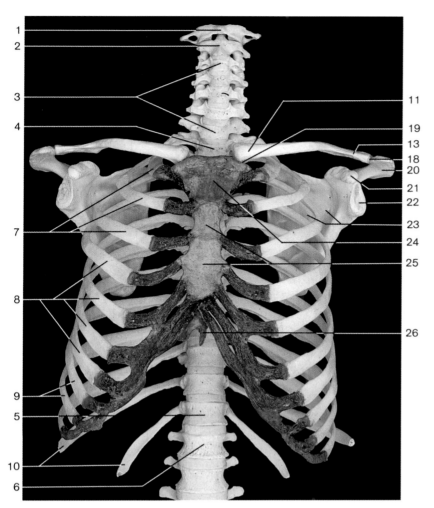

Vertebral column
1   Atlas
2   Axis
3   Third–seventh cervical vertebrae
4   First thoracic vertebra
5   Twelfth thoracic vertebra
6   First lumbar vertebra

Ribs
7   First–third ribs } True ribs
8   Fourth–seventh ribs }
9   Eighth–tenth ribs } False ribs
10 Eleventh and twelfth ribs }
    (floating ribs)

Clavicle
11 Sternal end
12 Articular facet for sternum
13 Acromial end
14 Articular facet for acromion
15 Impression for costoclavicular ligament
16 Conoid tubercle
17 Trapezoid line
18 Site of acromioclavicular joint
19 Site of sternoclavicular joint

Scapula
20 Acromion
21 Coracoid process
22 Glenoid cavity
23 Costal surface

Sternum
24 Manubrium
25 Body
26 Xiphoid process

Skeleton of shoulder girdle and thorax (anterior aspect).
The cartilaginous parts of the ribs appear dark brown.

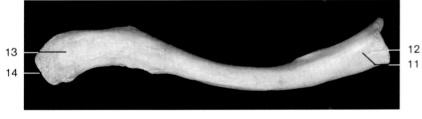

Right clavicle (superior aspect).

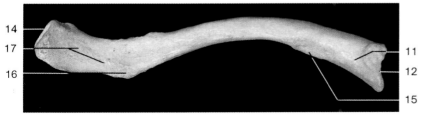

Right clavicle (inferior aspect).

Because of the human body's upright posture, the upper limb has developed a high degree of mobility. The shoulder girdle is to a great extent movable in the thorax and is connected with the trunk only by the sternoclavicular joint. A further characteristic of the forearm is the capacity for rotation (i.e., pronation and supination).

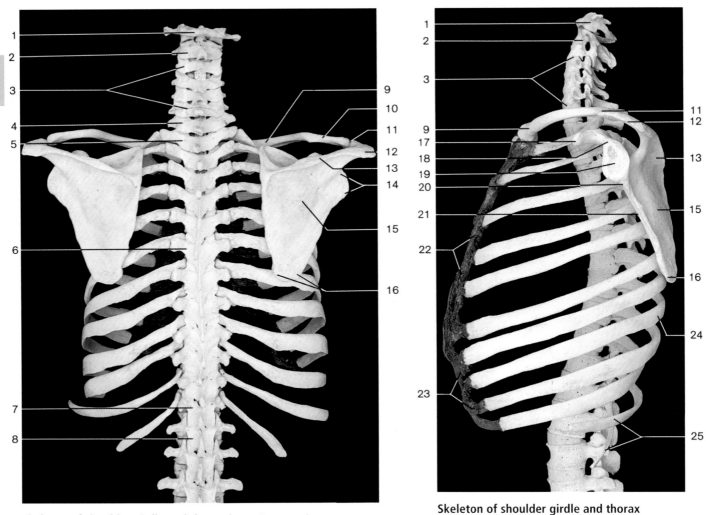

Skeleton of shoulder girdle and thorax (posterior aspect).

Skeleton of shoulder girdle and thorax
(lateral aspect).

Vertebral column
1 Atlas
2 Axis
3 Third–sixth cervical vertebrae
4 Seventh vertebra (vertebra prominens)
5 First thoracic vertebra
6 Sixth thoracic vertebra
7 Twelfth thoracic vertebra
8 First lumbar vertebra

Clavicle
9 Sternal end
10 Acromial end
11 Site of acromioclavicular joint

Scapula
12 Acromion
13 Spine of scapula
14 Lateral angle
15 Posterior surface
16 Inferior angle
17 Coracoid process
18 Supraglenoid tubercle
19 Glenoid cavity
20 Infraglenoid tubercle
21 Lateral margin

Thorax
22 Body of sternum
23 Costal arch
24 Angle of ribs
25 Floating ribs

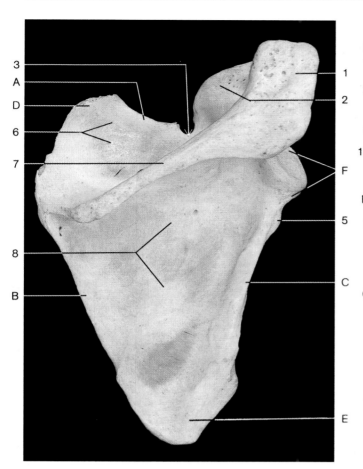

Right scapula (posterior aspect).

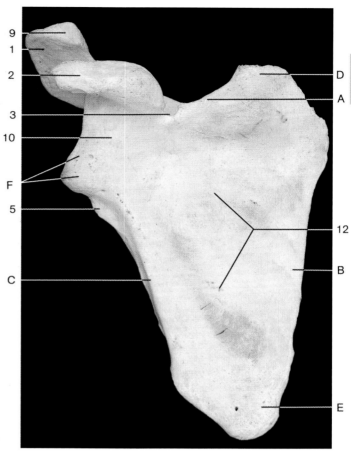

Right scapula (anterior aspect, costal surface).

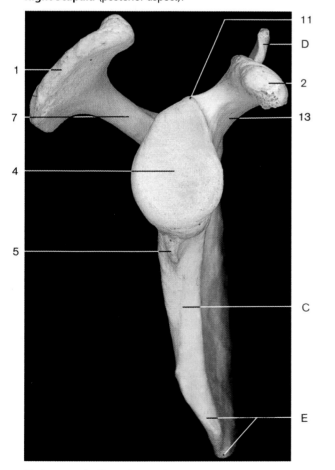

Right scapula (lateral aspect).

Scapula
A = superior border
B = medial border
C = lateral border
D = superior angle
E = inferior angle
F = lateral angle

1 Acromion
2 Coracoid process
3 Scapular notch
4 Glenoid cavity
5 Infraglenoid tubercle
6 Supraspinous fossa
7 Spine
8 Infraspinous fossa
9 Articular facet for acromion
10 Neck
11 Supraglenoid tubercle
12 Costal (anterior) surface
13 Base of coracoid process

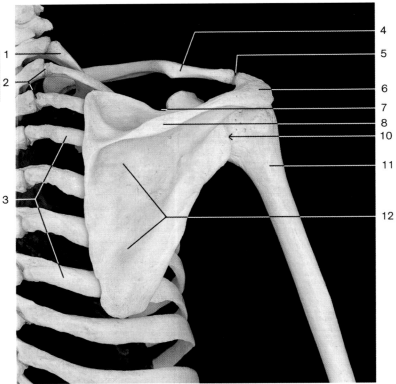

1   First rib
2   Position of costotransverse joints
3   Fourth–seventh ribs
4   Clavicle
5   Position of acromioclavicular joint
6   Acromion
7   Scapular notch
8   Spine of scapula
9   Head of humerus
10 Glenoid cavity
11 Surgical neck of humerus
12 Posterior surface of scapula
13 Coracoid process
14 Infraglenoid tubercle
15 Greater tubercle of humerus
16 Anatomical neck of humerus

Bones of shoulder joint (posterior aspect).

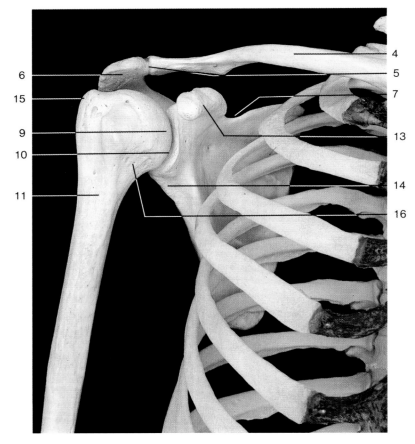

Bones of shoulder joint (anterior aspect).

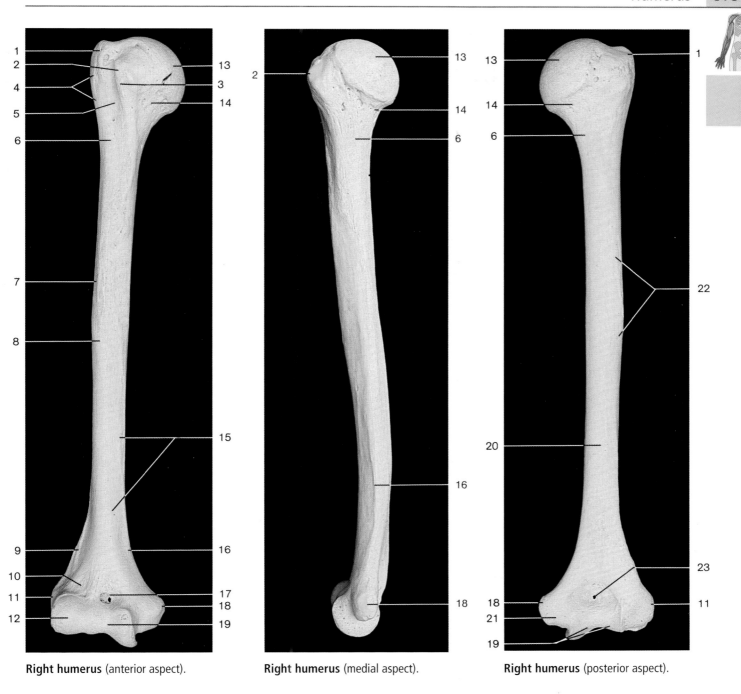

Right humerus (anterior aspect).

Right humerus (medial aspect).

Right humerus (posterior aspect).

Humerus

1	Greater tubercle	7	Deltoid tuberosity
2	Lesser tubercle	8	Anterolateral surface
3	Crest of lesser tubercle	9	Lateral supracondylar ridge
4	Crest of greater tubercle	10	Radial fossa
5	Intertubercular sulcus	11	Lateral epicondyle
6	Surgical neck	12	Capitulum

13	Head	19	Trochlea
14	Anatomical neck	20	Posterior surface
15	Anteromedial surface	21	Groove for ulnar nerve
16	Medial supracondylar ridge	22	Groove for radial nerve
17	Coronoid fossa	23	Olecranon fossa
18	Medial epicondyle		

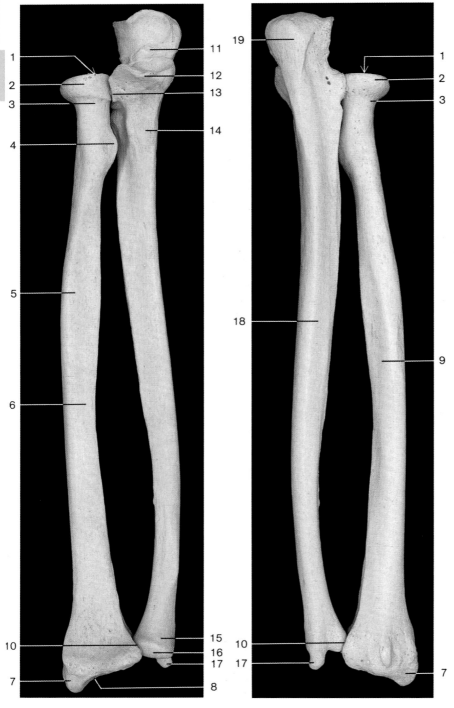

Bones of right forearm, radius, and ulna (anterior aspect).

Bones of right forearm, radius, and ulna (posterior aspect).

Radius
1 Head
2 Articular circumference
3 Neck
4 Radial tuberosity
5 Shaft
6 Anterior surface
7 Styloid process
8 Articular surface
9 Posterior surface
10 Ulnar notch

Ulna
11 Trochlear notch
12 Coronoid process
13 Radial notch
14 Ulnar tuberosity
15 Head
16 Articular circumference
17 Styloid process
18 Posterior surface
19 Olecranon

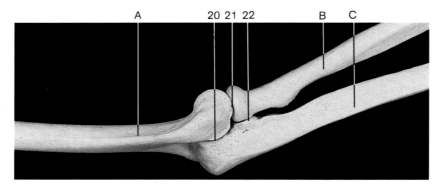

Bones of right elbow joint (lateral aspect).

Articulations at the right elbow
20 Site of humero-ulnar joint
21 Site of humeroradial joint
22 Site of proximal radio-ulnar joint

A = humerus
B = radius
C = ulna

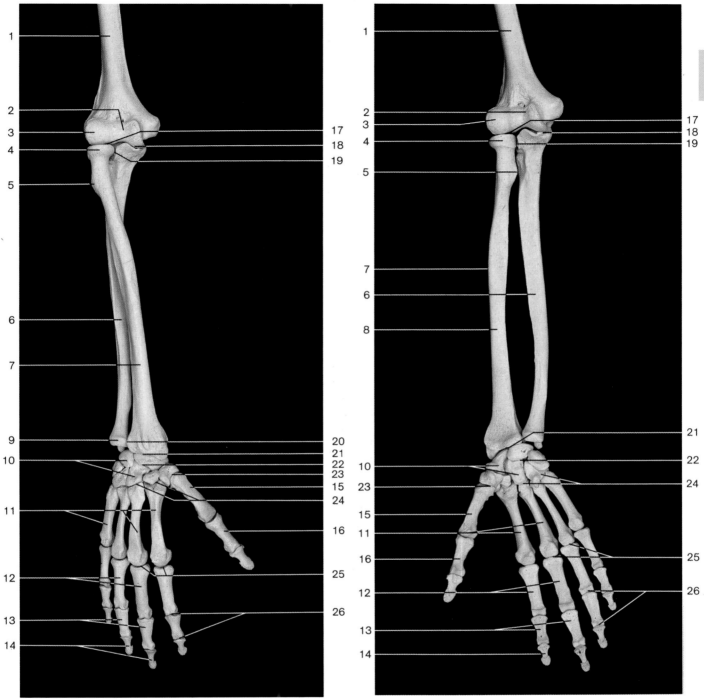

Skeleton of right forearm and hand in pronation.

Skeleton of right forearm and hand in supination.

1	Humerus	9	Articular circumference of ulna	**Sites of joints**	
2	Trochlea of humerus	10	Carpal bones	17	Humeroradial joint
3	Capitulum of humerus	11	Metacarpal bones	18	Humero-ulnar joint
4	Articular circumference of radius	12	Proximal phalanges	19	Proximal radio-ulnar joint
5	Radial tuberosity	13	Middle phalanges	20	Distal radio-ulnar joint
6	Anterior surface of ulna	14	Distal phalanges	21	Wrist joint
7	Posterior surface of radius	15	Metacarpal bone of thumb	22	Midcarpal joint
8	Anterior surface of radius	16	Proximal phalanx of thumb	23	Carpometacarpal joint of thumb
				24	Carpometacarpal joints
				25	Metacarpophalangeal joints
				26	Interphalangeal joints of the hand

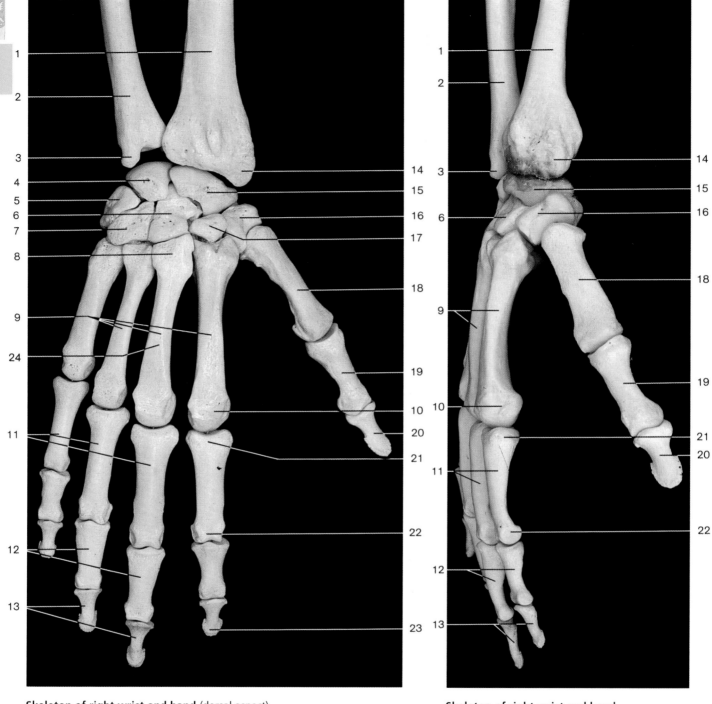

Skeleton of right wrist and hand (dorsal aspect).

Skeleton of right wrist and hand (medial aspect).

1	Radius	8	Base of third metacarpal bone	15	Scaphoid bone	22	Head of second proximal phalanx
2	Ulna	9	Metacarpal bones	16	Trapezium bone	Carpal bones	23	Tuberosity of distal phalanx
3	Styloid process of ulna	10	Head of metacarpal bone	17	Trapezoid bone		
4	Lunate bone	11	Proximal phalanges of hand	18	Metacarpal bone of thumb	24	Body of third metacarpal bone
5	Triquetral bone	Carpal bones	12	Middle phalanges of hand	19	Proximal phalanx of thumb		
6	Capitate bone	13	Distal phalanges of hand	20	Distal phalanx of thumb		
7	Hamate bone	14	Styloid process of radius	21	Base of second proximal phalanx		

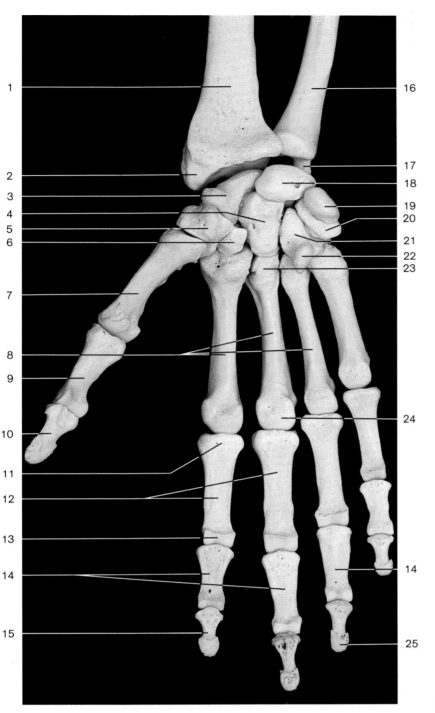

1   Radius
2   Styloid process of radius
3   Scaphoid bone ⎫
4   Capitate bone ⎬ Carpal bones
5   Trapezium   ⎪
6   Trapezoid bone ⎭
7   First metacarpal bone
8   Second to fourth metacarpal bones
9   Proximal phalanx of thumb
10 Distal phalanx of thumb
11 Base of second proximal phalanx
12 Proximal phalanges
13 Head of second proximal phalanx
14 Middle phalanges
15 Distal phalanx
16 Ulna
17 Styloid process of ulna
18 Lunate bone   ⎫
19 Pisiform bone ⎬ Carpal bones
20 Triquetral bone⎪
21 Hamate bone   ⎭
22 Hamulus or hook
    of hamate bone
23 Base of third metacarpal bone
24 Head of metacarpal bone
25 Tuberosity of distal phalanx

Skeleton of right wrist and hand (palmar aspect).

The human hand is one of the most admirable structures of the human body. The carpometacarpal joint of the thumb, a saddle joint, enjoys wide mobility so that the thumb can come into contact with all other fingers, thus enabling the hand to become an instrument for grasping and psychologic expression. During evolution, these newly developed functions appeared after the erect posture of the human body was achieved. An inevitable prerequisite for the development of human cultures is not only the differentiation of the brain but also the development of an organ capable of realizing its ideas: the human hand.

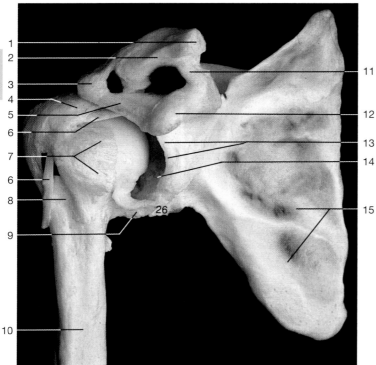

Right shoulder joint. The anterior part of the articular capsule has been removed and the head of the humerus has been slightly rotated outward to show the cavity of the joint.

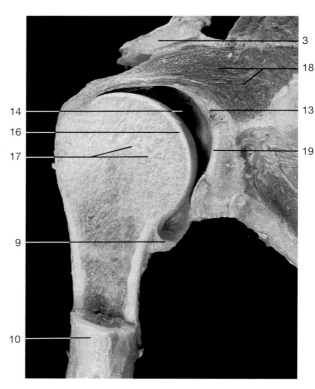

Coronal section of the right shoulder joint (anterior aspect).

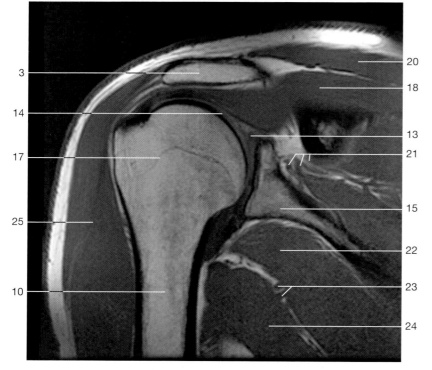

Coronal section of the right shoulder joint (MRI scan; from Heuck et al., MRT-Atlas, 2009).

1   Acromial end of clavicle
2   Acromioclavicular joint
3   Acromion
4   Tendon of supraspinatus muscle
    (attached to the articular capsule)
5   Coraco-acromial ligament
6   Tendon of long head of biceps brachii muscle
7   Tendon of subscapularis muscle
    (attached to the articular capsule)
8   Intertubercular sulcus
9   Articular capsule of shoulder joint
10 Humerus
11 Trapezoid ligament
12 Coracoid process
13 Glenoid labrum
14 Shoulder joint (joint cavity)
15 Scapula
16 Head of humerus
17 Epiphysial line
18 Supraspinatus muscle
19 Glenoid cavity
20 Trapezius muscle
21 Suprascapular artery, vein, and nerve
22 Teres major muscle
23 Circumflexa scapular artery and vein
24 Latissimus dorsi muscle
25 Deltoid muscle
26 Tendon of long head of triceps brachii muscle

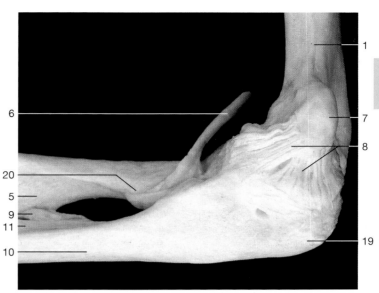

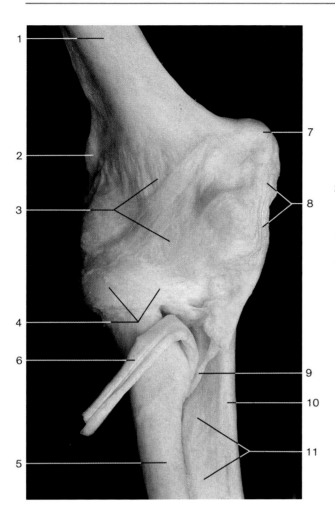

Elbow joint with collateral ligaments (medial aspect).

Ligaments of the elbow joint (anterior aspect).

1	Humerus	11	Interosseous membrane
2	Lateral epicondyle of humerus	12	Radial fossa
3	Articular capsule	13	Capitulum of humerus
4	Anular ligament of proximal radio-ulnar joint	14	Head of radius
5	Radius	15	Radial collateral ligament
6	Tendon of biceps brachii muscle	16	Coronoid fossa
7	Medial epicondyle of humerus	17	Trochlea of humerus
8	Ulnar collateral ligament	18	Coronoid process of ulna
9	Oblique chord	19	Olecranon
10	Ulna	20	Radial tuberosity

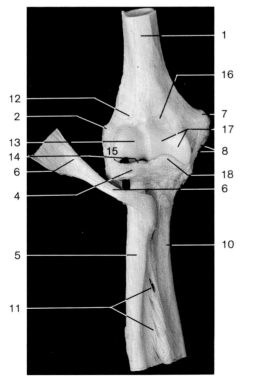

Elbow joint with ligaments (anterior aspect). Articular capsule has been removed to show the anular ligament.

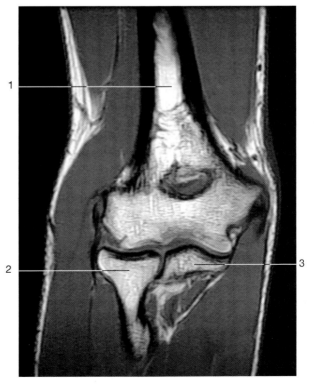

Coronal section of the elbow joint
(MRI scan, courtesy of Prof. Dr. A. Heuck, Munich).

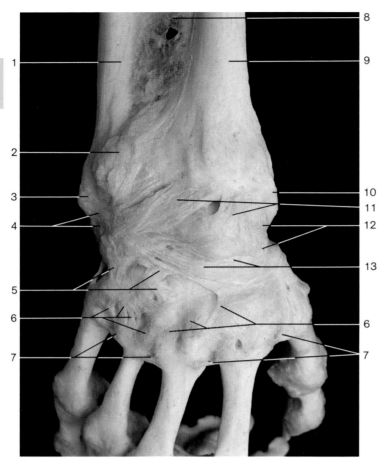

1   Ulna
2   Exostosis (pathological)
3   Head of ulna
4   Ulnar carpal collateral ligament
5   Deep intercarpal ligaments
6   Dorsal carpometacarpal ligaments
7   Dorsal metacarpal ligaments
8   Interosseous membrane
9   Radius
10   Styloid process of radius
11   Dorsal radiocarpal ligament
12   Radial collateral ligament
13   Articular capsule and dorsal intercarpal ligaments
14   Palmar radiocarpal ligament
15   Tendon of flexor carpi radialis muscle (cut)
16   Radiating carpal ligament
17   Palmar carpometacarpal ligaments
18   First metacarpal bone
19   Palmar ulnocarpal ligament
20   Tendon of flexor carpi ulnaris muscle (cut)
21   Pisohamate ligament
22   Pisometacarpal ligament
23   Palmar metacarpal ligaments
24   Fifth metacarpal bone
25   Articular disc (ulnocarpal)
26   Lunate bone
27   Triquetral bone
28   Hamate bone
29   Scaphoid bone (navicular)
30   Capitate bone
31   Trapezoid bone
32   Second and third metacarpal bones
33   Dorsal interosseus muscles

Ligaments of hand and wrist (dorsal aspect).

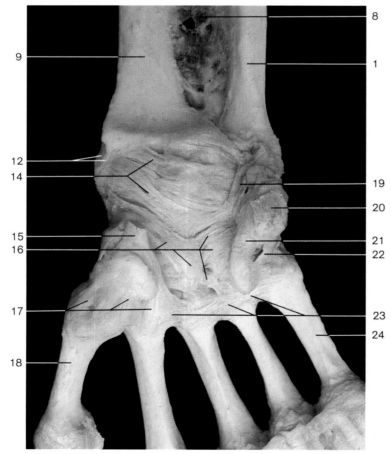

Ligaments of hand and wrist (palmar aspect).

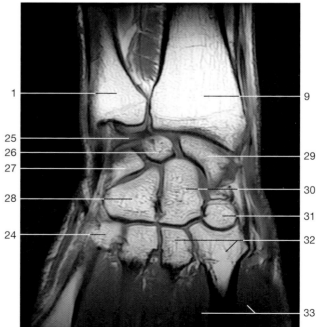

Coronal section of the hand and wrist (MRI scan; from Heuck et al., MRT-Atlas, 2009). Note the location of the wrist joint.

1   Radius
2   Styloid process of radius
3   Palmar radiocarpal ligament
4   Tendon of flexor carpi radialis muscle (cut)
5   Radiating carpal ligament
6   Articular capsule of carpometacarpal
    joint of thumb
7   Articular capsule of metacarpophalangeal
    joint of thumb
8   Palmar ligaments and articular capsule
    of metacarpophalangeal joints
9   Palmar ligaments and articular capsule
    of interphalangeal joints
10 Articular capsule
11 Interosseous membrane
12 Ulna
13 Distal radio-ulnar joint
14 Styloid process of ulna
15 Palmar ulnocarpal ligament
16 Pisiform bone with tendon of flexor
    carpi ulnaris muscle
17 Pisometacarpal ligament
18 Pisohamate ligament
19 Metacarpal bone
20 Deep transverse metacarpal ligament
21 Tendons of extensor muscles and
    articular capsule
22 Collateral ligament of interphalangeal joint
23 Collateral ligaments of
    metacarpophalangeal joints
24 Second metacarpal bone

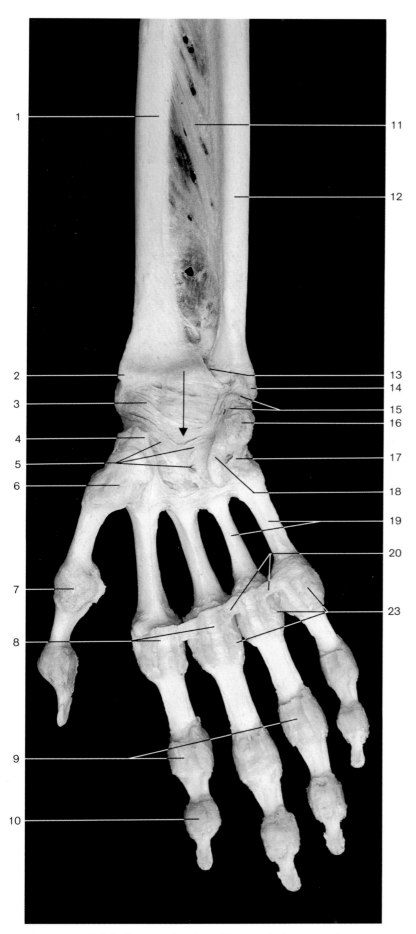

Ligaments of right forearm, hand, and fingers (palmar aspect).
The arrow indicates the location of the carpal tunnel.

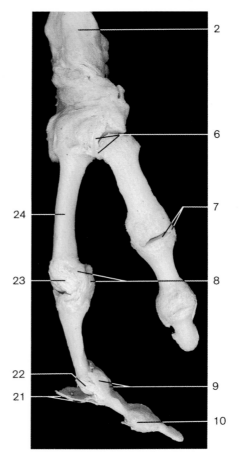

Ligaments of fingers
(lateral aspect).

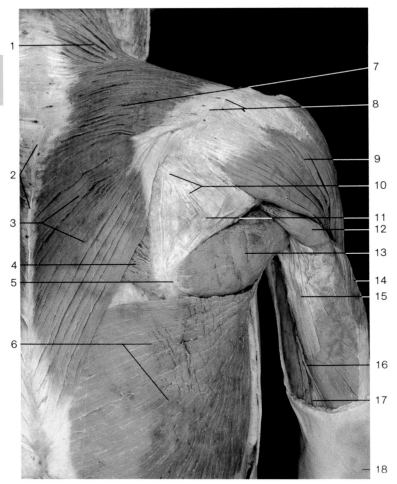

1. Descending fibers of trapezius muscle
2. Spinous processes of thoracic vertebrae
3. Ascending fibers of trapezius muscle
4. Rhomboid major muscle
5. Inferior angle of scapula
6. Latissimus dorsi muscle
7. Transverse fibers of trapezius muscle
8. Spine of scapula
9. Posterior fibers of deltoid muscle
10. Infraspinatus muscle and infraspinous fascia
11. Teres minor muscle and fascia
12. Long head of triceps brachii muscle
13. Teres major muscle
14. Lateral head of triceps brachii muscle
15. Medial head of triceps brachii muscle
16. Medial intermuscular septum
17. Ulnar nerve
18. Olecranon

Muscles of shoulder and arm, superficial layer (right side, dorsal aspect).

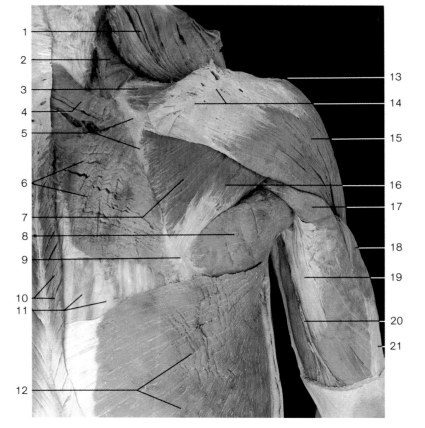

1. Trapezius muscle (reflected)
2. Levator scapulae muscle
3. Supraspinatus muscle
4. Rhomboid minor muscle
5. Medial border of scapula
6. Rhomboid major muscle
7. Infraspinatus muscle
8. Teres major muscle
9. Inferior angle of scapula
10. Cut edge of trapezius muscle
11. Intrinsic muscles of back with fascia
12. Latissimus dorsi muscle
13. Acromion
14. Spine of scapula
15. Deltoid muscle
16. Teres minor muscle
17. Long head of triceps brachii muscle
18. Lateral head of triceps brachii muscle
19. Medial head of triceps brachii muscle
20. Medial intermuscular septum
21. Tendon of triceps brachii muscle

Muscles of shoulder and arm, deeper layer (right side, dorsal aspect). The trapezius muscle has been cut near its origin at the vertebral column and reflected upward.

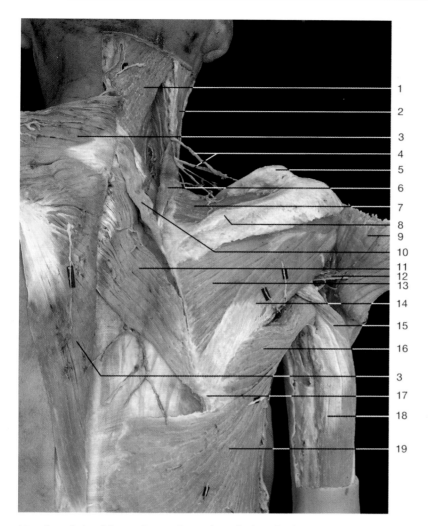

1 Splenius capitis muscle
2 Sternocleidomastoid muscle
3 Trapezius muscle (reflected)
4 Lateral supraclavicular nerves
5 Clavicle
6 Levator scapulae muscle
7 Supraspinatus muscle
8 Spine of scapula
9 Deltoid muscle (reflected)
10 Rhomboid minor muscle
11 Rhomboid major muscle
12 Axillary nerve and posterior
   circumflex humeral artery
13 Infraspinatus muscle
14 Teres minor muscle
15 Long head of triceps brachii muscle
16 Teres major muscle
17 Inferior angle of scapula
18 Triceps brachii muscle
19 Latissimus dorsi muscle

Muscles of shoulder and arm, deeper layer (right side, dorsal aspect).
The trapezius and deltoid muscles have been divided and reflected.

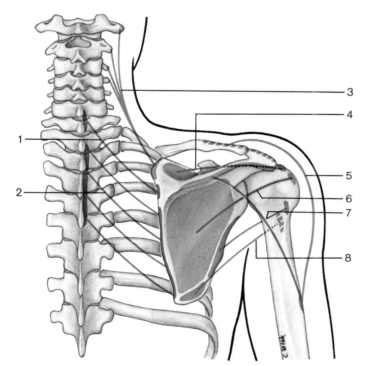

Shoulder muscles, schematic diagram illustrating the course of
the main muscles of the dorsal aspect of the shoulder.

1 Rhomboid minor muscle (red)
2 Rhomboid major muscle (red)
3 Levator scapulae muscle (red)
4 Supraspinatus muscle (blue)
5 Deltoid muscle (red)
6 Infraspinatus muscle (blue)
7 Teres minor muscle (red)
8 Teres major muscle (red)

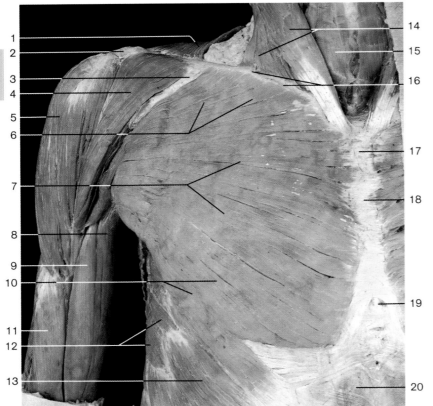

1   Trapezius muscle
2   Acromion
3   Deltopectoral triangle
4   Clavicular part of deltoid muscle
    (anterior fibers)
5   Acromial part of deltoid muscle
    (central fibers)
6   Clavicular part of pectoralis major muscle
7   Sternocostal part of pectoralis major muscle
8   Short head of biceps brachii muscle
9   Long head of biceps brachii muscle
10 Abdominal part of pectoralis major muscle
11 Brachialis muscle
12 Serratus anterior muscle
13 External abdominal oblique muscle
14 Sternocleidomastoid muscle
15 Infrahyoid muscles
16 Clavicle
17 Manubrium sterni
18 Body of sternum
19 Xiphoid process
20 Anterior layer of sheath of rectus
    abdominis muscle

Shoulder, arm, and pectoral muscles, superficial layer (ventral aspect).

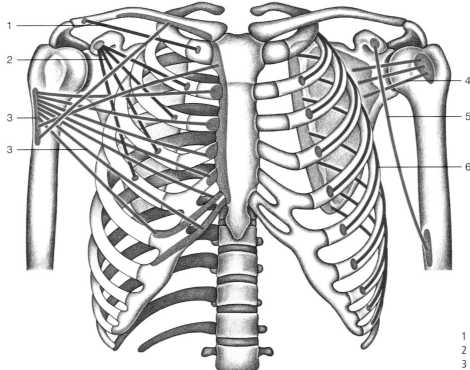

Arrangement of pectoral and shoulder muscles (ventral aspect).
(Schematic drawing.)

1   Subclavius muscle (blue)
2   Pectoralis minor muscle (blue)
3   Pectoralis major muscle (red)
4   Subscapularis muscle (red)
5   Coracobrachialis muscle (red)
6   Serratus anterior muscle (green)

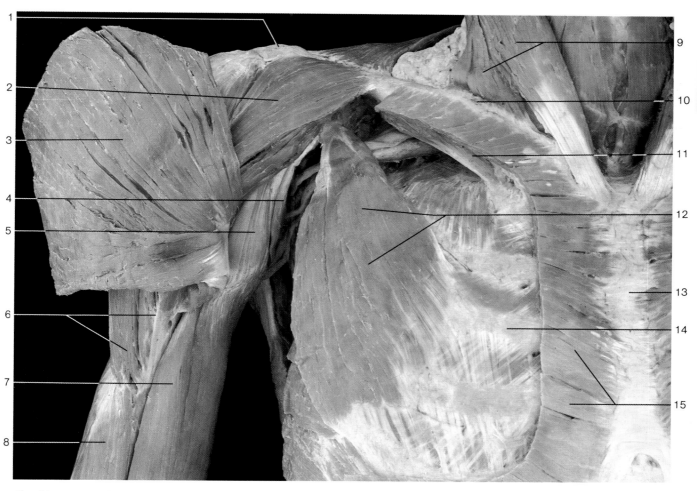

Shoulder, arm, and pectoral muscles, deep layer (ventral aspect).

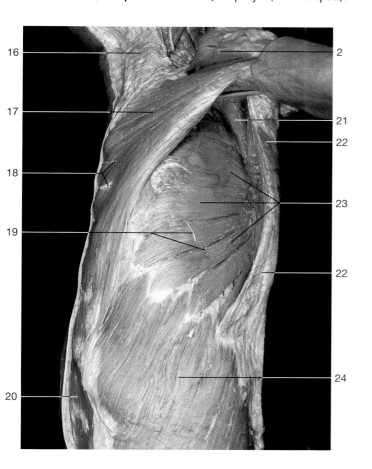

1   Acromion
2   Clavicular part of deltoid muscle
3   Pectoralis major muscle (reflected)
4   Coracobrachialis muscle
5   Short head of biceps brachii muscle
6   Deltoid muscle (insertion on humerus)
7   Long head of biceps brachii muscle
8   Brachialis muscle
9   Sternocleidomastoid muscle
10 Clavicle
11 Subclavius muscle
12 Pectoralis minor muscle
13 Sternum
14 Third rib
15 Pectoralis major muscle
16 Platysma muscle
17 Pectoralis major muscle forming the anterior axillary fold
18 Anterior cutaneous branches of intercostal nerves
19 Lateral cutaneous branches of intercostal nerves
20 Rectus abdominis muscle
21 Subscapularis muscle
22 Latissimus dorsi muscle forming the posterior axillary fold
23 Serratus anterior muscle forming the medial wall of the axilla
24 External abdominal oblique muscle

Axillary fossa and serratus anterior muscle
(left side, lateral aspect).

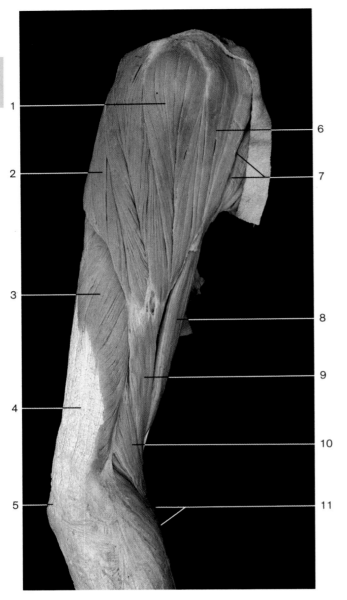

Muscles of the right arm (lateral aspect).

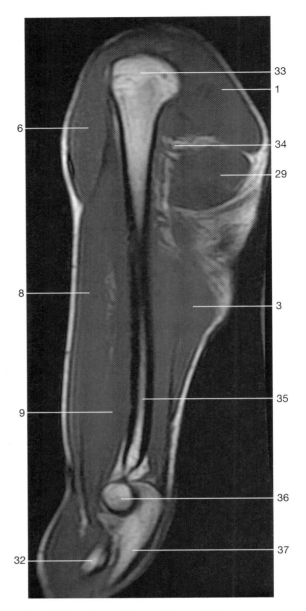

Sagittal section of the right arm (MRI scan; from Heuck et al., MRT-Atlas, 2009).

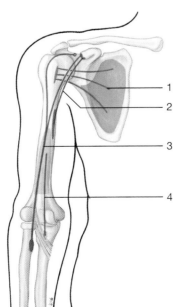

Position and course of flexors of arm (schematic drawing).

1   Subscapularis muscle (red)
2   Coracobrachialis muscle (blue)
3   Biceps brachii muscle (red)
4   Brachialis muscle (blue)

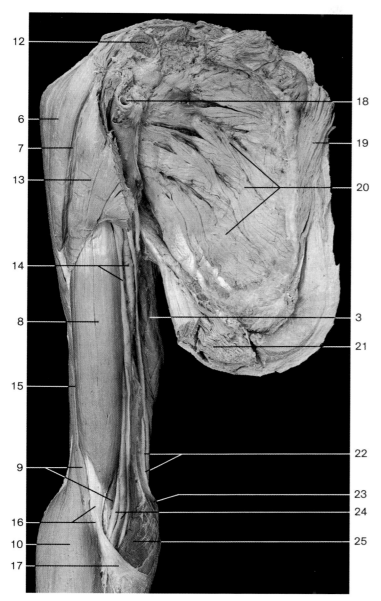

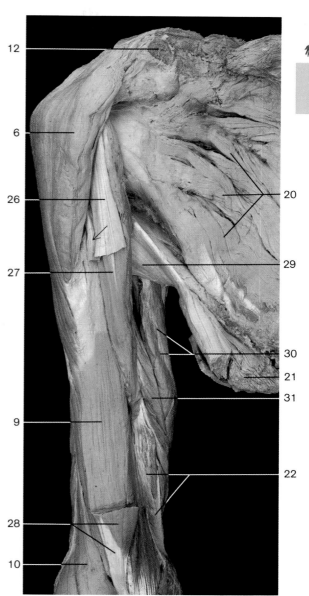

Muscles of the right arm (ventral aspect). The arm with the scapula and attached muscles has been removed from the trunk.

Muscles of the right arm (ventral aspect). Part of the biceps brachii muscle has been removed. Arrow: tendon of long head of biceps brachii muscle.

1 Acromial part of deltoid muscle (central fibers)
2 Scapular part of deltoid muscle (posterior fibers)
3 Triceps brachii muscle
4 Tendon of triceps brachii muscle
5 Olecranon
6 Clavicular part of deltoid muscle (anterior fibers)
7 Deltopectoral groove
8 Biceps brachii muscle
9 Brachialis muscle
10 Brachioradialis muscle
11 Extensor carpi radialis longus muscle
12 Clavicle (divided)
13 Pectoralis major muscle
14 Medial intermuscular septum with vessels and nerves
15 Lateral intermuscular septum
16 Tendon of biceps brachii muscle
17 Bicipital aponeurosis
18 Axillary artery
19 Rhomboid major muscle

20 Subscapularis muscle
21 Latissimus dorsi muscle (divided)
22 Medial intermuscular septum
23 Medial epicondyle of humerus
24 Brachial artery and median nerve
25 Pronator teres muscle
26 Tendon of short head of biceps
   brachii muscle
27 Coracobrachialis muscle
28 Distal part of biceps brachii muscle
29 Teres major muscle
30 Long head of triceps brachii muscle
31 Medial head of triceps brachii muscle
32 Radius
33 Head of humerus
34 Axillary nerve
35 Humerus
36 Trochlea
37 Ulna

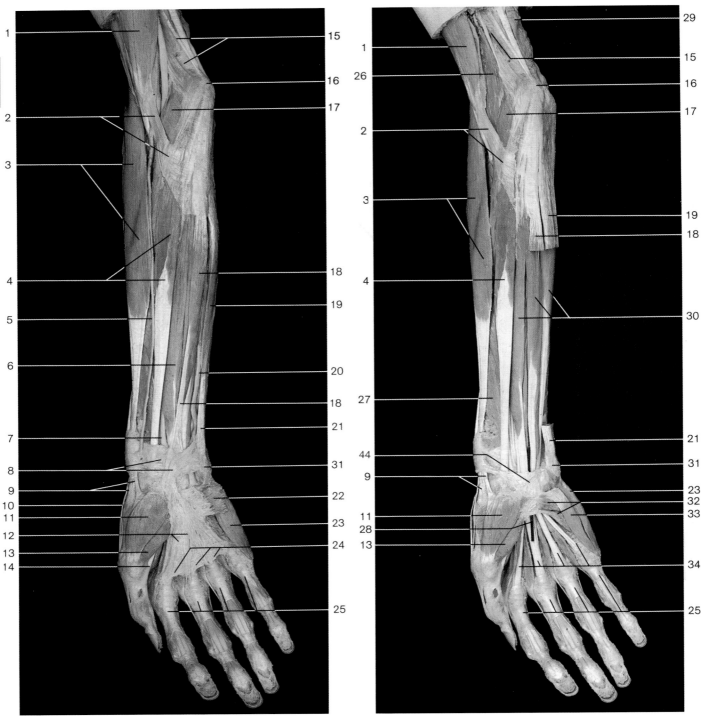

Flexor muscles of forearm and hand, superficial layer (ventral aspect).

Flexor muscles of forearm and hand, superficial layer (ventral aspect). The palmaris longus and flexor carpi ulnaris muscles have been removed.

1	Biceps brachii muscle
2	Bicipital aponeurosis
3	Brachioradialis muscle
4	Flexor carpi radialis muscle
5	Radial artery
6	Flexor digitorum superficialis muscle
7	Median nerve
8	Antebrachial fascia and tendon of palmaris longus muscle
9	Tendon of abductor pollicis longus muscle
10	Tendon of extensor pollicis brevis muscle
11	Abductor pollicis brevis muscle

12	Palmar aponeurosis
13	Superficial head of flexor pollicis brevis muscle
14	Tendon of flexor pollicis longus muscle
15	Medial intermuscular septum
16	Medial epicondyle of humerus
17	Humeral head of pronator teres muscle
18	Palmaris longus muscle
19	Flexor carpi ulnaris muscle
20	Ulnar artery
21	Tendon of flexor carpi ulnaris muscle
22	Palmaris brevis muscle

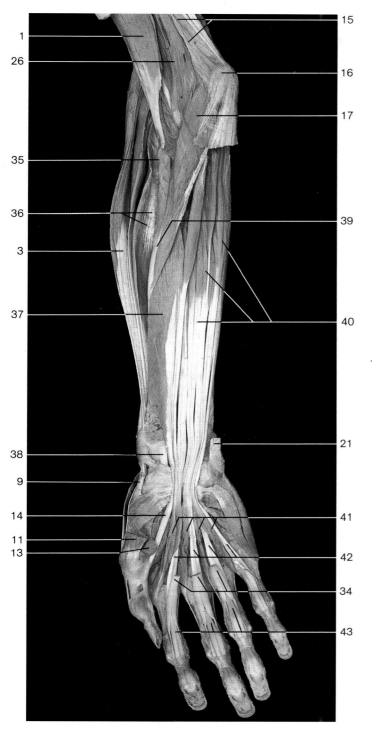

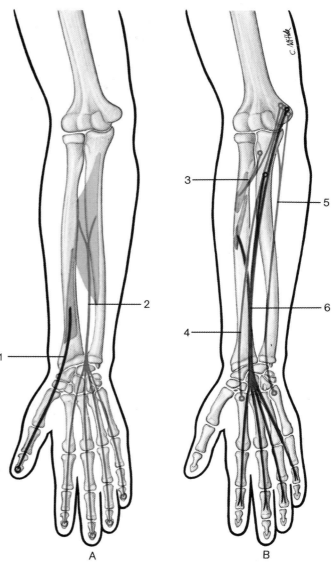

Flexor muscles of forearm and hand, middle layer (ventral aspect). The palmaris longus, flexor carpi radialis, and ulnaris muscles have been removed. The flexor retinaculum has been divided.

Position of flexors of fingers and hand (schematic drawing).

A   Deep layer

1   Flexor pollicis
     longus muscle (blue)
2   Flexor digitorum
     profundus muscle (red)

B   Superficial layer

3   Pronator teres muscle (red)
4   Flexor carpi radialis
     muscle (red)
5   Flexor carpi ulnaris
     muscle (red)
6   Flexor digitorum superficialis
     muscle (blue)

23   Abductor digiti minimi muscle
24   Transverse fasciculi of palmar aponeurosis
25   Digital fibrous sheaths of tendons of flexor digitorum muscle
26   Brachialis muscle
27   Flexor pollicis longus muscle
28   Carpal tunnel (canalis carpi, probe)
29   Triceps brachii muscle
30   Flexor digitorum superficialis muscle
31   Pisiform bone
32   Opponens digiti minimi muscle
33   Flexor digiti minimi brevis muscle
34   Tendons of flexor digitorum superficialis muscle

35   Supinator muscle
36   Extensor carpi radialis brevis muscle
37   Flexor pollicis longus muscle
38   Tendon of flexor carpi radialis muscle
39   Pronator teres muscle (insertion of radius)
40   Flexor digitorum profundus muscle
41   Lumbrical muscles
42   Tendons of flexor digitorum profundus muscle
43   Tendons of flexor digitorum profundus muscle having passed
      through the divided tendons of the flexor digitorum superficialis
      muscle
44   Flexor retinaculum

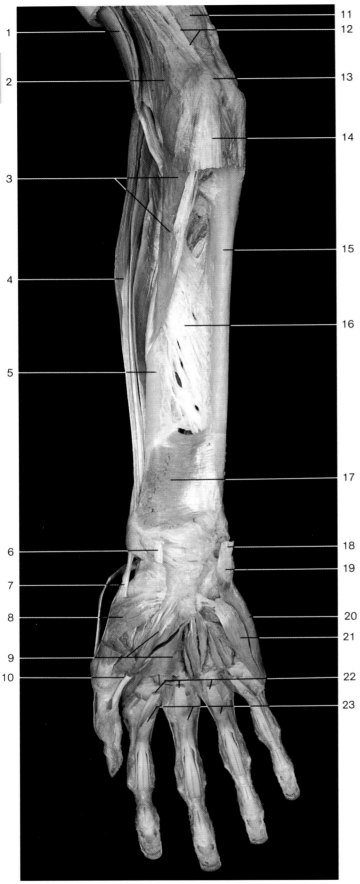

1 Biceps brachii muscle
2 Brachialis muscle
3 Pronator teres muscle
4 Brachioradialis muscle
5 Radius
6 Tendon of flexor carpi radialis muscle
7 Tendon of abductor pollicis longus muscle
8 Opponens pollicis muscle
9 Adductor pollicis muscle
10 Tendon of flexor pollicis longus muscle
11 Triceps brachii muscle
12 Medial intermuscular septum
13 Medial epicondyle of humerus
14 Common flexor mass (divided)
15 Ulna
16 Interosseous membrane
17 Pronator quadratus muscle
18 Tendon of flexor carpi ulnaris muscle
19 Pisiform bone
20 Abductor digiti minimi muscle
21 Flexor digiti minimi brevis muscle
22 Tendons of flexor digitorum profundus muscle
23 Tendons of flexor digitorum superficialis muscle
24 Flexor retinaculum
25 Hypothenar muscles
26 Thenar muscles
27 Common synovial sheath of flexor tendons
28 Synovial sheath of tendon of flexor pollicis longus muscle
29 Digital synovial sheaths of flexor tendons

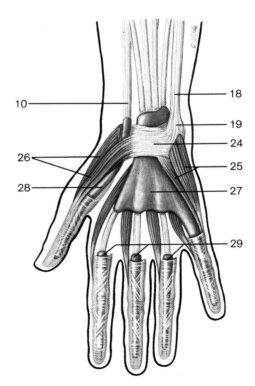

Flexor muscles of forearm and hand, deep layer (ventral aspect). All flexors have been removed to display the pronator quadratus and pronator teres muscles together with the interosseous membrane. Forearm in supination.

Synovial sheaths of flexor tendons (palmar aspect of right hand, semischematic drawing).

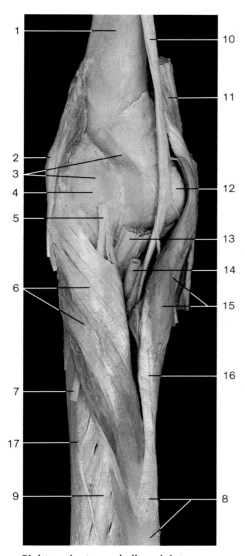

1   Humerus
2   Lateral epicondyle of humerus
3   Articular capsule
4   Position of capitulum of humerus
5   Deep branch of radial nerve
6   Supinator muscle
7   Entrance of deep branch of radial nerve to extensor muscles
8   Radius and insertion of pronator teres muscle
9   Interosseous membrane
10 Median nerve
11 Triceps brachii muscle
12 Trochlea of humerus
13 Tendon of biceps brachii muscle
14 Brachial artery
15 Pronator teres muscle
16 Tendon of pronator teres muscle
17 Ulna
18 Pronator quadratus muscle
19 Tendon of flexor carpi radialis muscle
20 Thenar muscles
21 Synovial sheath of tendon of flexor pollicis longus muscle
22 Fibrous sheath of flexor tendons
23 Digital synovial sheath of flexor tendons
24 Flexor digitorum superficialis muscle
25 Tendon of flexor carpi ulnaris muscle
26 Common synovial sheath of flexor tendons
27 Position of pisiform bone
28 Flexor retinaculum
29 Hypothenar muscles

Right supinator and elbow joint
(ventral aspect). Forearm in pronation.

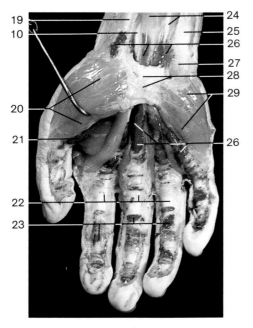

Synovial sheaths of flexor tendons
(palmar aspect of right hand). Blue PVA
solution has been injected into the sheaths.

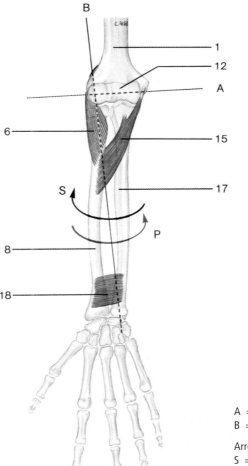

A = axis of flexion and extension
B = axis of rotation

Arrows:
S = supination
P = pronation

Diagram illustrating the two axes of the elbow joint.

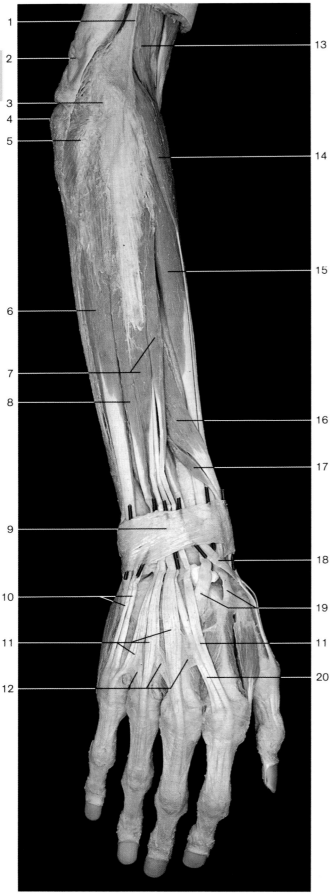

1 Lateral intermuscular septum
2 Tendon of triceps brachii muscle
3 Lateral epicondyle of humerus
4 Olecranon
5 Anconeus muscle
6 Extensor carpi ulnaris muscle
7 Extensor digitorum muscle
8 Extensor digiti minimi muscle
9 Extensor retinaculum
10 Tendons of extensor digiti minimi muscle
11 Tendons of extensor digitorum muscle
12 Intertendinous connections
13 Brachioradialis muscle
14 Extensor carpi radialis longus muscle
15 Extensor carpi radialis brevis muscle
16 Abductor pollicis longus muscle
17 Extensor pollicis brevis muscle
18 Tendon of extensor pollicis longus muscle
19 Tendons of both extensor carpi radialis longus
   and extensor carpi radialis brevis muscles
20 Tendon of extensor indicis muscle
21 First tunnel: Abductor pollicis longus muscle,
                    extensor pollicis brevis muscle
22 Second tunnel: Extensor carpi radialis longus and brevis muscles
23 Third tunnel: Extensor pollicis longus muscle
24 Fourth tunnel: Extensor digitorum muscle,
                   extensor indicis muscle
25 Fifth tunnel: Extensor digiti minimi muscle
26 Sixth tunnel: Extensor carpi ulnaris muscle

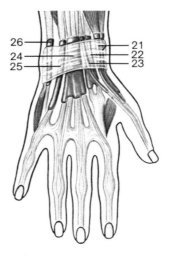

Synovial sheaths of extensor tendons on the back of the right wrist (indicated in blue). Notice the six tunnels for the passage of the extensor tendons beneath the extensor retinaculum (schematic drawing).

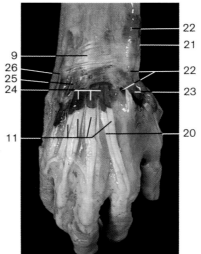

Extensor muscles of forearm and hand, superficial layer (dorsal aspect). Tunnels for extensor tendons indicated by probes.

Synovial sheaths of extensor tendons. The sheaths have been injected with blue gelatin.

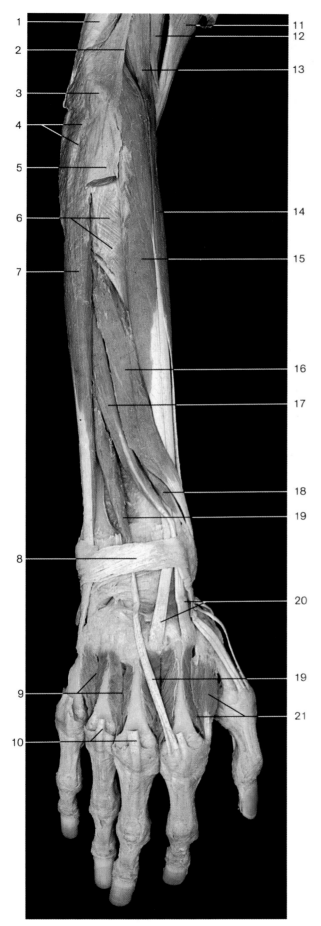

1 Triceps brachii muscle
2 Lateral intermuscular septum
3 Lateral epicondyle of humerus
4 Anconeus muscle
5 Extensor digitorum and extensor digiti minimi muscles (cut)
6 Supinator muscle
7 Extensor carpi ulnaris muscle
8 Extensor retinaculum
9 Third and fourth dorsal interosseous muscles
10 Tendons of extensor digitorum muscle (cut)
11 Biceps brachii muscle
12 Brachialis muscle
13 Brachioradialis muscle
14 Extensor carpi radialis longus muscle
15 Extensor carpi radialis brevis muscle
16 Abductor pollicis longus muscle
17 Extensor pollicis longus muscle
18 Extensor pollicis brevis muscle
19 Extensor indicis muscle
20 Tendons of the extensor carpi radialis longus and extensor carpi radialis brevis muscles
21 First dorsal interosseous muscle

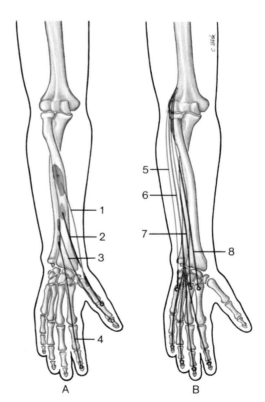

Position of extensor muscles of forearm and hand (schematic drawing).

A Extensors of thumb	**B Extensors of fingers and hand**
1 Abductor pollicis longus muscle (red)	5 Extensor carpi ulnaris muscle (blue)
2 Extensor pollicis brevis muscle (blue)	6 Extensor digitorum muscle (red)
3 Extensor pollicis longus muscle (red)	7 Extensor carpi radialis brevis muscle (blue)
4 Extensor indicis muscle (blue)	8 Extensor carpi radialis longus muscle (blue)

Extensor muscles of forearm and hand, deep layer (dorsal aspect).

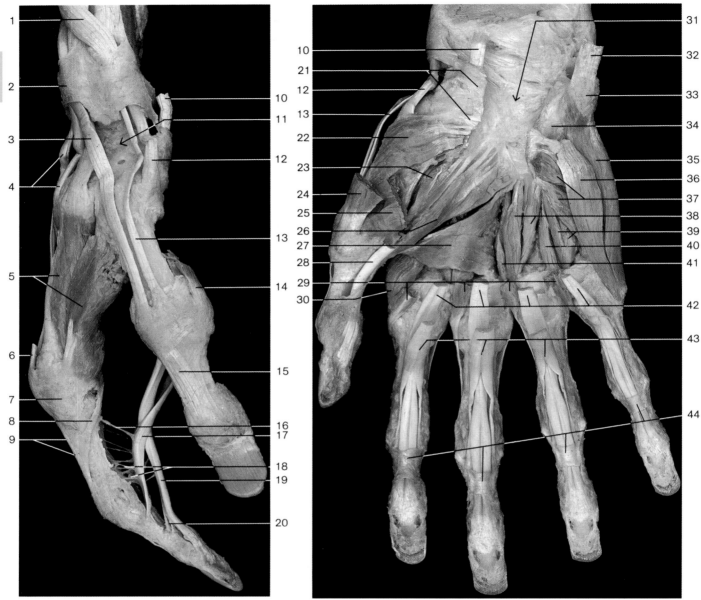

Muscles of thumb and index finger (medial aspect). The tendons of the extensor muscles of the thumb and the insertion of the flexor tendons of the index finger are displayed.

Muscles of right hand (palmar aspect). The tendons of the flexor muscles and parts of the thumb muscles have been removed. The carpal tunnel has been opened.

1	Tendons of extensor pollicis brevis and abductor pollicis longus muscle
2	Extensor retinaculum
3	Tendon of extensor pollicis longus muscle
4	Tendons of extensor carpi radialis longus and brevis muscles
5	First dorsal interosseous muscle
6	Tendon of extensor digitorum muscle for index finger
7	Location of metacarpophalangeal joint
8	Tendon of lumbrical muscle
9	Extensor expansion of index finger
10	Tendon of flexor carpi radialis muscle (cut)
11	Anatomical snuffbox
12	Tendon of abductor pollicis longus muscle
13	Tendon of extensor pollicis brevis muscle
14	Tendon of abductor pollicis brevis muscle
15	Extensor expansion of extensor of thumb
16	Vinculum longum
17	Tendons of flexor digitorum superficialis muscle dividing to allow passage of deep tendons
18	Vincula of flexor tendons
19	Tendon of flexor digitorum profundus muscle
20	Vinculum breve
21	Radial carpal eminence (cut edge of flexor retinaculum)
22	Opponens pollicis muscle
23	Deep head of flexor pollicis brevis muscle
24	Abductor pollicis brevis muscle (cut)
25	Superficial head of flexor pollicis brevis muscle (cut)
26	Oblique head of adductor pollicis muscle
27	Transverse head of adductor pollicis muscle
28	Tendon of flexor pollicis longus muscle (cut)
29	Lumbrical muscles (cut)
30	First dorsal interosseous muscle
31	Position of carpal tunnel
32	Tendon of flexor carpi ulnaris muscle
33	Location of pisiform bone
34	Hook of hamate bone
35	Abductor digiti minimi muscle
36	Flexor digiti minimi brevis muscle
37	Opponens digiti minimi muscle
38	Second palmar interosseous muscle
39	Third palmar interosseous muscle
40	Fourth dorsal interosseous muscle
41	Third dorsal interosseous muscle
42	Tendon of flexor digitorum profundus muscle (cut)
43	Tendons of flexor digitorum superficialis muscle (cut)
44	Fibrous flexor sheaths

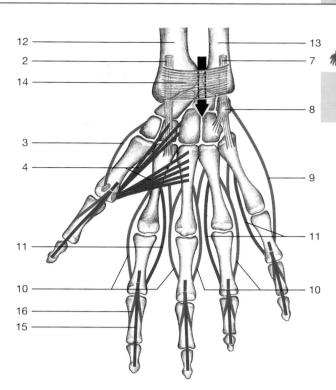

Actions of interosseous muscles in abduction and adduction of fingers (palmar aspect, schematic drawing).
Arrow: carpal tunnel.
Red = abduction (dorsal interosseous, abductor digiti minimi, and abductor pollicis brevis muscles)
Blue = adduction (palmar interosseous muscles, adductor pollicis muscle)

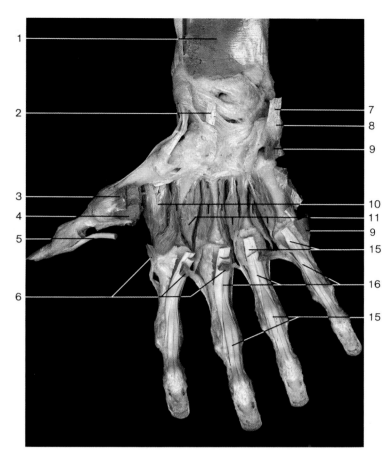

Muscles of right hand, deep layer (palmar aspect). The thenar and hypothenar muscles have been removed to display the interosseous muscles.

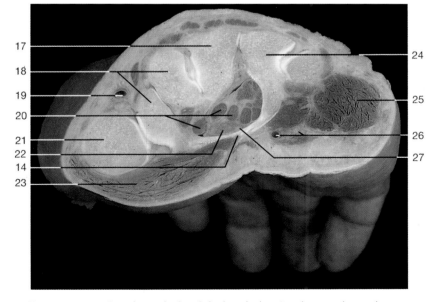

Transverse section through the right hand, showing the carpal tunnel (canalis carpi).

1   Pronator quadratus muscle
2   Tendon of flexor carpi radialis muscle
3   Abductor pollicis brevis muscle (divided)
4   Adductor pollicis muscle (divided)
5   Tendon of flexor pollicis longus muscle
6   Lumbrical muscles (cut)
7   Tendon of flexor carpi ulnaris muscle
8   Pisiform bone
9   Abductor digiti minimi muscle (divided)
10 Dorsal interosseous muscles
11 Palmar interosseous muscles
12 Radius
13 Ulna
14 Flexor retinaculum
15 Tendons of flexor digitorum profundus muscle
16 Tendons of flexor digitorum superficialis muscle
17 Capitate bone
18 Trapezium bone and trapezoid bone
19 Radial artery
20 Tendon of flexor muscles
21 First metacarpal bone
22 Median nerve
23 Thenar muscles
24 Hamate bone
25 Hypothenar muscles
26 Ulnar artery and nerve
27 Carpal tunnel (canalis carpi)

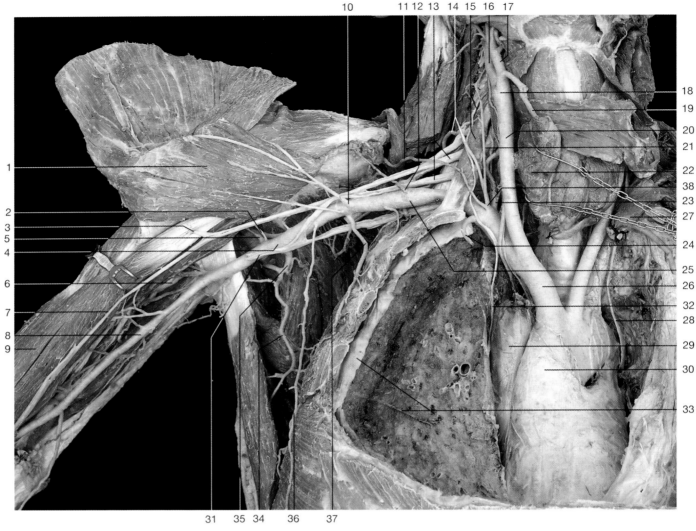

Main branches of right subclavian and axillary arteries (anterior aspect). Pectoralis muscles have been reflected, clavicle and anterior wall of thorax removed, and right lung divided. Left lung with pleura and thyroid gland have been reflected laterally to display aortic arch and common carotid artery with their branches.

1	Pectoralis minor muscle (reflected)	22	Thyroid gland
2	Anterior circumflex humeral artery	23	Inferior thyroid artery
3	Musculocutaneous nerve (divided)	24	Internal thoracic artery
4	Axillary artery	25	Right subclavian artery
5	Posterior circumflex humeral artery	26	Brachiocephalic trunk
6	Profunda brachii artery	27	Left brachiocephalic vein (divided)
7	Median nerve (var.)	28	Left vagus nerve
8	Brachial artery	29	Superior vena cava (divided)
9	Biceps brachii muscle	30	Ascending aorta
10	Thoraco-acromial artery	31	Median nerve (divided)
11	Suprascapular artery	32	Phrenic nerve
12	Descending scapular artery	33	Right lung (divided) and pulmonary pleura
13	Brachial plexus (middle trunk)	34	Thoracodorsal artery
14	Transverse cervical artery	35	Subscapular artery
15	Scalenus anterior muscle and phrenic nerve	36	Lateral mammary branches (variant)
16	Right internal carotid artery	37	Lateral thoracic artery
17	Right external carotid artery	38	Thyrocervical trunk
18	Carotid sinus	39	Superior thoracic artery
19	Superior thyroid artery	40	Superior ulnar collateral artery
20	Right common carotid artery	41	Inferior ulnar collateral artery
21	Ascending cervical artery	42	Middle collateral artery

43	Radial collateral artery
44	Radial recurrent artery
45	Radial artery
46	Anterior and posterior interosseous arteries
47	Princeps pollicis artery
48	Deep palmar arch
49	Common palmar digital arteries
50	Ulnar recurrent artery
51	Recurrent interosseous artery
52	Common interosseous artery
53	Ulnar artery
54	Superficial palmar arch
55	Median nerve and brachial artery
56	Biceps brachii muscle
57	Ulnar nerve
58	Flexor pollicis longus muscle
59	Palmar digital arteries
60	Anterior interosseous artery
61	Flexor carpi ulnaris muscle
62	Superficial palmar branch of radial artery

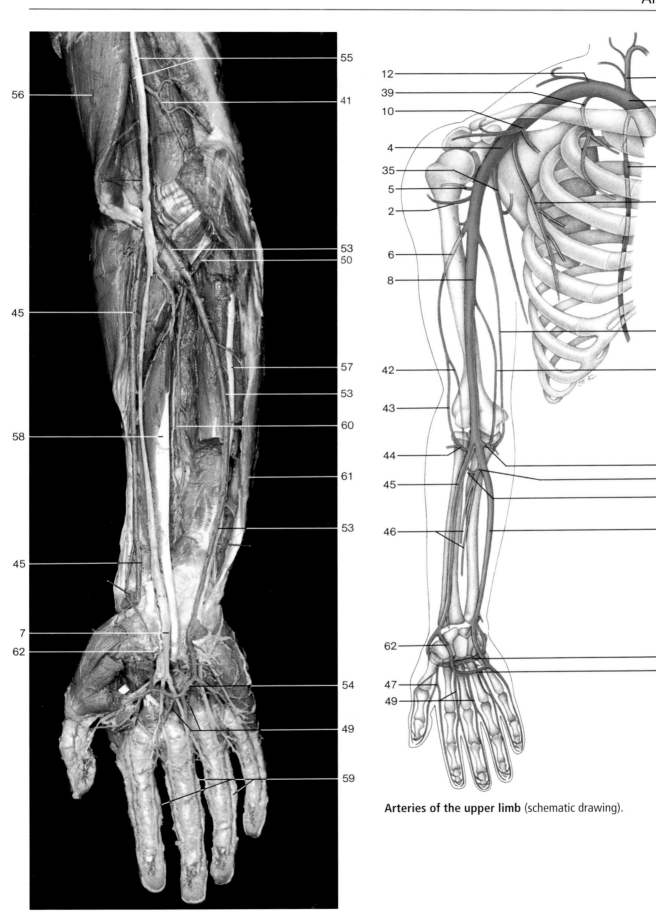

Dissection of the arteries of forearm and hand.
The superficial flexor muscles have been removed, the carpal tunnel opened, and the flexor retinaculum cut. The arteries have been filled with colored resin.

Arteries of the upper limb (schematic drawing).

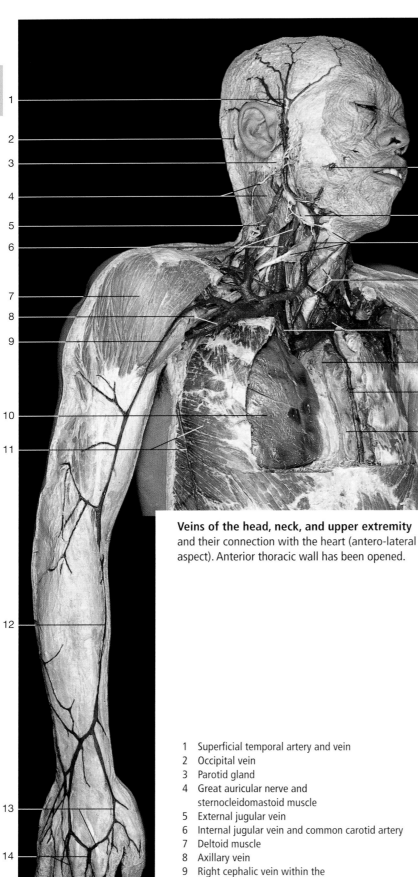

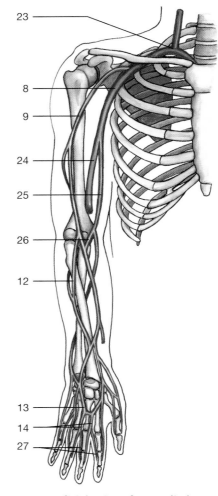

Veins of the head, neck, and upper extremity and their connection with the heart (antero-lateral aspect). Anterior thoracic wall has been opened.

Superficial veins of upper limb (schematic drawing).

1 Superficial temporal artery and vein
2 Occipital vein
3 Parotid gland
4 Great auricular nerve and sternocleidomastoid muscle
5 External jugular vein
6 Internal jugular vein and common carotid artery
7 Deltoid muscle
8 Axillary vein
9 Right cephalic vein within the deltopectoral groove
10 Right lung (middle lobe)
11 Serratus anterior muscle and lateral thoracic vein
12 Cephalic vein on forearm
13 Venous network on dorsum of hand

14 Dorsal metacarpal veins
15 Facial artery and vein
16 Submandibular gland
17 Anterior jugular vein, hyoid bone, and omohyoid muscle
18 Jugular venous arch and thyroid gland
19 Right and left brachiocephalic veins
20 Retrosternal body (remnant of thymus gland)
21 Internal thoracic artery and vein
22 Heart with pericardium
23 Right venous angle
24 Brachial vein
25 Basilic vein
26 Median cubital vein
27 Digital veins

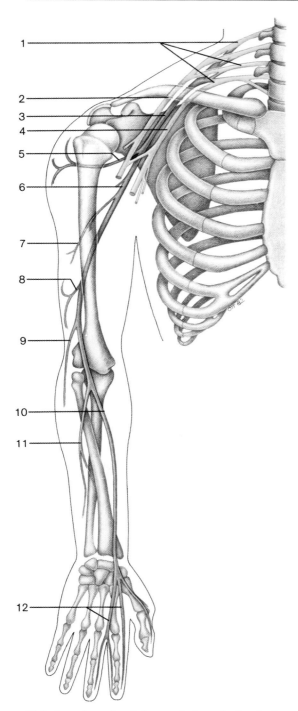

Main branches of radial nerve (schematic drawing). Posterior divisions of trunks and posterior cord and its branches are indicated in green.

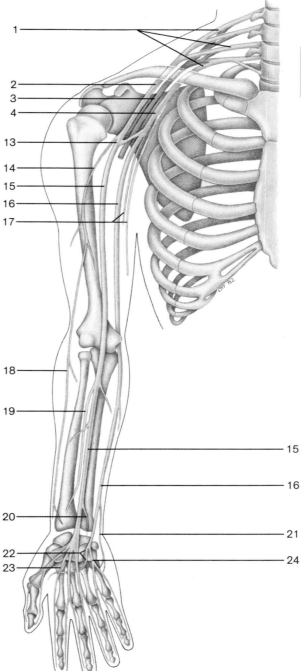

Main branches of musculocutaneous, median, and ulnar nerves (schematic drawing). Anterior divisions of the trunks and all the components arising from them are indicated in yellow.

1   Brachial plexus
2   Lateral cord of brachial plexus
3   Posterior cord of brachial plexus
4   Medial cord of brachial plexus
5   Axillary nerve
6   Radial nerve
7   Posterior cutaneous nerve of arm
8   Lower lateral cutaneous nerve of arm
9   Posterior cutaneous nerve of forearm
10 Superficial branch of radial nerve
11 Deep branch of radial nerve
12 Dorsal digital nerves

13 Roots of median nerve
14 Musculocutaneous nerve
15 Median nerve
16 Ulnar nerve
17 Medial cutaneous nerves of arm and forearm
18 Lateral cutaneous nerve of forearm
19 Anterior interosseous nerve
20 Palmar branch of median nerve
21 Dorsal branch of ulnar nerve
22 Deep branch of ulnar nerve
23 Common palmar digital nerves of median nerve
24 Superficial branch of ulnar nerve

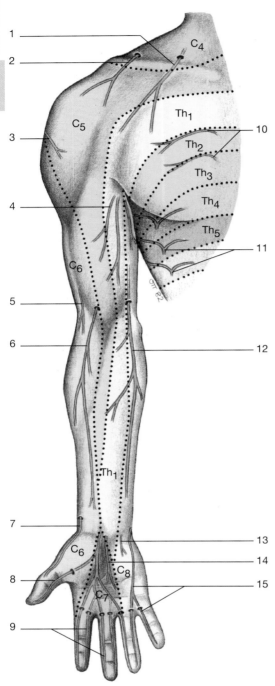

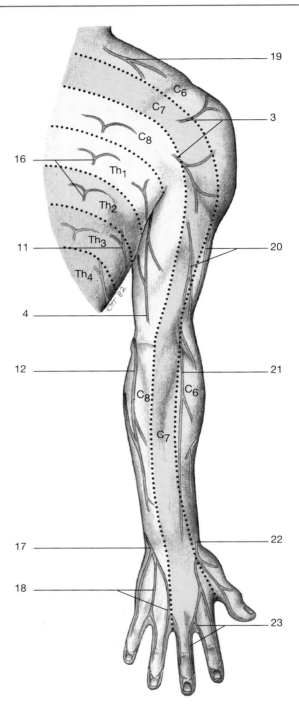

Cutaneous nerves of the right upper limb (ventral aspect, schematic drawing).

Cutaneous nerves of the right upper limb (dorsal aspect, schematic drawing).

1 Medial supraclavicular nerve
2 Intermediate supraclavicular nerve
3 Upper lateral cutaneous nerve of arm
4 Terminal branches of intercostobrachial nerves
5 Lower lateral cutaneous nerve of arm
6 Lateral cutaneous nerve of forearm
7 Terminal branch of superficial branch of radial nerve
8 Palmar digital nerve of thumb (branch of median nerve)
9 Palmar digital branches of median nerve
10 Anterior cutaneous branches of intercostal nerves
11 Lateral cutaneous branches of intercostal nerves
12 Medial cutaneous nerve of forearm

13 Palmar cutaneous branch of ulnar nerve
14 Palmar branch of median nerve
15 Palmar digital branches of ulnar nerve
16 Cutaneous branches of dorsal rami of spinal nerves
17 Dorsal branch of ulnar nerve
18 Dorsal digital nerves
19 Posterior supraclavicular nerve
20 Posterior cutaneous nerve of arm
21 Posterior cutaneous nerve of forearm
22 Superficial branch
23 Dorsal digital branches

from radial nerve

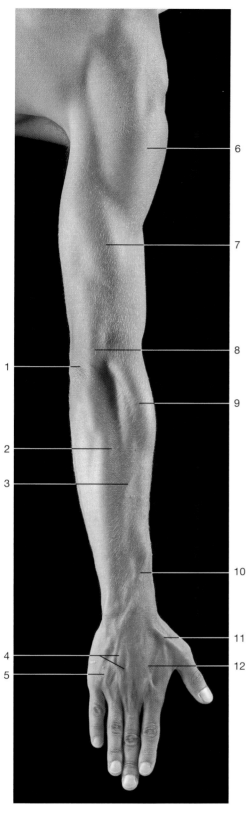

Surface anatomy of the right arm and hand (posterior aspect).

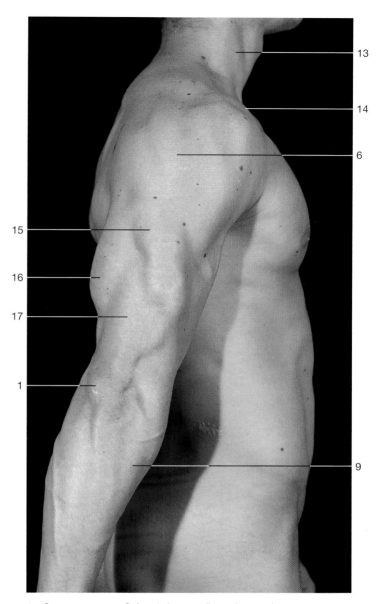

Surface anatomy of the right arm (lateral aspect).
Triceps brachii muscle is strongly contracted.

1	Olecranon	11	Tendon of abductor pollicis
2	Extensor muscles of forearm		longus muscle
3	Accessory cephalic vein	12	Tendon of extensor indicis
4	Tendons of extensor digitorum		muscle
	muscle	13	Sternocleidomastoid muscle
5	Dorsal venous network	14	Clavicle
	of hand	15	Lateral head of triceps
6	Deltoid muscle		brachii muscle
7	Triceps brachii muscle	16	Medial head of triceps
8	Lateral epicondyle of humerus		brachii muscle
9	Brachioradialis muscle	17	Tendon of triceps
10	Cephalic vein		brachii muscle

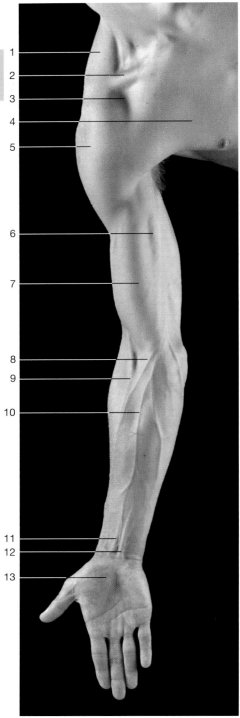

Surface anatomy of the right arm and hand (anterior aspect).

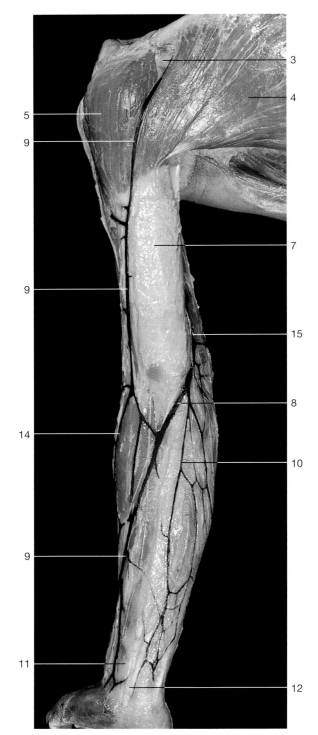

Superficial veins of the right arm, injected with blue gelatine (anterior aspect).

1   Trapezius muscle
2   Clavicle
3   Deltopectoral triangle
4   Pectoralis major muscle
5   Deltoid muscle
6   Brachial vein
7   Biceps brachii muscle

8   Median cubital vein
9   Cephalic vein
10 Median vein of forearm
11 Tendon of flexor carpi radialis
12 Tendon of palmaris longus muscle
13 Location of adductor pollicis muscle
14 Accessory cephalic vein
15 Basilic vein

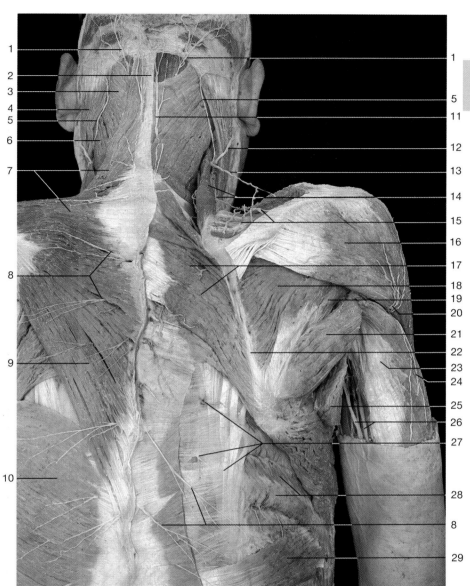

Posterior regions of neck and shoulder (dorsal aspect). Left side: superficial layer.
Right side: trapezius and latissimus dorsi muscles have been removed. Dissection of dorsal
branches of spinal nerves.

1 Greater occipital nerve	16 Deltoid muscle
2 Ligamentum nuchae	17 Rhomboid major muscle
3 Splenius capitis muscle	18 Infraspinatus muscle
4 Sternocleidomastoid muscle	19 Teres minor muscle
5 Lesser occipital nerve	20 Upper lateral cutaneous nerve of arm (branch of axillary nerve)
6 Splenius cervicis muscle	21 Teres major muscle
7 Descending and transverse fibers of trapezius muscle	22 Medial margin of scapula
8 Medial cutaneous branches of dorsal rami of spinal nerves	23 Long head of triceps muscle
9 Ascending fibers of trapezius muscle	24 Posterior cutaneous nerve of arm (branch of radial nerve)
10 Latissimus dorsi muscle	25 Latissimus dorsi muscle (divided)
11 Cutaneous branch of third occipital nerve	26 Ulnar nerve and brachial artery
12 Great auricular nerve	27 Lateral cutaneous branches of dorsal rami of spinal nerves and iliocostalis thoracis muscle
13 Accessory nerve (n. XI)	28 External intercostal muscle and seventh rib
14 Posterior supraclavicular nerve and levator scapulae muscle	29 Serratus posterior inferior muscle
15 Branches of suprascapular artery	

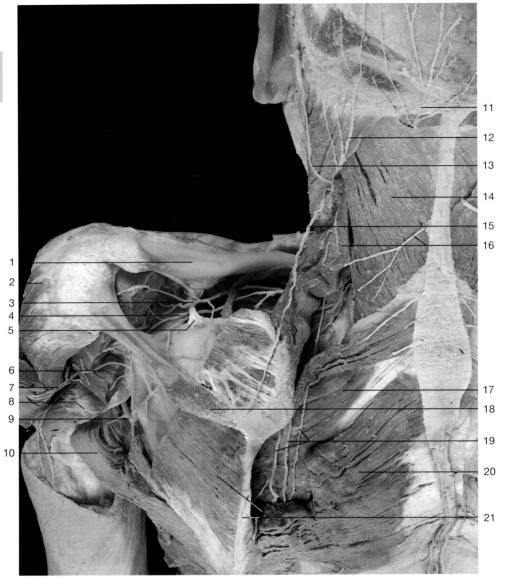

1	Clavicle
2	Deltoid muscle
3	Suprascapular artery
4	Suprascapular nerve
5	Superior transverse scapular ligament
6	Teres minor muscle
7	Axillary nerve and posterior circumflex humeral artery
8	Long head of triceps muscle
9	Circumflex scapular artery
10	Teres major muscle
11	Greater occipital nerve
12	Lesser occipital nerve
13	Great auricular nerve
14	Splenius capitis muscle
15	Accessory nerve (n. XI)
16	Third occipital nerve and levator scapulae muscle
17	Serratus posterior superior muscle
18	Spine of scapula
19	Descending scapular artery and dorsal scapular nerve
20	Rhomboid major muscle
21	Infraspinatus muscle and medial margin of scapula
22	Radial nerve and profunda brachii artery
23	Thoracodorsal artery
24	Thyrocervical trunk
25	Roots of brachial plexus

Posterior region of shoulder, deepest layer. Rhomboid and scapular muscles fenestrated; posterior part of deltoid muscle reflected.

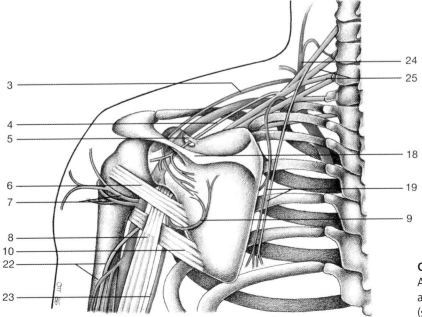

Collateral circulation of shoulder.
Anastomosis of suprascapular
and circumflex scapular arteries
(schematic drawing).

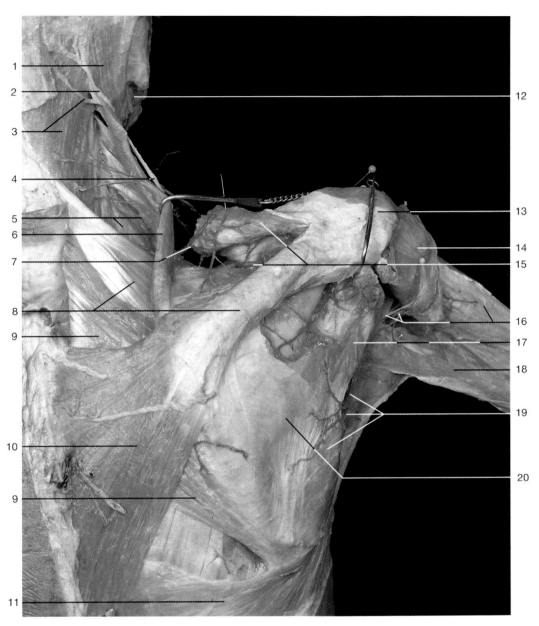

Posterior region of shoulder, deep layer. Arteries of scapular region are injected. Trapezius, deltoid, and infraspinatus muscles are partially removed or reflected.

1 Sternocleidomastoid muscle
2 Lesser occipital nerve
3 Splenius capitis muscle and third occipital nerve
4 Accessory nerve (n. XI)
5 Splenius cervicis muscle and transverse cervical artery (deep branch)
6 Levator of scapula muscle
7 Transverse cervical artery (superficial branch)
8 Spine of scapula and serratus posterior superior muscle
9 Rhomboid major muscle
10 Trapezius muscle
11 Latissimus dorsi muscle
12 Facial artery
13 Acromion
14 Deltoid muscle
15 Suprascapular artery and supraspinatus muscle (reflected)
16 Axillary nerve, posterior circumflex humeral artery, and lateral head of triceps brachii muscle
17 Teres minor muscle
18 Long head of triceps brachii muscle
19 Circumflex scapular artery and teres major
20 Infraspinatus muscle

1 Trapezius muscle
2 Posterior supraclavicular nerve
3 Middle supraclavicular nerve
4 Deltopectoral triangle
5 Deltoid muscle
6 Cephalic vein within the deltopectoral groove
7 Upper lateral cutaneous nerve of arm (branch of axillary nerve)
8 Latissimus dorsi muscle
9 Cephalic vein
10 Biceps brachii muscle
11 Triceps brachii muscle
12 Lateral cutaneous branches of intercostal nerves
13 Transverse cervical nerve and external jugular vein
14 Sternocleidomastoid muscle
15 Anterior jugular vein
16 Anterior supraclavicular nerve
17 Clavicle
18 Clavicular part of pectoralis major muscle
19 Sternocostal part of pectoralis major muscle
20 Perforating branch of internal thoracic artery
21 Anterior cutaneous branches of intercostal nerves
22 Abdominal part of pectoralis major muscle
23 Sternocleidomastoid muscle, cervical branch of facial nerve, and anterior jugular vein
24 External jugular vein and transverse cervical nerve (inferior branch)
25 Sternoclavicular joint (opened) with articular disc
26 Pectoralis major muscle
27 Omohyoid muscle and external jugular vein
28 Jugular venous arch and sternohyoid muscle
29 Sternoclavicular joint (not opened)

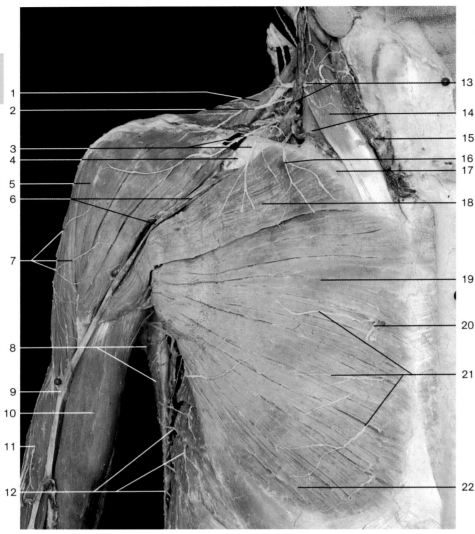

Right shoulder and thoracic wall, superficial layer (anterior aspect). Dissection of the cutaneous nerves and veins.

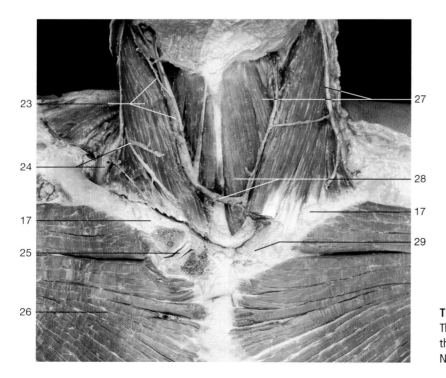

Thoracic wall with neck region (anterior aspect). The sternoclavicular joint is depicted. On the right side the joint has been opened by a coronal section. Note the articular disc.

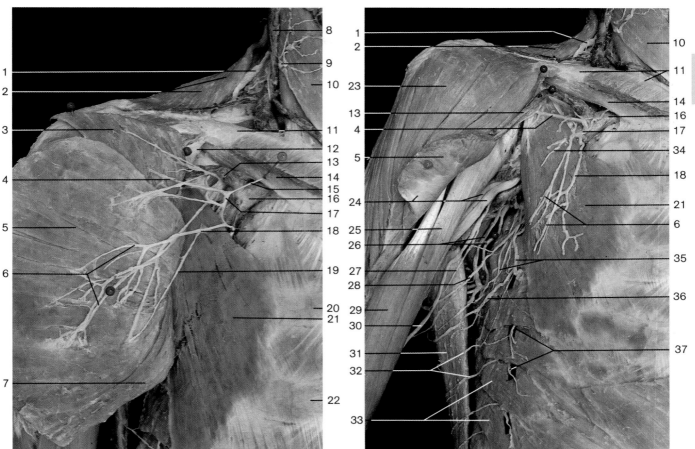

Right deltopectoral triangle, infraclavicular region
(anterior aspect). The pectoralis major muscle has been cut and reflected.

Right shoulder and thoracic wall with axillary region, deep layer (anterior aspect). The pectoralis major muscle has been cut and partly removed.

1 Accessory nerve
2 Trapezius muscle
3 Pectoralis major muscle (clavicular part)
4 Acromial branch of thoraco-acromial artery
5 Pectoralis major muscle
6 Lateral pectoral nerves
7 Abdominal part of pectoralis major muscle
8 External jugular vein
9 Cutaneous branches of cervical plexus
10 Sternocleidomastoid muscle
11 Clavicle
12 Clavipectoral fascia
13 Cephalic vein
14 Subclavius muscle
15 Clavicular branch of thoraco-acromial artery
16 Subclavian vein
17 Thoraco-acromial artery
18 Pectoral branch of thoraco-acromial artery
19 Medial pectoral nerve
20 Second rib

21 Pectoralis minor muscle
22 Third rib
23 Deltoid muscle
24 Pectoralis major muscle (reflected), brachial artery, and median nerve
25 Short head of biceps brachii muscle
26 Thoracodorsal artery and nerve
27 Medial cutaneous nerve of arm
28 Intercostobrachial nerve (T_2)
29 Long head of biceps brachii muscle
30 Medial cutaneous nerve of forearm
31 Latissimus dorsi muscle
32 Lateral cutaneous branches of intercostal nerves (posterior branches)
33 Serratus anterior muscle
34 Medial pectoral nerve
35 Long thoracic nerve and lateral thoracic artery
36 Intercostobrachial nerve (T_3)
37 Lateral cutaneous branches of intercostal nerves (anterior branches)

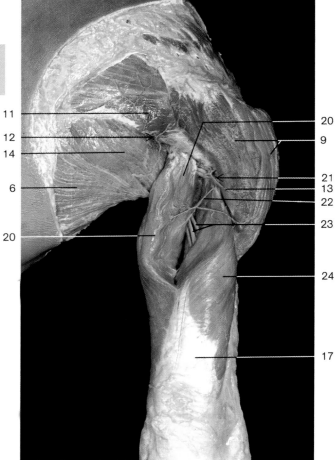

Shoulder and arm (dorsal aspect). Dissection of the quadrangular and triangular spaces of the axillary region.

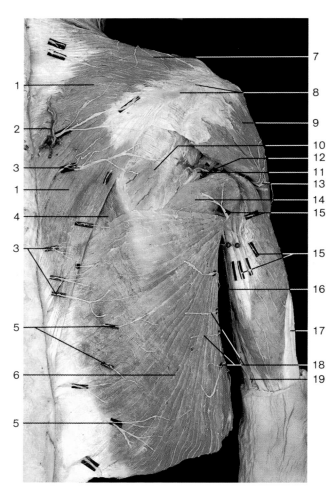

Posterior region of shoulder and arm, superficial layer. Note the segmental arrangement of the cutaneous nerves of the back.

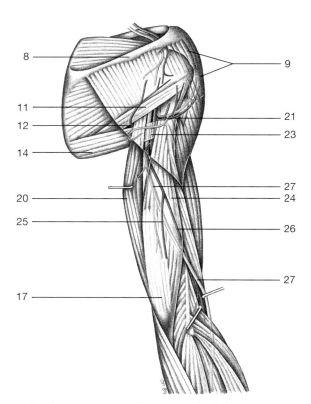

Regional anatomy of the upper limb (dorsal aspect). Localization of vessels and nerves.

1   Trapezius muscle
2   Dorsal branches of posterior intercostal artery and vein (medial cutaneous branches)
3   Medial branches of dorsal rami of spinal nerves
4   Rhomboid major muscle
5   Lateral branches of dorsal rami of spinal nerves
6   Latissimus dorsi muscle
7   Posterior supraclavicular nerves
8   Spine of scapula
9   Deltoid muscle
10   Infraspinatus muscle
11   Teres minor muscle
12   Triangular space with circumflex scapular artery and vein
13   Upper lateral cutaneous nerve of arm with artery
14   Teres major muscle
15   Terminal branches of intercostobrachial nerve
16   Medial cutaneous nerve of arm
17   Tendon of triceps brachii muscle
18   Lateral cutaneous branches of intercostal nerves
19   Medial cutaneous nerve of forearm
20   Long head of triceps brachii muscle
21   Quadrangular space with axillary nerve and posterior humeral circumflex artery
22   Anastomosis between profunda brachii artery and posterior humeral circumflex artery
23   Course of radial nerve and profunda brachii artery
24   Lateral head of triceps brachii muscle
25   Medial collateral artery
26   Radial collateral artery
27   Radial nerve

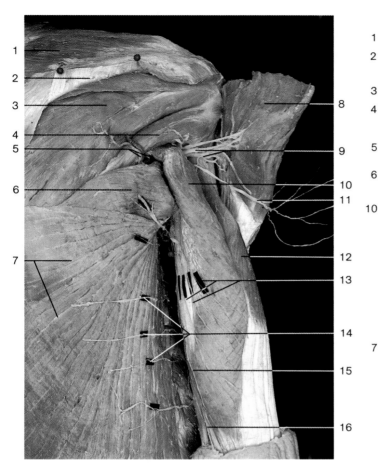

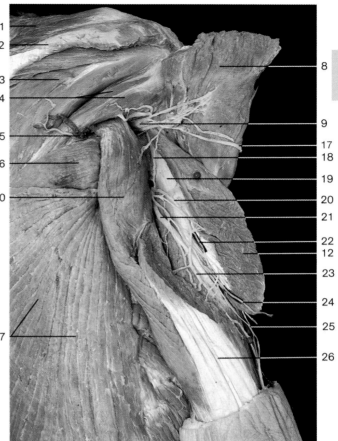

Scapular region, arm and shoulder, deep layer (dorsal aspect). Part of deltoid muscle has been cut and reflected to display the quadrangular and triangular spaces of the axillary region.

Scapular region, arm and shoulder, deep layer (dorsal aspect). The lateral head of the triceps brachii muscle has been cut to display the radial nerve and accompanying vessels.

1 Trapezius muscle
2 Spine of scapula
3 Infraspinatus muscle
4 Teres minor muscle
5 Triangular space containing circumflex scapular artery and vein
6 Teres major muscle
7 Latissimus dorsi muscle
8 Deltoid muscle (cut and reflected)
9 Quadrangular space containing axillary nerve and posterior circumflex humeral artery and vein
10 Long head of triceps brachii muscle
11 Cutaneous branch of axillary nerve
12 Lateral head of triceps brachii muscle
13 Terminal branches of intercostobrachial nerve

14 Lateral cutaneous branches of intercostal nerves
15 Medial cutaneous nerve of arm
16 Medial cutaneous nerve of forearm
17 Upper lateral cutaneous nerve of arm
18 Anastomosis between profunda brachii artery and posterior humeral circumflex artery
19 Humerus
20 Profunda brachii artery
21 Radial nerve
22 Radial collateral artery
23 Middle collateral artery
24 Lower lateral cutaneous nerve of arm
25 Posterior cutaneous nerve of forearm
26 Tendon of triceps brachii muscle

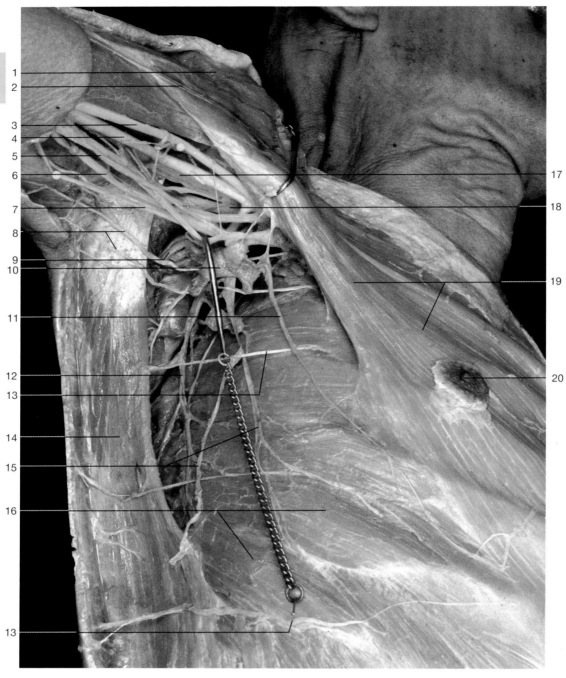

Right axillary region (inferior aspect). **Dissection of superficial axillary nodes and lymphatic vessels.**
The pectoralis major muscle has been slightly elevated.

1	Deltoid muscle	11	Lateral thoracic artery
2	Cephalic vein	12	Thoracodorsal artery
3	Median nerve	13	Lateral cutaneous branch of intercostal nerve
4	Brachial artery	14	Latissimus dorsi muscle
5	Medial cutaneous nerves of arm and forearm	15	Thoraco-epigastric vein
6	Ulnar nerve	16	Serratus anterior muscle
7	Basilic vein	17	Musculocutaneous nerve
8	Intercostobrachial nerves	18	Radial nerve
9	Circumflex scapular artery	19	Pectoralis major muscle
10	Superficial axillary nodes	20	Nipple

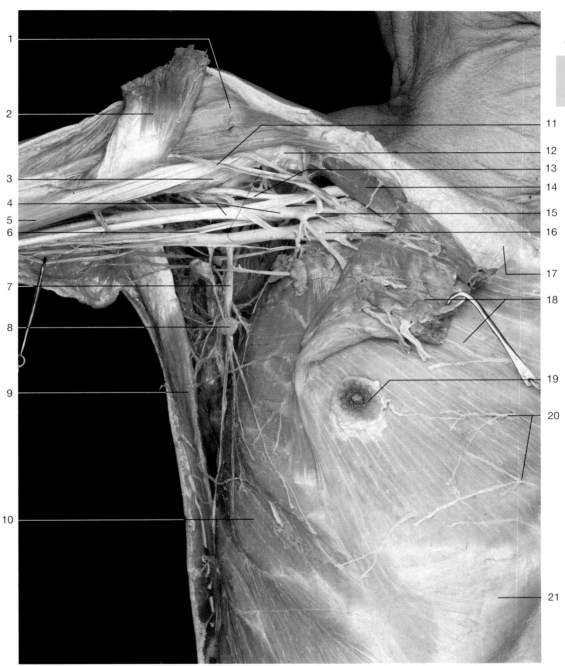

Right axillary region (anterior aspect). **Dissection of deep axillary nodes.** Pectoralis major and minor muscles divided and reflected. Shoulder girdle and arm elevated and reflected.

1 Deltoid muscle
2 Insertion of pectoralis major muscle
3 Coracobrachialis muscle
4 Roots of median nerve, axillary artery
5 Short head of biceps brachii muscle
6 Ulnar nerve and medial cutaneous nerve of forearm
7 Thoraco-epigastric vein
8 Deep axillary node
9 Latissimus dorsi muscle
10 Serratus anterior muscle

11 Cephalic vein
12 Insertion of pectoralis minor muscle (coracoid process)
13 Musculocutaneous nerve
14 Subclavius muscle
15 Thoraco-acromial artery
16 Axillary vein
17 Clavicle
18 Pectoralis major and minor muscles (reflected)
19 Nipple
20 Anterior cutaneous branches of intercostal nerves
21 Anterior layer of rectus sheath

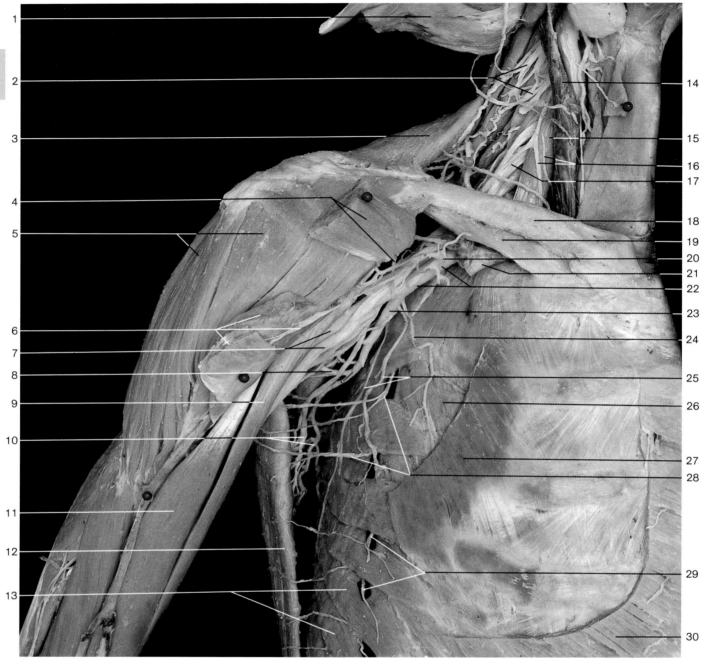

Right axillary region (anterior aspect). The pectoralis major and minor muscles have been cut and reflected to display the vessels and nerves of the axilla.

1 Sternocleidomastoid muscle (cut and reflected)
2 Cervical plexus
3 Trapezius muscle
4 Pectoralis minor muscle and medial pectoral nerve
5 Deltoid muscle
6 Pectoralis major muscle and lateral pectoral nerve
7 Median nerve and brachial artery
8 Circumflex scapular artery
9 Short head of biceps brachii muscle
10 Thoracodorsal artery and nerve
11 Long head of biceps brachii muscle
12 Latissimus dorsi muscle
13 Serratus anterior muscle
14 Internal jugular vein
15 Scalenus anterior muscle

16 Phrenic nerve and ascending cervical artery
17 Brachial plexus (at the levels of the trunks)
18 Clavicle
19 Subclavius muscle
20 Thoraco-acromial artery
21 Subclavian vein (cut)
22 Axillary artery
23 Subscapular artery
24 Superior thoracic artery
25 Lateral thoracic artery and long thoracic nerve
26 External intercostal muscle
27 Insertion of pectoralis minor muscle
28 Intercostobrachial nerves
29 Lateral cutaneous branches of intercostal nerves
30 Insertion of pectoralis major muscle

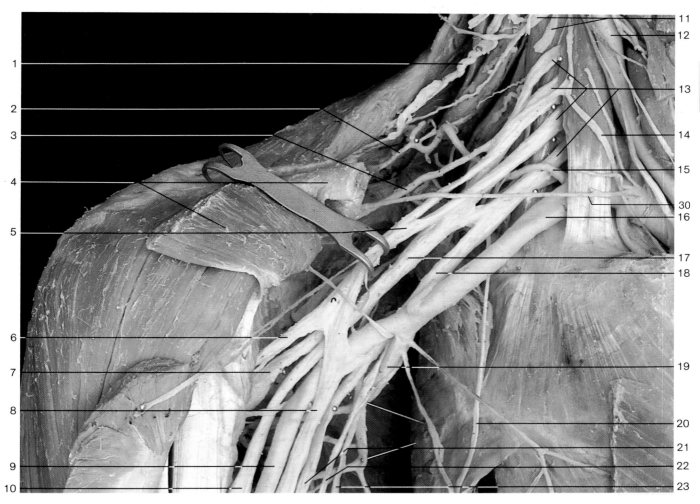

Brachial plexus (anterior aspect). Clavicle and the two pectoralis muscles have been partly removed.

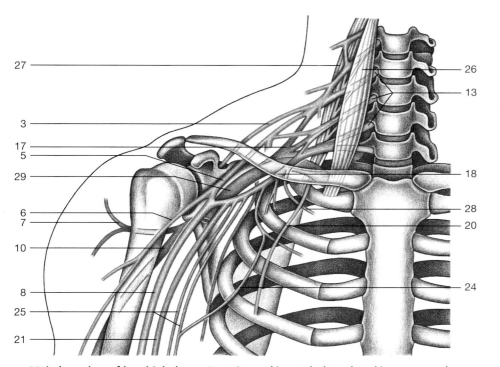

Main branches of brachial plexus. Posterior cord in purple, lateral cord in orange, and medial cord in green (schematic drawing).

1 Accessory nerve
2 Dorsal scapular artery
3 Suprascapular nerve
4 Clavicle and pectoralis minor muscle
5 Lateral cord of brachial plexus
6 Musculocutaneous nerve
7 Axillary nerve
8 Median nerve
9 Brachial artery
10 Radial nerve
11 Cervical plexus
12 Common carotid artery
13 Roots of brachial plexus (C_5–T_1)
14 Phrenic nerve
15 Transverse cervical artery
16 Subclavian artery
17 Posterior cord of brachial plexus
18 Medial cord of brachial plexus
19 Subscapular artery
20 Long thoracic nerve
21 Ulnar nerve
22 Medial cutaneous nerve of forearm
23 Thoracodorsal nerve
24 Intercostobrachial nerve
25 Medial cutaneous nerves of arm and forearm
26 Scalenus anterior muscle
27 Scalenus medius muscle
28 Intercostal nerve (T_1)
29 Axillary artery
30 Suprascapular artery

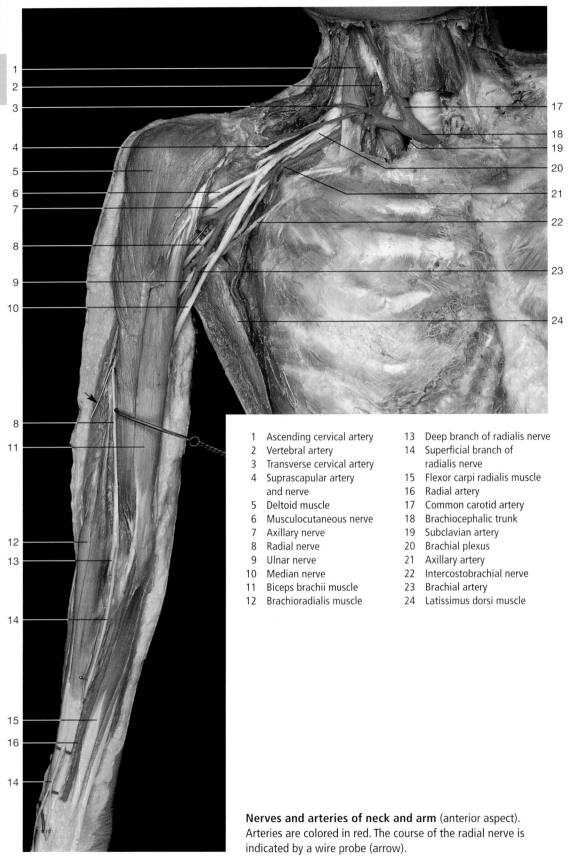

1 Ascending cervical artery	13 Deep branch of radialis nerve
2 Vertebral artery	14 Superficial branch of
3 Transverse cervical artery	radialis nerve
4 Suprascapular artery	15 Flexor carpi radialis muscle
and nerve	16 Radial artery
5 Deltoid muscle	17 Common carotid artery
6 Musculocutaneous nerve	18 Brachiocephalic trunk
7 Axillary nerve	19 Subclavian artery
8 Radial nerve	20 Brachial plexus
9 Ulnar nerve	21 Axillary artery
10 Median nerve	22 Intercostobrachial nerve
11 Biceps brachii muscle	23 Brachial artery
12 Brachioradialis muscle	24 Latissimus dorsi muscle

Nerves and arteries of neck and arm (anterior aspect).
Arteries are colored in red. The course of the radial nerve is
indicated by a wire probe (arrow).

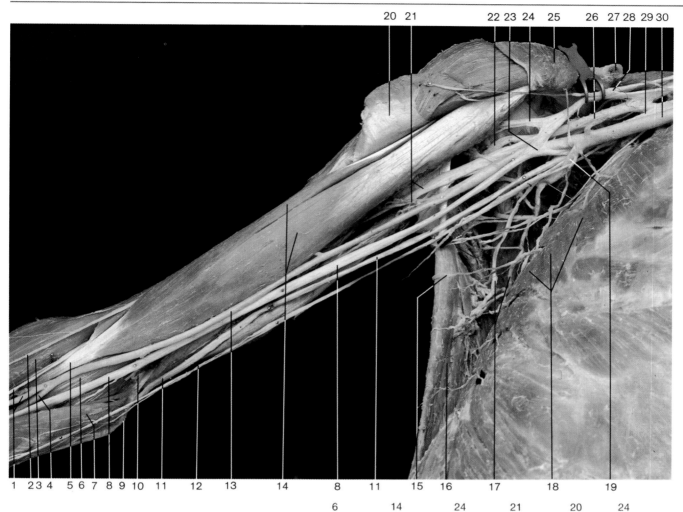

Right arm. Dissection of vessels and nerves (medial aspect). Shoulder girdle has been reflected slightly.

Right arm. Dissection of vessels and nerves, deeper layer. Biceps muscle has been reflected.

1	Radial artery and superficial branch of radial nerve	8	Median nerve
2	Lateral cutaneous nerve of forearm	9	Medial epicondyle of humerus
3	Brachioradialis muscle	10	Inferior ulnar collateral artery
4	Ulnar artery	11	Ulnar nerve
5	Tendon of biceps brachii muscle	12	Medial cutaneous nerve of forearm
6	Brachialis muscle	13	Brachial artery
7	Pronator teres muscle	14	Biceps brachii muscle
		15	Intercostobrachial nerve (T₃)
		16	Latissimus dorsi muscle

17 Thoracodorsal nerve and artery
18 Serratus anterior muscle
19 Subscapular artery
20 Pectoralis major muscle (reflected) and lateral pectoral nerve
21 Radial nerve and profunda brachii artery
22 Axillary nerve
23 Roots of the median nerve with axillary artery

24 Musculocutaneous nerve
25 Pectoralis minor muscle (reflected) and medial pectoral nerve
26 Posterior cord of brachial plexus
27 Clavicle (cut)
28 Lateral cord of brachial plexus
29 Medial cord of brachial plexus
30 Subclavian artery
31 Brachial vein

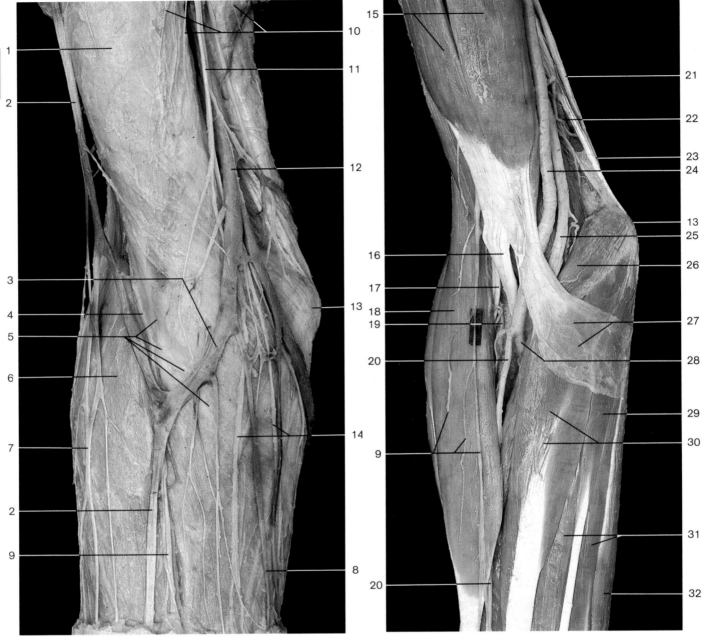

Cubital region (anterior aspect). Dissection of cutaneous nerves and veins.

Cubital region, superficial layer (anterior aspect). The fasciae of the muscles have been removed.

1   Biceps brachii muscle with fascia
2   Cephalic vein
3   Median cubital vein
4   Lateral cutaneous nerve of forearm
5   Tendon and aponeurosis of biceps brachii muscle (covered by the antebrachial fascia)
6   Brachioradialis muscle with fascia
7   Accessory cephalic vein
8   Median vein of forearm
9   Branches of lateral cutaneous nerve of forearm
10 Terminal branches of medial cutaneous nerve of arm
11 Medial cutaneous nerve of forearm
12 Basilic vein
13 Medial epicondyle of humerus
14 Terminal branches of medial cutaneous nerve of forearm
15 Biceps brachii muscle

16 Tendon of biceps brachii muscle
17 Radial nerve
18 Brachioradialis muscle
19 Radial recurrent artery
20 Radial artery
21 Ulnar nerve
22 Superior ulnar collateral artery
23 Medial intermuscular septum
24 Brachial artery
25 Median nerve
26 Pronator teres muscle
27 Bicipital aponeurosis
28 Ulnar artery
29 Palmaris longus muscle
30 Flexor carpi radialis muscle
31 Flexor digitorum superficialis muscle
32 Flexor carpi ulnaris muscle

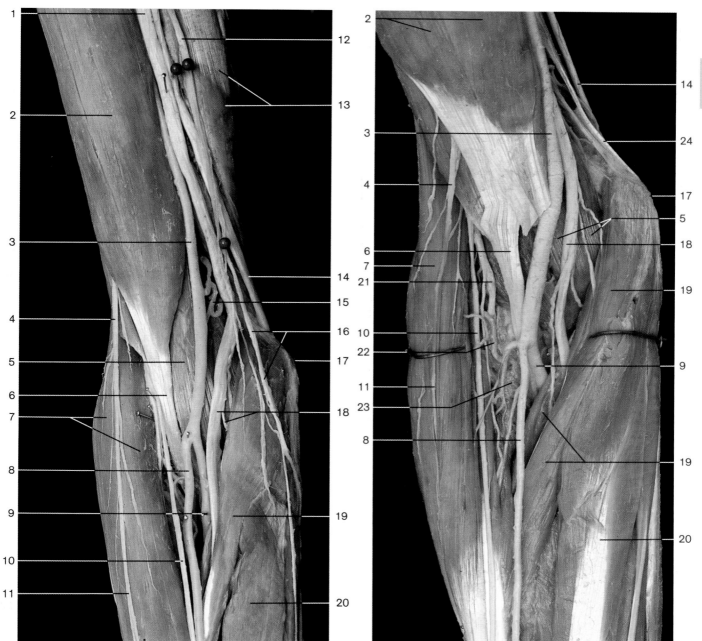

Cubital region, middle layer (anterior aspect). The bicipital aponeurosis has been removed.

Cubital region, middle layer (anterior aspect). The pronator teres and brachioradialis muscles have been slightly reflected.

1   Median nerve
2   Biceps brachii muscle
3   Brachial artery
4   Lateral cutaneous nerve of forearm
    (terminal branch of musculocutaneous nerve)
5   Brachialis muscle
6   Tendon of biceps brachii muscle
7   Brachioradialis muscle
8   Radial artery
9   Ulnar artery
10 Superficial branch of radial nerve
11 Lateral cutaneous nerve of forearm
12 Medial cutaneous nerve of forearm

13 Triceps brachii muscle
14 Ulnar nerve
15 Inferior ulnar collateral artery
16 Anterior branch of medial cutaneous nerve of forearm
17 Medial epicondyle of humerus
18 Median nerve with branches to pronator teres muscle
19 Pronator teres muscle
20 Flexor carpi radialis muscle
21 Deep branch of radial nerve
22 Radial recurrent artery
23 Supinator muscle
24 Medial intermuscular septum of arm

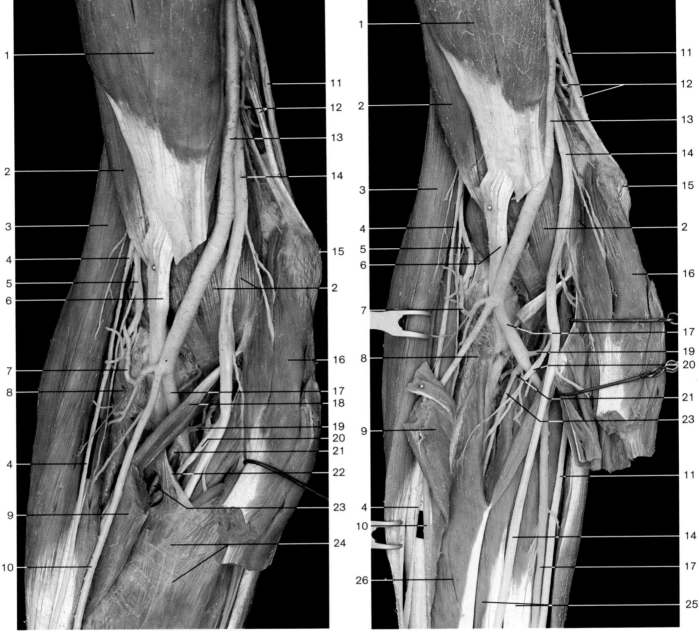

Cubital region, deep layer (anterior aspect). The pronator teres and flexor carpi ulnaris muscles have been cut and reflected.

Cubital region, deepest layer (anterior aspect). The flexor digitorum superficialis muscle and the ulnar head of the pronator teres muscle have been cut and reflected.

1   Biceps brachii muscle
2   Brachialis muscle
3   Brachioradialis muscle
4   Superficial branch of radial nerve
5   Deep branch of radial nerve
6   Tendon of biceps brachii muscle
7   Radial recurrent artery
8   Supinator muscle
9   Insertion of pronator teres muscle
10 Radial artery
11 Ulnar nerve
12 Medial intermuscular septum of arm and
    superior ulnar collateral artery
13 Brachial artery

14 Median nerve
15 Medial epicondyle of humerus
16 Humeral head of pronator teres muscle
17 Ulnar artery
18 Ulnar head of pronator teres muscle
19 Ulnar recurrent artery
20 Anterior interosseous nerve
21 Common interosseous artery
22 Tendinous arch of flexor digitorum superficialis muscle
23 Anterior interosseous artery
24 Flexor digitorum superficialis muscle
25 Flexor digitorum profundus muscle
26 Flexor pollicis longus muscle

1   Radial artery
2   Basilic vein
3   Pronator teres muscle
4   Flexor carpi radialis muscle
5   Ulnar artery
6   Palmaris longus muscle
7   Median nerve
8   Tendon of biceps brachii muscle
9   Flexor digitorum superficialis muscle
10 Ulnar nerve
11 Tendon of brachialis muscle
12 Flexor carpi ulnaris muscle
13 Flexor digitorum profundus muscle
14 Ulna
15 Median cubital vein
16 Cephalic antebrachii vein
17 Radial vein
18 Brachioradialis muscle
19 Superficial branch of radial nerve,
    radial artery and vein
20 Extensor carpi radialis longus muscle
21 Extensor carpi radialis brevis muscle
22 Supinator muscle
23 Deep branch of radial nerve
24 Radius
25 Extensor digitorum muscle
26 Extensor carpi ulnaris muscle
27 Anconeus muscle

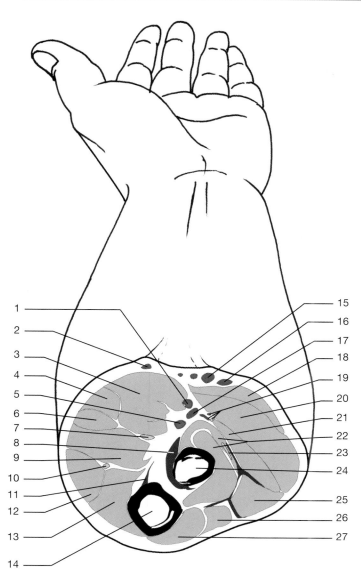

Muscles, nerves, and blood vessels of the forearm (axial section distally of the elbow joint, cf. MRI scan).

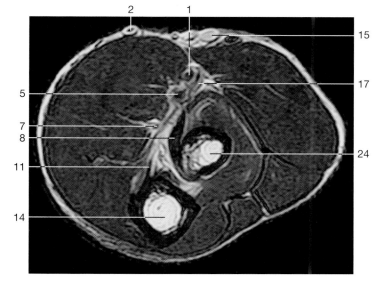

Axial section of the forearm (distally of the elbow joint, MRI scan; from Heuck et al., MRT-Atlas, 2009). For details see schematic drawing above.

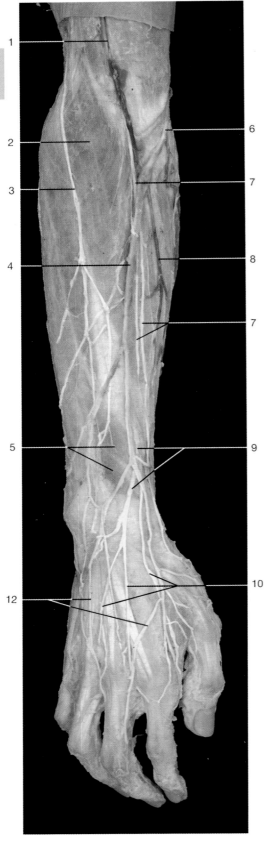

Superficial veins and cutaneous nerves of forearm and hand (posterior aspect).

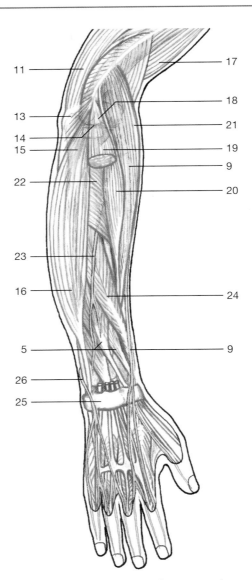

Course of the nerves to forearm and hand (posterior aspect).
Yellow = radial and ulnar nerves.

1	Cephalic vein
2	Brachioradialis muscle covered by its fascia
3	Posterior cutaneous nerve of forearm (branch of radialis nerve)
4	Cephalic vein of forearm
5	Extensor pollicis longus and brevis muscles covered by their fascia
6	Median cubital vein
7	Lateral cutaneous nerves of forearm (branch of musculocutaneous nerve)
8	Intermedian vein of forearm
9	Superficial branch of radial nerve
10	Dorsal digital branches of radial nerve
11	Triceps brachii muscle
12	Dorsal venous network of hand
13	Olecranon
14	Humeroradial joint
15	Ulna
16	Extensor carpi ulnaris muscle
17	Biceps brachii muscle
18	Trochlea of humerus
19	Extensor digitorum muscle
20	Extensor carpi radialis muscle
21	Brachioradialis muscle
22	Supinator muscle
23	Deep branch of radial nerve
24	Abductor pollicis longus muscle
25	Extensor retinaculum
26	Ulnar nerve

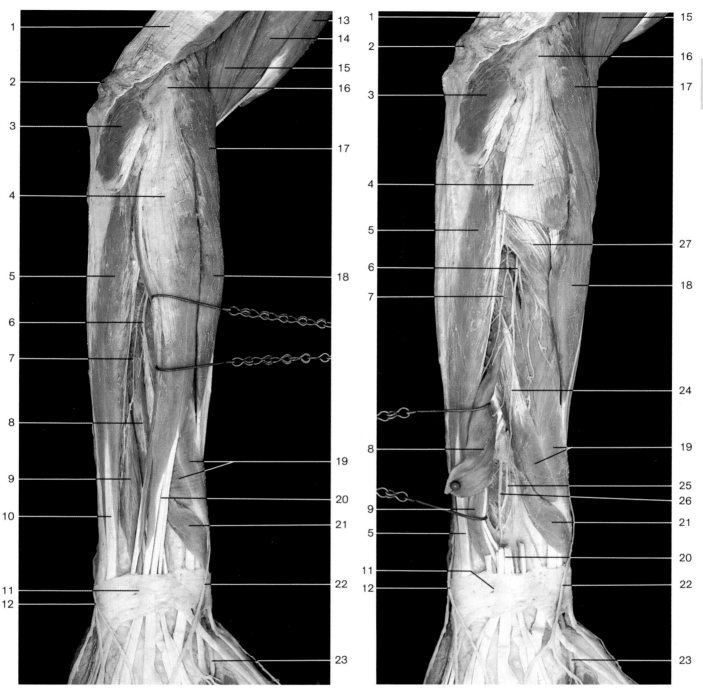

Vessels and nerves of right forearm, superficial layer
(posterior aspect).

Vessels and nerves of right forearm, deep layer
(posterior aspect).

1 Tendon of triceps brachii muscle	11 Extensor retinaculum	21 Extensor pollicis brevis muscle
2 Olecranon	12 Dorsal branch of ulnar nerve	22 Superficial branch of radial nerve
3 Anconeus muscle	13 Biceps brachii muscle	23 Radial artery
4 Extensor digitorum muscle	14 Brachialis muscle	24 Posterior interosseous nerve
5 Extensor carpi ulnaris muscle	15 Brachioradialis muscle	25 Posterior interosseous branch of
6 Deep branch of radial nerve	16 Lateral epicondyle of humerus	radial nerve
7 Posterior interosseous artery	17 Extensor carpi radialis longus muscle	26 Posterior branch of anterior
8 Extensor pollicis longus muscle	18 Extensor carpi radialis brevis muscle	interosseous artery
9 Extensor indicis muscle	19 Abductor pollicis longus muscle	27 Supinator muscle
10 Tendon of extensor carpi ulnaris muscle	20 Tendons of extensor digitorum muscle	

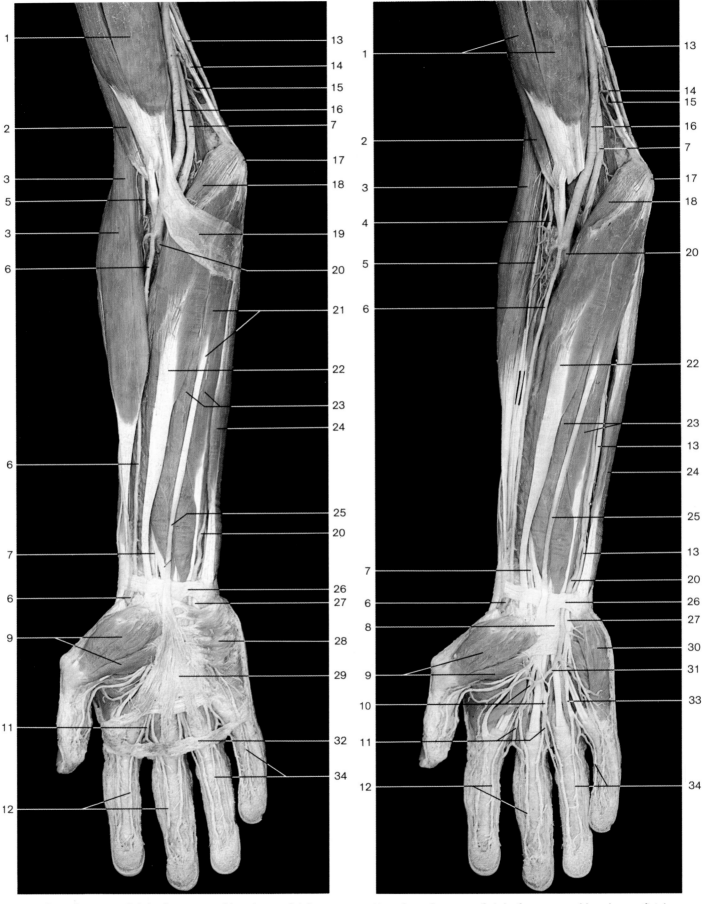

Vessels and nerves of right forearm and hand, superficial layer (palmar aspect).

Vessels and nerves of right forearm and hand, superficial layer (palmar aspect). The palmar aponeurosis of the hand and the bicipital aponeurosis have been removed.

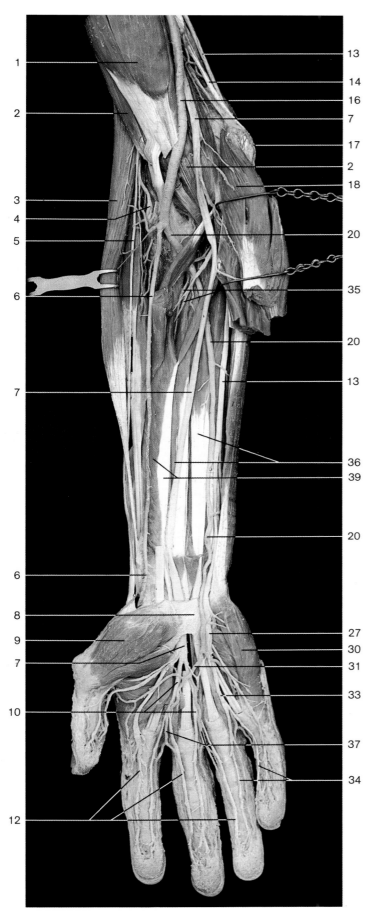

1   Biceps brachii muscle
2   Brachialis muscle
3   Brachioradialis muscle
4   Deep branch of radial nerve
5   Superficial branch of radial nerve
6   Radial artery
7   Median nerve
8   Flexor retinaculum
9   Thenar muscles
10 Common palmar digital branches of median nerve
11 Common palmar digital arteries
12 Proper palmar digital nerves (median nerve)
13 Ulnar nerve
14 Medial intermuscular septum of arm
15 Superior ulnar collateral artery
16 Brachial artery
17 Medial epicondyle of humerus
18 Pronator teres muscle
19 Bicipital aponeurosis
20 Ulnar artery
21 Palmaris longus muscle
22 Flexor carpi radialis muscle
23 Flexor digitorum superficialis muscle
24 Flexor carpi ulnaris muscle
25 Tendon of palmaris longus muscle
26 Remnant of antebrachial fascia
27 Superficial branch of ulnar nerve
28 Palmaris brevis muscle
29 Palmar aponeurosis
30 Hypothenar muscles
31 Superficial palmar arch
32 Superficial transverse metacarpal ligament
33 Common palmar digital branch of ulnar nerve
34 Proper palmar digital branches of ulnar nerve
35 Anterior interosseous artery and nerve
36 Flexor digitorum profundus muscle
37 Common palmar digital arteries
38 Palmar branch of median nerve
39 Flexor pollicis longus muscle
40 Palmar branch of ulnar nerve

Vessels and nerves of forearm and hand, deep layer (palmar aspect). The superficial layer of the flexor muscles has been removed.

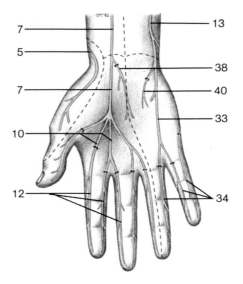

Innervation pattern of palmar surfaces of hand.
3½ digits by median nerve, 1½ digits by ulnar nerve.

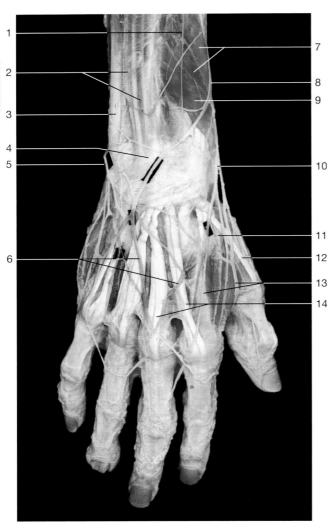

Posterior region of hand (superficial layer). Cutaneous nerves and veins are depicted.

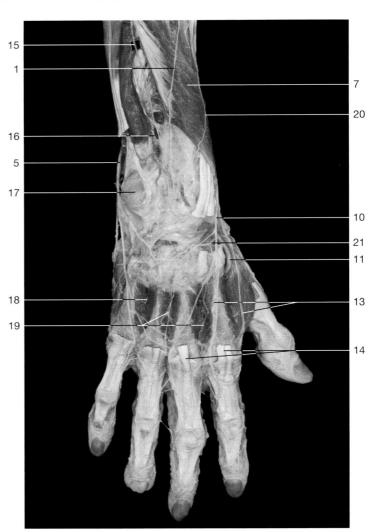

Posterior region of hand (deeper layer). Extensor digitorum muscle has been partly removed.

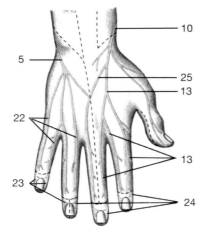

Innervation pattern of posterior surfaces of hand.
2¹/₂ digits by radial nerve, 2¹/₂ digits by ulnar nerve. Note that the terminal branches to the dorsal surfaces of the distal phalanges are derived from the palmar digital nerves. The cutaneous distribution varies; often 3¹/₂ digits are innervated by the radial and 1¹/₂ digits by the ulnar nerve.

1 Posterior cutaneous nerve of forearm (branch of radial nerve)
2 Extensor digitorum muscle
3 Tendon of extensor carpi ulnaris muscle
4 Extensor retinaculum
5 Ulnar nerve
6 Dorsal venous network of hand
7 Abductor pollicis longus muscle
8 Cephalic vein
9 Extensor pollicis brevis muscle
10 Radial nerve, superficial branch
11 Radial artery
12 Tendon of extensor pollicis longus muscle
13 Dorsal digital branches of radial nerve
14 Tendons of extensor digitorum muscle with intertendinous connections
15 Posterior interosseus nerve (branch of the deep radial nerve)
16 Posterior interosseous artery
17 Styloid process of ulna
18 Dorsal interosseus muscle IV
19 Dorsal carpal branch of radial artery
20 Lateral cutaneous nerve of forearm (branch of musculocutaneous nerve)
21 Dorsal metacarpal artery
22 Proper dorsal digital branches of ulnar nerve
23 Regions supplied by palmar digital nerves (ulnar nerve)
24 Regions supplied by palmar digital nerves (median nerve)
25 Communicating branch with ulnar nerve

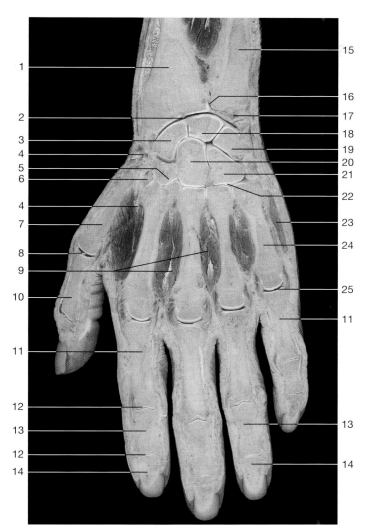

Coronal section through the left hand (posterior aspect).

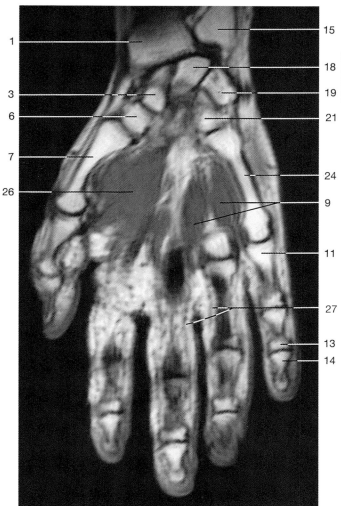

Coronal section through the left hand (posterior aspect)
(MRI scan, courtesy of Prof. Heuck, Munich).

Axial section through the left hand (MRI scan;
from Heuck et al., MRT-Atlas, 2009).

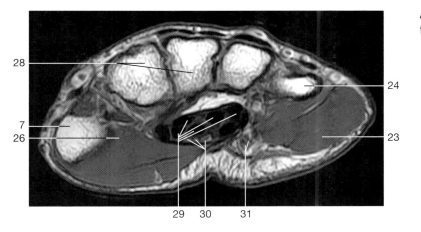

1	Radius
2	Wrist joint
3	Scaphoid (navicular) bone
4	Radial artery
5	Trapezoid bone
6	Trapezium bone
7	First metacarpal bone
8	Metacarpophalangeal joint of thumb
9	Interosseous muscles
10	Proximal phalanx of thumb
11	Proximal phalanx of fingers
12	Interphalangeal joints
13	Middle phalanx
14	Distal phalanx
15	Ulna
16	Distal radio-ulnar joint
17	Articular disc
18	Lunate bone
19	Triquetral bone
20	Capitate bone
21	Hamate bone
22	Carpometacarpal joints
23	Abductor digiti minimi muscle
24	Fifth metacarpal bone
25	Metacarpophalangeal joint
26	Adductor pollicis muscle
27	Proper palmar digital arteries
28	Second and third metacarpal bones
29	Tendons of flexor digitorum superficialis and profundus muscles
30	Median nerve
31	Ulnar artery and vein

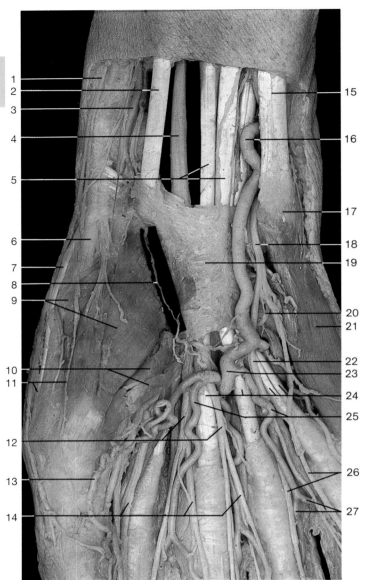

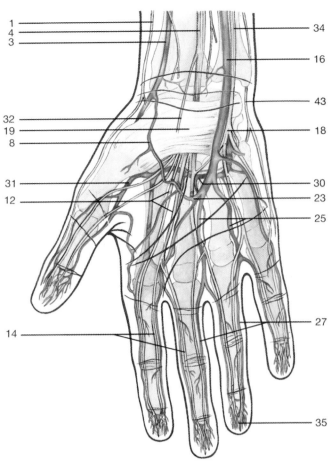

Arteries and nerves of the right hand
(palmar aspect, schematic drawing).

◁

Right hand, superficial layer (palmar aspect).
Dissection of the superficial palmar arch.

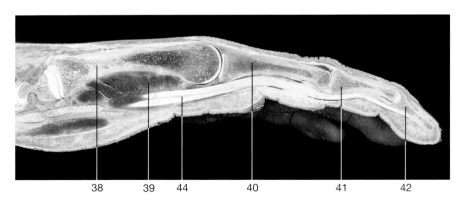

Longitudinal section through the hand
at the level of the third finger.

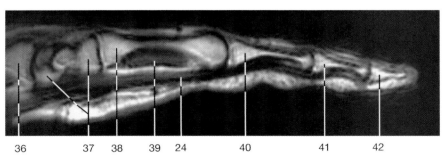

Longitudinal section through the hand
at the level of the third finger (MRI scan,
courtesy of Prof. Heuck, Munich).

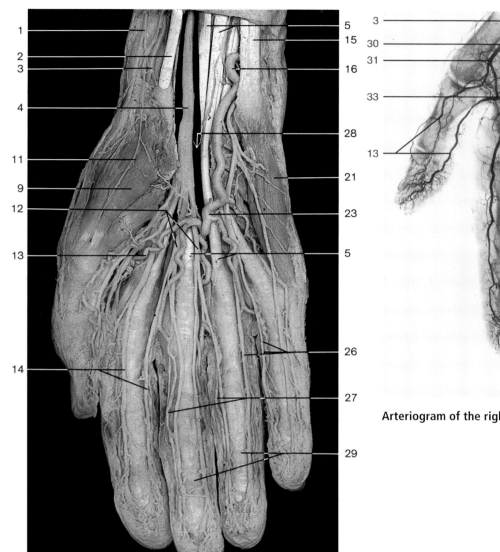

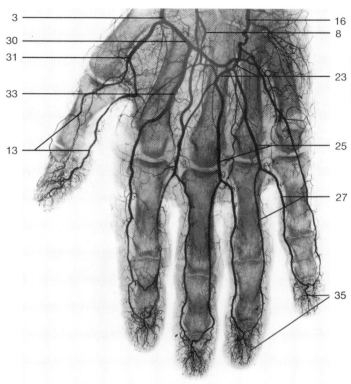

Arteriogram of the right hand (palmar aspect).

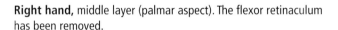

Right hand, middle layer (palmar aspect). The flexor retinaculum has been removed.

1   Superficial branch of radial nerve
2   Tendon of flexor carpi radialis muscle
3   Radial artery
4   Median nerve
5   Tendon of flexor digitorum superficialis muscle
6   Tendon of abductor pollicis longus muscle
7   Tendon of extensor pollicis brevis muscle
8   Superficial palmar branch of radial artery
9   Abductor pollicis brevis muscle
10 Superficial head of flexor pollicis brevis muscle
11 Terminal branches of superficial branch of radial nerve
12 Common palmar digital nerves (median nerve)
13 Proper palmar digital arteries of thumb
14 Proper palmar digital nerves (median nerve)
15 Tendon of flexor carpi ulnaris muscle
16 Ulnar artery
17 Position of pisiform bone
18 Superficial branch of ulnar nerve
19 Flexor retinaculum
20 Deep branch of ulnar nerve
21 Abductor digiti minimi muscle
22 Common palmar digital nerves (ulnar nerve)

23 Superficial palmar arch
24 Tendons of flexor digitorum muscles
25 Common palmar digital arteries
26 Palmar digital nerves (ulnar nerve)
27 Proper palmar digital arteries
28 Carpal tunnel
29 Fibrous sheaths for the tendons of flexor digitorum muscles
30 Deep palmar arch
31 Princeps pollicis artery
32 Palmar branch of median nerve
33 Common digital palmar artery
34 Ulnar nerve
35 Capillary network of finger
36 Radius
37 Carpal bones
38 Metacarpal bone
39 Interosseous muscles
40 Proximal phalanx
41 Middle phalanx
42 Distal phalanx
43 Dorsal branch of ulnar nerve
44 Tendons of flexor digitorum profundus (upper) and superficialis (lower) muscles

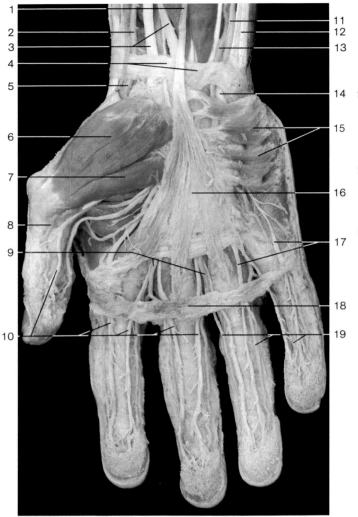

Right hand, superficial layer (palmar aspect). Dissection of vessels and nerves.

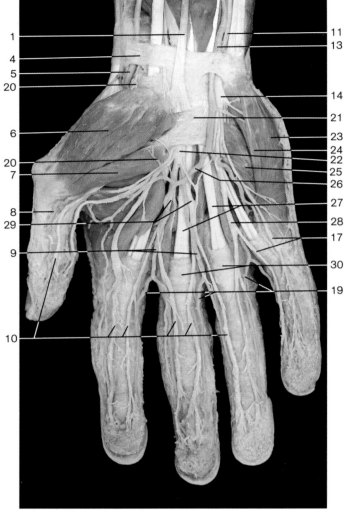

Right hand, superficial layer (palmar aspect). Dissection of vessels and nerves. The palmar aponeurosis has been removed to display the superficial palmar arch.

1	Tendon of palmaris longus muscle	17	Palmar digital nerves (ulnar nerve)
2	Radial artery	18	Superficial transverse metacarpal ligament
3	Tendon of flexor carpi radialis muscle and median nerve	19	Proper palmar digital arteries
4	Distal part of antebrachial fascia	20	Superficial palmar branch of radial artery
5	Radial artery passing into the anatomical snuffbox		(contributing to the superficial palmar arch)
6	Abductor pollicis brevis muscle	21	Flexor retinaculum
7	Superficial head of flexor pollicis brevis muscle	22	Median nerve
8	Palmar digital artery of thumb	23	Abductor digiti minimi muscle
9	Common palmar digital arteries	24	Flexor digiti minimi brevis muscle
10	Proper palmar digital nerves (median nerve)	25	Opponens digiti minimi muscle
11	Ulnar nerve	26	Superficial palmar arch
12	Tendon of flexor carpi ulnaris muscle	27	Tendons of flexor digitorum superficialis muscle
13	Ulnar artery	28	Common palmar digital branch of ulnar nerve
14	Superficial branch of ulnar nerve	29	Common palmar digital branch of median nerve
15	Palmaris brevis muscle	30	Fibrous sheath of flexor tendons
16	Palmar aponeurosis		

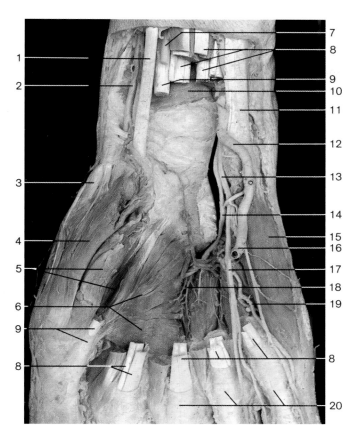

Right hand, deep layer (palmar aspect). The carpal tunnel has been opened, the tendons of the flexor muscles have been removed, and the superficial palmar arch has been cut.

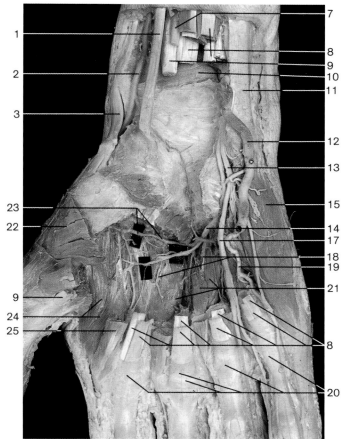

Right hand, deep layer (palmar aspect). Dissection of the deep palmar arch.

1	Tendon of flexor carpi radialis muscle	12	Ulnar artery
2	Radial artery	13	Superficial branch of ulnar nerve
3	Tendon of abductor pollicis longus muscle	14	Deep branch of ulnar nerve
4	Abductor pollicis brevis muscle	15	Abductor digiti minimi muscle
5	Superficial and deep heads of flexor pollicis brevis muscle	16	Superficial palmar arch (cut end)
6	Oblique and transverse heads of adductor pollicis muscle	17	Common palmar digital nerves (ulnar nerve)
7	Median nerve	18	Palmar metacarpal arteries of deep palmar arch
8	Tendons of flexor digitorum superficialis and profundus muscles	19	Palmar digital artery of the fifth finger
9	Tendon of flexor pollicis longus muscle	20	Fibrous sheaths of tendons of flexor muscles
10	Pronator quadratus muscle	21	Palmar interosseous muscles
11	Tendon of flexor carpi ulnaris muscle	22	Opponens pollicis muscle (cut)
		23	Deep palmar arch
		24	First dorsal interosseous muscle
		25	First lumbrical muscle

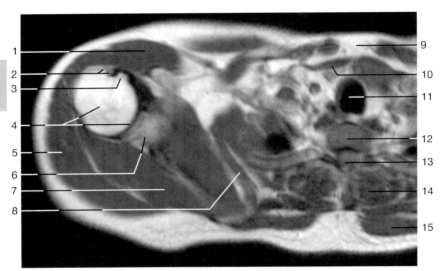

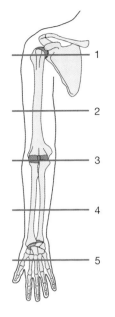

Horizontal section through the right shoulder joint (section 1; MRI scan; inferior aspect).

Upper limb, location of sections 1–5 (MRI scans, p. 430: courtesy of Prof. Heuck, Munich, Germany; MRI scans, p. 431: courtesy of Prof. Bautz and R. Janka, M. D., University of Erlangen, Germany).

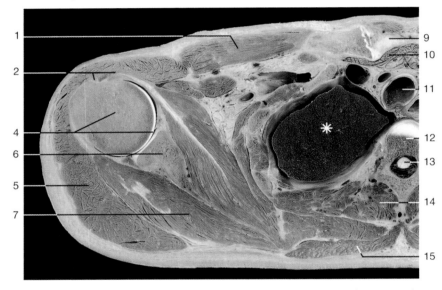

Horizontal section through the right shoulder joint (section 1; inferior aspect).
* = Upper lobe of lung.

1 Pectoralis major muscle
2 Greater tubercle and tendon of biceps muscle
3 Lesser tubercle
4 Head of humerus and articular cavity of shoulder joint
5 Deltoid muscle
6 Scapula
7 Infraspinatus muscle
8 Serratus anterior muscle
9 Sternum
10 Infrahyoid muscles
11 Trachea
12 Body of thoracic vertebra
13 Vertebral canal and spinal cord
14 Deep muscles of the back
15 Trapezius muscle
16 Brachialis muscle
17 Radial nerve and profunda brachii vessels

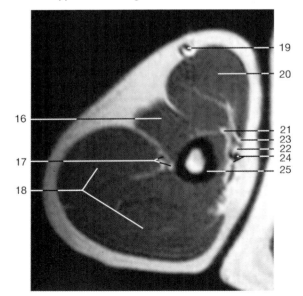

Axial section through the middle of the right arm (section 2; MRI scan; inferior aspect).

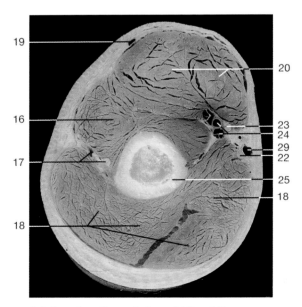

Axial section through the middle of the right arm (section 2; inferior aspect).

18 Triceps brachii muscle
19 Cephalic vein
20 Biceps brachii muscle
21 Musculocutaneous nerve
22 Ulnar nerve
23 Medianus nerve
24 Brachial artery and vein
25 Shaft of humerus
26 Brachioradialis muscle
27 Radial nerve
28 Olecranon and articular cavity
     of elbow joint
29 Basilic vein
30 Humerus
31 Pronator teres muscle
32 Extensor muscles of forearm
33 Ramus profundus of
     radialis nerve
34 Anterior interosseus
     vessels and nerve
35 Interosseous membrane
36 Ulna
37 Radius
38 Radial artery and superficial
     branch of radial nerve
39 Flexor pollicis longus muscle
40 Flexor digitorum
     superficialis and profundus
     muscles
41 Ulnar nerve, ulnar artery, and
     vein
42 Flexor carpi ulnaris muscle
43 Radial artery
44 Metacarpal bones III and IV
45 Carpal canal with tendons of
     flexor digitorum muscles
46 Hypothenar muscle
47 Median nerve
48 Interosseous muscles
49 First metacarpal bone
50 Thenar muscles
51 Articular cavity of
     humeroradial joint

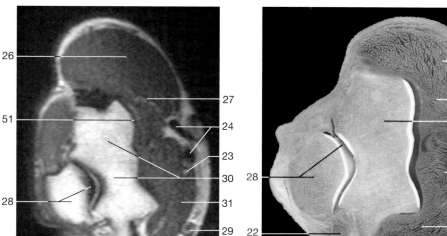

Axial section through the right elbow joint (section 3; MRI scan; inferior aspect).

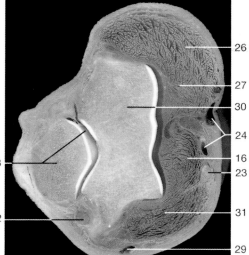

Axial section through the right elbow joint (section 3; inferior aspect).

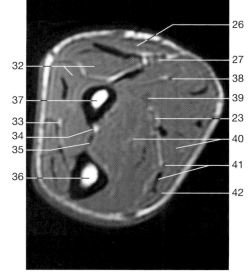

Axial section through the middle of the right forearm (section 4; MRI scan; inferior aspect).

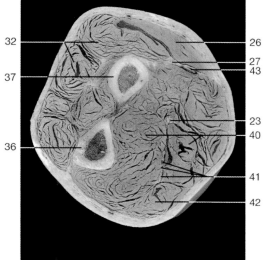

Axial section through the middle of the right forearm (section 4; inferior aspect).

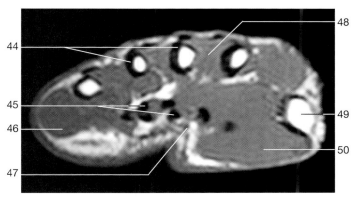

Axial section through the right hand at the level of the metacarpus (section 5; MRI scan; inferior aspect).

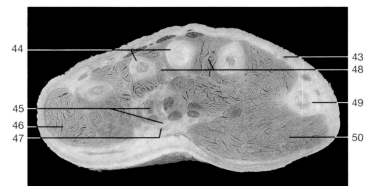

Axial section through the right hand at the level of the metacarpus (section 5; inferior aspect).

8 Lower Limb

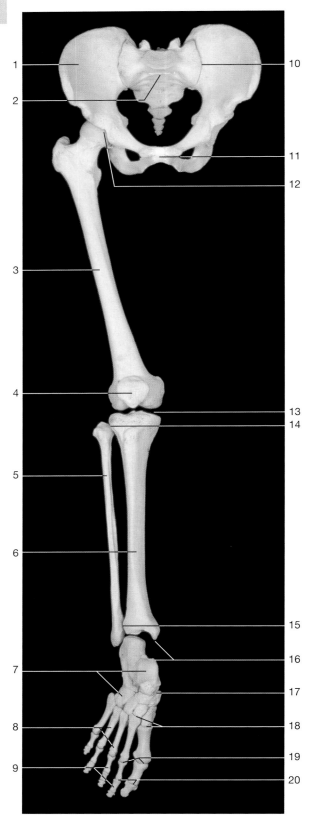

The lower limb (extremity) is specialized for support of the upright posture, locomotion, and maintaining balance. In contrast to the upper limb, the lower limb is more restricted in its movements, and the joints are tighter and fixed by strong ligaments. The hip joint is a ball-and-socket type of synovial joint between the head of the femur and acetabulum. The knee joint is a hinge type of synovial joint that permits only limited rotation. The talocrural joint is a hinge joint between the talus, fibula, and tibia, only allowing movements of flexion and extension.

The long axis of the foot is at a right angle to that of the leg, thus forming an effective arch for the upright stance of the body.

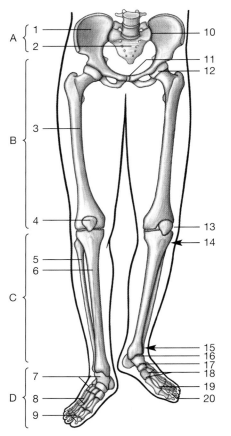

A = pelvic girdle
B = thigh
C = leg
D = foot

Organization of pelvic girdle and lower limb.

Skeleton of pelvic girdle and lower limb (anterior aspect). The ankle joint has been dislocated.

1	Right hip bone	11	Pubic symphysis
2	Sacrum	12	Hip joint
3	Femur	13	Knee joint
4	Patella	14	Proximal tibiofibular joint
5	Fibula	15	Distal tibiofibular joint
6	Tibia	16	Ankle joint
7	Tarsal bones	17	Talocalcaneonavicular joint
8	Metatarsal bones	18	Tarsometatarsal joints
9	Phalanges	19	Metatarsophalangeal joints
10	Sacro-iliac joint	20	Interphalangeal joints

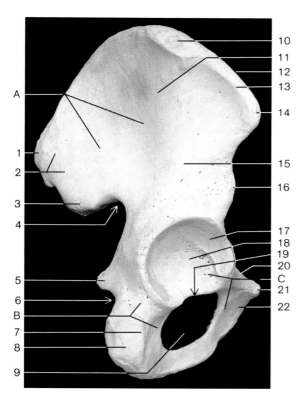

Right hip bone (lateral aspect).

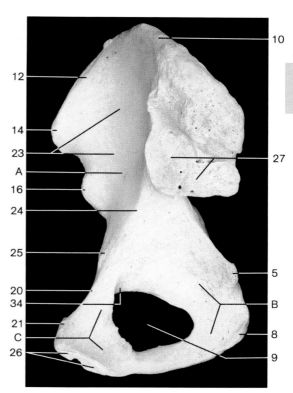

Right hip bone (medial aspect).

A = ilium
B = ischium
C = pubis

1   Posterior superior iliac spine
2   Posterior gluteal line
3   Posterior inferior iliac spine
4   Greater sciatic notch
5   Ischial spine
6   Lesser sciatic notch
7   Body of ischium
8   Ischial tuberosity
9   Obturator foramen
10   Iliac crest
11   Anterior gluteal line
12   Internal lip of iliac crest
13   External lip of iliac crest
14   Anterior superior iliac spine
15   Inferior gluteal line
16   Anterior inferior iliac spine
17   Lunate surface of acetabulum
18   Acetabular fossa
19   Acetabular notch
20   Pecten pubis
21   Pubic tubercle
22   Body of pubis
23   Iliac fossa
24   Arcuate line
25   Iliopubic eminence
26   Symphysial surface of pubis
27   Auricular surface
28   Pelvic surface of sacrum
29   Superior articular process of sacrum
30   Dorsal sacral foramina
31   Sacral tuberosity
32   Lateral sacral crest
33   Median sacral crest
34   Obturator groove
35   Coccyx

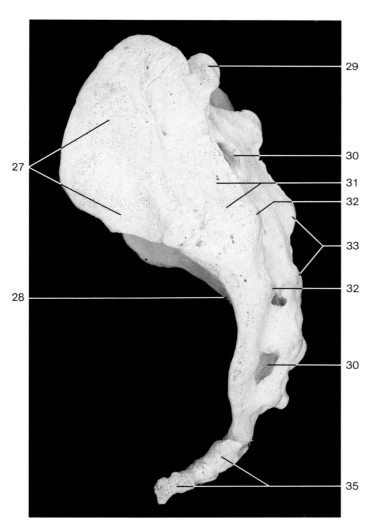

Sacrum and coccyx (lateral aspect).

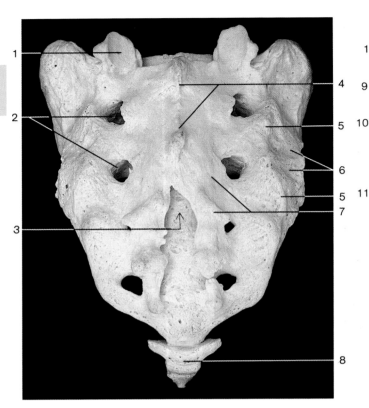

Sacrum (posterior aspect).

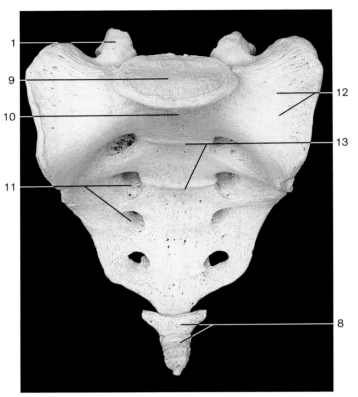

Sacrum (anterior aspect).

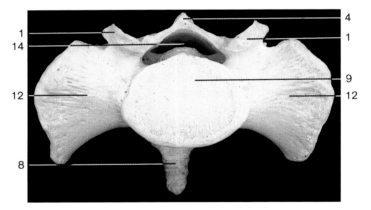

Sacrum (superior aspect).

1   Superior articular process of sacrum
2   Dorsal sacral foramina
3   Sacral hiatus
4   Median sacral crest
5   Lateral sacral crest
6   Sacral tuberosity
7   Intermediate sacral crest
8   Coccyx
9   Base of sacrum
10   Sacral promontory
11   Anterior sacral foramina
12   Lateral part of sacrum (ala)
13   Transverse line of sacrum
14   Sacral canal
15   Linea terminalis
16   True conjugate
17   Diagonal conjugate
18   Transverse diameter
19   Oblique diameter
20   Inferior pelvic aperture or outlet

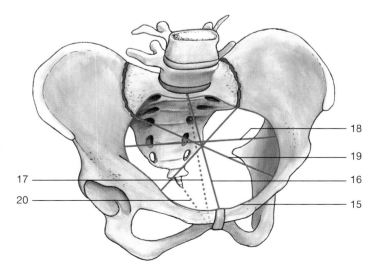

Diameters of pelvis (oblique superior aspect).
(Schematic drawing.)

The pelvic girdle is firmly connected to the vertebral column at the sacro-iliac joint. Therefore, the body can be kept upright more easily even if only one limb is used for support (as in walking). The mobility of the lower limb is more limited than that of the upper limb.

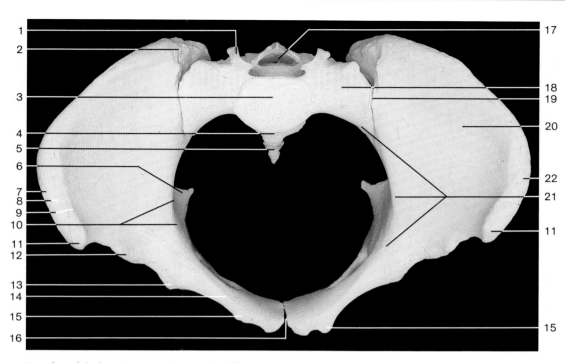

Female pelvis (superior aspect). Note the differences between the male and female pelvis, predominantly in the form and dimensions of the sacrum, the superior and inferior apertures, and the alae of the ilium.

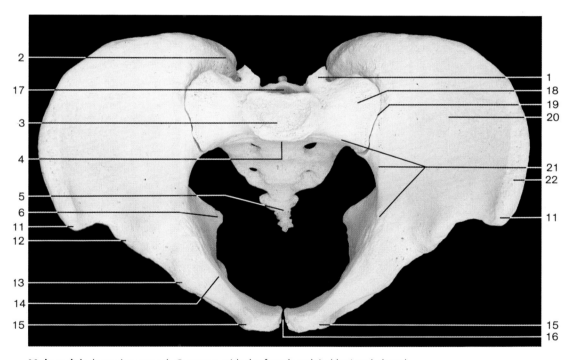

Male pelvis (superior aspect). Compare with the female pelvis (depicted above).

1	Superior articular process of sacrum	12	Anterior inferior iliac spine
2	Posterior superior iliac spine	13	Iliopubic eminence
3	Base of sacrum	14	Pecten pubis
4	Sacral promontory	15	Pubic tubercle
5	Coccyx	16	Pubic symphysis
6	Ischial spine	17	Sacral canal
7	External lip	18	Ala of sacrum
8	Intermediate line } of iliac crest	19	Position of sacro-iliac joint
9	Internal lip	20	Iliac fossa
10	Arcuate line	21	Linea terminalis
11	Anterior superior iliac spine	22	Iliac crest

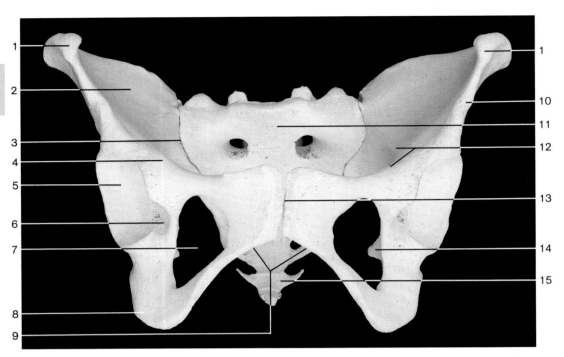

Female pelvis (anterior aspect). Note the differences between the form and dimensions of the male and female pelvis. The female pubic arch is wider than the male. The obturator foramen in the female pelvis is triangular, while that in the male pelvis is ovoid.

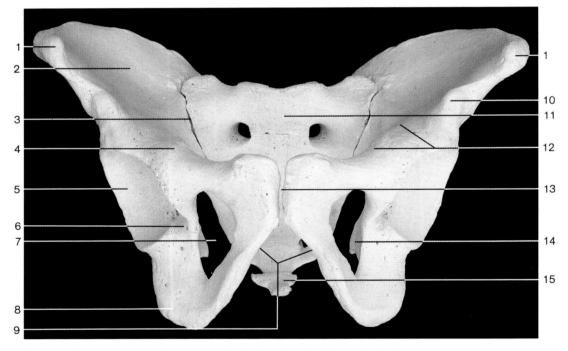

Male pelvis (anterior aspect). Compare with the female pelvis (depicted above).

1	Anterior superior iliac spine	9	Pubic arch
2	Iliac fossa	10	Anterior inferior iliac spine
3	Position of sacro-iliac joint	11	Sacrum
4	Iliopubic eminence	12	Linea terminalis (at margin of superior aperture)
5	Lunate surface of acetabulum	13	Pubic symphysis
6	Acetabular notch	14	Ischial spine
7	Obturator foramen	15	Coccyx
8	Ischial tuberosity		

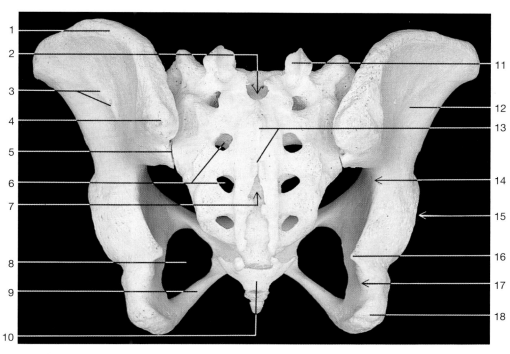

Female pelvis (posterior aspect). Note the differences between the female and male pelvis, especially with respect to the inferior aperture, the shape of the sacrum, the two sciatic notches, and the pubic arch.

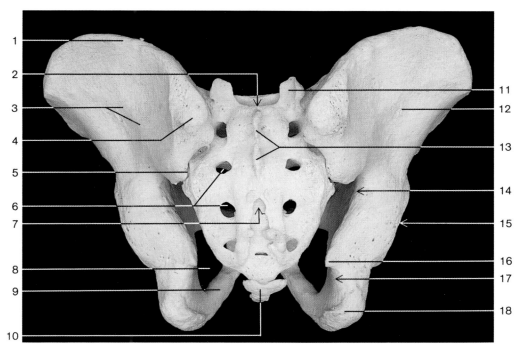

Male pelvis (posterior aspect). Compare with the female pelvis (depicted above).

1	Iliac crest	10	Coccyx
2	Sacral canal	11	Superior articular process of sacrum
3	Posterior gluteal line	12	Gluteal surface of ilium
4	Posterior superior iliac spine	13	Median sacral crest
5	Position of sacro-iliac joint	14	Greater sciatic notch
6	Dorsal sacral foramina	15	Position of acetabulum
7	Sacral hiatus	16	Ischial spine
8	Obturator foramen	17	Lesser sciatic notch
9	Ramus of ischium	18	Ischial tuberosity

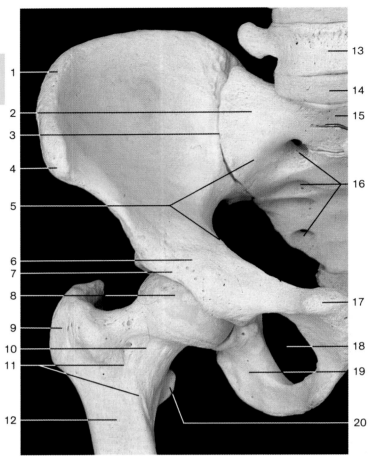

1. Iliac crest
2. Lateral part of sacrum (ala)
3. Position of sacro-iliac joint
4. Anterior superior iliac spine
5. Linea terminalis
6. Iliopubic eminence
7. Bony margin of acetabulum
8. Head of femur
9. Greater trochanter
10. Neck of femur
11. Intertrochanteric line
12. Shaft of femur
13. Fifth lumbar vertebra
14. Imitation intervertebral disc between fifth lumbar vertebra and sacrum
15. Sacral promontory
16. Anterior sacral foramina
17. Pubic tubercle
18. Obturator foramen
19. Ramus of ischium
20. Lesser trochanter
21. Dorsal sacral foramina
22. Greater sciatic notch
23. Ischial spine
24. Pubic symphysis
25. Pubis
26. Ischial tuberosity
27. Intertrochanteric crest
28. Symphysial surface

Bones of right hip joint (anterior aspect).

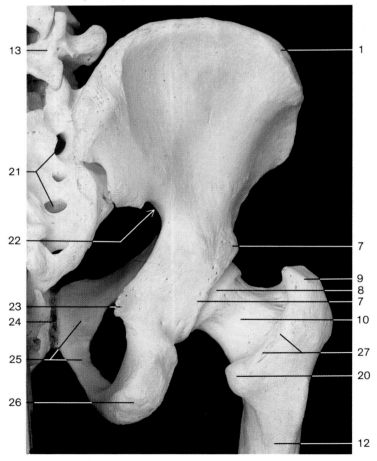

Bones of right hip joint (posterior aspect).

Diameters of the pelvis

A = true conjugate (11–11.5 cm) (conjugata vera)
B = diagonal conjugate (12.5–13 cm)
C = largest diameter of pelvis
D = inferior pelvic aperture
E = pelvic inclination (60°)

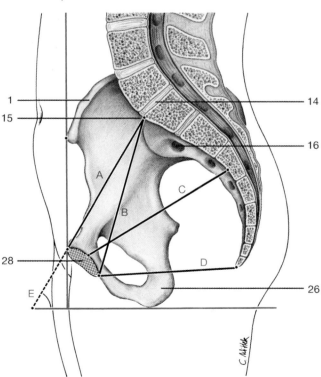

Inclination and diameters of the female pelvis, right half (medial aspect).

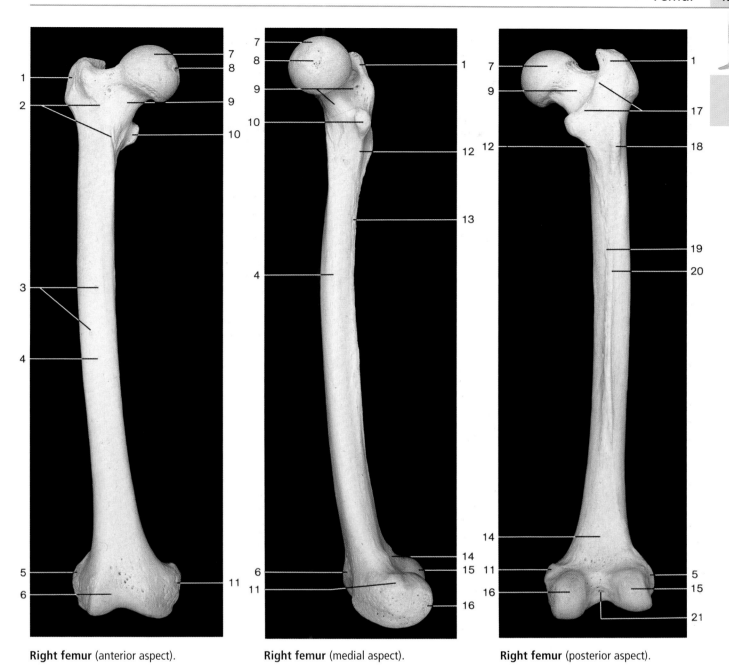

Right femur (anterior aspect).

Right femur (medial aspect).

Right femur (posterior aspect).

1 Greater trochanter	8 Fovea of head	15 Lateral condyle
2 Intertrochanteric line	9 Neck	16 Medial condyle
3 Nutrient foramina	10 Lesser trochanter	17 Intertrochanteric crest
4 Shaft of femur (diaphysis)	11 Medial epicondyle	18 Third trochanter
5 Lateral epicondyle	12 Pectineal line	19 Medial lip of linea aspera
6 Patellar surface	13 Linea aspera	20 Lateral lip of linea aspera
7 Head	14 Popliteal surface	21 Intercondylar fossa

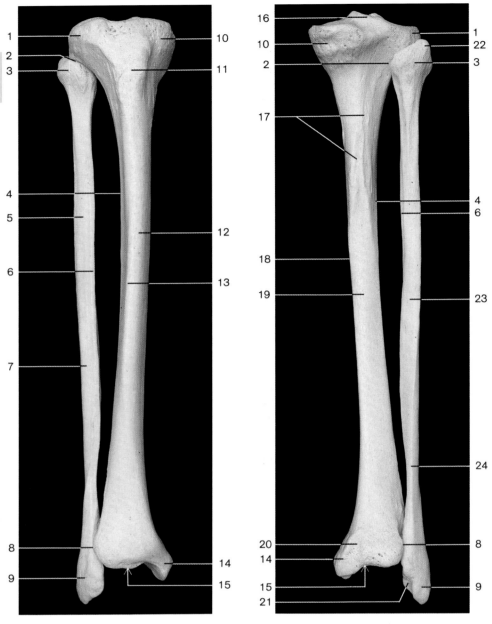

1   Lateral condyle of tibia
2   Position of tibiofibular joint
3   Head of fibula
4   Interosseous border of tibia
5   Shaft of fibula
6   Interosseous border of fibula
7   Lateral surface of fibula
8   Position of tibiofibular joint
9   Lateral malleolus
10 Medial condyle of tibia
11 Tuberosity of tibia
12 Shaft of tibia (diaphysis)
13 Anterior margin of tibia
14 Medial malleolus
15 Inferior articular surface
     of tibia
16 Intercondylar eminence
17 Soleal line
18 Medial border of tibia
19 Posterior surface of tibia
20 Malleolar sulcus of tibia
21 Malleolar articular surface
     of fibula
22 Apex of head of fibula
23 Posterior surface of fibula
24 Posterior border of fibula
25 Medial intercondylar tubercle
26 Posterior intercondylar area
27 Anterior intercondylar area
28 Lateral intercondylar tubercle

Bones of leg, right tibia, and fibula
(anterior aspect).

Bones of leg, right tibia, and fibula
(posterior aspect).

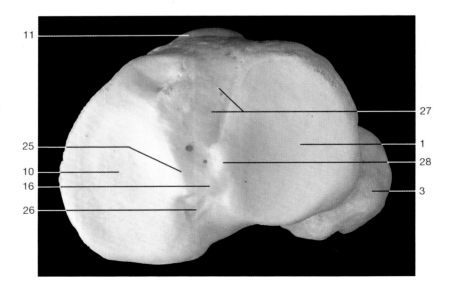

Upper end of right tibia with fibula
(from above), anterior margin of tibia above.
Superior articular surface of tibia.

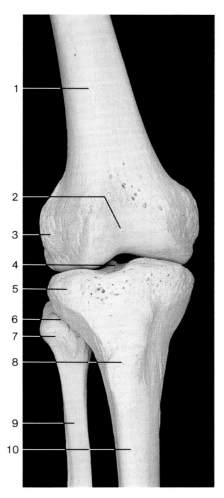

Bones of right knee joint
(anterior aspect).

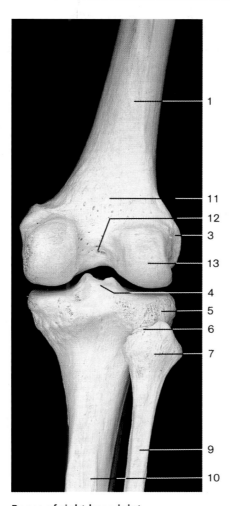

Bones of right knee joint
(posterior aspect).

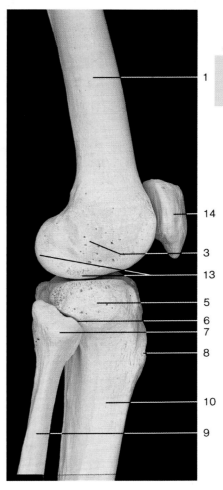

Bones of right knee joint
(lateral aspect).

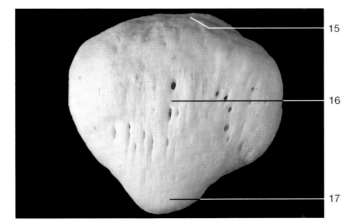

Right patella (anterior aspect).

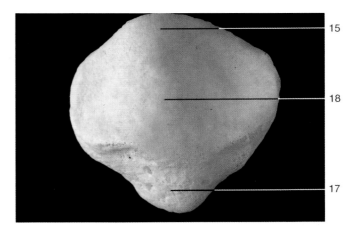

Right patella (posterior aspect).

1	Femur	10	Shaft of tibia
2	Patellar surface of femur	11	Popliteal surface of femur
3	Lateral epicondyle of femur	12	Intercondylar fossa of femur
4	Intercondylar eminence of tibia	13	Lateral condyle of femur
5	Lateral condyle of tibia	14	Patella
6	Position of tibiofibular joint	15	Base of patella
7	Head of fibula	16	Anterior surface of patella
8	Tuberosity of tibia	17	Apex of patella
9	Fibula	18	Articular surface of patella

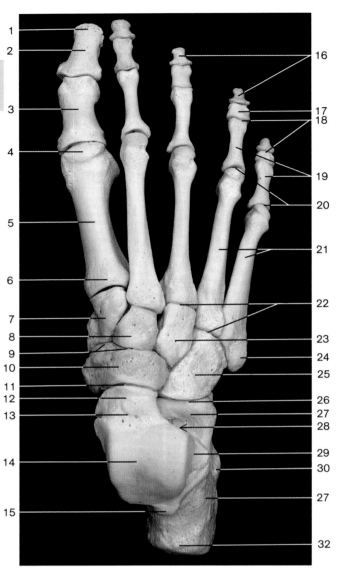

Bones of right foot (dorsal aspect).

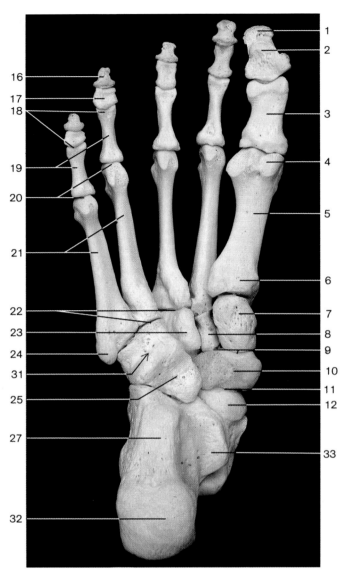

Bones of right foot (plantar aspect).

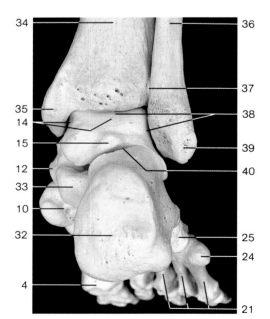

Bones of right foot together with tibia
and fibula (posterior aspect).

1 Tuberosity of distal phalanx of great toe
2 Distal phalanx of great toe
3 Proximal phalanx of great toe
4 Head of first metatarsal bone
5 First metatarsal bone
6 Base of first metatarsal bone
7 Medial cuneiform bone
8 Intermediate cuneiform bone
9 Position of cuneonavicular joint
10 Navicular bone

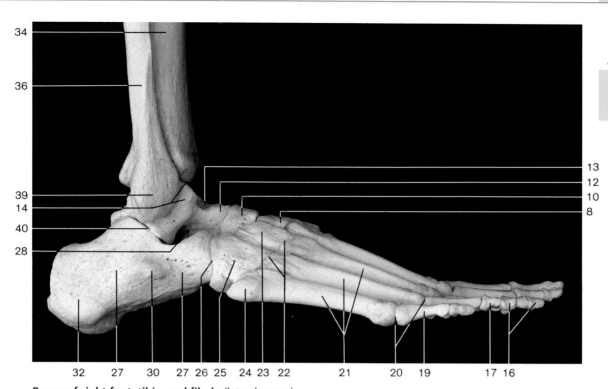

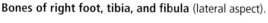

Bones of right foot, tibia, and fibula (lateral aspect).

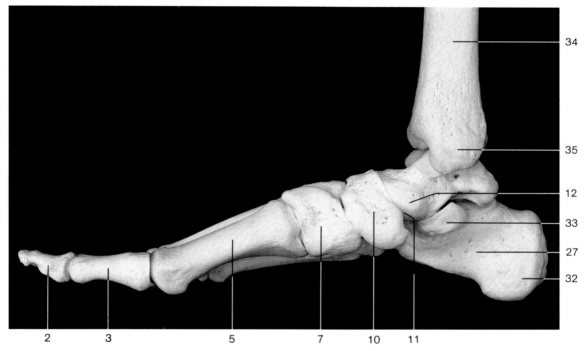

Bones of right foot, tibia, and fibula (medial aspect).

11	Position of talocalcaneonavicular joint	21	Metatarsal bones	31	Groove for tendon of peroneus longus
12	Head of talus	22	Position of tarsometatarsal joints	32	Calcaneal tuberosity
13	Neck of talus	23	Lateral cuneiform bone	33	Sustentaculum tali
14	Trochlea of talus	24	Tuberosity of fifth metatarsal bone	34	Tibia
15	Posterior talar process	25	Cuboid bone	35	Medial malleolus
16	Distal phalanges	26	Position of calcaneocuboid joint	36	Fibula
17	Middle phalanges	27	Calcaneus	37	Position of tibiofibular syndesmosis
18	Position of interphalangeal joints	28	Tarsal sinus	38	Position of ankle joint
19	Proximal phalanges	29	Lateral malleolar surface of talus	39	Lateral malleolus
20	Position of metatarsophalangeal joints	30	Peroneal trochlea of calcaneus	40	Position of subtalar joint

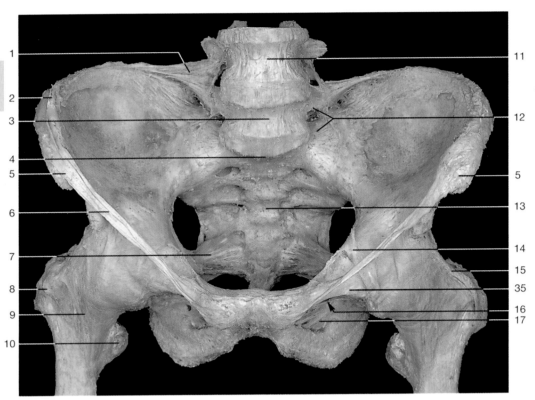

Ligaments of pelvis and hip joint (anterior aspect).

1 Iliolumbar ligament	13 Sacrum	26 Articular capsule of hip joint
2 Iliac crest	14 Iliopectineal arch	27 Dorsal sacro-iliac ligaments
3 Fifth lumbar vertebra	15 Iliofemoral ligament (horizontal band)	28 Coccyx with superficial dorsal
4 Sacral promontory	16 Obturator canal	sacrococcygeal ligament
5 Anterior superior iliac spine	17 Obturator membrane	29 Head of femur
6 Inguinal ligament	18 Greater sciatic foramen	30 Articular cartilage of head of femur
7 Sacrospinous ligament	19 Sacrospinous ligament	31 Articular cavity of hip joint
8 Greater trochanter	20 Sacrotuberous ligament	32 Acetabular lip
9 Iliofemoral ligament (vertical band)	21 Lesser sciatic foramen	33 Spongy bone
10 Lesser trochanter	22 Ischial tuberosity	34 Ligament of head of femur
11 Fourth lumbar vertebra	23 Ischiofemoral ligament	35 Pubofemoral ligament
12 Iliolumbar and ventral sacro-iliac	24 Intertrochanteric crest	36 Zona orbicularis
ligaments	25 Femur	

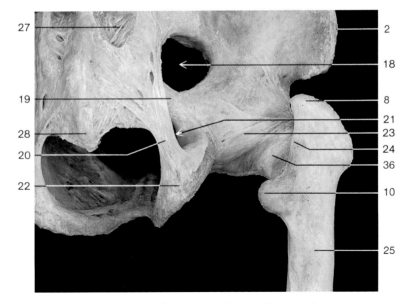

Ligaments of pelvis and hip joint (right posterior aspect).

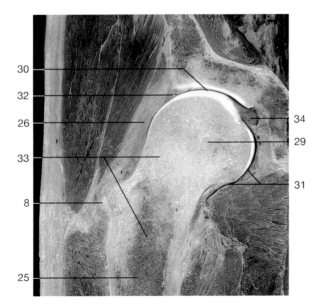

Coronal section of right hip joint (anterior aspect).

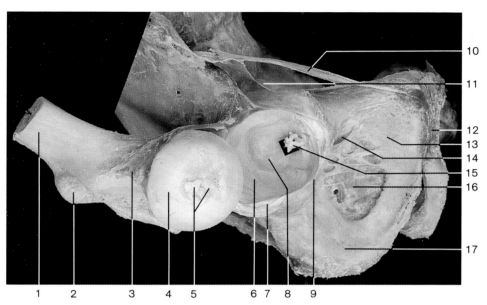

1   Femur
2   Lesser trochanter
3   Neck of femur
4   Head of femur
5   Fovea of head with cut edge of ligament of head
6   Lunate surface of acetabulum
7   Acetabular lip
8   Acetabular fossa
9   Transverse acetabular ligament
10 Inguinal ligament
11 Iliopectineal arch
12 Pubic symphysis
13 Pubic bone
14 Obturator canal
15 Ligament of head of femur
16 Obturator membrane
17 Ischium
18 Anterior longitudinal ligament (level of fifth lumbar vertebra)
19 Sacral promontory
20 Iliolumbar ligament
21 Iliac crest
22 Anterior superior iliac spine
23 Iliofemoral ligament (horizontal band)
24 Iliofemoral ligament (vertical band)
25 Greater trochanter
26 Pubofemoral ligament
27 Anterior inferior iliac spine
28 Ventral sacro-iliac ligaments
29 Sacrospinous ligament
30 Sacrotuberous ligament
31 Intertrochanteric line
32 Ischiofemoral ligament
33 Zona orbicularis

Right hip joint, opened (latero-anterior aspect). The ligament of the head of the femur has been divided, and the femur has been posteriorly reflected.

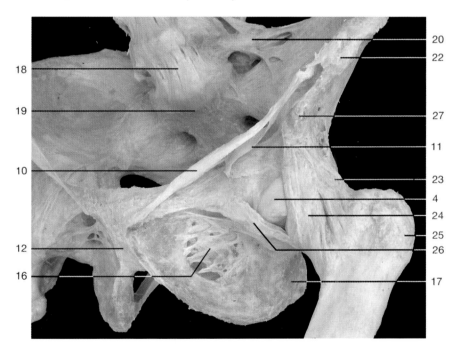

◁ **Ligaments of the pelvis and hip joint** (antero-lateral aspect).

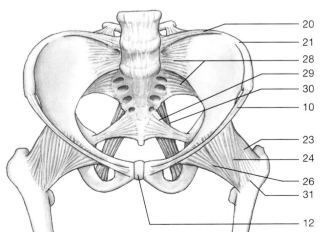

Ligaments of hip joint (anterior aspect, schematic drawing).

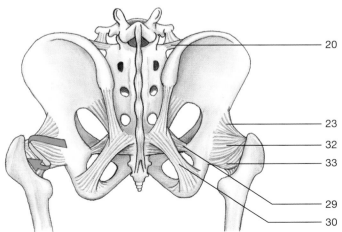

Ligaments of hip joint (posterior aspect, schematic drawing).

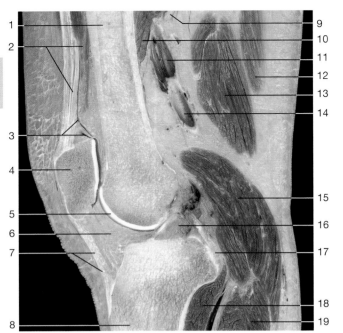

Sagittal section through the knee joint (lateral aspect). Anterior surface to the left.

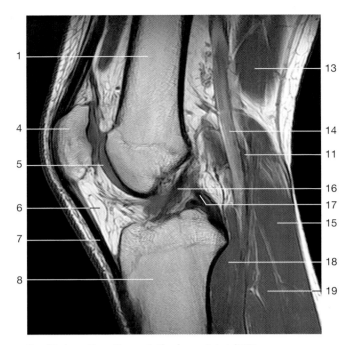

Sagittal section through the knee joint (MRI scan; from Heuck et al., MRT-Atlas, 2009).

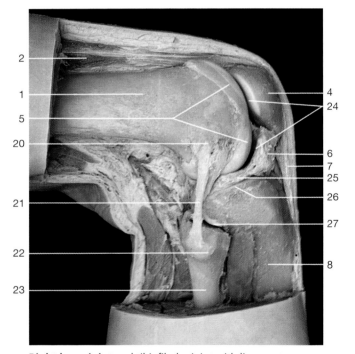

Right knee joint and tibiofibular joint with ligaments (lateral aspect). Note the position of the lateral meniscus.

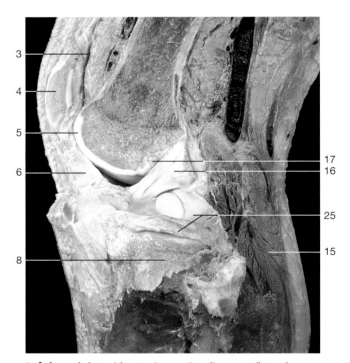

Left knee joint with anterior cruciate ligament (lateral aspect).

1 Femur	10 Adductor magnus muscle	19 Soleus muscle
2 Quadriceps femoris muscle	11 Popliteal vein	20 Lateral epicondyle of femur
3 Suprapatellar bursa and articular cavity	12 Semitendinosus muscle	21 Fibular collateral ligament
4 Patella	13 Semimembranosus muscle	22 Head of fibula
5 Articular cartilage of femur	14 Popliteal artery	23 Fibula
6 Infrapatellar fat pad	15 Gastrocnemius muscle	24 Articular cavity of knee joint
7 Patellar ligament	16 Anterior cruciate ligament	25 Lateral meniscus of knee joint
8 Tibia	17 Posterior cruciate ligament	26 Lateral condyle of tibia
9 Tibial nerve	18 Popliteus muscle	27 Tibiofibular joint

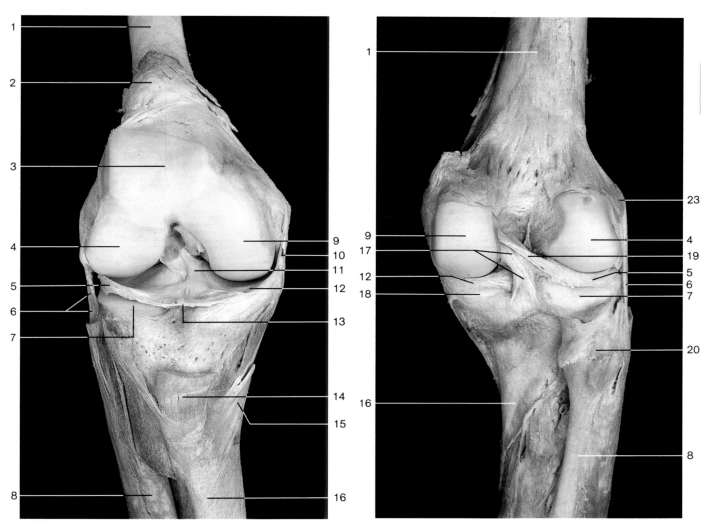

Right knee joint (opened) **with ligaments** (anterior aspect). The patella and articular capsule have been removed and the femur slightly flexed.

Right knee joint with ligaments (posterior aspect). The joint is extended and the articular capsule has been removed.

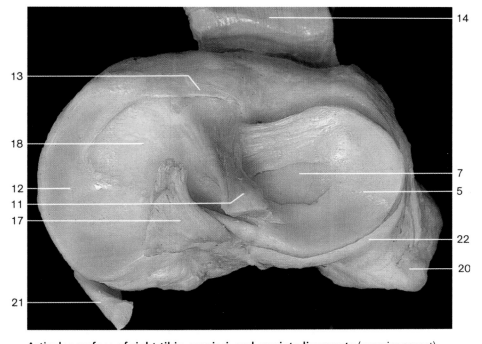

Articular surface of right tibia, menisci, and cruciate ligaments (superior aspect). Anterior margin of tibia above.

1   Femur
2   Articular capsule with suprapatellar bursa
3   Patellar surface
4   Lateral condyle of femur
5   Lateral meniscus of knee joint
6   Fibular collateral ligament
7   Lateral condyle of tibia (superior articular surface)
8   Fibula
9   Medial condyle of femur
10 Tibial collateral ligament
11 Anterior cruciate ligament
12 Medial meniscus of knee joint
13 Transverse ligament of knee
14 Patellar ligament
15 Common tendon of sartorius, semitendinosus, and gracilis muscles
16 Tibia
17 Posterior cruciate ligament
18 Medial condyle of tibia (superior articular surface)
19 Posterior meniscofemoral ligament
20 Head of fibula
21 Tendon of semimembranosus muscle
22 Posterior attachment of articular capsule of knee joint
23 Lateral epicondyle of femur

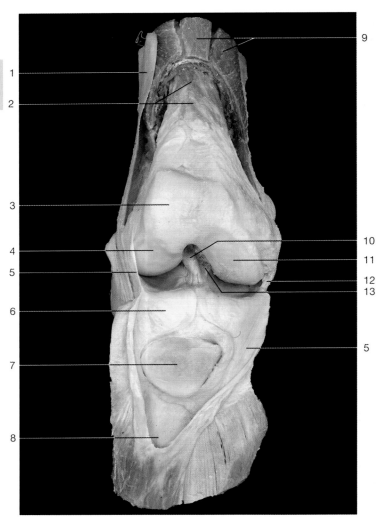

Right knee joint, opened (anterior aspect). Patellar ligament with patella reflected.

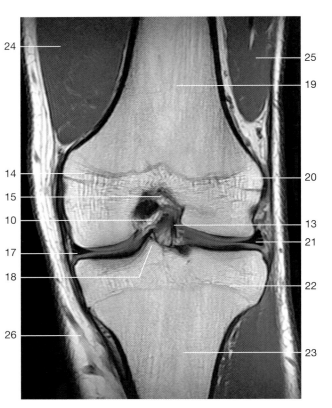

Coronal section through the knee joint (MRI scan; from Heuck et al., MRT-Atlas, 2009).

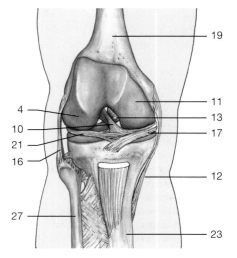

Ligaments of the right knee joint (anterior aspect).

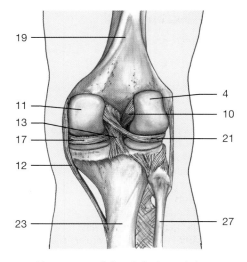

Ligaments of the right knee joint (posterior aspect).

1 Iliotibial tract
2 Articular muscle of knee
3 Patellar surface
4 Lateral condyle of femur
5 Articular capsule
6 Infrapatellar fat pad
7 Patella (articular surface)
8 Suprapatellar bursa
9 Quadriceps femoris muscle
10 Anterior cruciate ligament
11 Medial condyle of femur
12 Tibial collateral ligament
13 Posterior cruciate ligament
14 Medial epicondyle of femur
15 Intercondylar fossa of femur
16 Fibular collateral ligament
17 Medial meniscus of knee joint
18 Medial intercondylar tubercle
19 Femur
20 Lateral epicondyle of femur
21 Lateral meniscus of knee joint
22 Epiphysial line of tibia
23 Tibia
24 Vastus medialis muscle
25 Vastus lateralis muscle
26 Great saphenous vein
27 Fibula

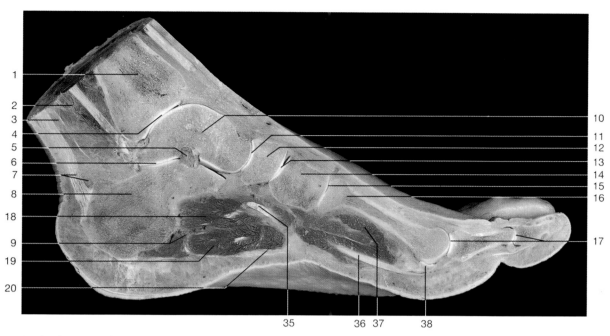

Sagittal section through the foot at the level of first phalanx.

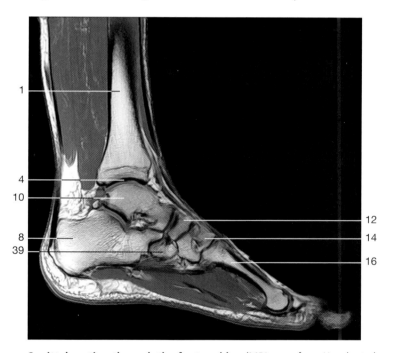

Sagittal section through the foot and leg (MRI scan; from Heuck et al., MRT-Atlas, 2009).

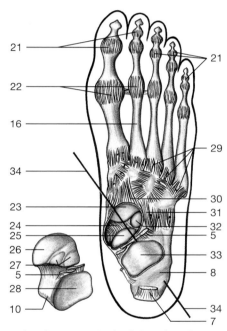

Talocalcaneonavicular joint. The talus has been rotated to show the articular surfaces of the joint.

1 Tibia	16 Metatarsal bones	27 Anterior and middle calcaneal surfaces of talus
2 Deep flexor muscles	17 Metatarsophalangeal and interphalangeal joints	28 Posterior calcaneal surface of talus
3 Superficial flexor muscles	18 Quadratus plantae muscle with flexor tendons	29 Dorsal tarsometatarsal ligaments
4 Ankle joint	19 Flexor digitorum brevis muscle	30 Talonavicular ligament
5 Interosseous talocalcaneal ligament	20 Plantar aponeurosis	31 Bifurcate ligament
6 Subtalar joint	21 Articular capsules of interphalangeal joints	32 Anterior talar articular surface of calcaneus
7 Calcaneal or Achilles tendon and bursa	22 Articular capsules of metatarsophalangeal joints	33 Posterior talar articular surface of calcaneus
8 Calcaneus	23 Articular surface of navicular bone	34 Axis for inversion and eversion
9 Vessels and nerves of foot	24 Plantar calcaneonavicular ligament	35 Tendon of tibialis posterior muscle
10 Talus	25 Middle talar articular surface of calcaneus	36 Tendon of flexor hallucis longus muscle
11 Talocalcaneonavicular joint	26 Navicular articular surface of talus	37 Flexor hallucis brevis muscle
12 Navicular bone		38 Sesamoid bone
13 Cuneonavicular joint		39 Cuboid bone
14 Intermediate cuneiform bone		
15 Tarsometatarsal joints		

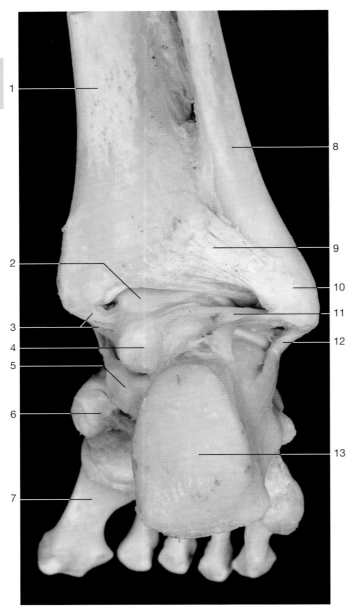

Ligaments of ankle joint, right foot (posterior aspect).

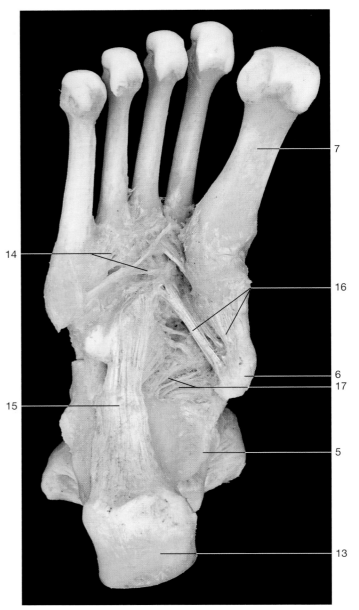

Deep ligaments of the foot, right foot (plantar aspect). The toes have been removed.

1	Tibia	9	Posterior tibiofibular ligament
2	Trochlea of talus	10	Lateral malleolus
3	Deltoid ligament of ankle (posterior tibiotalar part)	11	Posterior talofibular ligament
4	Talus	12	Calcaneofibular ligament
5	Sustentaculum tali	13	Calcaneal tuberosity
6	Navicular bone	14	Plantar tarsometatarsal ligaments
7	First metatarsal bone	15	Long plantar ligament
8	Fibula	16	Plantar cuneonavicular ligaments
		17	Plantar calcaneonavicular ligament

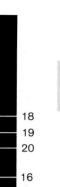

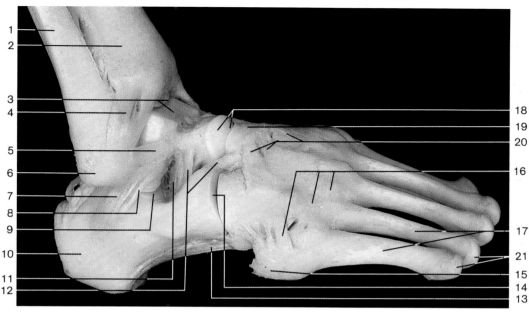

Ligaments of right foot (lateral aspect).

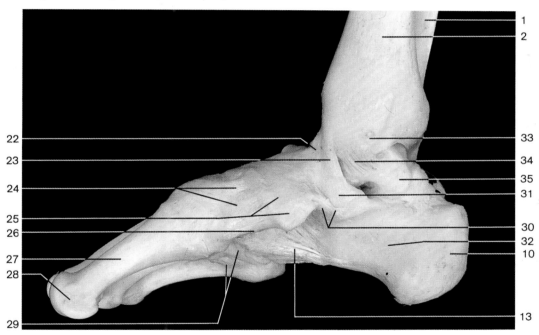

Ligaments of right foot (medial aspect).

1 Fibula	19 Navicular bone
2 Tibia	20 Dorsal cuneonavicular ligaments
3 Trochlea of talus and ankle joint	21 Heads of metatarsal bones
4 Anterior tibiofibular ligament	22 Medial or deltoid ligament of ankle (tibionavicular part)
5 Anterior talofibular ligament	23 Medial or deltoid ligament of ankle (tibiocalcaneal part)
6 Lateral malleolus	24 Dorsal cuneonavicular ligaments
7 Calcaneofibular ligament	25 Navicular bone
8 Lateral talocalcaneal ligament	26 Plantar cuneonavicular ligament
9 Subtalar joint	27 First metatarsal bone
10 Tuber calcanei	28 Head of first metatarsal bone
11 Interosseous talocalcaneal ligament	29 Plantar tarsometatarsal ligaments
12 Bifurcate ligament	30 Plantar calcaneonavicular ligament
13 Long plantar ligament	31 Sustentaculum tali
14 Calcaneocuboid joint	32 Calcaneus
15 Tuberosity of fifth metatarsal bone	33 Medial malleolus
16 Dorsal tarsometatarsal ligaments	34 Medial or deltoid ligament of ankle (posterior part)
17 Metatarsal bones	35 Talus
18 Head of talus and talocalcaneonavicular joint	

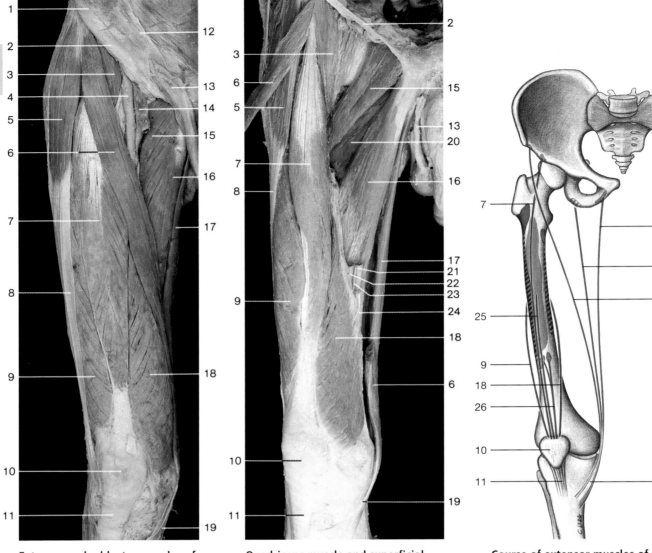

Extensor and adductor muscles of thigh, right thigh (anterior aspect).

Quadriceps muscle and superficial layer of adductor muscles, right thigh (anterior aspect). The sartorius muscle has been divided.

Course of extensor muscles of thigh and muscles inserting with common tendon on tibia (schematic drawing).

1	Anterior superior iliac spine	12	Aponeurosis of external abdominal
2	Inguinal ligament		oblique muscle
3	Iliopsoas muscle	13	Spermatic cord
4	Femoral artery	14	Femoral vein
5	Tensor fasciae latae muscle	15	Pectineus muscle
6	Sartorius muscle	16	Adductor longus muscle
7	Rectus femoris muscle	17	Gracilis muscle
8	Iliotibial tract	18	Vastus medialis muscle
9	Vastus lateralis muscle	19	Common tendon of sartorius, gracilis,
10	Patella		and semitendinosus muscles
11	Patellar ligament		(pes anserinus)

20	Adductor brevis muscle	
21	Femoral artery	} entering the
22	Femoral vein	} adductor canal
23	Saphenous nerve	}
24	Fascia of adductor canal	
25	Vastus intermedius muscle	
26	Articularis genus muscle	
27	Semitendinosus muscle	

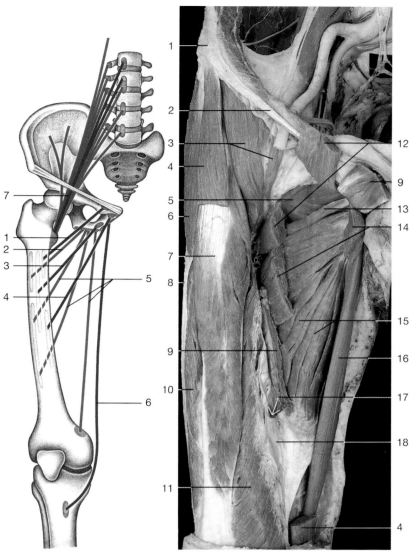

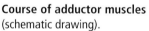

Course of adductor muscles
(schematic drawing).

1 Pectineus muscle (blue)
2 Adductor minimus muscle (red)
3 Adductor brevis muscle (blue)
4 Adductor longus muscle (blue)
5 Adductor magnus muscle (red)
6 Gracilis muscle (blue)
7 Iliopsoas muscle (red/blue)

**Adductor magnus muscle and deep layer
of adductor muscles,** right thigh (anterior
aspect). Pectineus, adductor longus, and
brevis muscles have been divided.

1 Anterior superior iliac spine
2 Inguinal ligament
3 Iliopsoas muscle
4 Sartorius muscle
5 Obturator externus muscle
6 Tensor fasciae latae muscle
7 Rectus femoris muscle
8 Iliotibial tract
9 Adductor longus muscle (divided)
10 Vastus lateralis muscle
11 Vastus medialis muscle
12 Pectineus muscle (divided)
13 Adductor minimus muscle
14 Adductor brevis muscle (cut)
15 Adductor magnus muscle
16 Gracilis muscle
17 Adductor hiatus
18 Vasto-adductor membrane
19 Diaphragm
20 Quadratus lumborum muscle
21 Iliacus muscle
22 Vastus intermedius muscle

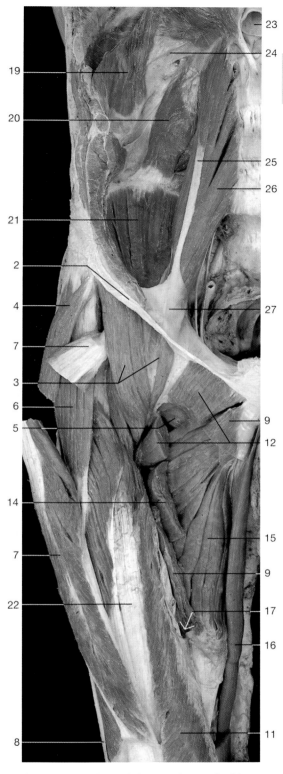

**Iliopsoas muscle and deepest layer of adductor
muscles,** right thigh (anterior aspect). Pectineus,
adductor longus and brevis, and rectus femoris
muscles have been divided.

23 Aorta in aortic hiatus
24 Twelfth rib
25 Psoas minor muscle
26 Psoas major muscle
27 Iliopectineal arch

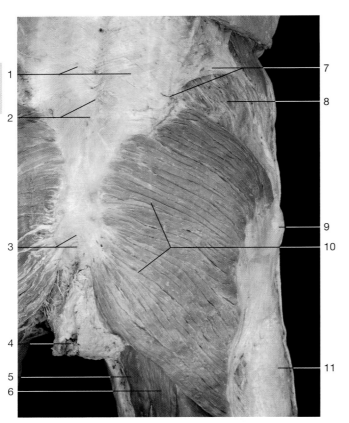

1
2
7
8
9
10
3
4
5
6
11

Gluteal muscles, superficial layer (posterior aspect).

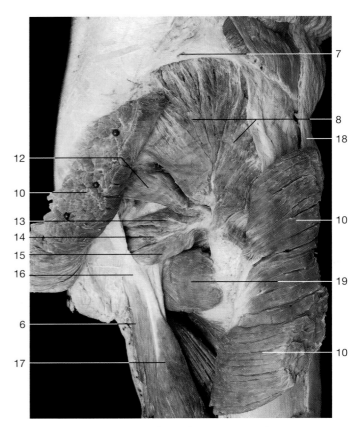

7
12
10
13
14
15
16
6
17
8
18
10
19
10

Gluteal muscles, deeper layer (posterior aspect).

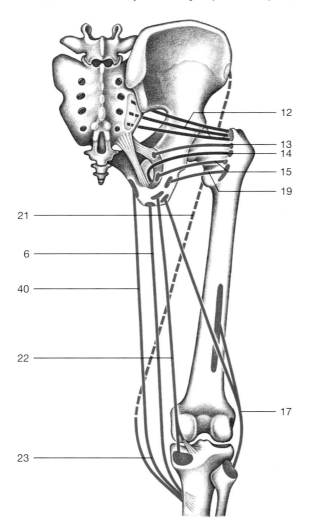

12
13
14
15
19
21
6
40
22
17
23

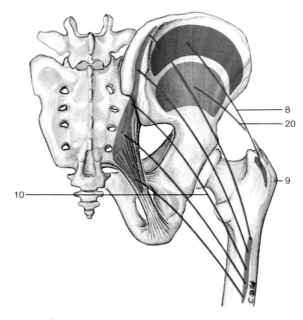

8
20
10
9

Course of gluteal muscles
(posterior aspect; schematic drawing).

◁

Course of gluteal muscles (deeper layer)
and of ischiocrural muscles (posterior aspect).
Sartorius muscle is indicated by a dotted line
(schematic drawing).

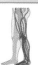

1 Thoracolumbar fascia
2 Spinous processes of lumbar vertebrae
3 Coccyx
4 Anus
5 Adductor magnus muscle
6 Semitendinosus muscle
7 Iliac crest
8 Gluteus medius muscle
9 Greater trochanter
10 Gluteus maximus muscle
11 Iliotibial tract
12 Piriformis muscle
13 Superior gemellus muscle
14 Obturator internus muscle
15 Inferior gemellus muscle
16 Ischial tuberosity
17 Biceps femoris muscle
18 Tensor fasciae latae muscle
19 Quadratus femoris muscle
20 Gluteus minimus muscle
21 Sartorius muscle
22 Semimembranosus muscle
23 Tendon of gracilis muscle
24 Tibial nerve
25 Medial head of gastrocnemius muscle
26 Common peroneal nerve
27 Tendon of biceps femoris muscle
28 Lateral head of gastrocnemius muscle
29 Rectus femoris muscle
30 Vastus medialis muscle
31 Vastus intermedius muscle
32 Vastus lateralis muscle
33 Sciatic nerve
34 Gluteus maximus muscle (insertion)
35 Great saphenous vein
36 Femoral artery
37 Femoral vein
38 Adductor longus muscle
39 Femur
40 Gracilis muscle
41 Septum between semitendinosus
    and semimembranosus muscles

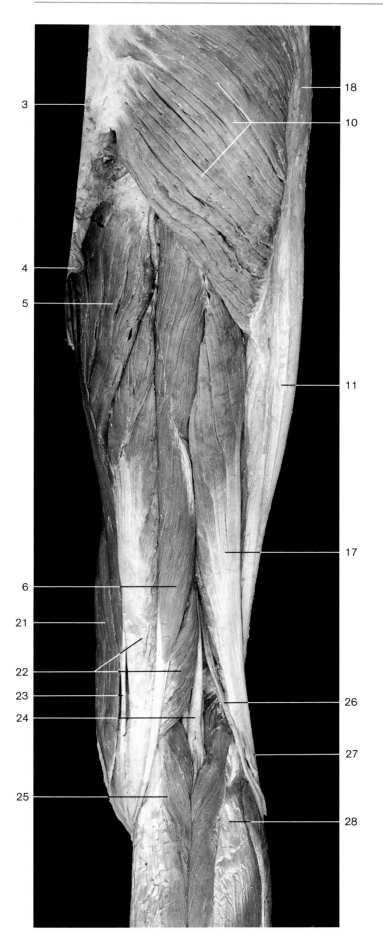

Flexors of the right thigh, superficial layer (posterior aspect).

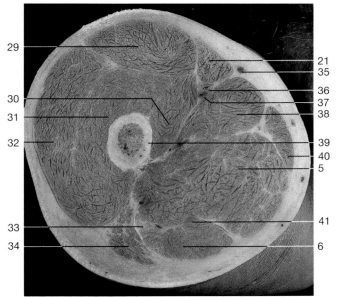

Cross section of right thigh (inferior aspect).
Anterior side on top.

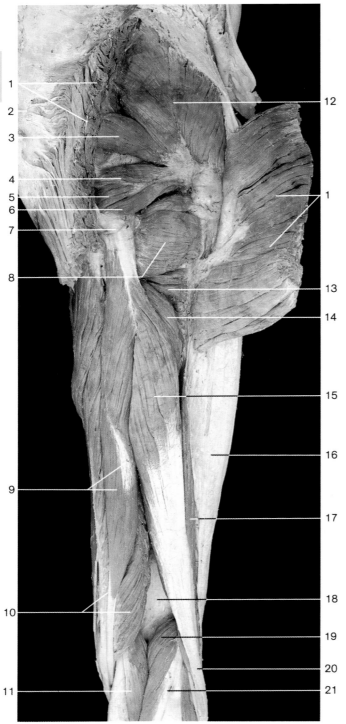

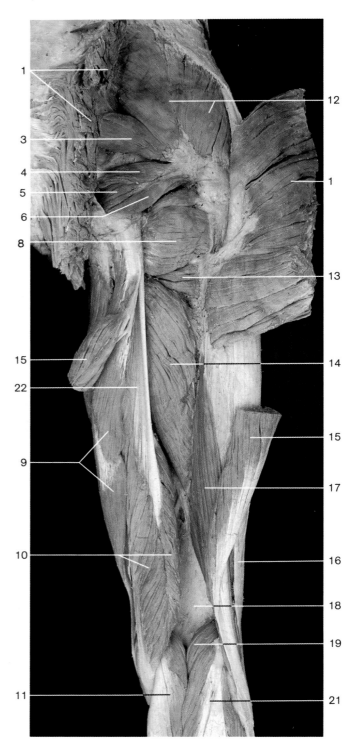

Dorsal muscles of right thigh (posterior aspect).
The gluteus maximus muscle has been cut and reflected.

Dorsal muscles of right thigh (posterior aspect).
The gluteus maximus muscle and the long head of biceps femoris muscle have been divided and displaced.

1 Gluteus maximus muscle (divided)	9 Semitendinosus muscle with intermediate tendon	17 Short head of biceps femoris muscle
2 Position of coccyx	10 Semimembranosus muscle	18 Popliteal surface of femur
3 Piriformis muscle	11 Medial head of gastrocnemius muscle	19 Plantaris muscle
4 Superior gemellus muscle	12 Gluteus medius muscle	20 Tendon of biceps femoris muscle
5 Obturator internus muscle	13 Adductor minimus muscle	21 Lateral head of gastrocnemius muscle
6 Inferior gemellus muscle	14 Adductor magnus muscle	22 Membranous part of
7 Ischial tuberosity	15 Long head of biceps femoris muscle	semimembranosus muscle
8 Quadratus femoris muscle	16 Iliotibial tract	

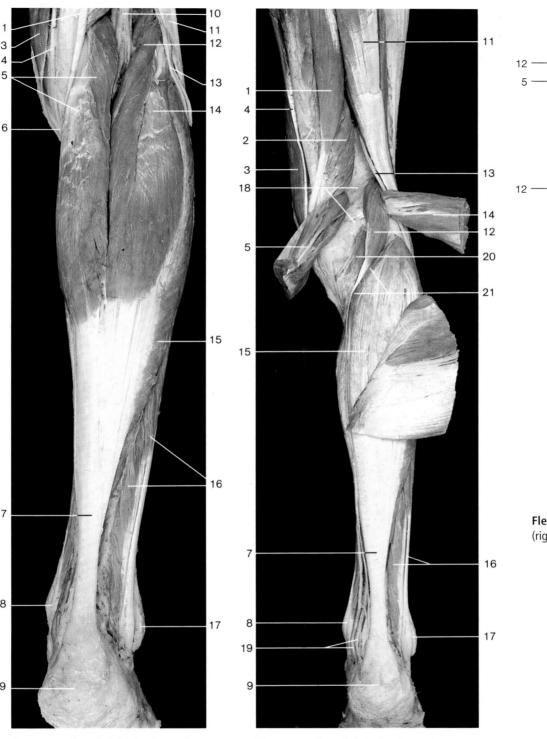

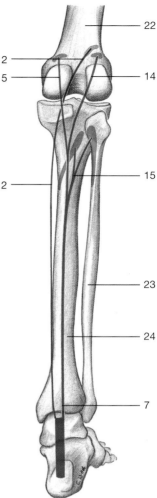

Flexor muscles of the leg (right side).

Flexor muscles of right leg (posterior aspect).

Flexor muscles of right leg (posterior aspect). Both heads of the gastrocnemius muscle have been cut and reflected.

1	Semitendinosus muscle	9	Calcaneal tuberosity	18	Popliteal fossa
2	Semimembranosus muscle	10	Tibial nerve	19	Tibial nerve and posterior tibial
3	Sartorius muscle	11	Biceps femoris muscle		artery
4	Tendon of gracilis muscle	12	Plantaris muscle	20	Popliteus muscle
5	Medial head of gastrocnemius muscle	13	Common peroneal nerve	21	Tendinous arch of soleus muscle
6	Common tendon of gracilis,	14	Lateral head of gastrocnemius muscle	22	Femur
	sartorius, and semitendinosus muscles	15	Soleus muscle	23	Fibula
7	Calcaneal or Achilles tendon	16	Peroneus longus and brevis muscles	24	Tibia
8	Medial malleolus	17	Lateral malleolus		

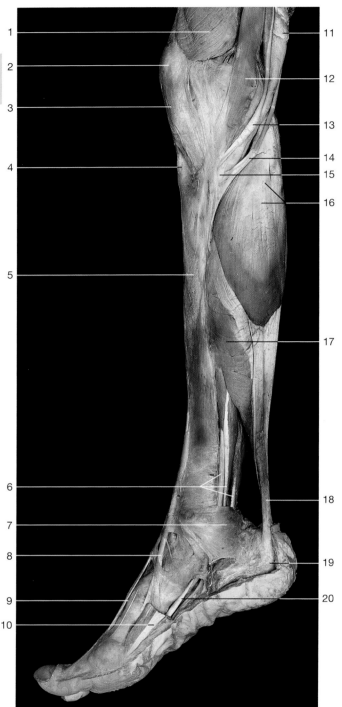

Muscles of right leg and foot (medial aspect).

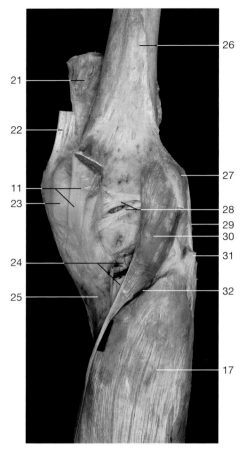

Popliteal region with plantaris and soleus muscles, right side (dorsal aspect). Notice the insertion of the tendon of semimembranosus muscle.

1 Vastus medialis muscle
2 Patella
3 Patellar ligament
4 Tibial tuberosity
5 Tibia
6 Tendons of deep flexor muscles (from anterior to posterior: 1. tibialis posterior; 2. flexor digitorum longus; 3. flexor hallucis longus muscles)
7 Flexor retinaculum
8 Tendon of tibialis anterior muscle
9 Tendon of extensor hallucis longus muscle
10 Abductor hallucis muscle

11 Semimembranosus muscle
12 Sartorius muscle
13 Tendon of gracilis muscle
14 Tendon of semitendinosus muscle
15 Common tendon of gracilis, semitendinosus, and sartorius muscles
16 Medial head of gastrocnemius muscle
17 Soleus muscle
18 Calcaneal or Achilles tendon
19 Calcaneus muscle
20 Tendon of flexor hallucis longus muscle
21 Quadriceps femoris muscle (divided)
22 Tendon of adductor magnus muscle (divided)

23 Medial condyle of femur
24 Popliteal artery and vein, tibial nerve
25 Tibia
26 Femur
27 Lateral epicondyle of femur
28 Oblique popliteal ligament
29 Lateral (fibular) collateral ligament
30 Plantaris muscle
31 Tendon of biceps femoris muscle (divided)
32 Tendinous arch of soleus muscle

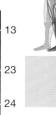

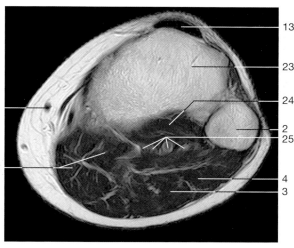

Axial section of the right leg distally of the knee joint (MRI scan; from Heuck et al., MRT-Atlas, 2009).

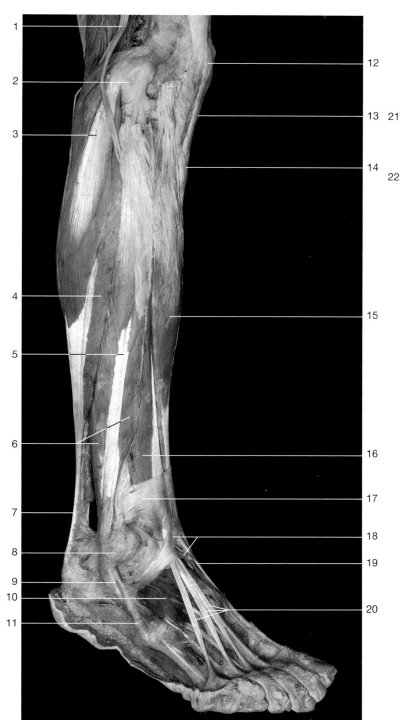

Muscles of right leg and foot (lateral aspect).

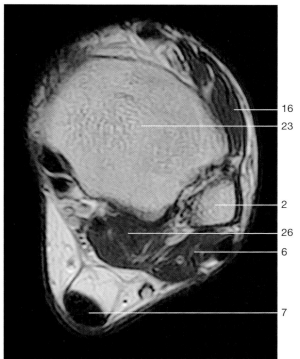

Axial section of the right leg cranially of the ankle joint (MRI scan; from Heuck et al., MRT-Atlas, 2009).

1 Common peroneal nerve	11 Tendon of peroneus brevis muscle	20 Tendons of extensor digitorum longus muscle
2 Head of fibula	12 Patella	21 Great saphenous vein
3 Lateral head of gastrocnemius muscle	13 Patellar ligament	22 Medial head of gastrocnemius muscle
4 Soleus muscle	14 Tuberosity of tibia	23 Tibia
5 Peroneus longus muscle	15 Tibialis anterior muscle	24 Popliteus muscle
6 Peroneus brevis muscle	16 Extensor digitorum longus muscle	25 Tibial nerve, popliteal artery, and veins
7 Calcaneal or Achilles tendon	17 Superior extensor retinaculum	26 Flexor hallucis longus muscle
8 Lateral malleolus muscle	18 Inferior extensor retinaculum	
9 Tendon of peroneus longus muscle	19 Tendon of extensor hallucis longus muscle	
10 Extensor digitorum brevis muscle		

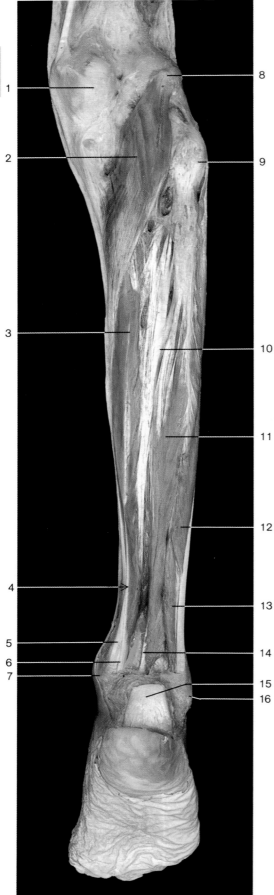

1   Medial condyle of femur
2   Popliteus muscle
3   Flexor digitorum longus muscle
4   Crossing of tendons in leg
5   Tendon of tibialis posterior muscle
6   Tendon of flexor digitorum longus muscle
7   Medial malleolus
8   Lateral condyle of femur
9   Head of fibula
10   Tibialis posterior muscle
11   Flexor hallucis longus muscle
12   Peroneus longus muscle
13   Peroneus brevis muscle
14   Tendon of flexor hallucis longus muscle
15   Calcaneal tendon (divided)
16   Lateral malleolus

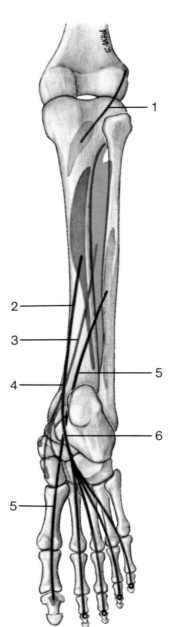

1   Popliteus muscle (blue)
2   Flexor digitorum longus muscle (blue)
3   Tibialis posterior muscle (red)
4   Crossing of tendons in leg
5   Flexor hallucis longus muscle (blue)
6   Crossing of tendons in sole

Deep flexor muscles of right leg and foot (posterior aspect).

Course of deep flexor muscles of leg (schematic drawing).

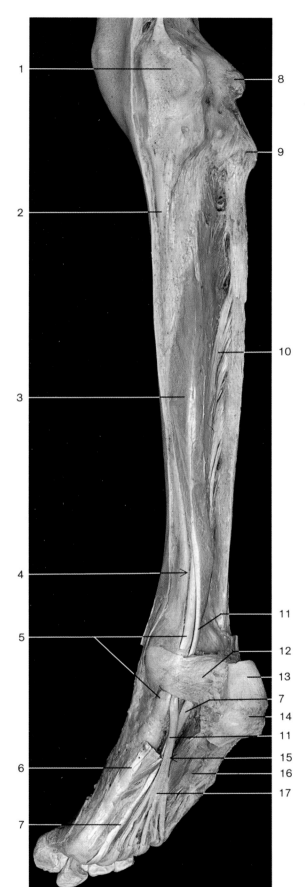

1   Medial condyle of femur
2   Tibia
3   Flexor digitorum longus muscle
4   Crossing of tendons in leg
5   Tendon of tibialis posterior muscle
6   Abductor hallucis muscle
7   Tendon of flexor hallucis longus
    muscle
8   Lateral condyle of femur
9   Head of fibula
10 Tibialis posterior muscle
11 Tendon of flexor digitorum longus
    muscle
12 Flexor retinaculum
13 Calcaneal tendon
14 Calcaneal tuberosity
15 Crossing of tendons in sole
16 Quadratus plantae muscle
17 Tendons of flexor digitorum
    longus muscle
18 Tendon of tibialis anterior muscle
19 Area of insertion of tibialis
    posterior muscle
20 Lumbrical muscles
21 Flexor hallucis longus muscle
22 Tibialis anterior muscle
23 Extensor hallucis longus muscle
24 Lateral malleolus of fibula
25 Trochlea of talus

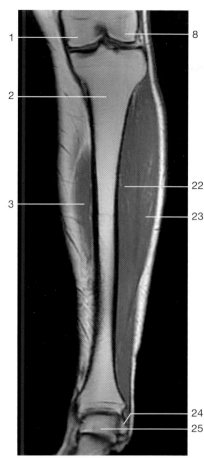

Coronal section of the leg
(MRI scan; from Heuck et al.,
MRT-Atlas, 2009).

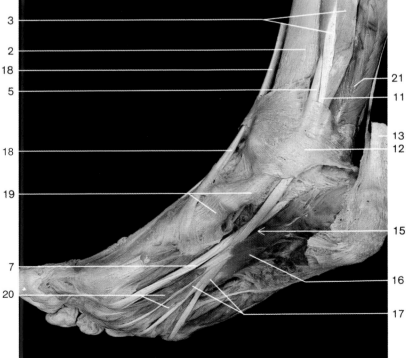

Deep flexor muscles of right leg and foot
(posterior oblique medial aspect). Flexor digitorum
brevis and flexor hallucis longus muscles have been
removed.

Sole of foot with tendons of long flexor muscles (oblique medial and
inferior aspect).

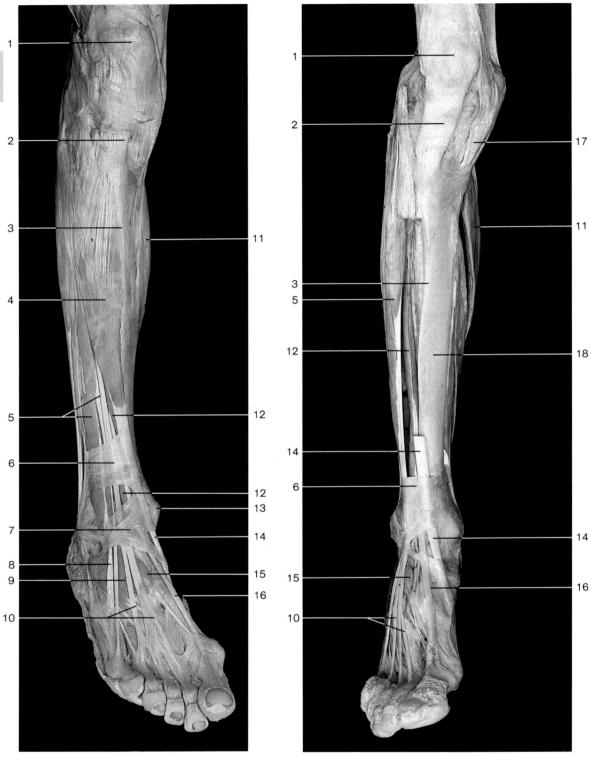

Extensor muscles of right leg and foot
(oblique antero-lateral aspect).

Extensor muscles of right leg and foot (anterior aspect). Part of the tibialis anterior muscle has been removed.

1	Patella	8	Tendon of peroneus tertius muscle	14	Tendon of tibialis anterior muscle
2	Patellar ligament	9	Extensor digitorum brevis muscle	15	Extensor hallucis brevis muscle
3	Anterior margin of tibia	10	Tendons of extensor digitorum longus muscle	16	Tendon of extensor hallucis longus muscle
4	Tibialis anterior muscle	11	Gastrocnemius muscle	17	Common tendon of gracilis, semitendinosus, and sartorius muscles
5	Extensor digitorum longus muscle	12	Extensor hallucis longus muscle		
6	Superior extensor retinaculum	13	Medial malleolus	18	Tibia
7	Inferior extensor retinaculum				

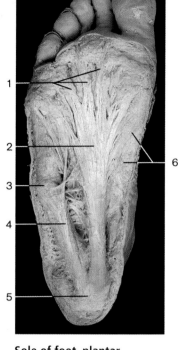

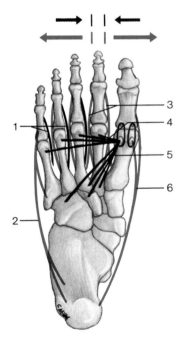

Sole of foot, plantar aponeurosis (from below).

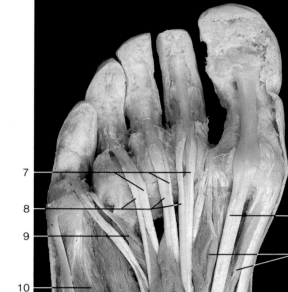

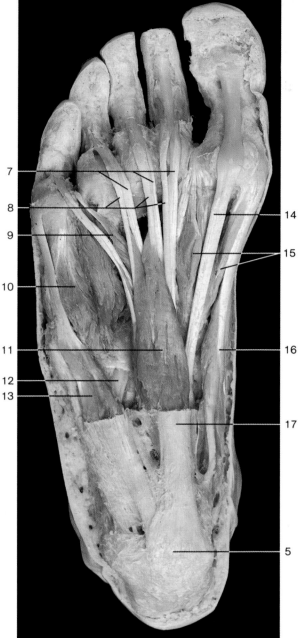

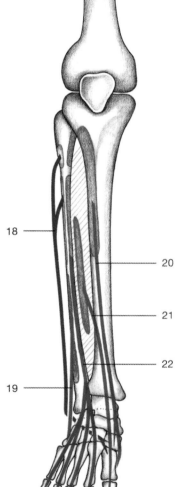

Extensor muscles of the leg (right side).

Muscles of sole of foot, first layer (from below). The plantar aponeurosis and the fasciae of the superficial muscles have been removed.

Course of abductor and adductor muscles of foot (schematic drawing).
Red arrows = abduction.
Black arrows = adduction.

1   Longitudinal bands of plantar aponeurosis
2   Plantar aponeurosis
3   Position of tuberosity of fifth metatarsal bone
4   Muscles of fifth toe with fascia
5   Calcaneal tuberosity
6   Muscles of great toe with fascia
7   Tendons of flexor digitorum longus muscle
8   Tendons of flexor digitorum brevis muscle
9   Lumbrical muscle
10   Flexor digiti minimi brevis muscle
11   Flexor digitorum brevis muscle

12   Tendon of peroneus longus muscle
13   Abductor digiti minimi muscle
14   Tendon of flexor hallucis longus muscle
15   Flexor hallucis brevis muscle
16   Abductor hallucis muscle
17   Plantar aponeurosis (cut)
18   Peroneus longus muscle
19   Peroneus brevis muscle
20   Tibialis anterior muscle
21   Extensor hallucis longus muscle
22   Extensor digitorum longus muscle

1   Plantar interossei muscles (black)
2   Abductor digiti minimi muscle (red)
3   Dorsal interosseous muscles (red)
4   Transverse head of adductor muscle (black)
5   Oblique head of adductor muscle (black)
6   Abductor hallucis muscle (red)

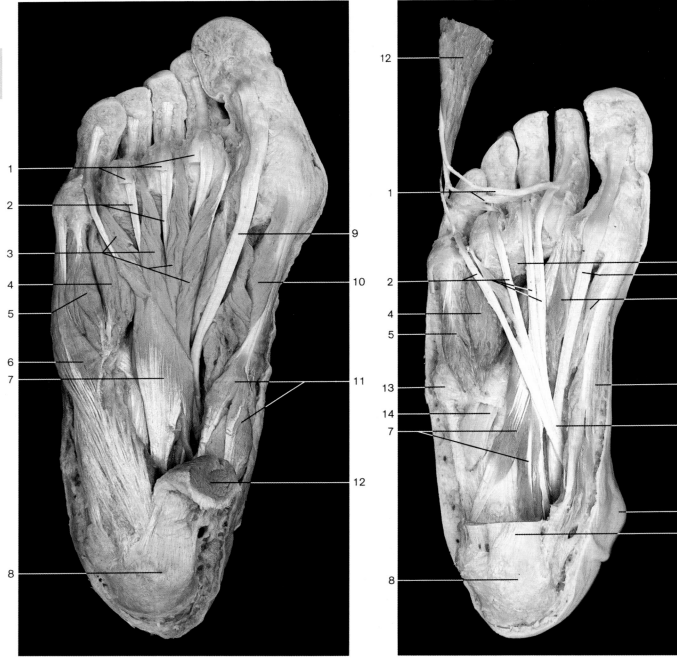

Muscles of sole of foot, second layer (from below). The flexor digitorum brevis muscle has been divided.

Muscles of sole of foot, second layer (from below). The tendons of the flexor muscles and the crossing of tendons are displayed. The flexor digitorum brevis muscle has been divided and reflected.

1 Tendons of flexor digitorum brevis muscle	6 Abductor digiti minimi muscle	13 Tuberosity of fifth metatarsal bone
2 Tendons of flexor digitorum longus muscle	7 Quadratus plantae muscle	14 Tendon of peroneus longus muscle
3 Lumbrical muscles	8 Calcaneal tuberosity	15 Transverse head of adductor hallucis muscle
4 Interossei muscles	9 Tendon of flexor hallucis longus muscle	16 Crossing of tendons in sole of foot
5 Flexor digiti minimi brevis muscle	10 Flexor hallucis brevis muscle	17 Medial malleolus
	11 Abductor hallucis muscle	18 Plantar aponeurosis (divided)
	12 Flexor digitorum brevis muscle (divided)	

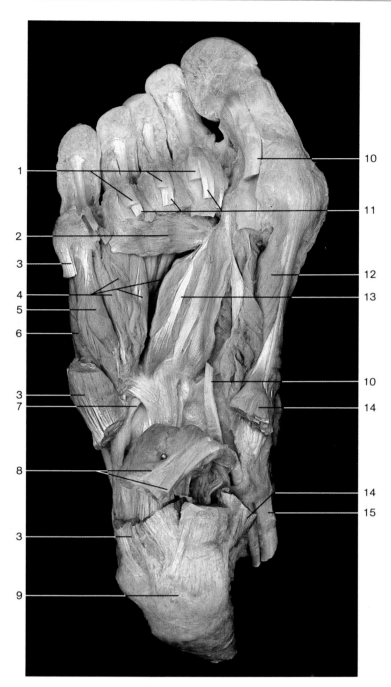

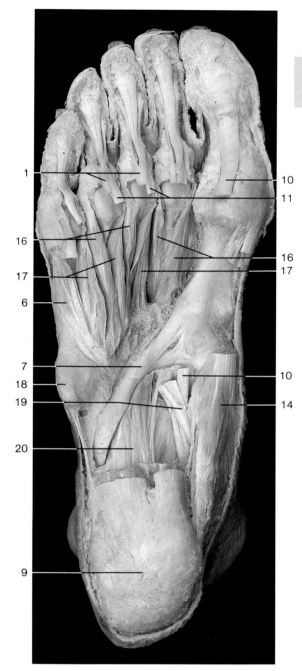

Muscles of sole of foot, third layer (from below). The flexor digitorum brevis muscle has been removed, and the quadratus plantae, abductor hallucis, and digiti minimi muscles have been divided.

Muscles of sole of foot, fourth layer (from below). The interosseous muscles and the canal for the tendon of peroneus longus muscle are shown.

1   Tendons of flexor digitorum brevis muscle
2   Transverse head of adductor hallucis muscle
3   Abductor digiti minimi muscle
4   Interossei muscles
5   Flexor digiti minimi brevis muscle
6   Opponens digiti minimi muscle
7   Tendon of peroneus longus muscle

8   Quadratus plantae muscle with tendon of flexor digitorum longus muscle
9   Calcaneal tuberosity
10 Tendons of flexor hallucis longus muscle (divided)
11 Tendon of flexor digitorum longus muscle
12 Flexor hallucis brevis muscle
13 Oblique head of adductor hallucis muscle
14 Abductor hallucis muscle (cut)

15 Tendon of tibialis posterior muscle
16 Dorsal interossei muscles
17 Plantar interossei muscles
18 Tuberosity of fifth metatarsal bone
19 Tendon of flexor digitorum longus muscle (crossing of plantar tendons)
20 Long plantar ligament

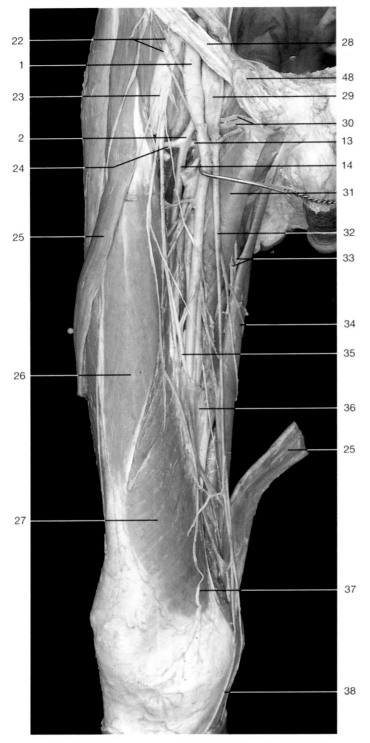

22
1
23
2
24
25
26
27

28
48
29
30
13
14
31
32
33
34
35
36
25
37
38

Main arteries and nerves of right thigh (anterior aspect).
Sartorius muscle has been divided and reflected. The femoral vein
has been partly removed to show the deep femoral artery.
Notice: the vessels enter the adductor canal to reach the popliteal
fossa.

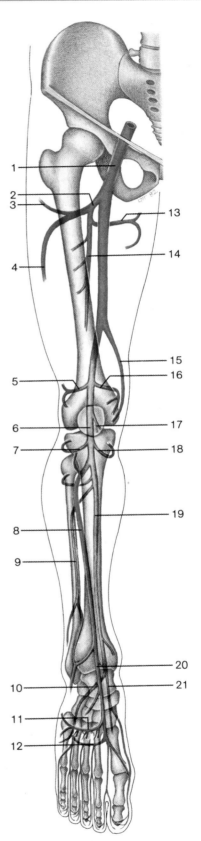

1
2
3
4
5
6
7
8
9
10
11
12

13
14
15
16
17
18
19
20
21

Main arteries of lower limb, right side
(anterior aspect, schematic drawing).

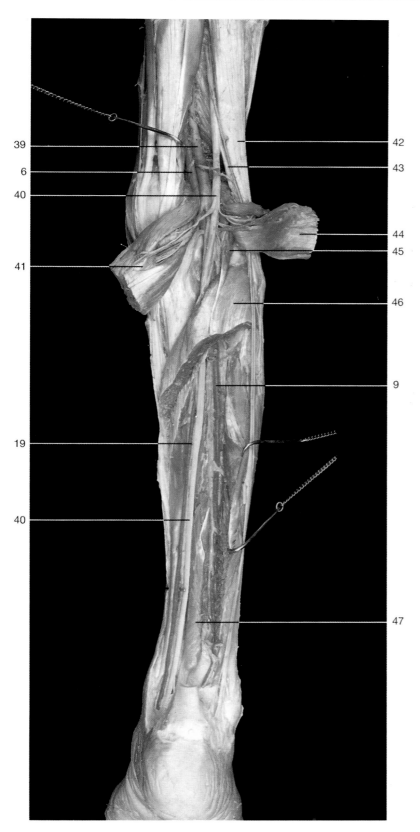

1   Femoral artery
2   Profunda femoris artery
3   Ascending branch of lateral circumflex
    femoral artery
4   Descending branch of lateral circumflex
    femoral artery
5   Lateral superior genicular artery
6   Popliteal artery
7   Lateral inferior genicular artery
8   Anterior tibial artery
9   Peroneal artery
10 Lateral plantar artery
11 Arcuate artery with dorsal metatarsal arteries
12 Plantar arch with plantar metatarsal arteries
13 Medial circumflex femoral artery
14 Profunda femoris artery with perforating
    arteries
15 Descending genicular artery
16 Medial superior genicular artery
17 Middle genicular artery
18 Medial inferior genicular artery
19 Posterior tibial artery
20 Dorsalis pedis artery
21 Medial plantar artery
22 Superficial and deep circumflex iliac arteries
23 Femoral nerve
24 Lateral circumflex femoral artery
25 Sartorius muscle (cut and reflected)
26 Rectus femoris muscle
27 Vastus medialis muscle
28 Inguinal ligament
29 Femoral vein (cut)
30 External pudendal artery and vein
31 Adductor longus muscle
32 Great saphenous vein
33 Obturator artery and nerve
34 Gracilis muscle
35 Saphenous nerve
36 Tendinous wall of adductor canal
37 Anterior cutaneous branch of femoral nerve
38 Infrapatellar branch of saphenous nerve
39 Popliteal vein
40 Tibial nerve
41 Medial head of gastrocnemius muscle
42 Biceps femoris muscle
43 Common peroneal nerve
44 Lateral head of gastrocnemius muscle
45 Plantaris muscle
46 Soleus muscle
47 Flexor hallucis longus muscle
48 Spermatic cord

Arteries of the right leg (posterior aspect).

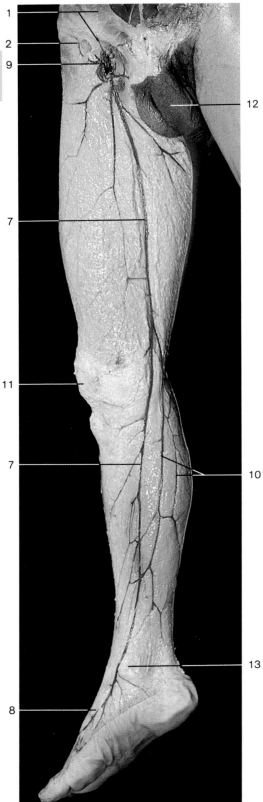

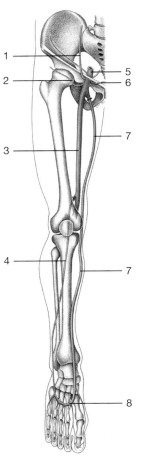

1 Superficial epigastric vein
2 Superficial circumflex iliac vein
3 Femoral vein
4 Small saphenous vein
5 External iliac vein
6 External pudendal vein
7 Great saphenous vein
8 Dorsal venous arch
9 Saphenous opening with femoral vein
10 Venous anastomoses of small saphenous vein with great saphenous vein
11 Patella
12 Penis
13 Medial malleolus
14 Popliteal fossa
15 Perforating veins
16 Lateral malleolus
17 Dorsal digital veins of foot
18 Dorsal venous arch of foot
19 Dorsal metatarsal veins
20 Anterior tibial artery and veins
21 Tibia
22 Posterior tibial artery and veins
23 Fibula
24 Peroneal artery and vein
25 Deep layer of crural fascia
26 Superficial layer of crural fascia
27 Perforating veins I–III (of Cockett)
28 Tibial nerve
29 Arcuate vein
30 Saphenous nerve
31 Medial dorsal cutaneous nerve (branch of superficial peroneal nerve)
32 Posterior tibial vein

Main veins of lower limb, right side (anterior aspect, schematic drawing).

Superficial veins of lower limb, right side (medio-anterior aspect). The veins have been injected with red solution.

Medial malleolar region. Dissection of tibial nerve, posterior tibial vessels, and great saphenous vein (veins injected with blue resin).

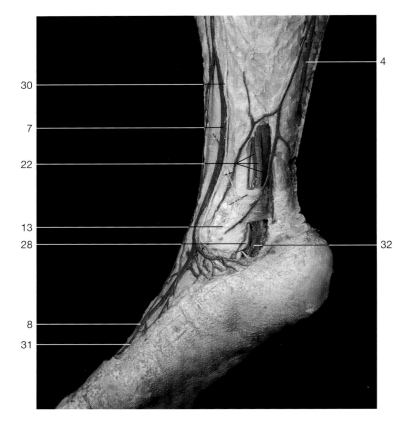

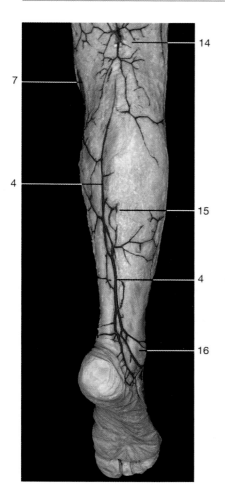

14
7
4
15
4
16

Superficial veins of leg (posterior aspect; veins injected with blue resin).

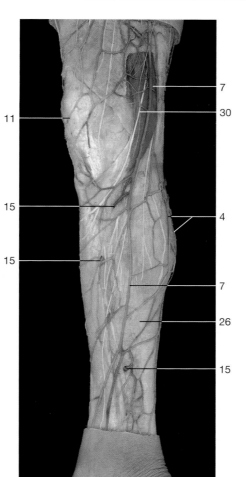

11
7
30
15
15
15
4
7
26
15

Superficial veins of leg. The perforating veins of Cockett have been dissected (left side, medial aspect).

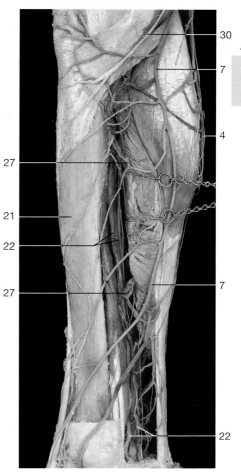

30
7
4
27
21
22
27
7
22

Veins of leg. The anastomoses between superficial and deeper veins are dissected (left side, medial aspect).

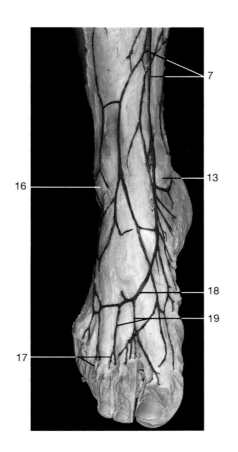

7
16
13
18
19
17

Anastomoses between superficial ▷ and deep veins of the leg (schematic drawing, after Aigner).
Arrows: directions of blood flow.

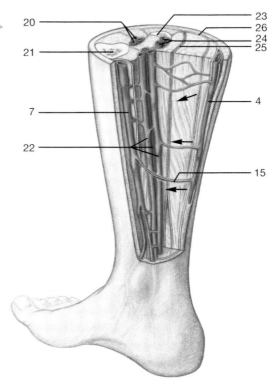

20
21
23
26
24
25
7
22
4
15

◁
Superficial veins on dorsum of foot (veins injected with blue resin).

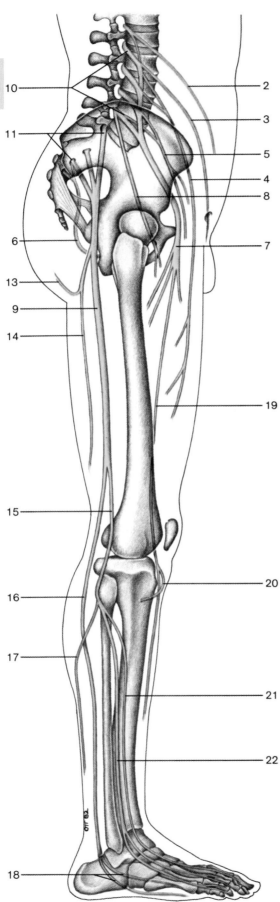

1   Subcostal nerve
2   Iliohypogastric nerve
3   Ilio-inguinal nerve
4   Lateral femoral cutaneous nerve
5   Genitofemoral nerve
6   Pudendal nerve
7   Femoral nerve
8   Obturator nerve
9   Sciatic nerve
10 Lumbar plexus (L₁–L₄)
11 Sacral plexus (L₄–S₄)   } lumbosacral plexus
12 "Pudendal" plexus (S₂–S₄)
13 Inferior cluneal nerves
14 Posterior femoral cutaneous nerve
15 Common peroneal nerve
16 Tibial nerve
17 Lateral sural cutaneous nerve
18 Medial and lateral plantar nerves
19 Saphenous nerve
20 Infrapatellar branch of saphenous nerve
21 Deep peroneal nerve
22 Superficial peroneal nerve
23 Anterior cutaneous branch of iliohypogastric nerve
24 Lateral cutaneous branch of iliohypogastric nerve
25 Femoral branch of genitofemoral nerve
26 Lateral cutaneous branches of intercostal nerve
27 Anterior cutaneous branches of intercostal nerve
28 Genital branch of genitofemoral nerve
29 Anterior scrotal nerve

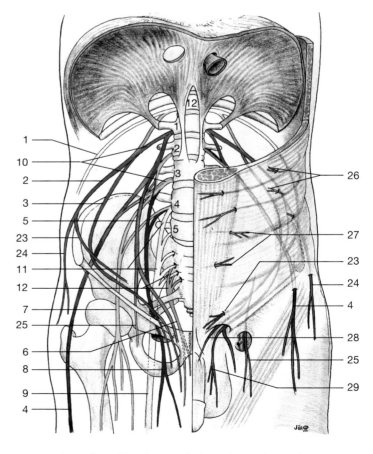

Nerves of lower limb, right side (lateral aspect).
(Schematic drawing.)

Main branches of lumbosacral plexus (ventral aspect).
(Schematic drawing.)

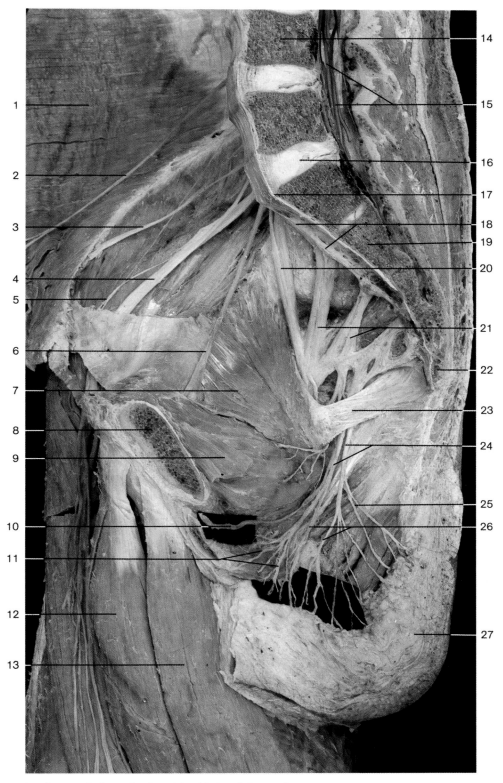

1 Transversus abdominis muscle
2 Iliohypogastric nerve
3 Ilio-inguinal nerve
4 Femoral nerve
5 Lateral femoral cutaneous nerve
6 Obturator nerve
7 Obturator internus muscle
8 Pubic bone (cut edge)
9 Levator ani muscle (remnant)
10 Dorsal nerve of penis
11 Posterior scrotal nerves
12 Adductor longus muscle
13 Gracilis muscle
14 Body of fourth lumbar vertebra
15 Cauda equina
16 Intervertebral disc
17 Sacral promontory
18 Sympathetic trunk
19 Sacrum
20 Lumbosacral trunk
21 Sacral plexus
22 Coccyx
23 Sacrospinous ligament
24 Pudendal nerve
25 Inferior rectal nerves
26 Perineal nerves
27 Subcutaneous fat tissue
   of gluteal region

Lumbosacral plexus in situ, right side (medial aspect).
Pelvic organs with peritoneum and part of the levator ani muscle have been removed.

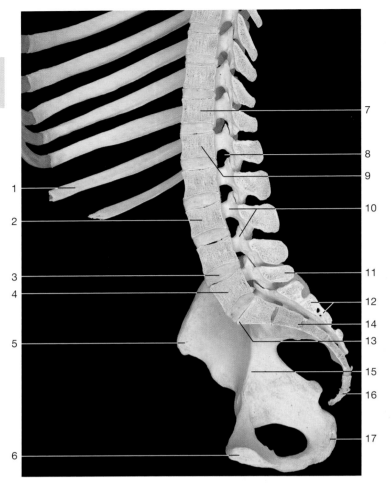

Lumbar part of vertebral column with pelvis (sagittal section, medial aspect).

1 Eleventh rib
2 Body of third lumbar vertebra
3 Intervertebral disc
4 Body of fifth lumbar vertebra
5 Anterior superior iliac spine
6 Symphysial surface
7 Body of twelfth thoracic vertebra
8 Intervertebral foramen
9 Body of first lumbar vertebra
10 Vertebral canal
11 Spinous process of fifth lumbar vertebra
12 Sacrum (median sacral crest)
13 Promontory (promontorium)
14 Sacrum
15 Arcuate line
16 Coccyx
17 Ischial tuberosity
18 Sympathetic trunk with ganglia
19 Ureter
20 Iliohypogastric nerve (Th_{12}, L_1)
21 Ilio-inguinal nerve (L_1)
22 Femoral nerve (L_2–L_4)
23 Genitofemoral nerve (L_1, L_2)
24 Inferior hypogastric plexus
25 Ductus deferens
26 Urinary bladder
27 Medullary cone of spinal cord
28 Root filaments of spinal nerves
29 Subarachnoid space
     (filled with cerebrospinal fluid) (blue)
30 Terminal filament of spinal cord
31 Sacral plexus
32 Pelvic splanchnic nerves (nervi erigentes)
33 Rectum

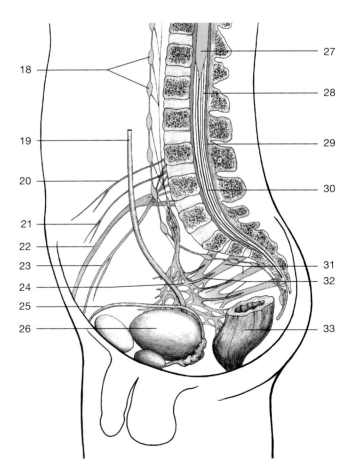

Vertebral canal with spinal cord and root filaments.
Note the high location of the medullary cone. Sacral plexus and inferior hypogastric plexus are schematically shown.

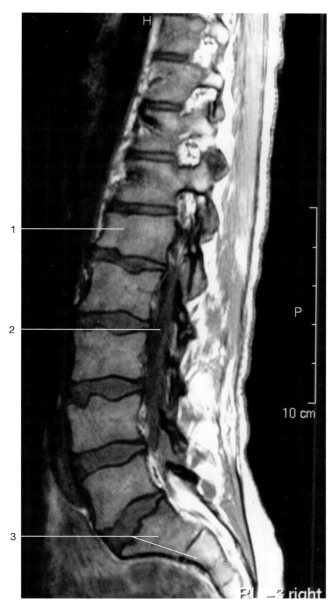

Paramedian section of lumbar part of vertebral canal
(MRI scan, dotted line in the schematic drawing below; courtesy
of Prof. Bautz, Erlangen, Germany).

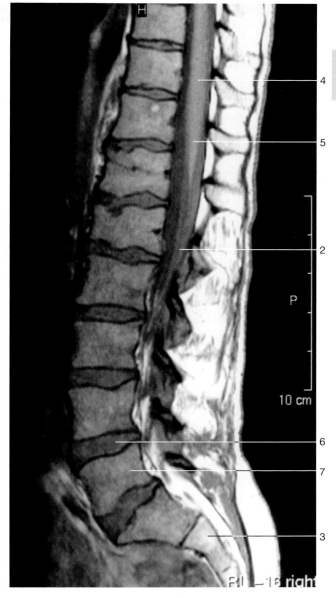

**Median section of lumbar part of vertebral canal at the
level of the medullary cone** (MRI scan, continuous line in the
schematic drawing below; courtesy of Prof. Bautz, Erlangen,
Germany).

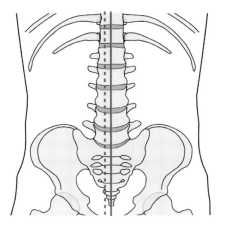

1   First lumbar vertebra
2   Root filaments of spinal nerves
3   Sacrum
4   Spinal cord
5   Medullary cone of spinal cord
6   Intervertebral disc between fourth and fifth
    lumbar vertebra
7   Fifth lumbar vertebra

**Location of the sections shown above through the
vertebral canal.**

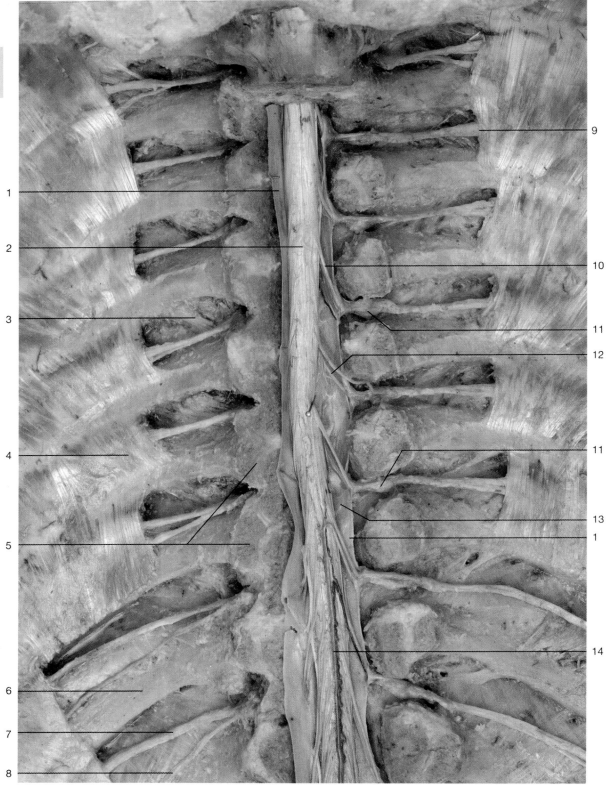

Spinal cord with intercostal nerves. Inferior thoracic region (anterior aspect). Anterior portion of thoracic vertebrae removed, dural sheath opened, and spinal cord slightly reflected to the right to display the dorsal and ventral roots.

1 Dura mater	6 Eleventh rib	10 Anterior root filaments
2 Spinal cord	7 Intercostal nerve	11 Spinal (dorsal root) ganglion
3 Costotransverse ligament	8 Collateral branch of intercostal nerve	12 Posterior root filaments
4 Innermost intercostal muscle	9 Intercostal nerve (entering the	13 Arachnoid mater and denticulate ligament
5 Vertebral arches (cut surfaces)	intermuscular interval)	14 Anterior spinal artery

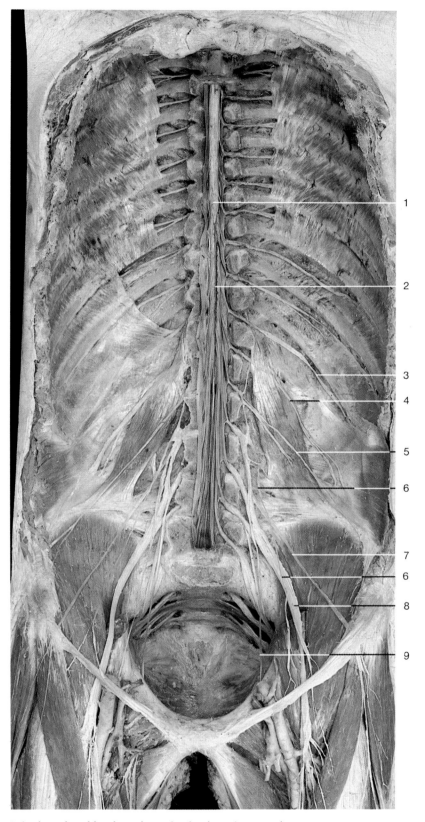

Spinal cord and lumbar plexus in situ (anterior aspect).

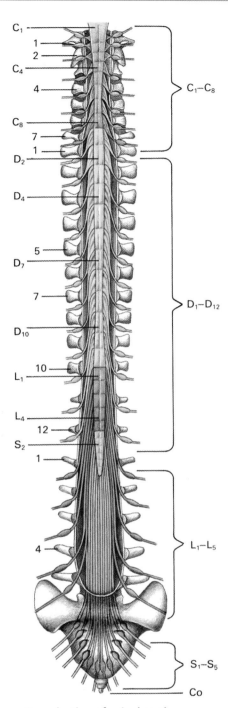

Organization of spinal cord segments in relation to the vertebral column (anterior aspect).
C = cervical; D = thoracic; L = lumbar; S = sacral segments; Co = coccygeal bone.
Numbers indicate the related vertebrae.

1 Conus medullaris	6 Genitofemoral nerve
2 Filum terminale	7 Lateral femoral cutaneous nerve
3 Subcostal nerve	8 Femoral nerve
4 Iliohypogastric nerve	9 Obturator nerve
5 Ilio-inguinal nerve	

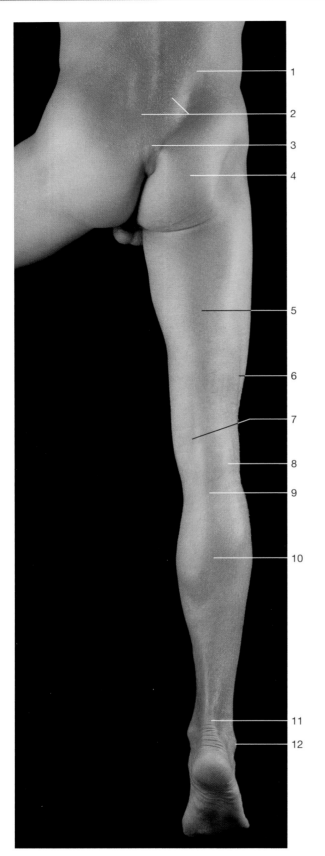

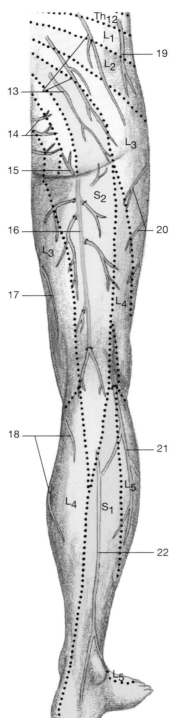

1 Iliac crest
2 Sacrum
3 Coccyx
4 Gluteus maximus muscle
5 Dorsal muscles of the leg
6 Iliotibial tract
7 Tendon of semimembranosus muscle
8 Tendon of biceps femoris muscle
9 Popliteal fossa
10 Triceps surae muscle
11 Calcaneal or Achilles tendon
12 Lateral malleolus
13 Superior cluneal nerves
14 Middle cluneal nerves
15 Inferior cluneal nerves
16 Posterior femoral cutaneous nerve
17 Obturator nerve
18 Saphenous nerve
19 Iliohypogastric nerve
20 Branch of lateral femoral cutaneous nerves
21 Common peroneal nerve
22 Sural nerve

Cutaneous nerves of the lower limb (posterior aspect). Dotted lines = border of segments.

Surface anatomy of the right leg (posterior aspect). Gluteal muscles contracted.

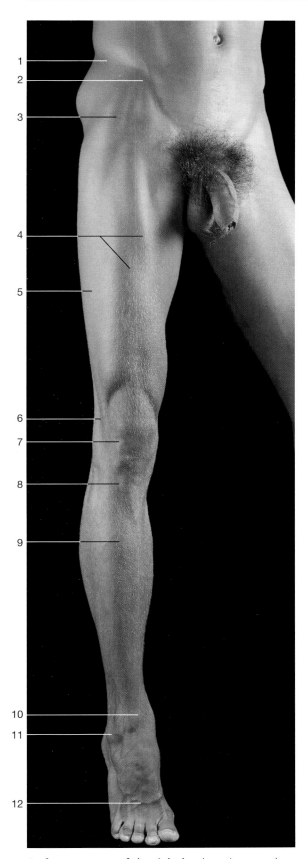

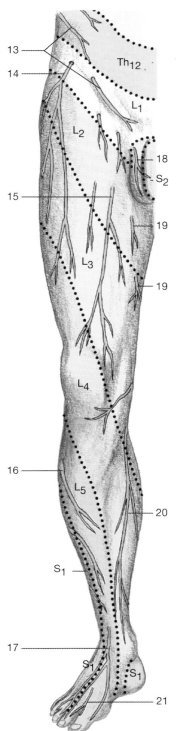

1   Iliac crest
2   Anterior superior iliac spine
3   Tensor fasciae latae muscle
4   Quadriceps femoris muscle
5   Iliotibial tract
6   Tendon of biceps femoris
     muscle
7   Patella
8   Patellar ligament
9   Tibia
10 Tendon of tibialis anterior
     muscle
11 Lateral malleolus
12 Venous network of dorsum
     of foot
13 Iliohypogastric nerve
14 Lateral femoral cutaneous
     nerve
15 Femoral nerve
16 Common peroneal nerve
17 Superficial peroneal nerve
18 Ilio-inguinal nerve
19 Obturator nerve
20 Saphenous nerve
21 Deep peroneal nerve

Cutaneous nerves of the lower limb (anterior aspect).
Dotted lines = border of segments.

Surface anatomy of the right leg (anterior aspect).

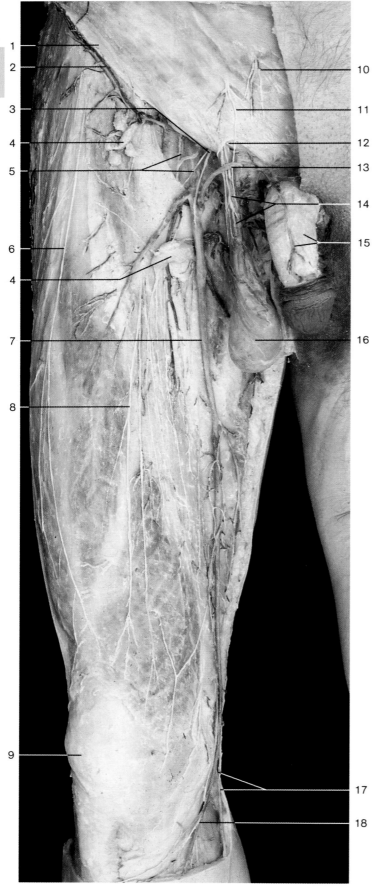

Cutaneous nerves and veins of thigh (anterior aspect).

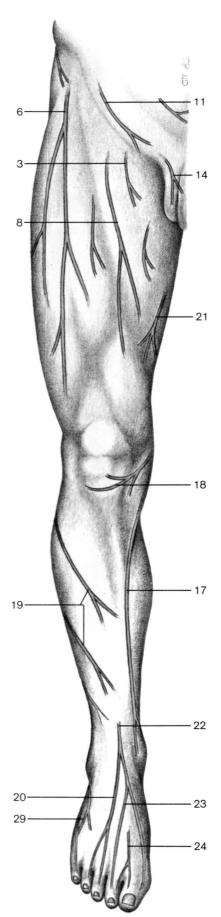

Cutaneous nerves of lower limb (anterior aspect). (Schematic drawing.)

1 Inguinal ligament
2 Superficial circumflex iliac vein
3 Femoral branch of genitofemoral nerve
4 Superficial inguinal lymph nodes
5 Saphenous opening with femoral artery and vein
6 Lateral femoral cutaneous nerve
7 Great saphenous vein
8 Anterior cutaneous branches of femoral nerve
9 Patella
10 Terminal branches of subcostal nerve
11 Terminal branches of iliohypogastric nerve
12 Superficial inguinal ring
13 External pudendal vein
14 Spermatic cord with genital branch of genitofemoral
     nerve
15 Penis with superficial dorsal vein of penis
16 Testis and its coverings
17 Saphenous nerve
18 Infrapatellar branch of saphenous nerve
19 Lateral sural cutaneous nerves
20 Intermediate dorsal cutaneous branch of superficial
     peroneal nerve
21 Cutaneous branch of obturator nerve
22 Superficial peroneal nerve
23 Medial dorsal cutaneous branch of superficial
     peroneal nerve
24 Deep peroneal nerve
25 Femoral nerve
26 Femoral artery
27 Superficial epigastric vein
28 Femoral vein
29 Lateral dorsal cutaneous branch of sural nerve
30 Inguinal nodes (enlarged)
31 Lympathic vessels
32 Sartorius muscle

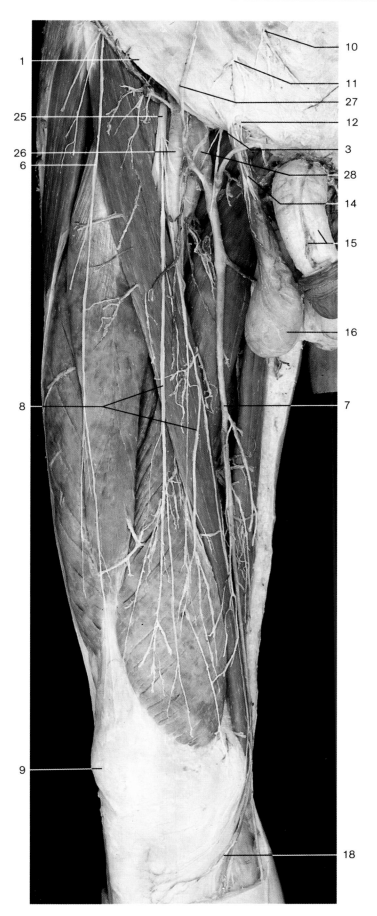

Cutaneous nerves and veins of thigh (anterior aspect). The
fascia lata and fasciae of the thigh muscles have been removed.

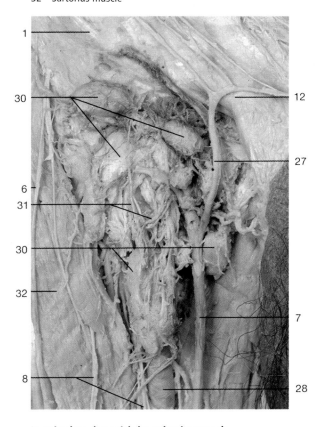

Inguinal nodes with lymphatic vessels
(anterior aspect).

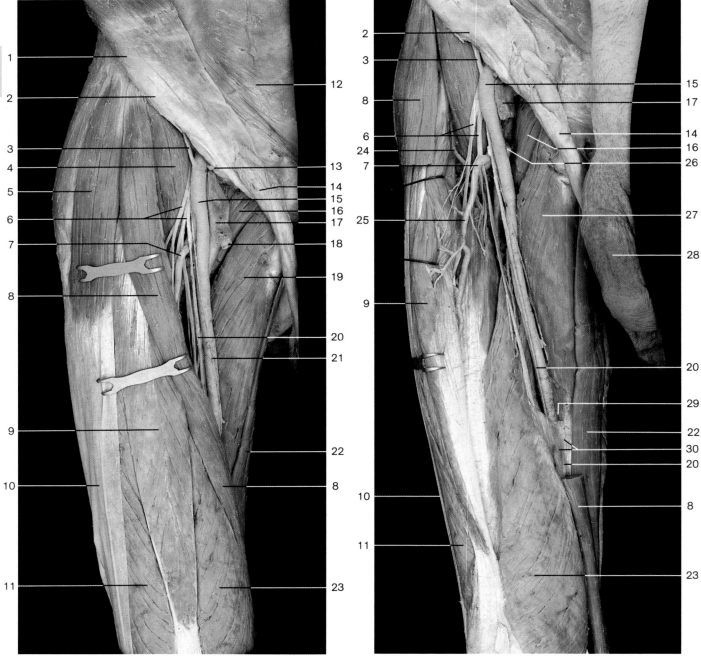

Anterior region of right thigh (anterior aspect). The fascia lata has been removed, and the sartorius muscle has been slightly reflected.

Anterior region of right thigh (anterior aspect). The fascia lata has been removed, and the sartorius muscle has been divided.

1   Anterior superior iliac spine
2   Inguinal ligament
3   Deep circumflex iliac artery
4   Iliopsoas muscle
5   Tensor fasciae latae muscle
6   Femoral nerve
7   Lateral circumflex femoral artery
8   Sartorius muscle
9   Rectus femoris muscle
10 Iliotibial tract
11 Vastus lateralis muscle
12 Anterior sheath of rectus abdominis muscle
13 Inferior epigastric artery
14 Spermatic cord
15 Femoral artery

16 Pectineus muscle
17 Femoral vein
18 Great saphenous vein (divided)
19 Adductor longus muscle
20 Saphenous nerve
21 Muscular branch of femoral nerve
22 Gracilis muscle
23 Vastus medialis muscle
24 Ascending branch of lateral circumflex femoral artery
25 Descending branch of lateral circumflex femoral artery
26 Medial circumflex femoral artery
27 Adductor longus muscle
28 Penis
29 Entrance to adductor canal
30 Vasto-adductor membrane of fascia beneath sartorius muscle

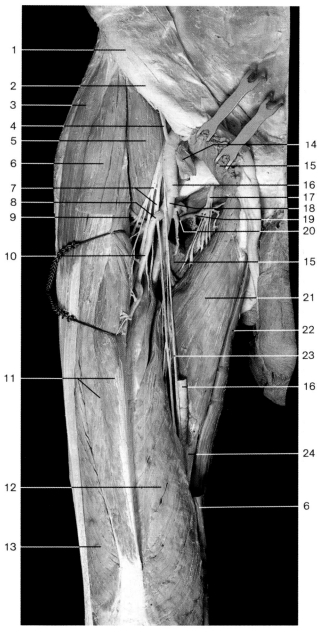

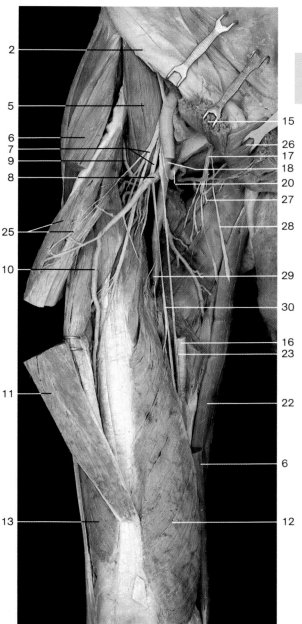

Anterior region of right thigh (anterior aspect).
The fascia lata has been removed. Sartorius muscle,
pectineus muscle, and femoral artery have been cut to
display the deep femoral artery with its branches.
The rectus femoris muscle has been slightly reflected.

Anterior region of right thigh (anterior aspect).
The sartorius, pectineus, adductor longus, and rectus
femoris muscles have been divided and reflected.
The greater part of the femoral artery has been
removed.

1	Anterior superior iliac spine
2	Inguinal ligament
3	Tensor fasciae latae muscle
4	Deep circumflex iliac artery
5	Iliopsoas muscle
6	Sartorius muscle (cut)
7	Femoral nerve
8	Lateral circumflex femoral artery
9	Ascending branch of lateral circumflex femoral artery
10	Descending branch of lateral circumflex femoral artery
11	Rectus femoris muscle
12	Vastus medialis muscle
13	Vastus lateralis muscle
14	Femoral vein
15	Pectineus muscle (cut)
16	Femoral artery (cut)

17	Obturator nerve
18	Profunda femoris artery
19	Ascending branch of medial circumflex femoral artery
20	Medial circumflex femoral artery
21	Adductor longus muscle
22	Gracilis muscle
23	Saphenous nerve
24	Distal part of vasto-adductor membrane
25	Rectus femoris muscle with muscular branch of femoral nerve
26	Adductor longus muscle (divided)
27	Posterior branch of obturator nerve
28	Anterior branch of obturator nerve
29	Point at which perforating artery branches off from profunda femoris artery
30	Muscular branch of femoral nerve to vastus medialis muscle

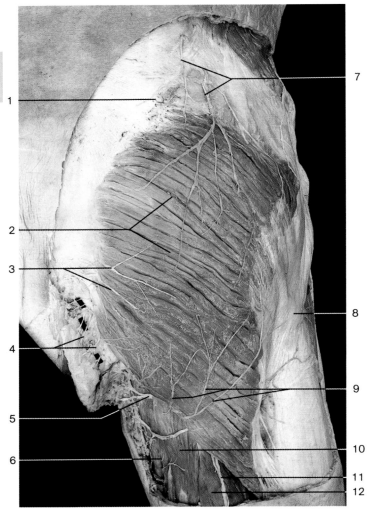

1 Iliac crest
2 Gluteus maximus muscle
3 Middle cluneal nerves
4 Anococcygeal nerves
5 Perineal branch of posterior femoral cutaneous nerve
6 Adductor magnus muscle
7 Superior cluneal nerves
8 Position of greater trochanter
9 Inferior cluneal nerves
10 Semitendinosus muscle
11 Posterior femoral cutaneous nerve
12 Long head of biceps femoris muscle

Gluteal region, right side (posterior aspect).

A	**Suprapiriform foramen** (of greater sciatic foramen)
	Superior gluteal artery, vein, and nerve
B	**Infrapiriform foramen** (of greater sciatic foramen)
	Sciatic nerve Inferior gluteal artery, vein, and nerve Posterior femoral cutaneous nerve Internal pudendal artery and vein Pudendal nerve
C	**Lesser sciatic foramen**
	Pudendal nerve Internal pudendal artery and vein

Red lines

1 Spine-tuber line:
   the infrapiriform foramen is situated in the middle of this line
2 Spine-trochanter line:
   the suprapiriform foramen is located in the upper third
3 Tuber-trochanter line:
   the ischiadic nerve can be found between the middle and posterior third

Other structures

4 Posterior superior iliac spine
5 Iliac crest
6 Greater trochanter
7 Ischial tuberosity
8 Sacrum

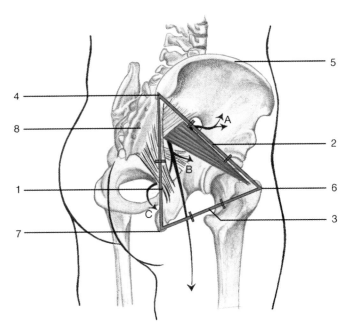

Gluteal region, right side (postero-lateral aspect). Location of sciatic foramina in relation to the bones (schematic drawing).

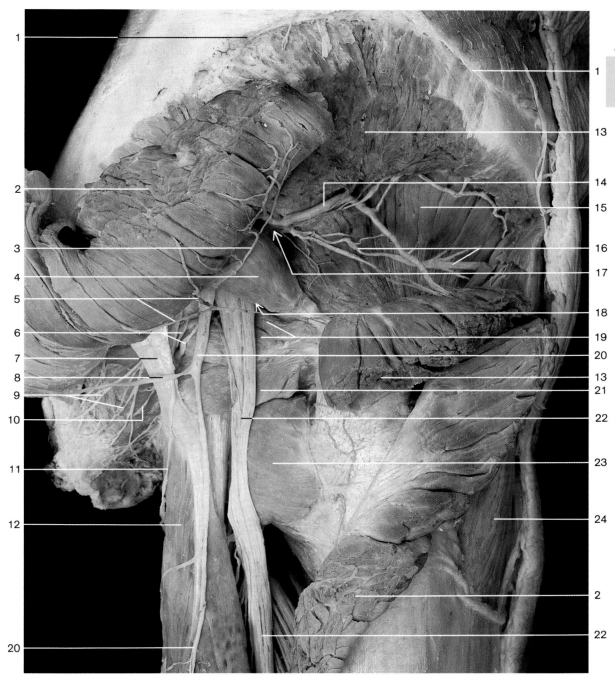

Gluteal region, right side (posterior aspect). The gluteus maximus and gluteus medius muscles have been divided and reflected. Notice the position of the foramina above and below the piriformis muscle and the lesser sciatic foramen.

1 Iliac crest	13 Gluteus medius muscle (cut)
2 Gluteus maximus muscle (cut)	14 Deep branch of superior gluteal artery
3 Inferior gluteal nerve	15 Gluteus minimus muscle
4 Piriformis muscle	16 Superior gluteal nerve
5 Muscular branches of inferior gluteal artery	17 Suprapiriform foramen ⎤ greater sciatic foramen
6 Pudendal nerve and internal pudendal artery within the lesser sciatic foramen (entrance to the pudendal canal)	18 Infrapiriform foramen ⎦
	19 Tendon of obturator internus and superior gemellus muscles
7 Sacrotuberous ligament	20 Posterior femoral cutaneous nerve
8 Inferior cluneal nerve	21 Inferior gemellus muscle
9 Inferior rectal nerves	22 Sciatic nerve
10 Inferior rectal arteries	23 Quadratus femoris muscle
11 Perforating cutaneous nerve	24 Tensor fasciae latae muscle
12 Long head of biceps femoris muscle	

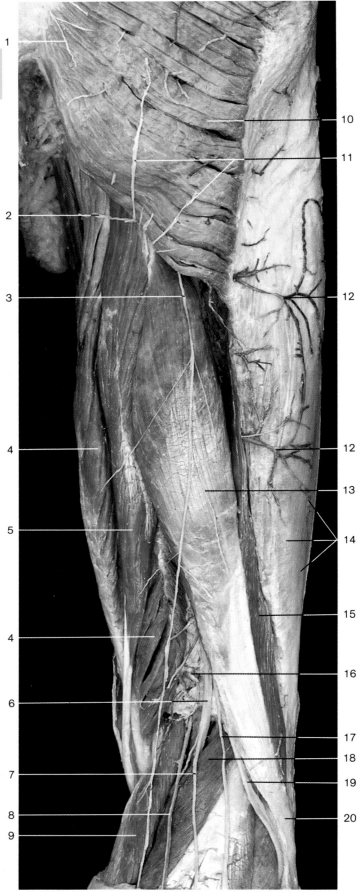

1   Middle cluneal nerves
2   Perineal branch of posterior femoral cutaneous nerve
3   Posterior femoral cutaneous nerve
4   Semimembranosus muscle
5   Semitendinosus muscle
6   Tibial nerve
7   Medial sural cutaneous nerve
8   Small saphenous vein
9   Medial head of gastrocnemius muscle
10 Gluteus maximus muscle
11 Inferior cluneal nerves
12 Cutaneous veins
13 Long head of biceps femoris muscle
14 Iliotibial tract
15 Short head of biceps femoris muscle
16 Popliteal fossa
17 Lateral sural cutaneous nerve
18 Lateral head of gastrocnemius muscle
19 Common peroneal nerve
20 Tendon of biceps femoris muscle
21 Inferior gluteal nerve
22 Sacrotuberous ligament
23 Inferior rectal branches of pudendal nerve
24 Anus
25 Gluteus medius muscle
26 Piriformis muscle
27 Sciatic nerve
28 Inferior gluteal artery
29 Gluteus maximus muscle (cut)
30 Quadratus femoris muscle
31 Sciatic nerve dividing into its two branches: the common
    peroneal nerve and the tibial nerve
32 Muscular branches of sciatic nerve to hamstring muscles
33 Popliteal artery
34 Popliteal vein
35 Small saphenous vein (cut)
36 Long head of biceps femoris muscle (cut)
37 Superficial peroneal nerve

Cutaneous nerves of thigh (posterior aspect).
The fascia lata and the fasciae of muscles have been removed.

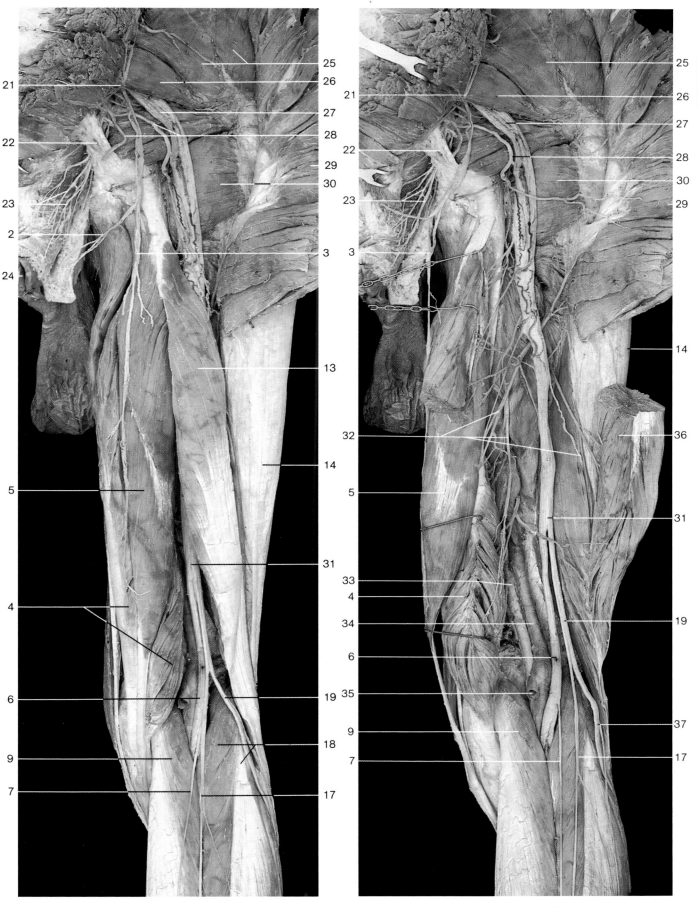

Gluteal region and posterior region of right thigh (posterior aspect). The gluteus maximus muscle has been divided and reflected.

Gluteal region and posterior region of right thigh (posterior aspect). The gluteus maximus muscle and the long head of the biceps femoris muscle have been divided and reflected.

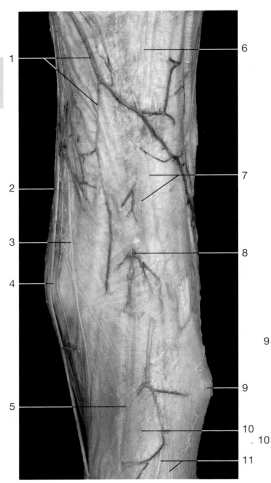

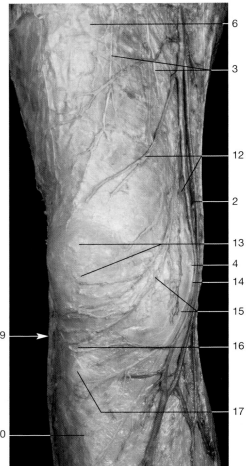

1   Cutaneous veins (tributaries of great saphenous vein)
2   Great saphenous vein
3   Cutaneous branch of femoral nerve
4   Position of medial condyle of femur
5   Position of small saphenous vein
6   Fascia lata
7   Terminal branches of posterior femoral cutaneous nerve
8   Cutaneous veins of popliteal fossa
9   Position of head of fibula
10 Superficial layer of fascia cruris
11 Lateral sural cutaneous nerve
12 Venous network around knee
13 Patella
14 Saphenous nerve
15 Infrapatellar branch of saphenous nerve
16 Patellar ligament
17 Position of tuberosity of tibia
18 Sartorius muscle
19 Semimembranosus muscle
20 Gastrocnemius muscle
21 Popliteal vein
22 Tibial nerve
23 Biceps femoris muscle
24 Popliteal artery
25 Lateral inferior genicular artery
26 Fibula

Posterior region of right knee, cutaneous nerves and veins (posterior aspect).

Anterior region of right knee, cutaneous nerves and veins (anterior aspect).

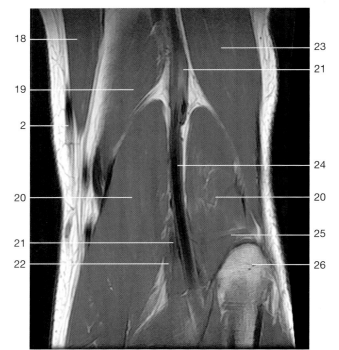

Coronal section of popliteal fossa (MRI scan; from Heuck et al., MRT-Atlas, 2009).

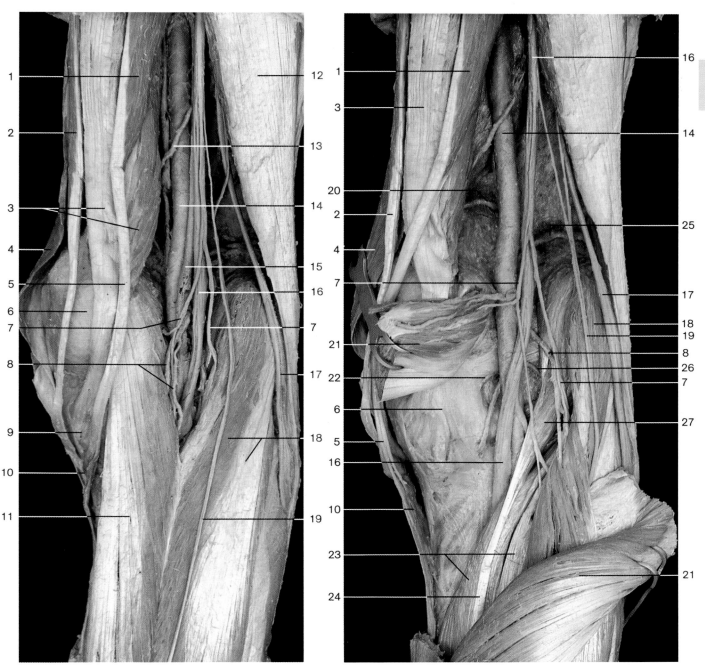

Right leg, popliteal fossa, middle layer (posterior aspect). The gastrocnemius muscle has been divided and reflected.

Right leg, popliteal fossa, deep layer (posterior aspect). The gastrocnemius and the soleus muscles have been divided and reflected.

1 Semitendinosus muscle
2 Gracilis muscle
3 Semimembranosus muscle
4 Sartorius muscle
5 Tendon of semitendinosus muscle
6 Position of medial condyle of femur
7 Muscular branches of tibial nerve
8 Sural arteries and veins
9 Tendon of semimembranosus muscle
10 Common tendon of gracilis, semitendinosus, and sartorius muscles
11 Medial head of gastrocnemius muscle
12 Biceps femoris muscle
13 Muscular branch of popliteal artery

14 Popliteal artery
15 Popliteal vein
16 Tibial nerve
17 Common peroneal nerve
18 Lateral head of gastrocnemius muscle
19 Medial sural cutaneous nerve
20 Medial superior genicular artery
21 Medial head of gastrocnemius muscle (cut and reflected)
22 Medial inferior genicular artery
23 Soleus muscle
24 Tendon of plantaris muscle
25 Lateral superior genicular artery
26 Lateral inferior genicular artery
27 Plantaris muscle

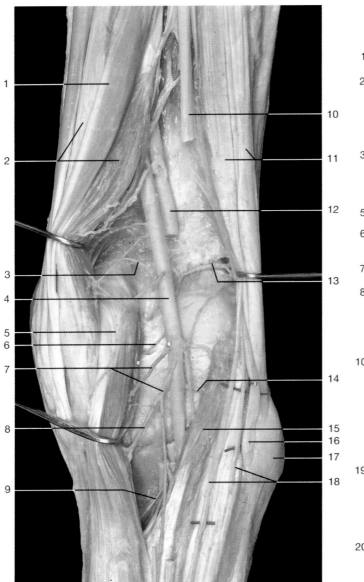

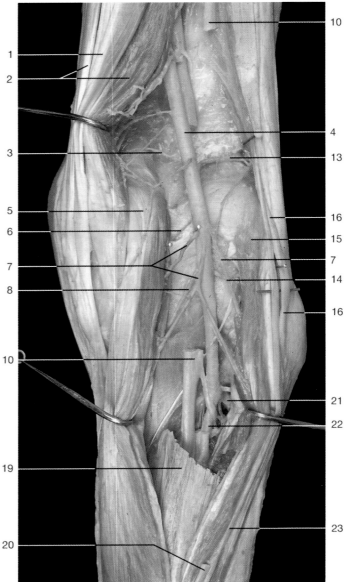

Right leg, popliteal fossa, deep layer (posterior aspect).
The muscles have been reflected to display the genicular arteries.

Right leg, popliteal fossa, deepest layer (posterior aspect).
Tibial nerve and popliteal vein have been partly removed
and a portion of the soleus muscle was cut away to display the
anterior tibial artery.

1	Semitendinosus muscle
2	Semimembranosus muscle
3	Medial superior genicular artery
4	Popliteal artery
5	Medial head of gastrocnemius muscle
6	Middle genicular artery
7	Muscular branches
8	Medial inferior genicular artery
9	Tendon of plantaris muscle
10	Tibial nerve (cut)
11	Biceps femoris muscle

12	Popliteal vein (cut)
13	Lateral superior genicular artery
14	Lateral inferior genicular artery
15	Lateral head of gastrocnemius muscle
16	Common peroneal nerve
17	Head of fibula
18	Lateral sural cutaneous nerves
19	Soleus muscle
20	Medial sural cutaneous nerve
21	Anterior tibial artery
22	Posterior tibial artery
23	Lateral sural cutaneous nerve

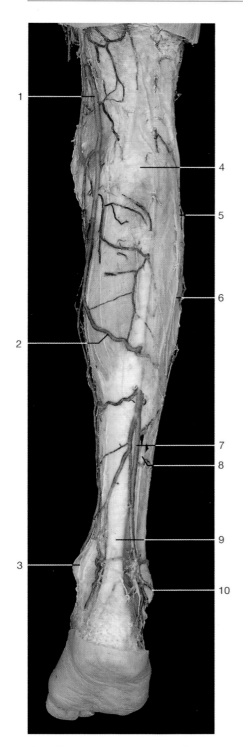

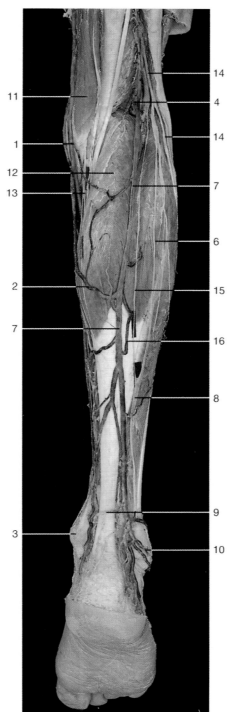

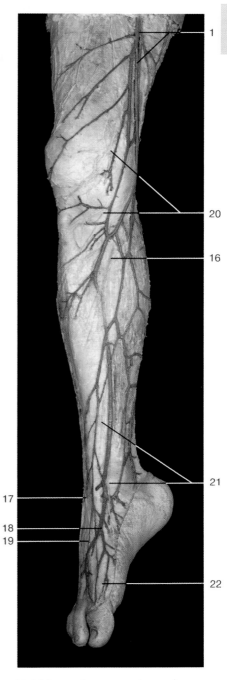

Right leg, cutaneous veins and nerves (posterior aspect).

Right leg, cutaneous veins and nerves (posterior aspect). The superficial layer of the crural fascia has been removed.

Right leg, cutaneous veins and nerves (antero-medial aspect).

1	Great saphenous vein
2	Venous anastomosis between small and great saphenous veins
3	Medial malleolus
4	Popliteal fossa
5	Position of head of fibula
6	Lateral sural cutaneous nerve
7	Small saphenous vein
8	Sural nerve
9	Calcaneal tendon
10	Lateral malleolus
11	Semitendinosus muscle
12	Medial head of gastrocnemius muscle
13	Saphenous nerve
14	Common peroneal nerve
15	Medial sural cutaneous nerve
16	Perforating veins
17	Superficial peroneal nerve
18	Dorsal venous arch
19	Intermediate dorsal cutaneous nerve
20	Infrapatellar branches of saphenous nerve
21	Terminal branches of saphenous nerve
22	Medial dorsal cutaneous nerve

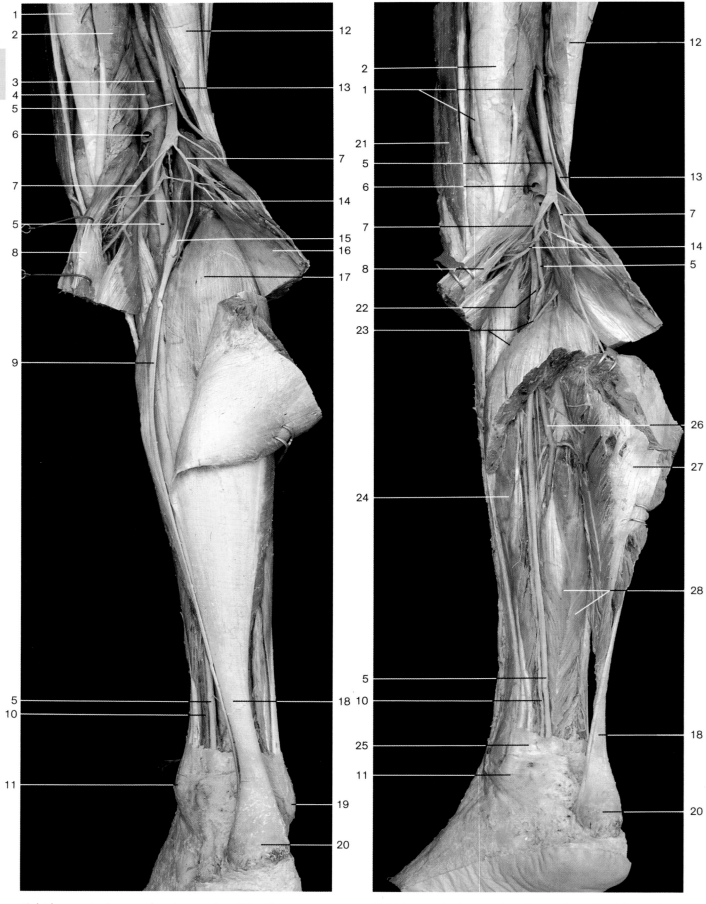

Right leg, posterior crural region, and popliteal fossa, middle layer (posterior aspect). The cutaneous veins and nerves have been removed.

Right leg, posterior crural region, and popliteal fossa, deep layer (posterior aspect). The medial head of gastrocnemius muscle has been divided and reflected.

1   Semimembranosus muscle
2   Semitendinosus muscle
3   Popliteal vein
4   Popliteal artery
5   Tibial nerve
6   Small saphenous vein (cut)
7   Muscular branch of tibial nerve
8   Medial head of gastrocnemius muscle
9   Tendon of plantaris muscle
10 Posterior tibial artery
11 Medial malleolus
12 Biceps femoris muscle
13 Common peroneal nerve
14 Sural arteries
15 Plantaris muscle
16 Lateral head of gastrocnemius muscle
17 Soleus muscle
18 Calcaneal tendon
19 Lateral malleolus
20 Calcaneal tuberosity
21 Sartorius muscle
22 Popliteal artery
23 Tendinous arch of soleus muscle
24 Flexor digitorum longus muscle
25 Flexor retinaculum
26 Peroneal artery
27 Soleus muscle
28 Flexor hallucis longus muscle
29 Anterior tibial artery
30 Muscular branches of tibial nerve
31 Tibialis posterior muscle
32 Communicating branch of peroneal artery
33 Tendon of tibialis anterior muscle
34 Tibia
35 Tendon of extensor hallucis longus muscle
36 Tendons of extensor digitorum longus muscle
37 Anterior tibialis artery
38 Fibula
39 Tendons of peroneus longus and brevis muscles

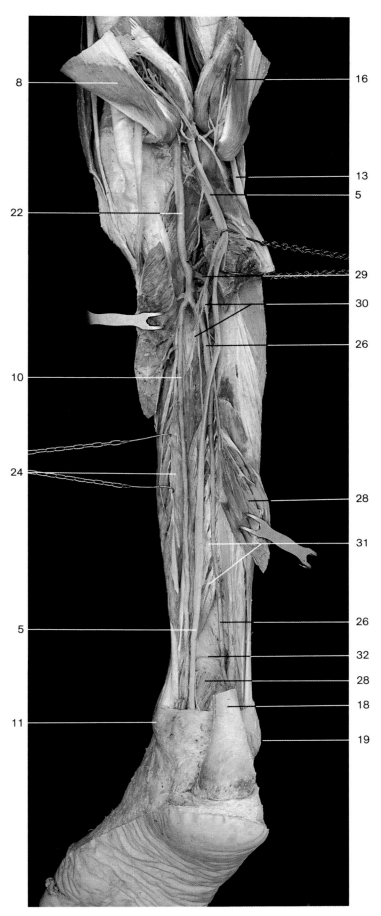

Right leg, posterior crural region, deepest layer (posterior aspect). Triceps surae (gastrocnemius and soleus) and flexor hallucis longus muscles have been cut and reflected.

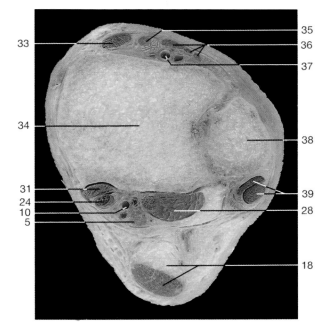

Cross section of the leg, superior to the malleoli (from below).

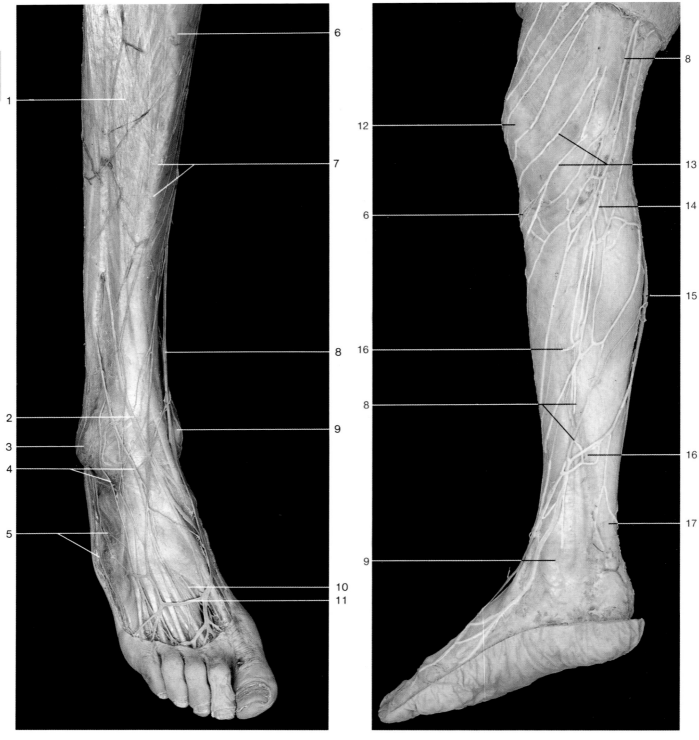

Right leg and foot, anterior crural region and dorsum of foot (anterior aspect). Cutaneous nerves and veins.

Right leg and foot (medial aspect). Cutaneous nerves and veins.

1   Superficial crural fascia
2   Medial cutaneous branch of superficial peroneal nerve
3   Lateral malleolus
4   Lateral cutaneous branch of superficial peroneal nerve
5   Cutaneous branch of sural nerve
6   Position of tuberosity of tibia
7   Anterior margin of tibia
8   Great saphenous vein
9   Medial malleolus

10   Deep peroneal nerve
11   Venous arch of dorsum of foot
12   Position of patella
13   Infrapatellar branches of saphenous nerve
14   Saphenous nerve
15   Small saphenous vein
16   Perforating vein
17   Calcaneal tendon

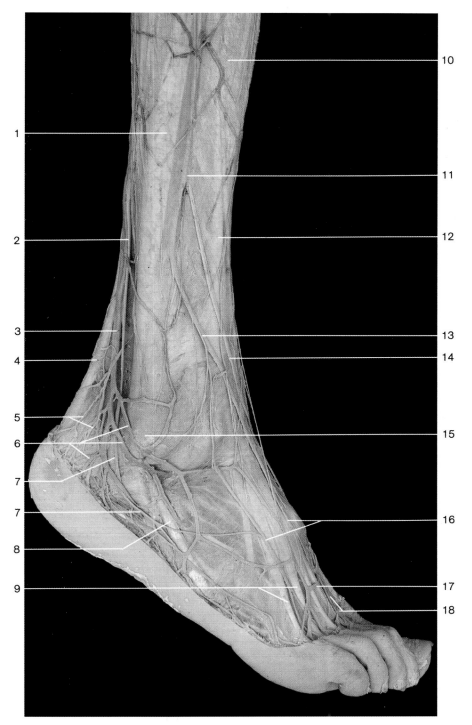

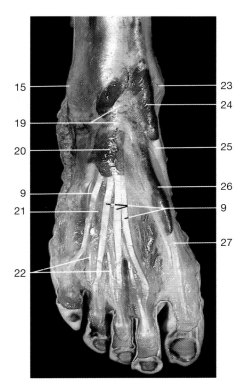

Right leg and foot (lateral aspect). Cutaneous nerves and veins.

Right foot with synovial sheaths of extensor muscles (dorsal aspect). The synovial sheaths have been injected with blue solution.

1   Position of fibula
2   Sural nerve
3   Small saphenous vein
4   Calcaneal tendon
5   Lateral calcaneal branches of sural nerve
6   Venous network at lateral malleolus
7   Cutaneous branch of sural nerve
8   Tendon of peroneus brevis muscle
9   Tendons of extensor digitorum longus muscle
10 Fascia cruris

11 Superficial peroneal nerve
12 Position of tibia
13 Lateral cutaneous branch ⎤ of superficial
14 Medial cutaneous branch ⎦ peroneal nerve
15 Lateral malleolus
16 Dorsal digital nerves
17 Dorsal venous arch
18 Deep peroneal nerve
19 Inferior extensor retinaculum
20 Common synovial sheath of extensor digitorum longus muscle
21 Extensor digitorum brevis muscle

22 Tendons of extensor digitorum brevis muscle
23 Medial malleolus
24 Synovial sheath of tendon of tibialis anterior muscle
25 Tendon of tibialis anterior muscle
26 Synovial sheath of tendon of extensor hallucis longus muscle
27 Tendon of extensor hallucis longus muscle

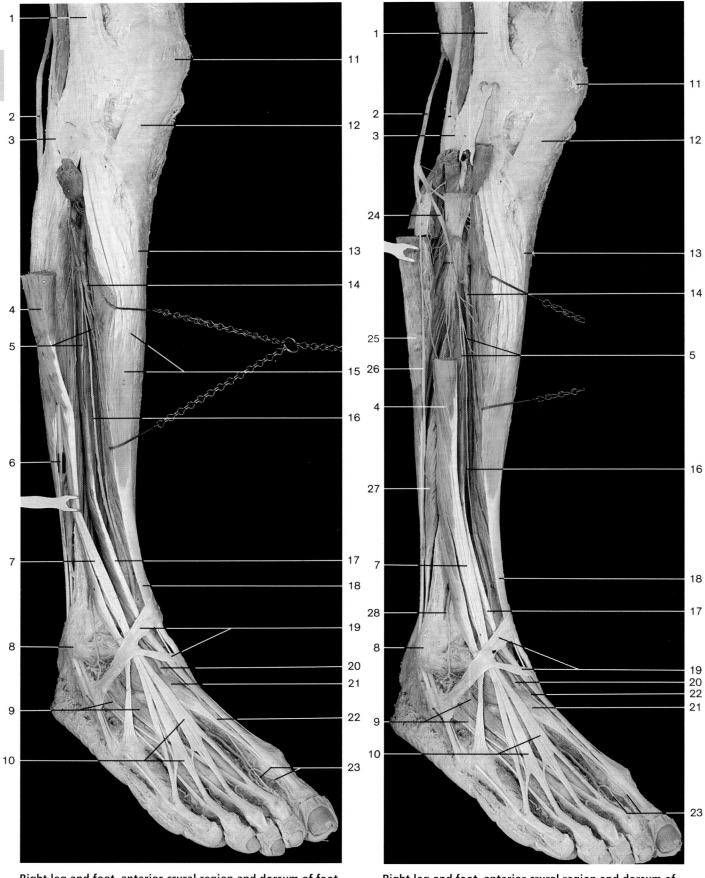

Right leg and foot, anterior crural region and dorsum of foot, middle layer (antero-lateral aspect). The extensor digitorum longus muscle has been divided and reflected laterally.

Right leg and foot, anterior crural region and dorsum of foot, deep layer (antero-lateral aspect). The extensor digitorum longus and peroneus longus muscles have been divided or removed. The common peroneal nerve has been elevated to show its course around the head of fibula.

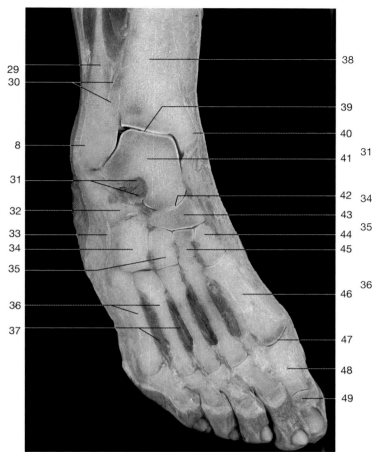

Coronal section through the foot and ankle joint (anterior aspect).

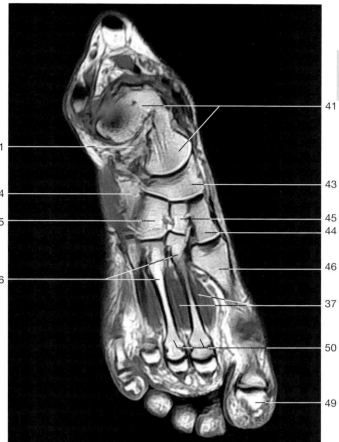

Coronal section through the foot and ankle joint (MRI scan; from Heuck et al., MRT-Atlas, 2009).

1   Iliotibial tract
2   Common peroneal nerve
3   Position of head of fibula
4   Extensor digitorum longus muscle
5   Muscular branches of deep peroneal nerve
6   Superficial peroneal nerve
7   Tendon of extensor digitorum longus muscle
8   Lateral malleolus
9   Extensor digitorum brevis muscle
10 Tendons of extensor digitorum longus muscle
11 Patella
12 Patellar ligament
13 Anterior margin of tibia
14 Anterior tibial artery
15 Tibialis anterior muscle
16 Deep peroneal nerve
17 Extensor hallucis longus muscle
18 Tendon of tibialis anterior muscle
19 Extensor retinaculum
20 Dorsalis pedis artery
21 Extensor hallucis brevis muscle
22 Deep peroneal nerve (on dorsum of foot)
23 Dorsal digital nerves (terminal branches of deep peroneal nerve)
24 Deep peroneal nerve
25 Peroneus longus muscle (cut)

26 Superficial peroneal nerve (with peroneal muscles laterally reflected)
27 Peroneus brevis muscle
28 Lateral anterior malleolar artery
29 Fibula
30 Distal tibiofibular joint (syndesmosis)
31 Talocalcaneal interosseous ligament
32 Calcaneus
33 Tendon of peroneus brevis muscle
34 Cuboid bone
35 Lateral cuneiform bone
36 Metatarsal bones
37 Dorsal interosseous muscles
38 Tibia
39 Ankle joint
40 Medial malleolus
41 Talus
42 Talocalcaneonavicular joint
43 Navicular bone
44 Medial cuneiform bone
45 Intermediate cuneiform bone
46 First metatarsal bone
47 Metatarsophalangeal joint of great toe
48 Proximal phalanx of great toe
49 Distal phalanx of great toe
50 Heads of metatarsal bones II–III

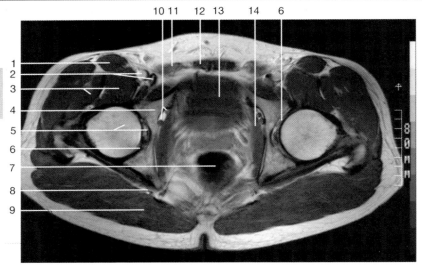

Axial section through the pelvis and the hip joints
(section 1; MRI scan; inferior aspect).

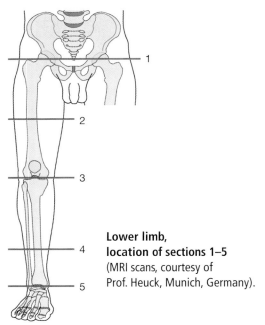

**Lower limb,
location of sections 1–5**
(MRI scans, courtesy of
Prof. Heuck, Munich, Germany).

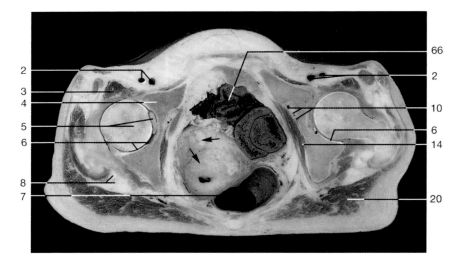

Axial section through the pelvis and the hip joints in the female
(section 1; inferior aspect). Arrows: uterus, myometrium with myoma.

1 Sartorius muscle
2 Femoral artery and vein
3 Iliopsoas muscle
4 Pubis (os pubis)
5 Femoral head with ligament of femoral
   head
6 Articular cavity
7 Rectum
8 Sciatic nerve and accompanying artery
9 Gluteus maximus muscle
10 Obturator vessels and obturator nerve
11 Rectus abdominis muscle
12 Pyramidalis muscle
13 Urinary bladder
14 Obturator internus muscle
15 Rectus femoris muscle
16 Vastus intermedius and vastus lateralis
   of quadriceps femoris muscle

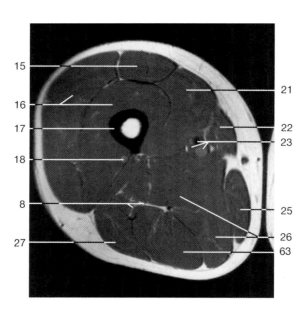

Axial section through the middle of the right
thigh (section 2; MRI scan; inferior aspect).

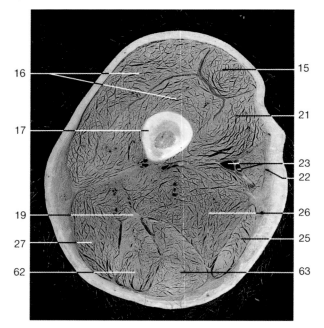

Axial section through the middle of the right
thigh (section 2; inferior aspect).

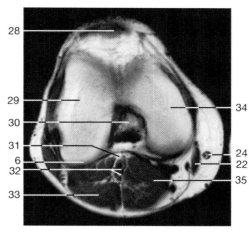

Axial section through the right knee joint (section 3; MRI scan; inferior aspect).

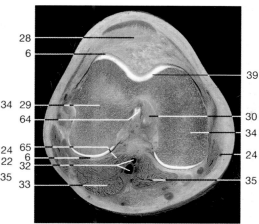

Axial section through the right knee joint (section 3; inferior aspect).

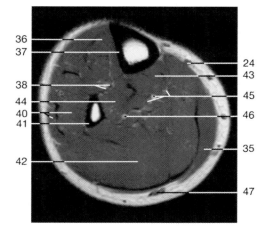

Axial section through the middle of the right leg (section 4; MRI scan; inferior aspect).

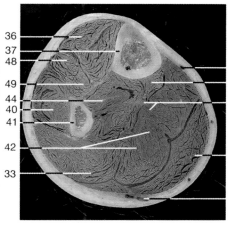

Axial section through the middle of the right leg (section 4; inferior aspect).

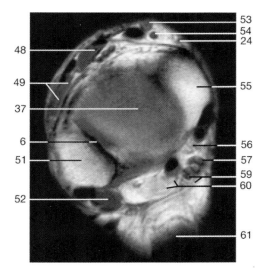

Axial section through the end of the right leg (section 5; MRI scan; inferior aspect).

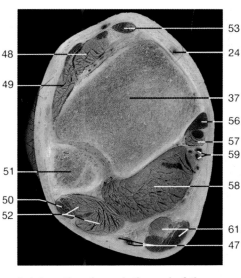

Axial section through the end of the right leg (section 5; inferior aspect).

17 Femur
18 Perforating artery
19 Sciatic nerve
20 Gluteus maximus muscle (insertion)
21 Vastus medialis muscle
22 Sartorius muscle
23 Femoral artery and vein
24 Great saphenous vein
25 Gracilis muscle
26 Adductor muscles
27 Biceps femoris muscle
28 Patellar ligament
29 Lateral condyle of femur
30 Posterior cruciate ligament
31 Tibial nerve
32 Popliteal artery and vein
33 Lateral head of gastrocnemius muscle
34 Medial condyle of femur
35 Medial head of gastrocnemius muscle
36 Tibialis anterior muscle
37 Tibia
38 Deep peroneal nerve, anterior tibial artery, and vein
39 Patellar surface
40 Peroneus longus and brevis muscles
41 Fibula
42 Soleus muscle
43 Flexor digitorum longus muscle
44 Tibialis posterior muscle
45 Posterior tibial artery and vein and tibial nerve
46 Peroneal artery
47 Small saphenous vein and sural nerve
48 Extensor hallucis longus muscle
49 Extensor digitorum longus muscle
50 Tendon of peroneus longus muscle
51 Lateral malleolus (fibula)
52 Peroneus brevis muscle
53 Tibialis anterior muscle (tendon)
54 Dorsalis pedis artery
55 Medial malleolus (tibia)
56 Tibialis posterior muscle (tendon)
57 Flexor digitorum longus muscle (tendon with synovial sheath)
58 Flexor hallucis longus muscle
59 Posterior tibial artery and vein
60 Lateral and medial plantar nerves
61 Calcaneal tendon
62 Semitendinosus muscle
63 Semimembranosus muscle
64 Anterior cruciate ligament
65 Plantaris muscle
66 Small intestine

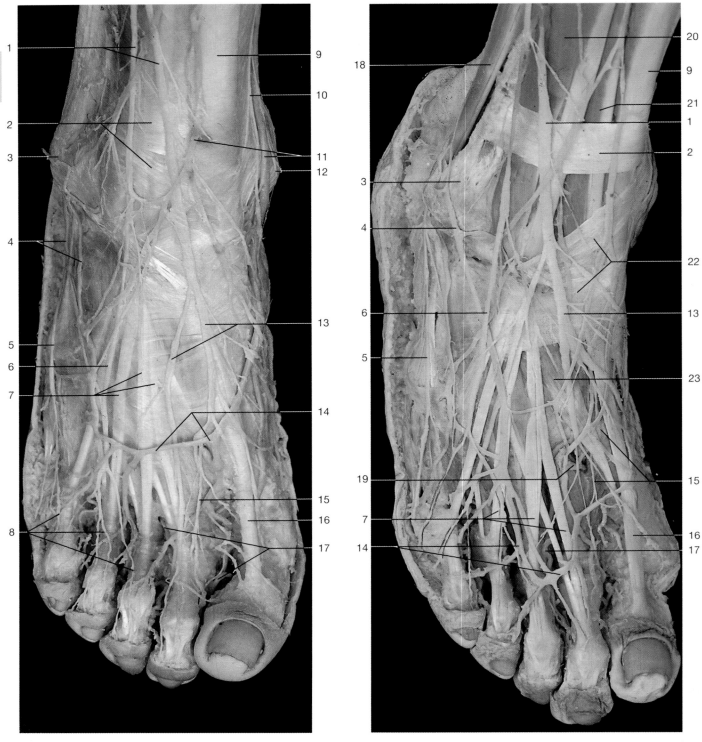

Dorsum of the right foot, superficial layer (anterior aspect).

Dorsum of the right foot, superficial layer (anterior aspect). The fascia of the dorsum has been removed.

1	Superficial peroneal nerve	9	Tendon of tibialis anterior muscle	17	Dorsal digital arteries
2	Superior extensor retinaculum	10	Saphenous nerve	18	Peroneal muscles
3	Lateral malleolus	11	Venous network of medial malleolus and	19	Deep plantar branch of dorsalis pedis
4	Venous network of lateral malleolus and		tributaries of great saphenous vein		artery anastomosing with plantar arch
	tributaries of small saphenous vein	12	Medial malleolus	20	Extensor digitorum longus muscle
5	Lateral dorsal cutaneous nerve (branch of	13	Medial dorsal cutaneous nerves	21	Extensor hallucis longus muscle
	sural nerve)	14	Dorsal venous arch	22	Inferior extensor retinaculum
6	Intermediate dorsal cutaneous nerve	15	Dorsal digital nerve (of deep peroneal	23	Extensor hallucis brevis muscle
7	Tendons of extensor digitorum longus muscle		nerve)		
8	Dorsal digital nerves	16	Tendon of extensor hallucis longus muscle		

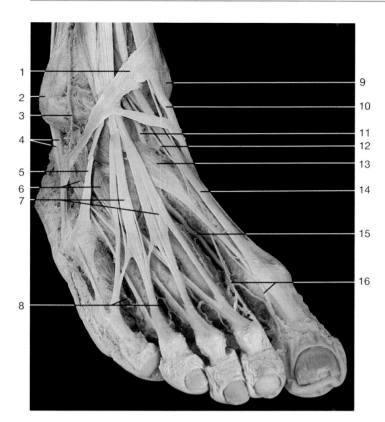

1 Extensor retinaculum
2 Lateral malleolus
3 Lateral anterior malleolar artery
4 Tendons of peroneal muscles
5 Tendon of peroneus tertius muscle
6 Extensor digitorum brevis muscle
7 Tendons of extensor digitorum longus muscle
8 Dorsal metatarsal arteries
9 Medial malleolus
10 Tendon of tibialis anterior muscle
11 Dorsalis pedis artery
12 Deep peroneal nerve (on dorsum of foot)
13 Extensor hallucis brevis muscle
14 Tendon of extensor hallucis longus muscle
15 Dorsalis pedis artery with deep plantar branch to the plantar arch
16 Dorsal digital nerves (terminal branches of deep peroneal nerve)
17 Lateral tarsal artery
18 Extensor digitorum brevis muscle (divided)
19 Arcuate artery
20 Dorsal interosseous muscles
21 Deep peroneal nerve
22 Medial cuneiform and first metatarsal bone
23 Tendon of peroneus longus muscle
24 Abductor hallucis and flexor hallucis brevis muscles
25 Medial plantar artery, vein, and nerve
26 Fourth and fifth metatarsal bone
27 Adductor hallucis muscle (oblique head)
28 Tendons of flexor digitorum longus muscle
29 Lateral plantar artery, vein, and nerve
30 Flexor digitorum brevis muscle
31 Plantar aponeurosis

Dorsum of the right foot, middle layer (antero-lateral aspect). The cutaneous nerves have been removed.

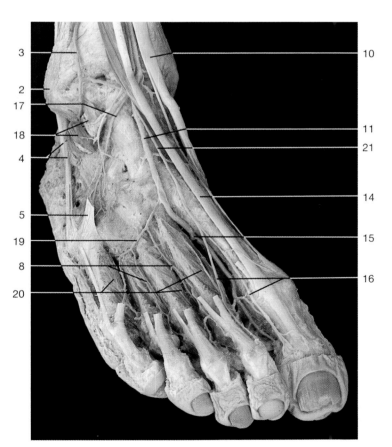

Dorsum of the right foot, deep layer (antero-lateral aspect). The extensor digitorum and hallucis brevis muscles have been removed.

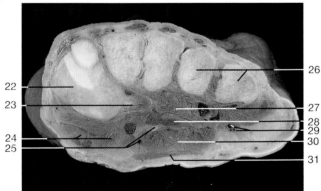

Cross section of the right foot at the level of the metatarsal bones (posterior aspect).

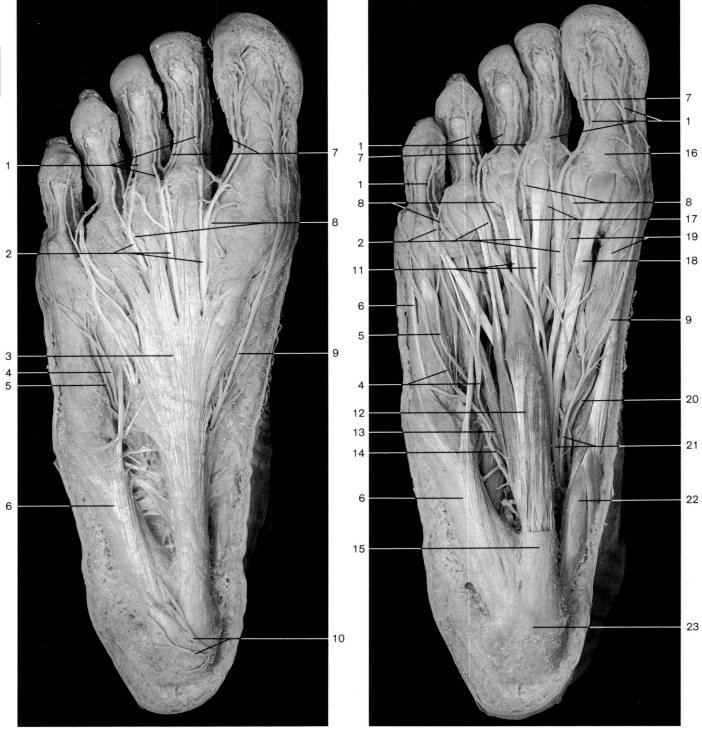

Sole of the right foot, superficial layer (from below).
Dissection of cutaneous nerves and vessels.

Sole of the right foot, middle layer (from below).
The plantar aponeurosis has been removed.

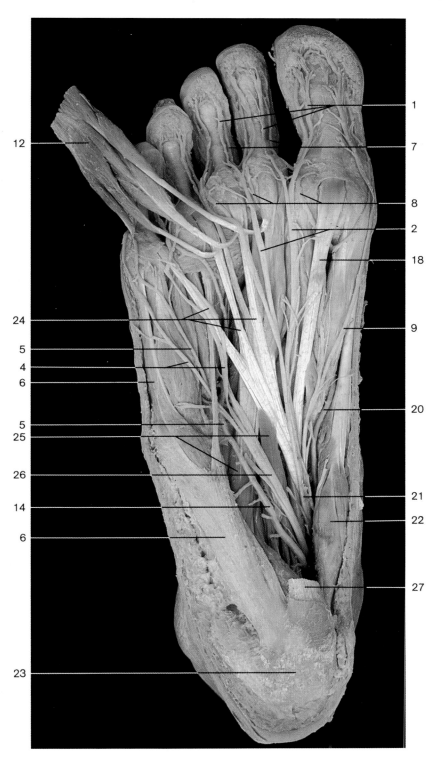

1 Proper plantar digital nerves
2 Common plantar digital nerves
3 Plantar aponeurosis
4 Superficial branch of lateral plantar nerve
5 Superficial branch of lateral plantar artery
6 Abductor digiti minimi
7 Proper plantar digital arteries
8 Common plantar digital arteries
9 Digital branch of medial plantar nerve to great toe
10 Medial calcaneal branches
11 Tendons of flexor digitorum brevis muscle
12 Flexor digitorum brevis muscle
13 Superficial branch of lateral plantar nerve
14 Lateral plantar artery
15 Plantar aponeurosis (remnant)
16 Digital synovial sheath
17 Lumbrical muscles
18 Tendon of flexor hallucis longus muscle
19 Flexor hallucis brevis muscle
20 Medial plantar artery
21 Medial plantar nerve
22 Abductor hallucis muscle
23 Calcaneal tuberosity
24 Tendons of flexor digitorum longus muscle
25 Quadratus plantae muscle
26 Lateral plantar nerve
27 Flexor digitorum brevis muscle (cut)
28 Synovial sheaths
29 Plantar arch

Sole of the right foot, middle layer (from below). Dissection of vessels and nerves. The flexor digitorum brevis muscle has been divided and anteriorly reflected.

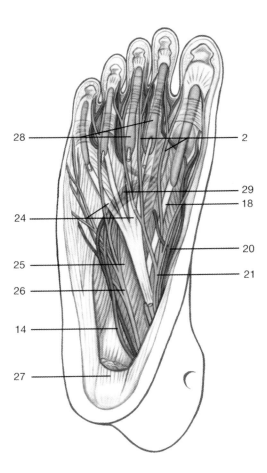

Sole of the right foot. Synovial sheaths of flexor tendons indicated in light blue (schematic drawing).

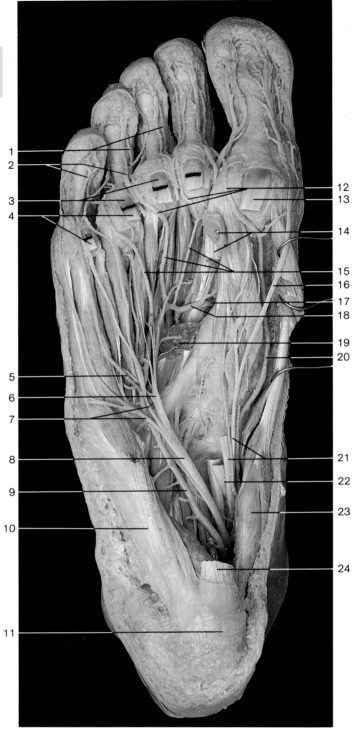

1   Proper plantar digital arteries
2   Proper plantar digital nerves
3   Tendons of flexor digitorum brevis muscle
4   Tendons of flexor digitorum longus muscle
5   Superficial branch of lateral plantar artery
6   Deep branch of lateral plantar nerve
7   Superficial branch of lateral plantar nerve
8   Lateral plantar nerve
9   Lateral plantar artery
10 Abductor digiti minimi muscle
11 Calcaneal tuberosity
12 Common plantar digital arteries
13 Tendon of flexor hallucis longus muscle
14 Insertion of both heads of adductor hallucis muscle
15 Plantar metatarsal arteries
16 Medial plantar nerve of great toe
17 Deep plantar branch of dorsalis pedis artery
    (perforating branch)
18 Plantar arch
19 Oblique head of adductor hallucis muscle (cut)
20 Medial plantar artery
21 Medial plantar nerve
22 Crossing of tendons in sole of foot (flexor hallucis
    longus and flexor digitorum longus muscles)
23 Abductor hallucis muscle
24 Origin of flexor digitorum brevis muscle

Sole of the right foot, deep layer (from below). Dissection
of vessels and nerves. The flexor digitorum brevis muscle, the
quadratus plantae muscle with the tendons of the flexor digitorum
longus muscle, and some branches of the medial plantar nerve
have been removed. The flexor hallucis brevis and adductor
hallucis muscles have been cut and portions removed to show the
somewhat atypical course of the medial plantar artery and deep
muscles of the foot.

Index

Page numbers in **bold** indicate main discussions.

A

Abdomen, parasagittal section 298
Abdominal organs 291 ff
− position 292, 306
− upper 301, 312 ff
− − arteries 314 f
− − blood supply 316
− vessels 302 ff
Abduction of fingers 395
Acetabulum 188, 345, 432
− bony margin 438
− lunate surface 433, **436**, 445
Achilles tendon 449, **457 ff**, 489, 491 ff
− surface anatomy 476
Acromion 15, 188 f, **369 ff**, 378, 382, 384 f
Adduction of fingers 395
Adductor hiatus 453
Adhesion, interthalamic 86, **107**
Adnexa of uterus 359 ff
Air cells
− ethmoidal 28, 36, **38**, 41 f, 44 f, **48**, 53, 135
− − openings 144
− mastoid 70, 125 ff
Ala s. also Wing
− of central lobule of vermis 102
− of ilium 435
− of sacrum **434 f**, 438
− of vomer 37, 45, **48 f**
Amnion 359
Ampulla 128 f
− bony 129
− of ductus deferens **336 ff**, 342, 344
− of rectum 342, 354
− of uterine tube 358, 361, 366
Amygdala (amygdaloid body) **107**, 110 f, **114 f**, 116
Anastomoses, portocaval 303
Aneurysm, infrarenal, of aorta 348
Angiogram(-graphy)
− fluorescent, of eye 134
− internal carotid artery 95 f
Angle
− costal 192
− inferior, of scapula **370 f**, 382 f
− infrasternal 7, 192, 248
− − surface anatomy 204
− lateral, of scapula 188, **370 f**
− of mandible 21, **52**
− of ribs 370
− sphenoidal, of parietal bone 29
− sternal 192 f
− superior, of scapula 371
− venous

− − left 17
− − right 17, 398
Ankle joint 432, **443**, **449 ff**, 495
Ansa
− cervicalis 71, **163**, 177, **181 f**, 266
− − muscular branches 181, 265
− − root
− − − inferior 184
− − − superior 69, 71, **82 f**, 152, 179
− lenticular 116
− subclavia of sympathetic trunk 169
− thyroid, of sympathetic trunk 169
Antihelix 124
Antitragus 124
Antrum
− mastoid 127
− pyloric 294, 324
− tympanic 126
Anulus
− fibrosus 198
− inguinalis s. Ring, inguinal
− tympanic, of newborn 33
Anus 350 ff, 354, 361 ff, 366
Aorta 16 f
− abdominal 16, 210, **245**, 256, 278, 292, 296, 300, 302, 329 ff, **348**, 359 f
− − subtraktion angiography 328
− ascending 243, 245, **252 ff**, 260, 266, 272, 284, 396
− − bypass vessel 263
− − of fetus 288
− − horizontal section 286
− descending 244, 252 f, 276
− − of fetus 288 f
− − horizontal section 286
− − main branches 281
− relation to bronchial tree 275
− thoracic 253, 274, **281**
Aperture
− lateral, of fourth ventricle 112
− of Luschka 112
− of Magendie 94, **112**
− median, of fourth ventricle 94, **112**
− nasal, anterior 22 f, 45
− pelvic, inferior 434, **438**
Apex
− of cochlea 125
− of head of fibula 440
− of heart **252**, 257 f, 262 f
− of lung 248 f, 271
− of patella 441
− of petrous part of temporal bone 27, 127
− of sacrum 191
− of urinary bladder 337, 339, 357
Aponeurosis 388 ff
− of abdominal wall 187
− bicipital **387 f**, 416, 423
− of external abdominal oblique muscle 217, 362

− of levator palpebrae superioris muscle 142
− palmar 388, 423
− − transverse fasciculi 388
− plantar 449, **463**, 499, 501
− − longitudinal bands 463
Apparatus
− auditory 22, **122 ff**, 129
− lacrimal 142
− masticatory 22
− vestibular **122 ff**, 129
− visual 132 ff
Appendix(-ces) 304
− of epididymis 343
− epiploicae 306
− fibrosa 299
− of testis 343
− vermiform 291, 304, **306 f**, 310, 318, 324
− − Head's area 205
− − orifice 310
− − variations in the position 307
Aqueduct
− cerebral 65, 73 ff, **86**, 90, 94, 99, **112**, 116, 121
− of cochlea 129
− of vestibule 27, **129**
Arachnoid mater 84 f, **89**, **92**, 100, 118
− spinal 230, **232**, 474
Arbor vitae of cerebellum 94, 116
Arch
− anterior, of atlas 165, 200, 203
− aortic 95, 154, 169, 177, **245**, 253, 256 f, 273 f, 279, **284**
− − of fetus 288 f
− azygos 273 f, 276, 283
− of cervical vertebra 239 f
− costal 3 f, 188, **192 ff**, 196, 212 f, 243 f, 264 f, **370**
− − surface anatomy 204
− of cricoid cartilage 158
− dental 52
− iliopectineal 444 f, **453**
− palatoglossal 147
− palatopharyngeal 147
− palmar
− − deep 427, **429**
− − superficial 396, 423, **426 ff**
− plantar 467, 501 f
− posterior
− − of atlas **200**, 239
− − of axis 239
− pubic 436 f
− tendinous
− − of flexor digitorum superficialis muscle 418
− − of soleus muscle 457, 491
− venous
− − dorsal, of foot **468**, 489, 492 f, 498
− − jugular 170, **172**, 398, 406
− of vertebra 191, 231, 474

Page numbers in **bold** indicate main discussions.

Page numbers in **bold** indicate main discussions.

Page numbers in **bold** indicate main discussions.

Page numbers in **bold** indicate main discussions.

Page numbers in **bold** indicate main discussions.

Page numbers in **bold** indicate main discussions.

Page numbers in **bold** indicate main discussions.

Page numbers in **bold** indicate main discussions.

Page numbers in **bold** indicate main discussions.

Page numbers in **bold** indicate main discussions.

Page numbers in **bold** indicate main discussions.

Page numbers in **bold** indicate main discussions.

Page numbers in **bold** indicate main discussions.

Page numbers in **bold** indicate main discussions.

Page numbers in **bold** indicate main discussions.

Page numbers in **bold** indicate main discussions.

Page numbers in **bold** indicate main discussions.

Page numbers in **bold** indicate main discussions.

Page numbers in **bold** indicate main discussions.

Page numbers in **bold** indicate main discussions.

O

Page numbers in **bold** indicate main discussions.

Page numbers in **bold** indicate main discussions.

Page numbers in **bold** indicate main discussions.

Page numbers in **bold** indicate main discussions.

Page numbers in **bold** indicate main discussions.

Page numbers in **bold** indicate main discussions.

Page numbers in **bold** indicate main discussions.

Page numbers in **bold** indicate main discussions.

Page numbers in **bold** indicate main discussions.

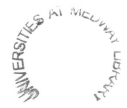